Epilepsy

ADVANCES IN EPILEPTOLOGY: THE Xth EPILEPSY INTERNATIONAL SYMPOSIUM

ADVANCES IN EPILEPTOLOGY SERIES

Advances in Epileptology: The XIth Epilepsy International Symposium, *R. Canger, F. Angeleri, and J. K. Penry, editors; 512 pp., 1980.*

Advances in Epileptology: The Xth Epilepsy International Symposium, *J. Wada and J. K. Penry, editors; 568 pp., 1980.*

Epilepsy: The Eighth International Symposium, *J. K. Penry, editor; 432 pp., 1977.*

Advances in Epileptology

The Xth Epilepsy
International Symposium

Editors

Juhn A. Wada, M.D.
Professor of Neurological Sciences
Director, Neurology Unit EEG
Department
Health Sciences Center Hospital
The University of British Columbia
Vancouver, British Columbia, Canada

J. Kiffin Penry, M.D.
Professor of Neurology
Associate Dean for Neurosciences
Development
Wake Forest University
Bowman Gray School of Medicine
Winston-Salem, North Carolina
and President, International Epilepsy
League

Raven Press ■ New York

Raven Press, 1140 Avenue of the Americas, New York, New York 10036

Great care has been taken to maintain the accuracy of the information contained in the volume. However, Raven Press cannot be held responsible for errors or for any consequences arising from the use of the information contained herein.

Materials appearing in this book prepared by individuals as part of their official duties as U.S. Government employees are not covered by the above-mentioned copyright.

Library of Congress Cataloging in Publication Data

International Symposium on Epilepsy, 10th,
      Vancouver, B.C., 1978.
      The Xth epilepsy international symposium.

      (Advances in epileptology)
      Includes bibliographies and index.
      1. Epilepsy—Congresses. I. Wada, Juhn A.
II. Penry, J. Kiffin, 1929–   III. Series.
(DNLM: 1. Epilepsy—Congresses. W1 AD556M / WL385
E6425 1978t)
RC372.I47 1978   616.8'53   80-20162
ISBN 0-89004-511-9

Preface

The planning of the Epilepsy International Symposium held in Vancouver in 1978 began in the summer of 1975. Since the Xth Epilepsy International Symposium was the first of this series of International Symposia to be hosted on the North American continent, specifically on the Pacific West Coast, it was considered important to join the resources and forces of professionals interested in epilepsy from among the Pacific rim countries. Thus, the American Epilepsy Society, the Canadian League Against Epilepsy, the Japanese Epilepsy Society and the Western Institute on Epilepsy (U.S.A.) became the moving force to which additional professional as well as lay organization's support was added from the British Columbia Epilepsy Society, the Canadian Association of EEG Technologists, Canadian Epilepsy Association, Canadian Neurological Society, Epilepsy Foundation of America and the University of British Columbia.

As the planning progressed, plenary themes of "Intensive Monitoring" became the major theme of the American Epilepsy Society, "Natural History and Prognosis" that of the Japanese Epilepsy Society, "New Surgical Treatment through Experimental Models" of the Canadian League Against Epilepsy, "New Drug Testing, Marketing and Availability" of the International League Against Epilepsy, and the final major theme of "Comprehensive Care of Epilepsy" became the joint effort of the British Columbia Epilepsy Society, the Canadian Epilepsy Association, the Epilepsy Foundation of America, and the Western Institute on Epilepsy. In addition, special events traditional to each participating organization and society were included. For example, the Lennox Lectures of the American Epilepsy Society and Western Institute on Epilepsy were delivered and special sessions such as Neurotransmitter Up-Date, Teratogenicity of Antiepileptic Drugs, Epilepsy and Behavior, and Pregnancy and Epilepsy* were arranged to meet special needs of certain aspects of the problems of epilepsy.

The response to this program was overwhelming, and more than 350 papers were submitted which covered all facets of the problems of epilepsy. In order to reach far beyond the immediate participants of the symposium, for educational purposes, we made an effort to assemble critical information and new knowledge produced as of September 1978. Since it would not be feasible to publish an expansion of all abstracts in a single volume, as many abstracts as possible were chosen to be expanded tenfold. Each of these

---

*For those who are interested in the topics of the special sessions, this information is available in a joint publication of the Canadian League Against Epilepsy and the Western Insitute on Epilepsy.

longer articles presents the essence of the subject without the details of methodology and complete discussion that would pre-empt the publication of a full length scientific paper. It is hoped that each contribution represents an abbreviated account of the essentials commensurate with the quality of the usual scientific literature. For those who could not attend the symposium and for the sake of completeness, those abstracts not chosen for expansion have been included in a brief form. Thus, the reader of this volume should be able to obtain information on practically every aspect covering the problems and frontiers of epilepsy.

Juhn A. Wada
J. Kiffin Penry

Acknowledgments

The Editors gratefully acknowledge the efficient secretarial assistance of Mary Mann, Betty Canning, and Linda Dixon, as well as the meticulous editorial assistance of Sue Calthrop. We are most grateful to Raven Press and especially to Rita Scheman for making the publication of this proceedings a reality.

Contents

Abstracts

CONTENTS

New Surgical Treatment Through Experimental Models

New Drug Testing, Marketing, and Availability

Abstracts

Comprehensive Care

Abstracts

Experimental Seizures and Mechanisms

Abstracts

Antiepileptic Drug Treatment

Abstracts

Side Effects of Drugs

Abstracts

Behavior, Performance, and Seizures

Abstracts

Clinical and Electrographic Aspects of Epilepsy

Abstracts

Contributors

Advances in Epileptology:
The Xth Epilepsy International Symposium,
edited by J. A. Wada and J. K. Penry.
Raven Press, New York © 1980.

Limits and Perspectives of Our Knowledge of Epilepsy: Progress from Research

R. Naquet

Departement de Neurophysiologie Appliquée Laboratoire de Physiologie Nerveuse,
92290 Gif-sur-Yvette, France

The title of this chapter corresponds only approximately to my intended subject. It will not be an exhaustive review of the progress made in recent years by various neurophysiological, neuroanatomical, neuropharmacological, or neurochemical techniques. Nor will it be a summary of future perspectives made possible by application of these techniques.

Rather, I wish to discuss some observations and conclusions based on my own experience and on a survey of the recent literature on various experimental models of epilepsy that basic researchers and clinical epileptologists have described in recent years to try to understand and treat the numerous forms of epilepsy in humans.

The first observation regards the increasing number of models of experimental epilepsy. Each year scientific publications are full of presentations of new models that their inventors consider best for explaining certain forms of epilepsy and its consequences. However, few withstand the test of time as models, despite the undeniable value of some in the comprehension of the functioning of the nervous system.

Among the models that seem to have attracted the most work in recent years, with the exception of epilepsy induced by alumina cream or cobalt (see Ward, 1972) (which have been known for a much longer time), we can mention the photosensitive epilepsy of *Papio papio* (Killam et al., 1966, 1967), generalized penicillin epilepsy of the cat (Prince and Farrell, 1969), and the kindling phenomenon (Goddard et al., 1969). In spite of the possible future interest in the model of Lennox-Gastaut syndrome that occurs in the Rhesus monkey (Bert et al., 1978) with certain forms of experimental Kuru, it seems too early to evaluate its importance.

A second point, closely related to the first, concerns the great variety of expression of the epileptic symptoms. A given model can be excellent for explaining certain signs and useless in explaining others.

1. There is reason to differentiate between the models of generalized epilepsy (reflex or not) from those of focal epilepsy, i.e., those that reproduce paroxysmal elements that characterize the interictal discharges (ID), from

those that induce seizure discharges (SD). There is also a reason to distinguish between generalized spike-and-wave discharges (GSWD) whether or not accompanied by clinical manifestations, from the generalized tonic-clonic seizures (GTCS), even when the latter follow the GSWD. The two are not regulated by the same mechanisms. It is not rare, however, that interictal focal discharges and even bursts of GSWD should be similarly governed.

(a) On the one hand, bursts of spike-and-waves (SW) or polyspike-and-waves (PSW) of the absence of myoclonic petit mal in the human, bursts of PSW in the *Papio papio* whether or not induced by intermittent light stimulation (ILS) (see Naquet and Meldrum, 1972), bursts of SW of generalized penicillin epilepsy of the cat (Gloor and Testa, 1974; Guberman and Gloor, 1974) and on the other hand, ID of the kindling (Wada and Sato 1974; Tanaka et al., 1975) are frequently blocked by anything that induces an activation pattern of the EEG. In fact, they are blocked during active wakening as during paradoxical sleep, and are, on the contrary, enhanced by "synchronization": relaxed awakening, drowsiness, and slow wave sleep (SWS).

(b) Conversely, one does not find such a singularity of reactivity to the variations of the level of vigilance for the SD of another type. For example, if the generalized secondary seizures (GSS) induced by amygdaloid stimulation during kindling (stage V of Racine, 1972) are identical regardless of the level of vigilance of the animal, and if the intensity of the electric stimulation necessary to induce them remains unchanged regardless of the level of vigilance of the animal, certain GTCSs, especially the tonic seizures of Lennox-Gastaut syndrome, as in those of the experimental Kuru, are definitely facilitated by SWS and particularly by stage II (Bert et al., 1978). Immediately prior to the onset of these seizures we found frequency potential analogous to V wave or K complex and this has led us to suppose that the attack could often be produced by arrival afferent messages as an expression of a seizure discharge of the internal face of the hemispheres (Naquet and Menini, 1978).

(c) Furthermore, whereas the GSWDs, even those accompanied by myoclonus, do not modify at all the organization of sleep of *Papio papio*, the GTCSs induced in the same by ILS (Tanaka and Naquet, 1976) or by other causes (see Naquet, 1977) do modify the sleep patterns, as do, however, the GSSs of kindling in the cat (Tanaka and Naquet, 1975).

(d) Finally, these two types of discharges do not propagate in the same manner. One must assume normal neuroanatomic connections for the transmission of bursts of GSWD (as well as for ID), whereas for the GTCS or for the GSS, all the modes of transmission and development of the discharge are possible (Green and Naquet, 1957). In general the section of a pathway, the destruction of nuclei considered as "essential" by some researchers for the genesis of SD, is ineffective (Bach-y-Rita et al., 1969; Lanoir, 1972; McCaughram et al., 1978a). Conversely, commissural sections modify the propagation from one hemisphere to the other and very often originally generalized seizures become predominantly unilateral (Naquet et al., 1972; McCaughram et al., 1978*b*).

2. It is normal to dissociate the isolated GTCS whether "primary" or secondary, from repetitive seizures building up to a true status epilepticus (SE). The consequences for the whole brain are completely different in the two cases.

For example, GTCSs induced frequently during several months, but with the necessary and sufficient interval between two stimulations in order for them to be effective, do not induce, with a few exceptions, any secondary lesions in different parts of the brain and particularly at the level of the hippocampus either in the rat or in the cat during kindling (Goddard et al., 1969) or in the photosensitive *Papio papio* (Riche et al., 1971). On the other hand, less than 2 hr of generalized SE induced by systemic injection of allylglycine or bicuculline in the rat or the primate (Meldrum and Brierley 1973; Meldrum et al., 1974; Meldrum and Nilsson, 1976) or secondary generalized SE after implantation of alumina cream on the amygdala of the cat (Naquet et al., 1962) or of microdoses of kainic acid in the same nuclei in the rat (Ben Ari and Lagowska, 1978), provoke very definite lesions of the hippocampus. These lesions are bilateral in the case of the former, unilateral and on the side of the injection in the latter. These secondary lesions do not appear to be the result of a cerebral edema, as has been suggested in the child after an hemiclonus SE (Gastaut, 1954; Gastaut et al., 1977); they are also unlikely to be the result of "an additional metabolic stress" as Meldrum and Nilsson (1976) reviewed. Such metabolic stress could be caused by cerebral hypoxia, arterial hypotension, hyperpyrexia, or hypoglycemia frequently found in SE. There is another associated or independent etiology yet to be found and recently Blennow et al. (1978) "proposed that neuronal damage in animals with unrestricted cerebral oxygen and glucose availability is due to oxidative mechanisms in cells with excessively enhanced neuronal activity."

A third subject for consideration is the following. Since no model is perfect, it is necessary to make numerous reservations before any extrapolation can be made with regard to the human subject, as the phylogenetic, ontogenetic, and susceptibility conditions of an individual or of a group of individuals intervene continuously to modify the data. Of the many examples meriting attention, one finds:

(a) The problems raised by peptides, i.e., the isolation from brain of peptides (enkephalins) (Hughes, 1975; Hughes et al., 1975) and endorphins (Lazarus et al., 1976; Ling and Guillemin, 1976) that interact with opiate receptors and manifest narcotic and analgesic actions similar to morphine raised the question of a role of such peptides in the modulation of seizure threshold. Urca et al. (1977) and Frenk et al. (1978) described transient epileptiform discharges on the EEG occurring shortly after the intracerebral ventricular injection of morphine or Leu or Met enkephalin in rats.

Moreover, Le Gal La Salle et al. (1977) have shown that injections of morphine, which were already known to be epileptogenic in heavy doses (Verdeaux and Marty, 1954) could in weak doses and by intramuscular injection considerably increase the length and strength of the seizures in kindled rats and increase in the same preparation ID frequency. The effects are stereospecific and reversed by naloxone. Urca et al. (1977) and Le Gal La Salle et al. (1977) concluded that "presumed endogenous opiate-like substances may well play a significant role in the susceptibility of various brain structures to epileptogenic procedures."

More recent works (see Bloom et al., 1978) have shown that β-endorphin, like the enkephalins, provoked the appearance of SD at the level of the limbic system in the rat (particularly hippocampus) but equally registered on the EEG even though there are none accompanied by motor phenomenon. Its action seems weaker in the monkey, in which it induces only isolated ID at the level of the hippocampus (F. E. Bloom, *personal communication*).

The use of these peptides in *Papio papio* has on the whole been disappointing (Meldrum et al., 1979). Neither the Met, nor the Leu-enkephalin nor β-endorphin intracerebroventricularly modify the degree of photosensitivity of the animals. Morphine intracerebroventricularly or intramuscularly reduces the photosensitivity of the animals and this effect is reversed by naloxone. FK 33.824 blocks the photosensitivity of the animals for a long time, especially intracerebroventricularly, but it also provokes a depression of respiration for an equally long period and consequently slows down considerably the background of the EEG. The effects are blocked, at least temporarily, by naloxone, to such an extent that one cannot affirm that the anticonvulsant action of the drug is not the consequence of the two last effects.

Based on these results, we should make some reservations concerning the epileptogenic role of these peptides in humans, in any case, and especially in generalized epilepsy. At the present state of our knowledge, their therapeutic role seems nil, at least for epilepsy.

(b) The problems raised by PM absence epilepsy, as it exists in humans, has, in our opinion, never been exactly reproduced in the animal. The models that come the closest are generalized penicillin epilepsy in the cat [which cannot be reproduced in the *Papio papio* (Meldrum et al., 1978)] and photosensitive epilepsy of the *Papio papio*. However, in both cases it is related more to myoclonic PM than PM absence. Furthermore, before extrapolating to man from data gathered from these two models, one must remember that they are not exactly equivalent even to the human myoclonic PM.

The topography of the SWDs, especially of those registered in the subcortical structures, varies according to whether the penicillin is applied largely on the cortex or injected intramuscularly (Fischer and Prince, 1977; Quesney et al., 1977; Gloor et al., 1977). One wonders then which of these two preparations comes closest to the human PM.

The frequency of ILS capable of inducing paroxysmal discharges (PD) accompanied by myoclonus, followed or not by GTCS, is more rapid in the *Papio papio* (25 cs) than in humans (15 cs). In the former, the ILS never induces posterior PD as it frequently does in humans, and frontorolandic PD which it provokes is of the type photomyologic or photoparoxystic associated (according to the terms of Klass and Fischer-Williams, 1976) and not dissociated, as is most often the case in humans (see Naquet, 1973; Naquet, 1977). Animals that possess a stable and high degree of photosensitivity are rare (Wada et al., 1972), and the curarization of animals blocks the apparition of PD (Naquet and Menini, 1972). The addition of an appropriate dose of allylglycine IV (Horton and Meldrum, 1973) increases the photosensitivity of animals and it remains constant during several hours, even under curarization. Despite the pharmacological interest of this model (allylglycine + ILS in baboons), from a purely neurophysiological point of view we must make the same restrictions as those already applied to generalized penicillin epilepsy of the cat. Genetics data are irrelevant in generalized epilepsy in the cat; on the other hand some genetic data may be expected from the *Papio papio* (Balzamo et al., 1975).

Despite these reservations concerning the validity of these models, they have helped to prove "that bilateral synchronous SWD and so-called "generalized seizures" start at the cortical level" (see Naquet and Menini, 1978). We do not yet know precisely the cause of the cortical hyperexcitability or the role of the subcortical structures in the regulation of this hyperexcitability. It has been shown that a role is played by certain thalamic nuclei responsible for the spindles of sleep in the generation of SW in generalized penicillin epilepsy in the cat (Quesney et al., 1977; Gloor et al., 1977). The spindles occupy the same territory as the SW in this form of epilepsy (P. Gloor, *personal communication*) as in the *Papio papio* (Naquet and Menini, 1978) and the two may be related as formulated by Bancaud et al. (1953). But one must remember that thalamus is not necessary for the appearance of GS (Bach-y-Rita et al., 1969; Lanoir, 1972). Others have suggested that the origin of the cortical hyperexcitability is the consequence of a disturbance of the GABAergic or catecholaminergic inhibitor mechanisms (see Naquet and Menini, 1978) or in glutamic acid metabolism (see Van Gelder, 1978), which would bring into question the structures of brainstem as well as the cortex.

Finally, the discovery of a particular thermolability of the benzodiazepine receptors in a *Papio papio* presenting not only an excessive photosensitivity but also spontaneous GTCS opens a whole new field of investigation (Squires et al., 1979) especially inasmuch as these receptors, in contrast to the naloxone receptors, are localized at the cortical level in the rat or in the *Papio papio* as well as in humans (Squires and Braestrup, 1977; Braestrup et al., 1977; Mohler and Okada, 1977; Squires et al. 1978). These data are of particular interest because, as we have seen before, at the present time one must admit that this form of epilepsy is of cortical rather than centrencephalic origin.

(c) The problem of the kindling phenomenon: It was known that electrical stimulation of the amygdala or the implantation of alumina cream at this level (Gastaut et al., 1952 *a* and *b*, Gastaut et al., 1953; Naquet, 1953) brought on a whole series of behavioral symptoms representing true focal epileptic seizures or GSS in the nonanesthetized cat. The knowledge gained from this experiment has been extrapolated to humans (Castells et al., 1952; Gastaut et al., 1952*c*; Gastaut et al., 1953*b*; Penfield and Jasper, 1956; Baldwin and Bailey, 1958) and has allowed to explain, at least in part, the complex symptomatology of psychomotor or temporal epilepsy. The discovery of the kindling phenomenon (Goddard et al., 1969) was subsequently to show that:

(a) The behavioral symptomatology induced by repeated electrical stimulation of amygdala varied from the rat to the cat, but even more so in the primate (Goddard et al. 1969; Wada and Osawa, 1976; Wada et al., 1978).

(b) The induction of GSS took much longer in the primate than in the rat or the cat, true GSS being particularly difficult to obtain in the Rhesus monkey (Wada et al., 1978).

(c) Up until the present, regardless of the species, stimulation of the amygdala is most apt to induce this type of GSS, the number of stimulations necessary to obtain such seizures being clearly greater for other structures (Goddard et al., 1969).

(d) It is necessary to stimulate rats nearly 300 times at a rate of several stimulations per day in order to induce spontaneous seizures identical to those set off by repeated electrical stimulation of this nucleus (Pinel and Rovner, 1978), whereas to kindle a rat, 15 stimulations are sufficient (Goddard et al., 1969). Spontaneous seizures have been noted in the literature in other species with a fewer number of stimulations; however, these are exceptions (Wada and Osawa, 1976).

During this same period, the development of stereotaxic surgery in humans, especially for temporal lobe epilepsy permitted a better analysis of the associated behavioral symptoms, SD initiated at the level of the amygdala (spontaneous seizures, electrical stimulations). From this exploration it was learned that the seizures starting from the amygdala in humans have a symptomatology very different from that observed in the cat and the rat, particularly in that the amygdala, exceptionally, is at the origin of the temporal SD, that it is most often invaded secondarily, the SD beginning more easily at the level of the hippocampus or of the inferior face of the frontal lobe, and finally that the SDs that initiate in this territory are exceptionally followed by GSS (Bancaud, *personal communication*).

All of these considerations call for great care in extrapolation to humans, in the genesis of GSS, of the mechanisms that underlie the institution of the kindling phenomenon by amygdaloid stimulation in the rat, the cat, and eventually even in certain baboons (Wada, 1978). These few restrictions do not minimize the importance of this model and the many perspectives it offers for a better understanding of the generalization of the epileptic phenomena from a histochemical as well as from a neurochemical or neuropharmacological point of view. It has allowed emphasis of the very important role of the repetition of seizures at given intervals in maintaining a certain level of cerebral hyperexcitability. Once the kindling is established, the animal for each stimulation is no longer capable of making focal seizures, but only GSS, a true "all or nothing" phenomenon (Wada and Sato, 1974). However, this is the rule only for the intervals of limited time (albeit several months). This property can disappear afterwards; the animal then reacts with only focal seizures to isolated stimulations, a very small number of new repetitive stimulations reestablishing the GSS. Conversely, the administration of certain substances with anticonvulsant properties, such as valproic acid, can hinder the appearance of GSS for periods largely exceeding their disappearance in the blood (Leviel and Naquet, 1977). Their mechanism of action is not yet known, but one wonders if it might be analogous to that envisioned by some authors for taurine, with presumed long-term effects on the metabolism of amino acids, "and consequent stabilization of neuronal activity" (Van Gelder et al., 1977; Van Gelder, 1978).

I would like to add a final point concerning the choice of examples used to illustrate this chapter. Most of them come from subjects having no cerebral-organic lesions at their origin. This is true for generalized penicillin epilepsy of the cat by definition, for photosensitive epilepsy in the *Papio papio* (Fischer-Williams et al., 1968), as well as for the kindling phenomenon (Goddard et al., 1969; Brotchi et al., 1978).

One might ask whether a spike appearing on a healthy cortex is governed by the same production mechanisms as on a damaged cortex. The hypersensitivity of deafferentation observed by Ward (1969) at the level of the cortical focus by alumina cream was of little value for the aforementioned models and for other models such as focal epilepsy with penicillin; it was necessary to look for other hypotheses to explain them (see Ajmone-Marsan, 1978). Bert et al. (1978*a*) were correct to wonder, in view of the importance of the cortical lesions particularly at the level of the internal face of the hemispheres during experimental Kuru, if one should also equate the hypersensitivity of deafferentation with the action of alumina cream to explain the ID and the tonic seizures they observed.

Clearly, everything has not yet been resolved and we are far from a solution. In spite of the importance of recent neurophysiological discoveries, notably at the unitary level (see Chalazonitis and Boisson, 1978), or neurochemical discoveries [close relationship between content of specific amino acid in blood, CSF or epileptogenic cortex and severity of epilepsy in humans as well as in animals (Van Gelder and Courtois (1972); Mutani et al. 1974; Van Gelder et al., 1972)], the problems that remain unsolved are not simple. The multiplicity of the data that we can expect to gain in the future from the application of a whole series of new sophisticated methods of investigation will not simplify them. It will be more than ever necessary to establish permanent contacts between basic investigators and epileptologists if we are to avoid hasty generalizations and/or experiments of little interest to the understanding of the multiple aspects of human epilepsy.

REFERENCES

Ajmone Marsan, C. (1978): An experimental model to investigate disinhibitory mechanisms in penicillin epileptogenesis. In: Experimental models for the development of an interictal focus. *Electroencephalogr. Clin. Neurophysiol. (Suppl.)*, 34:285–287.

Bach-y-Rita, G., Poncet, M., and Naquet, R. (1969): Morphology and spatio-temporal evolution of ictal discharges induced by cardiazol in the presence of various cortico diencephalic lesions in the cat. In: *The Physiopathogenesis of the Epilepsies*, edited by H. Gastaut, H. Jasper, J. Bancaud, and A. Waltregny, pp. 256–267. Charles C Thomas, Springfield, Illinois.

Baldwin, M., and Bailey, P. (1958): *Temporal Lobe Epilepsy*, p. 587. Charles C Thomas, Springfield, Illinois.

Balzamo, E., Bert, J., Menini, Ch., and Vanquet, R. (1975): Excessive light sensitivity in *Papio papio*: Its variation with age, sex, and geographic origin. *Epilepsia*, 16:269–276.

Bancaud, J., Bloch, V., and Paillard, J. (1953): Contribution E.E.G. à l'étude des potentiels évoqués chez l'homme au niveau du vertex. *Rev. Neurol.*, 89:399–418.

Ben-Ari, Y., and Lagowska, Y. (1978): L'acide kaïnique, un nouveau modèle d'épilepsie expérimentale: Son application au niveau de l'amygdale chez le rat. *C.R. Acad. Sci. Paris*, 287:813–816.

Bert, J., Vuillon-Cacciuttolo, G., Balzamo, E., Comte-Devolx, J., Gambarelli, D., de Mico, P., Tamalet, J., and Gastaut, H. (1978a): Données electroencéphalographiques sur le Kuru expérimental chez le singe Rhésus. *Rev. EEG Neurophysiol.*, 8:617–625.

Bert, J., Vuillon-Cacciuttolo, G., Balzamo, E., de Mico, P., Gambarelli, D., Tamalet, J., and Gastaut, H. (1978b): Appearance of E.E.G. changes reminiscent of a secondary generalized epilepsy in a Rhesus monkey inoculated with a strain of Kuru. *Epilepsia*, 19:257–264.

Blennow G., Brierley, J. B., Meldrum, B. S., and Siesjö, B. K. (1978): Epileptic brain damage: the role of systemic factors that modify cerebral energy metabolism. *Brain*, 101:687–700.

Bloom, F. E., Rossier, J., Battenberg, E. L. F., Bayon, A., French, E., Henriksen, S. J., Siggins, G. R., Segal, D., Browne, R., Ling, N., and Guillemin, R. (1978): β-Endorphin: cellular localization, electrophysiological and behavioral effects. In: *Advances in Biochemical Psychopharmacology*, edited by E. Costa and M. Trabucchi. Raven Press, New York.

Braestrup, C., Albrechtsen, R., and Squires, R. F. (1977): High densities of benzodiazepine receptors in human cortical areas. *Nature*, 269:702–704.

Brotchi, J., Tanaka, T., and Leviel, V. (1978): Lack of activated astrocytes in the kindling phenomenon. *Exp. Neurol.*, 58:119–125.

Castells, C., Gastaut, H. Vigouroux, R., and Ferrer, S. (1952): Etude des réactions déviationnelles au cours des crises temporales. *Rev. Neurol.*, 86:674–678.

Chalazonitis, N., and Boisson, M. (1978): *Abnormal Neuronal Discharges*. Raven Press, New York.

Fischer, R. S., and Prince, D. A. (1977): Spike-wave rhythms in cat cortex induced by parenteral penicillin. I: Electroencephalographic features. *Electroencephalogr. Clin. Neurophysiol.*, 42:608–624.

Fischer-Williams, M., Poncet, M., Riche, D., and Naquet, R. (1968): Light induced epilepsy in the baboon *Papio papio*: Cortical and depth recording. *Electroencephalogr. Clin. Neurophysiol.*, 25:557–569.

Frenk, H., Urca, G., and Liebeskind, J. C. (1978): Epileptic properties of leucine and methionine-enkephalin: Comparison with morphine and reversibility by naloxone. *Brain Res.*, 147:327–337.

Gastaut, H. (1954): Etat actuel des connaissances sur l'anatomie pathologique des épilepsies. In: Colloque sur les problèmes d'anatomie normale et pathologique posés par les décharges épileptiques. *Acta Medica Belgi.*, 5–20.

Gastaut, H., Naquet, R., and Roger, A. (1952b): Etude des postdécharges électriques provoquées par stimulation du complexe nucléaire amygdalien chez le chat. *Rev. Neurol.*, 87:224–231.

Gastaut, H., Naquet, R., and Vigouroux, R. (1953*a*): Un cas d'épilepsie amygdalienne expérimentale chez le chat. *Electroencephalogr. Clin. Neurophysiol.*, 5:291–294.

Gastaut, H., Naquet, R., Vigouroux, R., Roger, A., and Badier, M. (1953*b*): Etude electrographique chez l'homme et chez l'animal des décharges épileptiques dites "psychomotrices." *Rev. Neurol.*, 88:310–354.

Gastaut, H., Pinsard, N., Gastaut, J. L., Régis, H., Michel, B., Roger, J., and Dravet, Ch. (1977): Etude tomodensitométrique des accidents cérébraux responsables des hémiplégies aigües de l'enfant. *Rev. Neurol.*, 133:595–607.

Gastaut, H., Terzian, H., Naquet, R., and Luschnat, K. (1952*c*): Corrélations entre les "automatismes" des crises temporales et les phénomènes électroencephalographiques qui les accompagnent. *Rev. Neurol.*, 86:678–682.

Gastaut, H., Vigouroux, R., and Naquet, R. (1952*a*): Lésions épileptogènes amygdalohippocampiques provoquées chez le chat par injection de "crème d'alumine." *Rev. Neurol.*, 87:607–609.

Gloor, P., Quesney, L. F., and Zumstein, H. (1977): Pathophysiology of generalized penicillin epilepsy in the cat: The role of cortical and subcortical structures. II: Topical application of penicillin to the cerebral cortex and to subcortical structures. *Electroencephalogr. Clin. Neurophysiol.*, 43:79–94.

Gloor, P., and Testa, G. (1979): Generalized penicillin epilepsy in the cat: Effects of intracarotid and intravertebral pentylenetetrazol and amobarbital injections. *Electroencephalogr. Clin. Neurophysiol.*, 36:499–575.

Goddard, G. V., McIntyre, D. C., and Leech, C. R. (1969): A permanent change in brain function resulting from daily electrical stimulation. *Exp. Neurol.*, 25:295–330.

Green, J. B., and Naquet, R. (1957): Etude de la propagation locale et à distance des décharges épileptiques. *Acta Medica Belg.*, 226–249.

Guberman, A., and Gloor, P. (1974): Cholinergic drug studies of generalized penicillin epilepsy in the cat. *Brain Res.*, 78:203–222.

Horton, R. W., and Meldrum, B. S. (1973): Seizures induced by allylglycine, 3-mercaptopropionic acid and 4-deoxypyridoxine in mice and photosensitive baboon, and different mode of inhibition of cerebral glutamic acid decarboxylase. *Br. J. Pharmacol.*, 49:52–63.

Hughes, J. (1975): Isolation of an endogenous compound from the brain with pharmacological properties similar to morphine. *Brain Res.*, 88:295–308.

Hughes, J., Smith, T. W., Kosterlitz, H. W., Fothergill, L. A., Morgan, B. A., and Morris, H. R. (1975): Identification of two related pentapeptides from the brain with potent opiate agonist activity. *Nature (Lond.)*, 258:577–579.

Killam, K. F., Killam, E. K., and Naquet, R. (1966): Mise en évidence chez certains singes d'un syndrome photomyoclonique. *C.R. Acad. Sci. Paris.*, 262:1010–1012.

Killam, K. F., Killam, E. K., and Naquet, R. (1967): An animal model of light sensitive epilepsy. *Electroencephalogr. Clin. Neurophysiol.*, 22:497–513.

Klass, D. W., and Fischer-Williams, M. (1976): Sensory stimulation, sleep and sleep deprivation. In: *Handbook of Electroencephalography and Clinical Neurophysiology.*, Vol. 3, Part D, edited by A. Remond. Elsevier, Amsterdam.

Lanoir, J. (1972): Etude electrocorticographique de la veille et du sommeil chez le chat. Thèse de science, Marseille.

Lazarus, L. H., Ling, N., and Guillemin, R. (1976): β-lipotrophin as a prohormone for the morphinomimetic peptides endorphins and enkephalins. *Proc. Natl. Acad. Sci. USA*, 73:2156–2159.

Le Gal La Salle, G., Calvino, B., and Ben-Ari, Y. (1977): Morphine enhances amygdaloïd seizures and increases interictal spike frequency in kindled rats. *Neurosci. Lett.*, 6:255–260.

Leviel, V., and Naquet, R. (1977): A study of the action of valproic acid on the kindling effect. *Epilepsia*, 18:229–234.

Ling, N., and Guillemin, R. (1976): Morphinomimetic activity of synthetic fragments of β-lipotrophin and analogs. *Proc. Natl. Acad. Sci. USA*, 73:3308–3310.

McCaughran, J. A., Corcoran, M. E., and Wada, J. (1978*a*): Role of the nonspecific thalamus in amygdaloid kindling. *Exp. Neurol.*, 58:471–485.

McCaughran, J. A., Corcoran, M. E., and Wada, J. (1978*b*): Role of the forebrain commissures in amygdaloid kindling in rats. *Epilepsia*, 19:19–33.

Meldrum, B. S., Braïlowsky, S., and Naquet, R. (1978): Approche pharmacologique de l'épilepsie photosensible du *Papio papio*. In: *Actualités pharmacologiques, 30e série*, edited by J. Cheymol, J. R. Boissier and P. Le Chat. Masson, Paris.

Meldrum, B. S., and Brierley, J. B. (1973): Prolonged epileptic seizures in primates: Ischemic cell change and its relation to ictal physiological events. *Arch. Neurol.*, 78:10–17.

Meldrum, B. S., Horton, R. W., and Brierley, J. B. (1974): Epileptic brain damage in adolescent baboons following seizures induced by allylglycine. *Brain*, 97:407–418.

Meldrum, B. S., Menini, Ch., Stutzmann, J. M., and Naquet, R. (1979): Effects of opiate-like peptides, morphine and naloxone in the photosensitive baboon, *Papio papio*. *Brain Res.*, 170:333–348.

Meldrum, B. S., and Nilsson, B. (1976): Cerebral blood flow and metabolic rate early and late in prolonged epileptic seizures induced in rats by bicuculline. *Brain*, 99:523–542.

Ménini, Ch., Stutzmann, J. M., and Valin, A. (1979): Localisation topographique comparée des décharges paroxystiques et des fuseaux chez le *Papio papio*. *Rev. Neurol.* (*in press*).

Mohler, H., and Okada, T. (1977): Benzodiazepine receptor: Demonstration in the central nervous system. *Science*, 198–849.

Mutani, R., Monaco, F., Durelli, L., and Delsedime, M. (1974): The free amino acids in the SCF of epileptic subjects. *Epilepsia*, 15:593–597.

Naquet, R. (1953): Sur les fonctions du rhinencéphale d'après les résultats de sa stimulation chez le chat. Thèse de doctorat en Médecine, Marseille.

Naquet, R. (1973): L'épilepsie photosensible du Papio papio. Un modèle de l'épilepsie photosensible de l'homme. *Arch. Ital. Biol.*, 111:516–526.

Naquet, R. (1977): Sleep and experimental epilepsy. In: *Sleep, 1976, Third European Congress of Sleep Research*, Montpellier, 1976, edited by W. P. Koella and P. Levin. S. Karger AG., Basel.

Naquet, R. (1977): L'épilepsie photosensible, données humaines et expérimentales. *Neurobiol. Recife*, 40:145–180.

Naquet, R., and Meldrum, B. S. (1972): Photogenic seizures in baboon. In: *Experimental Models of Epilepsy. A Manual for the Laboratory Worker*, edited by D. P. Purpura, J. K. Penry, D. B. Tower, D. M. Woodbury, and R. D. Walter. Raven Press, New York.

Naquet, R., and Menini, Ch. (1972): La photosensibilité excessive du *Papio papio:* Approches neurophysiologiques et pharmacologiques de ses mécanismes. *Electroencephalogr. Clin. Neurophysiol.* (*Suppl.*), 31:13–26.

Naquet, R., and Menini, Ch. (1978): New data on the physiopathogeny of experimental generalized epilepsies. *Electroencephalogr. Clin. Neurophysiol.* (*Suppl.*), 34:277–284.

Naquet, R., Menini, Ch., and Catier, J. (1972): Photically induced epilepsy in *Papio papio:* The initiation of discharges and the role of the frontal cortex and of the corpus callosum. In: *Synchronisation of E.E.G. Activity in Epilepsies*, edited by H. Petsche and M. A. B. Brazier. Springer Verlag, Vienna, New York.

Naquet, R., Tiberin, P., Toga, M., and Vigouroux, R. (1962): Rhinencéphale et épilepsie expérimentale. Rôles respectifs du siège de la lésion cicatricielle primitive et des lésions secondaires de l'hippocampe. In: *Physiologie de l'Hippocampe*, edited by P. Passouant. Editions du C.N.R., Paris.

Penfield, W., and Jasper, H. (1956): *Epilepsy and the Functional Anatomy of the Human Brain*. Churchill, London.

Pinel, J. P. J., and Rovner, L. I.: (1978): Experimental epileptogenesis: kindling induced epilepsy in rats. *Exp. Neurol.*, 58:190–202.

Prince, D. A., and Farrell, D. (1969): ''Centrencephalic'' spike and wave discharges following parenteral penicillin injection in the cat. *Neurology* (*Minneap.*), 19:309–310.

Quesney, L. F., Gloor, P., Kratzenberg, E., and Zumstein, H. (1977): Pathophysiology of generalized penicillin epilepsy in the cat: The role of cortical and subcortical structure. I: Systemic application of penicillin. *Electroencephalogr. Clin. Neurophysiol.*, 42:640–655.

Racine, R. (1972): Modification of seizure activity by electrical stimulation. II: Motor seizure. *Electroencephalogr. Clin. Neurophysiol.*, 32:269–279.

Riche, D., Gambarelli-Dubois, D., Dam, M., and Naquet, R. (1971): Repeated seizures and cerebral lesions in photosensitive baboons (*Papio papio*). A preliminary report. In: *Brain Hypoxia*, edited by J. B. Brierley and B. S. Meldrum. Spastics International Medical Publishers, London.

Squires, R. F., and Braestrup, C. (1977): Benzodiazepine receptors in rat brain. *Nature*, 266:732–734.

Squires, R., Naquet, R., Riche, D., and Braestrup, C. (1979): Increased thermolability of benzodiazepine receptors in cerebral cortex of a baboon with spontaneous seizures. *Epilepsia*, 20:215–221.

Tanaka, T., Lange, H., and Naquet, R. (1975): Sleep, subcortical stimulation and kindling in the cat. *Can. J. Neurol. Sciences*, 2:447–455.

Tanaka, T., and Naquet, R. (1975): Kindling effect and sleep organization in cats. *Electroencephalogr. Clin. Neurophysiol.*, 39:449–454.

Tanaka, T., and Naquet, R. (1976): Epilepsy and sleep organization in the baboon *Papio papio*. *Electroencephalogr. Clin. Neurophysiol.*, 41:580–586.

Urca, G., Frenk, H., Liebeskind, J. C., and Taylor, A. N. (1977): Morphine and enkephalin: Analgesic and epileptic properties. *Science*, 197:83–86.

Van Gelder, N. M. (1978): Glutamic acid and epilepsy: the action of taurine. In: *Taurine and Neurological Disorders*, edited by A. Barbeau and R. J. Huxtable. Raven Press, New York.

Van Gelder, N. M., and Courtois, A. (1972): Close relation between changing content of specific amino acids in epileptogenic cortex of cats, and severity of epilepsy. *Brain*, 43:477–484.

Van Gelder, N. M., Koyama, I., and Jasper, H. H. (1977): Taurine treatment of spontaneous chronic epilepsy in a cat. *Epilepsia*, 18:45–54.

Van Gelder, N. M., Sherwin, A. L., and Rasmussen, T. (1972): Amino acid content of epileptogenic human brain: Focal versus surrounding regions. *Brain*, 40:385–393.

Verdeaux, G., and Marty, R. (1954): Action sur l'électroencephalogramme de substances pharmacodynamiques d'intérêt clinique. *Rev. Neurol.*, 91:405–427.

Wada, J. A. (1978): Kindling as a model of epilepsy. *Electroencephalogr. Clin. Neurophysiol.* (*Suppl.*), 34:309–316.

Wada, J. A., Miroguchi, T., and Osawa, T. (1978): Secondarily generalized convulsive seizure induced by daily amygdaloid stimulation in rhesus monkeys. *Neurology (Minneap.)*, 28:1026–1036.

Wada, J. A., and Osawa, T. (1976): Spontaneous recurrent seizure state induced by daily electric amygdaloïd stimulation in senegalese baboons (*Papio papio*). *Neurology (Minneap.)*, 26:273–286.

Wada, J. A., and Sato, M. (1974): Generalized convulsive seizures induced by daily electrical stimulation of the amygdala in cats. *Neurology (Minneap.)*, 24:565–574.

Wada, J. A., Terao, A., and Booker, H. E. (1972): Longitudinal correlative analysis of epileptic baboon, *Papio papio. Neurology (Minneap.)*, 22:1272–1285.

Ward, A. A. Jr. (1969): The epileptic neuron: chronic foci in animals and man. In: *Basic Mechanisms of the Epilepsies*, edited by H. H. Jasper, A. A. Ward, Jr., and A. Pope. Little, Brown and Company, Boston.

Ward, A. A. Jr. (1972): Topical convulsant metals. In: *Experimental Models of Epilepsy. A Manual for the Laboratory Worker*, edited by D. P. Purpura, J. K. Penry, D. B. Tower, D. M. Woodbury, and R. D. Walter. Raven Press, New York.

Advances in Epileptology:
The Xth Epilepsy International Symposium,
edited by J. A. Wada and J. K. Penry.
Raven Press, New York © 1980.

Control of Epilepsy and Its Consequences

Richard L. Masland

*Neurological Institute, College of Physicians and Surgeons of Columbia University,
New York, New York 10032*

In presenting the William Lennox lecture this year, it is appropriate to review the findings of the National Commission for the Control of Epilepsy and its Consequences, for such a commission had been one of Dr. Lennox's long-sought goals. Another—the establishment of a unified voluntary effort for epilepsy—has been achieved both at the national and the international level this year.

The establishment of such an effort could do much to correct a major problem presented to the commission by persons with epilepsy, that is, failure of human communication. Patients complain that neither they nor their families, nor their physicians, nor the public understood their problems; would listen to their concerns; or could talk freely to them about themselves. They sensed a similar lack of communication and knowledge to exist also between professionals. The social isolation of persons with epilepsy, and possibly of some of those who care for them, manifests itself at all levels—failure of drug compliance; denial of employment; and isolation in large institutions. This failure of human communication is related not only to the epileptic person: How else can one explain our failure to adhere to strict programs of prophylactic vaccination and highway safety? As I review some of the highlights of the commission's report, ignorance and failure of communication are found to be a constant theme.

The major focus of the commission's effort was on prevention—prevention of epilepsy, prevention of seizures in those with epilepsy, and prevention of disability in those with uncontrollable seizures.

Regarding the prevention of epilepsy, a reported decline in the annual incidence of epilepsy is a hopeful sign that encourages further prevention efforts. Hauser et al. (1977) report that from 1964 to 1974 the annual incidence of epilepsy dropped 28%. The cause of this decline is uncertain. It could reflect an observed tendency of physicians to start prophylactic treatment after a single seizure. However, the decline in epilepsy parallels a decline in cerebral palsy (Hagberg et al., 1975) and in neonatal death rate, both attributable to a decline in adverse perinatal factors that also relate to epilepsy (Davis, 1978).

In fact, among known causes of epilepsy, the leaders are perinatal factors (18%), infections of the central nervous system (CNS) (12%), and head injury (12%) (Bergamini et al., 1977). Measures for the control of infections and of head injury are the subject of a special report at this meeting by Mrs. Ellen Grass, chairman of the commission. Their importance is enhanced because they are so clearly preventable. Our failure to utilize currently available methods for their control is a national and an international disgrace and should be the focus of an intensive public education effort.

But known or "organic" causes of epilepsy account for less than 50%. For example, computerized transverse axial tomographic (CAT) scan is abnormal in only 50% of cases, ranging from 4% in primary generalized absence to 60% in partial epilepsy (Gastaut and Gastaut, 1976). Granted that minor structural changes could be undetected, the varying ratios indicate that for many, especially the primary generalized epilepsies, other factors are responsible.

A genetic factor has been assumed. Fortunately, we are getting a clearer picture of the role of inheritance. Over 100 single-gene disorders have epilepsy as a symptom (Anderson, 1977); most have other gross characteristics. Together, they account for less than 2% of cases of epilepsy.

Inheritance in epilepsy is more commonly complex and multifactorial. We must rely on empiric risk figures. These vary greatly, depending on the nature of the epilepsy and the known family history.

For counseling, the key questions are: For the person with epilepsy, "What are the chances my child would have epilepsy?" For the parent with an epileptic child, "What are the chances that my next child will have epilepsy?" In some instances, the enhanced risk is zero; in others it may approach 20% (Tsuboi and Endo, 1977). For such a complex picture, counseling must be highly specialized and individualized.

An additional complication is that "familial" does not always mean "genetic." Still unexplained, for example, is that children of epileptic mothers are more likely to have epilepsy than are children of epileptic fathers (Annegers et al., 1976). This suggests an environmental nongenetic factor. Surprisingly, not until the late 1960s (Massey, 1966) was the teratogenic role of anticonvulsant drugs discovered. Recognition of the fetal hydantoin syndrome is even more recent, yet evidence of this trait may appear in up to 44%. Its full impact, including lowered I.Q. scores, is only beginning to be appreciated (Hanson et al., 1976). In addition, one might postulate that exposure of the embryo to drugs would modify enzyme development in the CNS and cause seizure susceptibility after delivery. However, data to support this speculation are lacking.

Clearly, however, the epileptic woman and her child are at risk from many adverse factors. New knowledge brings new responsibilities. First, regarding the question of eugenics, we have passed from the days of indiscriminate sterilization. We now have the information and the resources to permit each individual to make his or her own decision. Sometimes in our desire not to offend, we may avoid the truth. For an enlightened decision, our patients deserve the facts.

Beyond that, there must be a broader recognition that the epileptic gravida has special problems. She must be provided with the special supervision and counseling that she requires. In the future, we must intensify the study of epilepsy and pregnancy and our search for new nonteratogenic anticonvulsants.

The second level of prevention is the prevention of seizures through anticonvulsant medication and other measures. Since the passage of drug control legislation in 1962, drug development in the United States has lagged behind other countries. For example, there are four anticonvulsants now marketed in Great Britain unavailable in the United States. Valproic acid, now recognized as a major advance, was first marketed in France in 1967. Authorization for testing in the United States was not requested by any drug company until 1974. It was released in 1978. Eleven years had elapsed, 13 years from the first report of clinical effectiveness (Carraz et al., 1965).

Part of the blame may rest with the Food and Drug Administration (FDA). Their failure to accept the data developed in France (which were acceptable to the British Drug Committee in 1972) suggests either that the French certification was lax, that United States certification is too restrictive, or that there was a lack of communication.

However, the more important lag was the 9 years from the discovery of the drug's effectiveness to the initial investigations in the United States. For this, the United States drug companies and the scientific community are responsible.

Legislation is pending (HR11611) to reform the drug regulation program. It provides for increased flexibility for FDA and the investigators in the initial testing of drugs. In addition, it proposes to establish a "National Center for Clinical Pharmacology" for new drug development.

Many feel that the function of drug development could be done better through increased funding and a broadened mandate for the National Institutes of Health, and that there are other defects in this proposed legislation that might enhance rather than relax the bureaucratic delays of FDA. The American Epilepsy Society should study this legislation carefully, and all of us should be prepared to speak for a program that will enhance new drug development in this country.

Clearly, we need stronger advocacy and a more powerful international program for anticonvulsant drug development. This could be a role for Epilepsy International. The establishment of a worldwide drug development and evaluation program is already a program of The International League, which has approved a uniform terminology and published agreed-on standards for clinical investigation. A next step might be use of uniform data collection forms, and even cooperative trials. For uncommon complications such as congenital malformation, data from a number of institutions will be required. Meanwhile, this annual meeting provides a forum within which all can keep abreast of the latest new developments.

But there still remains that shrinking group for whom medication is ineffective. For them, we still have the responsibility to prevent or minimize the social and emotional consequences.

The most bitter complaint of epileptic persons is their inability to find work. The average employer in the United States will reject an applicant known to have had a seizure within 1 year. Even employment agencies for the handicapped require 6 months of freedom from seizures, yet the Training and Placement Services (TAPS) Program under Epilepsy Foundation of America (EFA) is demonstrating that epileptic persons can be placed and work well.

New legislation in the United States (PL503-PL504) requires government grantees and contractors to employ qualified handicapped persons and not to discriminate against them in providing services. The long-delayed regulations to implement these laws are still being drafted. They require close scrutiny, for their effectiveness will depend on the definition of what is a "qualified" applicant, and even more, what constitutes the "reasonable" accommodations that the employer must make in order for his place of employment to be "accessible and usable" for handicapped persons.

More important than the direct legal impact of this legislation through the courts is its educational value. Much more will be accomplished by education and demonstration, as in the TAPS Program, for in the last analysis, epilepsy will be accepted on the assembly line only when within the work place irrational fear of the epileptic person and his seizures has been overcome by knowledge and understanding.

Closely related to the problems of unemployment are those of transportation and driver's licenses. Most states will now permit persons with epilepsy to drive after they have been free of seizures for 1 or 2 years. In some states the application of these laws has been inflexible and arbitrary; others have established a mechanism for individual review and adjudication on the basis of overall reliability and individual needs. It is disturbing that surveys reveal that a large proportion of epileptic drivers are not licensed. As a result, nine states require a physician to report cases of epilepsy in persons of driving age. If this trend is to be stopped, physicians must to a greater extent impress on their patients their responsibility for self-reporting.

A great opportunity exists to improve the living conditions of persons with epilepsy who because of incompletely controlled seizures or related disabilities are incapable of independent living. The day of the epileptic colony is past; improved seizure control made it unnecessary for the majority of persons with epilepsy. However, there are still an estimated 58,000 epileptic residents of institutions for developmentally disabled persons, and 20,000 in neuropsychiatric hospitals. Often these institutions suffer from the dehumanizing effect of large size, and from geographic and administrative isolation from home and community. Improved transportation and a fresh outlook are now encouraging the integration of these previously isolated populations into the community through the establishment of integrated medical, educational, and vocational services. A project in six large institutions demonstrated spectacular improvement of seizure control through intervention by a well-trained team of specialists. Other institutions are seeking cooperative and consultative arrangements with university medical centers, a trend that should have important impact both on the institution and on future physicians.

Even more exciting is the present opportunity for the development of supervised and cooperative small community-based homes. Newly passed legislation in the United States (the 1978 Amendments to the Housing and Community Development Act of 1974) authorizes the Department of Housing and Urban Development to finance 3- to 5-year renewable contracts for supplying services to elderly and disabled persons residing in public or private non-profit housing projects. Included also are funds for loans to establish community based facilities. Also provided are rent subsidies for handicapped persons living in the community who otherwise might require institutional care (Section 8).

From this brief chapter, touching on only a few highlights of the Commission's report, it is evident great opportunities exist at the present time. At no other time has the scientific community enjoyed such support for its research efforts. Never in the past has there been such worldwide concern for the rights of the underprivileged, including those handicapped by epilepsy.

The potential exists, but these opportunities will be exploited in the United States only if there is leadership. This leadership must come from a strong, unified, national organization operating at every level of the national, state, and local structure. Its educational campaign must reach the patient, the physician, the public, and the legislature. On the international scene, the creation of Epilepsy International provides the means through which laymen and professionals may join forces for a cooperative effort through which the best in each country may be made available to all. It could be a new day for epilepsy.

REFERENCES

Anderson, E. (1977): *"Genetic Counselling for Epilepsy," Report of the Commission for the Control of Epilepsy and its Consequences*, 2:141–174.

Annegers, J. F., Hauser, W. A., and Kurland, L. T. (1976): Seizure disorders in offspring of parents with a history of seizures. *Epilepsia*, 17:1–10.

Bergamini, L., Bergomasco, B., Benna, P., and Gilli, M. (1977): Acquired etiologic factors in 1,785 epileptic subjects. *Epilepsia*, 18:437–444.

Davis, J. (1978): Neonatal convulsions: Etiology, late neonatal status and long-term outcome. *Dev. Med. Child. Neurol.*, 20:143–158.

Carraz, G., Fau, R., Chateau, R., and Bonnin, J. (1965): Communication a propos des Premiers

Essais Cliniques Sur L'Activite Antiepileptique de L'Acide N-dipropyl Acetique (Sel de Na). *Ann. Med. Psychol. (Paris)*, 122:577–585.

Gastaut, H., and Gastaut, J. L. (1976): Computerized transverse axial tomography in epilepsy. *Epilepsia*, 17:325–336.

Hagberg, B., Hagberg, G., and Olow, I. (1975): The changing panorama of cerebral palsy. *Acta Paediatr. Scand.*, 64:185–192.

Hanson, J. W., Myrianthopoulos, M. D., Sedgwick Harvey, M. A., and Smith, D. W. (1976): Risks to the offspring of women treated with hydantoin anticonvulsants, with emphasis on the fetal hydantoin syndrome. *J. Pediatr.*, 89:662–668.

Hauser, W. A., Annegers, J. S., and Kurland, L. T. (1977): Is the incidence of epilepsy declining? *Am. J. Epidemiol.*, 106:264–276.

Massey, K. M. (1966): Teratogenic effects of diphenyl hydantoin sodium. *J. Oral Ther. Pharmacol.*, 2:380–385.

Tsuboi, T., and Endo, S. (1977): Incidence of seizures and EEG abnormalities among offspring of epileptic patients. *Humangenetik*, 36:173–189.

Advances in Epileptology:
The Xth Epilepsy International Symposium,
edited by J. A. Wada and J. K. Penry.
Raven Press, New York © 1980.

Seizure-Related Changes in Brain Structures

Arnold B. Scheibel

Departments of Anatomy and Psychiatry; and Brain Research Institute, UCLA
Center for the Health Sciences, Los Angeles, California 90024

The studies reported here represent another phase in the century-long quest for visible evidence of change in epileptogenic cortex. Over the years, evidence has developed documenting the loss of nerve cells and the appearance of reactive gliosis as pathological changes frequently related to the chronic seizure state (Sommer, 1880; Pfleger, 1880; Spielmeyer, 1927; Earle et al., 1953; Penfield, 1956; Falconer, 1971). With the exception of Demoor's (1898) virtually forgotten clinicopathological study, and the recent investigations of Westrum et al. (1964) evaluating lesions associated with experimentally induced epilepsy, all previous reports were based on staining methods that did not allow visualization of the neuronal dendritic domain. Since this may constitute 80 to 90% of the surface area of the neuron, it is clear that much had still to be learned through the application of appropriate techniques such as the methods of Golgi. The use of Golgi impregnation methods by Demoor (1898) first implicated dendritic tissue in the ictal process. He described diffuse spine loss and moniliform deformities of almost all of the dendrite shafts he examined. These changes were related, by implication at least, to problems in blood supply or metabolic support. Golgi studies of the environs of experimental alumina cream lesions by Westrum et al. (1964) showed even more dramatic changes in dendritic morphology, although the comparative contributions of the irritative substance itself and of the electrical storms that followed remain unclear.

METHODS

The present study is based on examination of pes hippocampus and adjacent temporal lobe tissue surgically removed by Dr. Paul Crandall from 11 patients with intractable temporal lobe epilepsy. The patients had been followed clinically from 1 to 4 years and, prior to surgery, had undergone extensive periods of chronic recording from cortical surface and/or depth arrays of electrodes. Studies with implanted electrode ensembles were carried out for 3 to 4 weeks and seizure activity was monitored by radiotelemetry through at least several spontaneous clinical seizures. The anterior temporal lobes resected were the most frequent sites of autonomous epileptiform potentials, periodic paroxysms of sustained seizure activity, and rhythmic EEG waves preceding the onset of the clinical seizure. After removal of small tissue slabs for Golgi, electron microscopy, and histochemical studies, the anterior lobe was resected en bloc, including amygdala, uncus, and parahippocampal gyrus, and fixed in formalin for routine pathological studies.

Our Golgi material was prefixed immediately after surgical excision in buffered 10% formalin solution for 1 to 3 hr, then placed in osmic dichromate (rapid Golgi) solution for 5 to 10 days and impregnated in 0.75% silver nitrate solution for 24 to 48 hr. Specimens were blocked in paraffin without dehydration, cut at 100 to 150 μm, dehydrated, cleared, and mounted under a neutral synthetic medium such as Permount without coverslips for study, photography, and drawing.

RESULTS

In 7 of the 11 cases studied, changes of varying intensity have been noted in the cell dendrite systems of hippocampus and dentate gyrus. The degree of change has shown remarkable latitude, and although some cases seem more pathologically involved than others, there is a tendency for considerable variation of pathological alterations in the individual case.

(a) *Minimal changes:* The most subtle variations noted include local loss of dendrite spines over portions of an individual dendrite, either with or without nodulation of the denuded shaft. The silhouette of the dendrite shaft may also become lumpy or irregular. Although patchy spine loss may be seen anywhere along the apical or basilar shafts of hippocampal pyramids, changes are most often seen initially toward the periphery and at the tips of the shafts, the basilar dendrites being particularly involved.

(b) *More serious changes:* In addition to loss of spines and nodulation that gradually becomes generalized along the entire dendrite domain of the cell, long segments of shaft may now appear swollen and develop leaf-like excrescences followed by distortion and shrinkage (Fig. 1). Dendrites progressively shrivel, eventually becoming distorted stumps and then disappear entirely. The cell bodies may either swell and lose their capacity to stain or else shrink and fragment.

Many cases of surgically excised hippocampus show dense fields of fibrillary astrocytes. Since these are usually found in areas unusually poor in neurons, it is assumed that these represent the fields of gliosis described by other investigators. Many of these glial cells show changes not ordinarily found in gliocytes. Principal among them is the presence of nodular enlargements along the individual stalks or at their terminals. These enlargements do not have the regularity of arrangement characteristic of dendritic nodulation, which we have called the "string of beads" deformity (Scheibel and

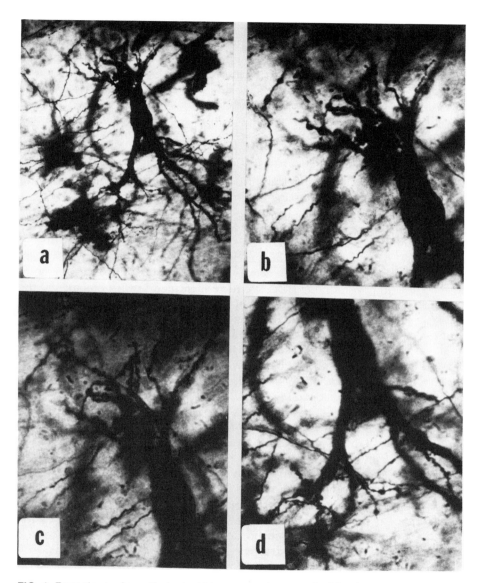

FIG. 1. Four views of a pathological hippocampal neuron in CA_2 of a temporal lobe epilepsy patient. In **a,** the entire neuron is viewed at low power ($\times150$) while the changes on the various dendrite systems are seen at higher power ($\times400$) in **b, c,** and **d,** at slightly different planes of focus. The primary changes include loss of spines, development of nodulation, and loss of the majority of the dendrite shafts. Modified rapid Golgi stain.

Scheibel, 1973). They are highly variable in size and shape, often approaching 3 to 5 μm in size and usually irregularly arranged along the glial fibers.

(c) *Pathological changes in dentate granules:* The human dentate granule cell normally shows a wider range of morphological variation than those of rodents, carnivores, or even primates. It is therefore necessary to exercise caution in identifying changes of pathological significance. Two general categories of change have been found with reasonable regularity in tissue from patients with temporal lobe disease. The first type includes those that can be found throughout neocortex and archicortex subject to pathological processes. It encompasses loss of dendrite spines, development of nodules along the dendritic shafts, and progressive distortion in the appearance of the dendritic domain culminating in shrinkage and atrophy.

The second group of changes includes variations in appearance of the entire dendrite system and is probably related to pathological processes although, of course, appropriate control specimens are not easily available. On the other hand, study of human autopsy tissue seldom reveals such changes, providing at least some degree of confidence that the changes are of pathological import. Among these we have identified inward collapse of the dentate cell dendrite tree onto the central axis of the dendritic domain producing a long, thin, tightly packed dendrite array. We have called this the "folded parasol deformity" (Scheibel and Scheibel, 1973). A second structural variation that appears more or less unique to tissue from seizured patients consists of a lateral bending or distortion of the dendrite systems of a number of adjacent cells. This "windblown look" frequently appears adjacent to areas of cell loss and gliosis.

These dentate-specific changes exist in varying combinations; the previous section has alluded to the more widely observed alterations. As dentate granule cells lose their spine systems and appear to contract in on the central axis of the domain, the shafts also may become thinner, taking on a glial-like appearance. These elements apparently disappear with time, to be replaced by proliferating astrocytes as noted in the pes hippocampus.

The initially localized or spotty nature of pathological change seen in hippocampus is repeated in the dentate. However, one gains the impression that dentate pathology may proceed faster or generalize sooner since in a few cases with long-standing histories of ictal episodes, the great majority of dentate cells show pathological changes with little in the way of intact islands of neural tissue so characteristic of the pes hippocampus.

The mossy tuft-bearing axons of the dentate cells that project onto the hippocampal pyramids also show marked changes in the majority of cases so far studied. These variations include beading and fragmentation of the axon stalks and replacement of the familiar lobulated or tufted profiles of the terminal structures with clusters or bunches of nodes often larger than the original tufts. The broad dispersion of such pathological structures, even when the zones of dentate cell involvement are still limited, bear witness to the extensive course and multiple terminal systems provided by the axon of each dentate granule cell.

In conjunction with these studies on the structural substrates of temporal lobe epilepsy in man, we have used two animal models for their possible correlative value. Mongolian gerbils are small rat-like rodents, a substantial number of which exhibit naturally occurring seizures. Although a wide range of ictal patterns may be seen, they frequently start with twitching of nostrils and/or vibrissae, then progressively involve the entire animal in a grand mal-like convulsion. Using animals provided by Drs. Richard Schain and James Diaz; Linda Paul, Itzhak Fried, and I have studied approximately 500 Golgi-stained brain sections from 40 gerbils, equally divided between seizured and nonseizured animals (Paul et al., 1978). Concentrating on the hippocampal-dentate complex and adjacent entorhinal cortex, we have found several features that may be related to the seizured state although the correlation is, so far, only tentative. In many, but not all of the seizured animals, mossy tufts appear swollen and shapeless, compared with their more intricate and convoluted appearance in nonseizured animals. The mossy axons themselves often appear irregular in silhouette and loaded with nodules, a feature also common to the perinatal rapid growth state.

Most interesting from our point of view is the terminal distribution of tufts on the receptive hippocampal pyramids of CA4, CA3, and CA2. The usual terminal site for these powerfully facilitative axon streams (Andersen and Lomo, 1966; Yamamoto, 1972) is on the apical shaft of the CA2 and CA3 pyramid, approximately one-quarter to one-third of the way from soma to terminal dendritic arches (Lorente de No, 1934). In many of our seizured animals, tufts appear more widely spread along the proximal portions of the apical *and* the basilar shafts, and sometimes applied directly to soma and even to the axon hillock-initial segment. Recent evidence identifies soma and axon hillock as preferential synaptic sites for the strongly inhibitory basket cell system (Andersen et al., 1963). This area has been proposed as the locus for most effective inhibitory control of the entire cell-dendrite complex. Its apparent invasion by a population of strongly facilitatory terminals might drastically alter the balance of mechanisms controlling firing patterns, thereby further enhancing the already low threshold of hippocampus to the generation and spread of ictal activity. Electron microscopic studies are in an early stage, and at this point we are comparing mossy tuft size, shape, number of synaptic specializations, and the density and distribution patterns of synaptic vesicles within the tufts.

The kindled rat has also been studied as a possible model of the human epileptic state. Since the initial description by Goddard et al. (1969) that brief subconvulsive stimuli delivered chronically to various parts of the brain result eventually in generalized convulsive seizures, the substrate mechanisms have been sought. We examined brain tissue from approximately 50 kindled rats and an equal number of controls supplied to us by Drs. John

Pinel of Vancouver and Jerome Engel of Los Angeles (Engel et al., 1978). The study is based on Golgi stained sections prepared for light microscopy. In addition some of the material is being studied with the electron microscope in collaboration with Drs. W. Jann Brown and Elizabeth Lu. The enormous variation in morphology of mossy tufts and the regional differences within the pes hippocampus have made establishment of correlations difficult so far. The gross morphology of hippocampal cell dendrites and the structure and density patterns of dendrite spines are also being examined.

DISCUSSION

No consensus exists as to pathogenesis of the ictal process or to the nature of the relationship between these recently recognized pathoanatomic changes (Scheibel and Scheibel, 1973) and the underlying seizure mechanisms. We previously summarized three current working hypotheses on the genesis of lesions in temporal lobe disease. The first envisions stepwise development of the characteristic lesion as a result of vascular spasm assumed to accompany each ictal episode (Spielmeyer, 1927). Direct observation of cortical vessels during seizures has not confirmed the presence of such spasms, however. The second, developed by Earle et al. (1953), attributes the primary lesion to compression of the fetal head during passage down the birth canal with resultant herniation of uncus and hippocampus under the tentorium. The third, suggested by Falconer (1971), looks to early asphyxial episodes such as febrile convulsions or status epilepticus occurring at a period of life when hippocampus and other mesial structures are particularly vulnerable to anoxia. The resultant damage during infancy is conceived as developing into a sclerosing lesion that serves as the epileptogenic focus. In Falconer's experiments, approximately one-half of his cases seemed based on such lesions. In the 11 cases studied in this chapter, there is no history of birth injury or infantile seizures in any patient, although two were known to have suffered head trauma and subsequent unconsciousness during childhood or early adolescence.

It has been observed that deafferentation leads to loss of dendrite spines (Colonnier, 1964). In view of the apparently early, if patchy, loss of spines noted before, antecedent destruction of axons must be considered as a putative pathogenic factor, especially in light of Brown's (1973) observations with the electron microscope on the degenerative changes in small hippocampal axon systems. On the other hand, there are no data to indicate that axonal (presynaptic) changes regularly antedate alterations in dendrite spines and dendrites. Both, in fact, may be the result of ongoing pathogenic processes in the parent neurons. Several investigators have suggested that the gliosis characteristic of advanced epileptic foci may form a barrier that progressively isolates neuronal assemblies both from sources of metabolic supply and from afferent input (Pfleger, 1880; Spielmeyer, 1927; Earle et al.,

1953; Westrum et al., 1964; Falconer, 1971). Once again, there is no clear indication whether this is an etiologic factor or a consequence of the primary process.

We have been impressed by the generally spotty nature of the pathology. In most of the cases examined with Golgi methods, some cellular elements show only the earliest stages of pathological change, i.e., spine loss and/or nodulation along one segment of a single dendrite, frequently alongside neurons with far advanced alterations involving the entire dendritic tree and soma. This may go on to complete cell loss and replacement gliosis. Even cases with clinical histories measured in years or decades may have this combination of very "old" and very "new" lesions, a fact confirmed by electron microscopy. For this reason, we have suggested the possibility that, at least for the temporal lobe syndromes studied in this report, the active process represents ongoing focal brain disease secondary to some slow progressive process, whether infectious (slow virus?) or genetic-enzymatic in nature. This concept stands in considerable contrast to the more usually acceptable view of the epileptic syndromes as the consequence of a single insult at birth or during infancy.

The experimental models on which we have briefly reported stress the difficulty in establishing a visibly recognizable substrate. Studies now in progress are considering the possibility of both pre- and postsynaptic structures as central to the epileptogenic process. At present, while our search is centered in the hippocampus-dentate complex of the limbic lobe, we are studying the size, shape, and internal structure of mossy tufts and their distribution patterns on hippocampal pyramids. At the same time, we are examining the receptive structures—dendrites and dendrite spines—for morphological and quantitative changes.

It seems likely that there may be multiple etiological factors involved in the genesis of electrical storms in the nervous system. Alumina cream, penicillin, asphyxia, physical trauma, and electrical kindling procedures would seem, at first glance, to invoke widely different pathogenetic sequences in the ultimate development of an electrical and behavioral fit. It remains to be seen whether common mechanisms and common morphological criteria can be established for all.

REFERENCES

Andersen, P., Eccles, J. C., and Løyning, Y. (1963): Recurrent inhibition in the hippocampus with identification of the inhibitory cell and its synapses. *Nature (Lond.),* 198:540–542.
Andersen, P., and Lomo, T. (1966): Mode of activation of hippocampal pyramids by excitatory synapses on dendrites. *Exp. Brain Res.,* 2:247–260.
Brown, W. J. (1973): Structural substrates of seizure foci in the human temporal lobe. In: *Epilepsy, Its Phenomena in Man,* edited by M. A. B. Brazier, pp. 339–374. Academic Press, New York.
Colonnier, M. (1964): Experimental degeneration in the cerebral cortex. *J. Anat.,* 98:47–53.
Demoor, J. (1898): La mecanisme et la signification de l'état moniliforme des neurones. *Ann. Soc. Roy. Sci. Med. Nat. Brux.,* 7:205–250.

Earle, K., Baldwin, M., and Penfield, W. (1953): Incisural sclerosis and temporal lobe seizures produced by hippocampal herniation at birth. *Arch. Neurol. Psychiatr.*, 69:27–42.

Engel, Jr., J., Wolfson, L., and Brown, L. (1978): Anatomical correlates of electrical and behavioral events related to amygdaloid kindling. *Ann. Neurol.*, 3:538–544.

Falconer, M. A. (1971): Genetic and related aetiological factors in temporal lobe epilepsy. A review. *Epilepsia*, 12:13–31.

Goddard, G. V., McIntyre, D., and Leech, C. (1969): A permanent change in brain function resulting from daily electrical stimulation. *Exp. Neurol.*, 25:295–330.

Lorente de No., R. (1934): Studies on the structure of the cerebral cortex. II. Continuation of ammonic system. *J. Psychol. Neurol.*, 46:113–177.

Paul, L., Fried, I., Watanabe, K., Diez, J., and Scheibel, A. B. (1978): Possible structural correlates of spontaneous seizures in Mongolian gerbils. *Soc. for Neuroscience* (abstr.) In press.

Penfield, W. (1956): Epileptogenic lesions. *Acta Neurol. Belg.*, 56:75–88.

Pfleger, L. (1880): Beobachtung über Schrumpfung und Sclerose des Ammonshornes bei Epilepsie. *Allg. Z. Psychiat.*, 36:359–365.

Scheibel, M. E., and Scheibel, A. B. (1973): Hippocampal pathology in temporal lobe epilepsy. A Golgi survey. In: *Epilepsy, Its Phenomena in Man.* M. A. B. Brasier (ed.), Academic Press, Inc., New York, pp. 311–337.

Sommer, W. (1880): Erkrankung des Ammonshorns als aetiologisches Moment der Epilepsie. *Arch. Psychiat.*, 10:631–675.

Spielmeyer, W. (1927): Die Pathogenese des epileptichen Krampfes. *Z. Ges. Neurol. Psychiat.*, 109:501–515.

Westrum, L., White, L., and Ward, A. (1964): Morphology of the experimental epileptic focus. *J. Neurosurg.*, 21:1033–1046.

Yamamoto, C. (1972): Activation of hippocampal neurons by mossy fiber stimulation in thin brain sections *in vitro. Exp. Brain Res.*, 14:423–435.

INTENSIVE MONITORING

Advances in Epileptology:
The Xth Epilepsy International Symposium,
edited by J. A. Wada and J. K. Penry.
Raven Press, New York © 1980.

Intensive Monitoring of Epileptic Patients

J. Kiffin Penry

Epilepsy Branch, Neurological Disorders Program, National Institute of
Neurological and Communicative Disorders and Stroke, National
Institutes of Health, Bethesda, Maryland 20205

Intensive monitoring of epileptic patients requires detailed, frequent, and accurate quantitative observations and determinations; it is invaluable in the differentiation of psychogenic seizures from epileptic seizures and is indicated in patients who have intractable seizures. Information otherwise unavailable is provided through intensive monitoring so that diagnosis and appropriate treatment can be initiated. Quantitation of the frequency, magnitude, and duration of seizures along with determination of the concentration of prescribed antiepileptic medications in the blood provides the necessary guides to successful treatment. Prolonged videotape recording, along with prolonged EEG recording and frequent simultaneous determination of antiepileptic drug concentrations, have resulted in significant improvement in the majority (61%) of selected patients with long-standing intractable seizures (Porter et al., 1977). Since this subject was reviewed (Penry and Porter, 1977), capability for intensive monitoring of epileptic patients has been developed in numerous centers around the world where many studies are now in progress.

Although most centers are capable of making prolonged recordings of videotape and EEG simultaneously along with antiepileptic drug level determinations, the evaluation of patient performance during an epileptic seizure varies widely from one center to another. Although it is important to have spontaneously recorded seizures without external intervention and stimuli, it is likewise important to demonstrate the level of comprehension and performance during epileptic seizures, especially prolonged complex partial seizures involving psychomotor symptomatology.

PLAN OF INTERVENTION

Intensive monitoring is not a routine test that can be ordered like a blood sample. A technician must be continuously present to make sure that quality data is being recorded, to administer to any needs that may arise with the patient, to maintain a routine behavioral activity record by hourly or half-hourly intervals, and to be prepared to intervene to determine the patient's level of comprehension and performance during the seizures. The physician supervising the intensive monitoring unit should make a plan of monitoring and discuss it with the technician according to the historical features of the patient's seizures. When the patient's seizures are frequent (several times daily) and last for more than 10 sec, rather elaborate plans of intervention may be devised. Although the individual is never completely free of environmental stimuli, it is better to allow the first seizure to occur spontaneously without active intervention. On the other hand, if seizures are infrequent and a psychogenic mechanism is suspected, it may be necessary to intervene during the first recorded seizure. Individuals with seizure-free intervals of 3 or more days are not cost-effective candidates for intensive monitoring unless their seizures have a trigger mechanism or history where the seizures occur in clusters with a long history of many years of intractable seizures.

When the single seizure has been recorded without active intervention, the technician and supervising physician should review the seizure together to discuss the plan of intervention. There are different levels of information to be obtained. What are the spontaneous manifestations of the seizure without intervention? Is there drooping of the eyelids, an arrest of activity, focal motor components of clonic movements, or posturing? Does the patient appear to lose contact with his environment? The alteration of consciousness or the impairment of performance during a seizure may be very subtle, requiring a comparison with normal function. Therefore, it is important to demonstrate perceptiveness and performance during interictal recordings. The patient should be interviewed to determine his mental status and motor performance. Some of the parameters checked during the interictal recording should be repeated during the ictus. Does the patient have a warning or aura? When the patient returns to consciousness, is he confused or fully alert? Is there a subtle dysphasia that may last for seconds or minutes? In the case of psychogenic seizures, it is often possible to interrupt the seizures and produce normal performance with the patient returning into and completing his seizure.

AWARENESS, PERCEPTION

When studying the videotape recorded seizure of spontaneous onset, it may not be apparent that there is any alteration of consciousness, or there may be only a blank stare with loss of visual fixation. The object of intervention is to determine how much awareness or perception are altered, if any. The only possible clue to alteration would be raised in some cases by the presence of abnormal paroxysmal discharges in the EEG without any clinical evidence. A verbal stimulation in the form of numbers, words, word combinations, phrases, or poems may be given during the seizure to see if the patient can recall these items after the seizure. If the verbal stimulation is recalled accurately, a higher level function must be tested through reaction time or multiple-choice reaction times during the paroxysm with either auditory or visual stimulation. Visual surveillance interictally may suppress the occurrence of abnormal paroxysmal discharges. On the other hand, if verbal stimuli are partially or completely unrecalled, verbal commands may be tried during the attack, asking the patient either to close his eyes or raise his hands. It should be noted whether a single command in a normal voice evokes a normal response, or whether repeated commands and loud voices must be used to get a response, or whether there is no response at all. Altered responses must be pursued to define their alteration, and unresponsiveness to commands must result in further types of stimuli. Visual threat stimuli, touching, posturing the patient, or normal tactile responses may be attempted. If these fail, such responses as pinprick may be utilized to measure responsiveness during an attack. Although some standard stimuli should be given to every patient for the purposes of comparison, these alterations must be appraised in each individual.

PERFORMANCE

For those individuals with slight diminution of awareness or distortion of perception, high-level performance should be evaluated. Such individuals can be asked to do multiple choice reaction times, simple reaction times, mental arithmetic, or read a paragraph from a magazine. They should be asked to remember phrases and words to be repeated after the seizure. Individuals who follow commands readily without repetition should be asked to write something on paper and should be given complicated requests for performance, for example, "Touch your right index finger to your nose and your left thumb to your left ear." For individuals who have significant impairment requiring repeated commands to get motion, the technician may tactically move the patients about or lead them around in front of the camera, or assist their performance tactically to see what the limits of their activity may be.

It is important to know when the patient has returned to normal functioning. Frequently this is obvious when the patient says "I feel fine" and can engage in rapid, accurate conversation. If the seizure has lasted for several minutes, the patient is often dull for a long period of time and may remain slow or inaccurate with mental arithmetic. After appearance of normal performance, the patient again may appear to be confused and the technician will note on the EEG that the patient is again in another seizure.

EVALUATION OF AWARENESS, PERCEPTION, AND PERFORMANCE

If there has been no intervention during a seizure, even though it may be possible to review it several times on videotape recording, there are limitations to interpretation or prophesy. It is not fair to speculate about a function that has not been tested or appraised. On the other hand, skilled intervention may answer a great number of questions. Even then, there may still be uncertainties. In individuals with minimal impairment, it may be necessary to compare their responses during the seizure with their response to the same stimulus during an earlier interictal period. At the present time, it is important to determine if there is an abrupt onset and an abrupt cessation of impaired awareness, perception, and performance.

HOW LONG SHOULD A PATIENT BE MONITORED?

Although there are exceptions, a minimum of 6 hr is required for most patients. It is a mistake to have the patient ready for monitoring, and then discontinue the monitoring after 1 hr because a single seizure is recorded. The majority of individuals coming to intensive monitoring have a history of more than one type of seizure. Even for a single seizure type, there are variations on the theme. One of our patients serves as an example—a young boy who had many attacks each day with slow spike-and-wave in the ictal EEG, but often with only slow wave activity. Two seizures monitored 1 hr apart varied in duration. The first seizure was very brief, and had only slow spike-and-wave with minimal clonic movements, suggesting an absence attack. There was a sudden onset to the seizure and a very rapid recovery at the end of the seizure. The second seizure recorded during the same monitoring period was much longer, consisting of focal jerking of the left lower extremity and a slow return to full awareness during a period of generalized slow wave activity after the slow spike-and-wave. In general, intensive monitoring should be for a minimum of 6 hr, with the hope of recording as many seizures as possible. If the seizures are brief, intervention may be poor, with the need for further intensive monitoring sessions. Each case must be individualized as mentioned above in the Plan for Intervention. Where response to medication is being evaluated with frequent determinations of antiepileptic drug concentration, comparable serial recordings may be necessary, including some attempt to control environmental stimuli. The technician's behavioral record is very important to standardize a routine of daily living during comparable recordings.

DETERMINATION OF ANTIEPILEPTIC DRUG CONCENTRATIONS IN THE BLOOD

The frequency of blood sampling depends on the antiepileptic drug involved and the need for monitoring. If the patient is uncontrolled, the number of fluctuations of the concentration with dose and trough level may be more important. It could be that metabolites would have to be sampled as well as the free and bound components of the antiepileptic drug. If the question of toxicity must be solved by the monitoring, it may be important to have one or more samples around the peaks after absorption. When the patient is taking more than one antiepileptic drug, it is necessary to monitor the levels of all of these drugs because of differential effects and interactions. It is rarely necessary to sample more than every 30 min (Rowan et al., 1979) or less than once every 24 hr when the patient is on constant dosage of medication. The interpretation of these values requires a complete knowledge of the pharmacokinetics of each antiepileptic drug or its metabolite.

CONCLUSIONS

Intensive monitoring of epileptic patients is of great value in the differential diagnosis of epileptic seizures versus psychogenic seizures and in the classification of patients suffering from intractable seizures. Accurate diagnosis of complex partial seizures and the differentiation between complex partial seizures and absence seizures often requires intervention by a technician during the seizure. Ideally, planned intervention should accurately appraise awareness, perception, and performance during and after seizures so that an accurate classification is possible. Speculation concerning awareness, perception, and performance without intervention is usually unsuccessful.

REFERENCES

Penry, J. K., and Porter, R. J. (1977): Intensive monitoring of patients with intractable seizures. In: *Epilepsy: The Eighth International Symposium,* edited by J. K. Penry, pp. 95–101. Raven Press, New York.

Porter, R. J., Penry, J. K., and Lacy, J. R. (1977): Diagnostic and therapeutic re-evaluation of patients with intractable epilepsy. *Neurology (Minneap.),* 27:1006–1011.

Rowan, A. J., Binnie, C. D., de Beer-Pawlikowski, N. K. B., et al. (1979): Sodium valproate: Serial monitoring of EEG and serum levels. *Neurology,* 29:1450–1459.

Advances in Epileptology:
The Xth Epilepsy International Symposium,
edited by J. A. Wada and J. K. Penry.
Raven Press, New York © 1980.

Methodology of Continuous Monitoring with Videotape Recording and Electroencephalography

Roger J. Porter

Epilepsy Branch and Clinical Epilepsy Section of the Experimental Therapeutics Branch, National Institute of Neurological and Communicative Disorders and Stroke, National Institutes of Health, Bethesda, Maryland 20205

The characteristics of any intensive monitoring system largely depend on two major factors: (a) the kind of data needed for analysis, and (b) the availability of equipment, trained personnel, and space. It seems clear that the more such systems are utilized, the more we can learn about the patients we treat; this in turn helps us realize that an ever-increasing number of patients may benefit from intensive monitoring. The electroencephalographic (EEG) and video systems for monitoring patients with epilepsy are first discussed independently and then as an integrated system.

ELECTROENCEPHALOGRAPHY

Prolonged monitoring of the EEG is not new. Many clinicians and investigators have advocated a departure from the routine 20-min recording, and good laboratories are as flexible with the amount of recording time as they are with modification of montages. Prolongation of a routine recording, however, has such limitations and disadvantages that special techniques of obtaining the long-term EEG have been developed. The disadvantages include (a) artificial environment, (b) confined observation space, (c) limited ability of patient to move about without risking prominent artifact, (d) electrode problems, and (e) excessive accumulation of paper records. In order to collect long-term EEG data for quantitation, classification, and localization, two acceptable alternatives have been devised to alleviate these problems.

The simplest alternative is merely a modification of the "front end" of the recording system that allows the patient to move about while attached to a 7 to 10 meter cable. Low-voltage scalp potentials cannot be measured over these distances, however, and modification at the source is essential. Successful systems of this type are in use at the Montreal Neurological Institute (Ives et al., 1976) and at the Institute voor Epilepsiebestrijding in The Netherlands (A. Kamp, *personal communication*). Both of these systems utilize preamplification at the head to increase the signal strength for transmission in relatively low-impedance cables. This decreases the likelihood of interference from extraneous sources and presents a reasonable voltage to the recording system. One system (Ives et al., 1976) multiplexes the signal at the head so that only one channel of information need be carried to a decoder. The other system uses a multichannel cable with appropriate connections directly to the recording system. Multiplexing at the head and reducing the data to a single channel has the advantage of allowing a hospital unit to be wired with relatively inexpensive cable, using multiple inputs throughout the unit occupied by the patient. The advantage of the unmultiplexed system is its relative simplicity, with absence of the difficulties inherent in encoding and decoding. Both systems are effective.

The alternative to direct, "hard-wired" EEG recording is the radio-telemetered EEG. The patient is allowed much greater freedom of movement because the "umbilical cord" is absent. Preamplification at the head is an integral part of the system, and the major problems are related to the actual transmitter-receiver characteristics. The systems have been reviewed (Porter et al., 1971, 1976), and only the critical features are outlined here. First, the preamplifiers must be sensitive enough to recognize the low-voltage scalp potentials. Second, for multichannel recording, multiplexing is virtually mandatory because it requires only one transmitter and receiver. Third, crystal control is highly desirable to avoid drift in both the transmitter and receiver. Fourth, the transmitted signal should be frequency modulated. Finally, some system of dual antenna-receivers is recommended (Porter et al., 1971). All of the above will greatly enhance the quality of the recording and decrease the likelihood of outside interference.

Scalp recordings require good technique of electrode application, with impedances below 5,000 ohms per pair. We use silver, 10-mm, cup electrodes with a 2-mm hole, which can be refilled with a blunt needle as required; our newest telemetry system sounds an alarm when an electrode develops high impedance. Collodion is used to apply the electrodes, sometimes with double layers of gauze for recordings longer than 6 hr. Electrode wires should be trimmed short to decrease artifact from movement and extraneous electrical sources.

Aside from computer analysis, the final step is the recording of the EEG itself. Both the "hard-wired" and the telemetered systems are capable of sending the EEG data to a tape recorder or to a standard EEG machine. The advantages of a tape recorder are simplicity of operation and compactness of data storage. Disadvantages are the need for expensive multichannel FM recorders if the signal is not already multiplexed, inability to see the EEG as it is being recorded (an oscilloscope may be added for this purpose), and the need for a time-code generator so that recording time can be multiplexed onto the tape; this is very useful when a certain moment in time is sought for playback onto paper.

The usefulness of intensive, telemetered EEG monitoring has been clearly demonstrated, for example, in investigations of the absence seizure. Although various drugs had been utilized for many years in the treatment of absence seizures, quantitative data on efficacy was singularly lacking. A series of studies demonstrated the high correlation of generalized spike wave discharges with decrement in mental function (Goode et al., 1970; Porter et al., 1973; Browne et al., 1974), and quantitative determinations of generalized spike wave discharges were begun (Penry et al., 1971a, 1971b). Ethosuximide was shown to be effective for the treatment of absence seizures, but attacks were completely controlled in only 19% of the patients (Browne et al., 1975). Excellent information regarding the efficacy of this drug is now available, and other drugs can be tested in the absence model. This has been done for clonazepam (Sato et al., 1977) and valproic acid (Redenbaugh et al., 1977). Intensive EEG monitoring of the absence seizure, therefore, has greatly enhanced our ability to determine which drugs are effective and allows us to evaluate new and promising agents when they appear.

VIDEOTAPE RECORDING

Intensive monitoring with video recording is a more recent advance than EEG monitoring, but it has added a very significant dimension to our understanding of seizures. The usefulness of video recording has been demonstrated in the definition and classification of seizure types for nosologic purposes, the classification of seizures in individual patients for diagnostic and therapeutic purposes, and the selection of patient populations for pharmacologic studies. There are three basic elements of any video system: cameras, tape recorders, and video monitors. A number of integrated systems are available for monochromatic (black and white) recordings, and many are relatively inexpensive. Unfortunately, the less expensive systems usually have the least resolution and the least flexibility. The best systems are of modular construction, utilizing the best model and manufacturer for each piece of equipment. Cameras should be reasonably sensitive, and the following features are desirable, although not mandatory: (a) zoom lens, either hand or remote controlled, (b) remote focus, (c) automatic iris and other automatic black and white level controls (highly desirable when light may change, for example, as when a nurse in a white uniform walks in front of the camera), and (d) remote pan-tilt for aiming the camera.

Videotape recorders are an important link and, to a large extent, determine the quality of the resulting recording. As a rule, there is a direct relationship between the width of the tape and the resultant quality. The most inexpensive machines use $\frac{1}{2}$-inch tape. The standard U-matic cassettes use $\frac{3}{4}$-inch tape. The better, industrial open-reel machines use 1-inch tape. Broadcast quality, in most cases, requires 2-inch tape. Clearly, the most expensive machines use the widest tape and obtain the best resolution. Several factors determine what type of machine is required. Expense is a major consideration. The need for transfer and editing will be discussed below. Ease of operation and the possibility of remote operation should be considered, as should the value of a second audio track. One of the most difficult decisions regards the use of open-reel versus cassette video systems. The better open-reel systems offer superior recording characteristics, but the cassettes are relatively convenient, easily stored, and if the U-matic format is chosen, have the advantage of being played on multiple machines with little difficulty. The disadvantages of cassettes are related to the complex mechanisms in the recorder. They are very difficult to "cue" properly, a severe problem for intensive monitoring. Reviewing a seizure multiple times can be time-consuming and frustrating because the simple "rewind" procedure is made complex.

Two little-publicized facts about video recording are worth emphasizing. The first relates to information transfer. Many investigators occasionally videotape record seizures and then later wish to show them at a different location on a different machine; disappointment is the usual result. First, except for the very best, well-aligned machines, the original tape will almost always play best on the machine used for recording. Even an identical machine may have subtle (or severe) differences in mechanical alignment that will affect the reproduction. Even differences in line voltage, temperature, or humidity may cause a decrement in reproduction quality. This whole problem becomes especially severe when a tape is transferred to another, or "edited." Since video tape cannot be spliced, the transfer is electronic; 20 to 30% degradation of quality in the electronic copy is the rule, and more severe degradation occurs with less expensive machines, different types of machines, original recordings of poor quality, and poorly aligned machines. It is no surprise to the experienced technician to see a tape play perfectly on the original machine but very poorly (or not at all) on a similar machine; electronic transfer of the information on such a tape is difficult or impossible. The way to avoid this problem is to use high quality, well-aligned machines for both recording and playback.

The second fact about video recording that is not widely appreciated is the need for a highly qualified technician, on at least a part-time basis, to keep the various components in good order. Video systems are not merely "on" or "off," but are capable of functioning at many levels of efficiency; only the optimal level will give good recordings. Cameras and tape recorders require periodic, expert maintenance to achieve this level of performance, and electronic technicians who have only a passing familiarity with video technology (an electronic world of its own) will likely not provide the expertise needed.

The only other mandatory piece of equipment for video recording is the monitor, which resembles a television set without a receiver. The simplest monitor will give only a view of the video information. More sophisticated monitors can help analyze the recorded signal and are extremely useful to the experienced technician.

Other equipment may be very useful in video recordings. A time-code generator that projects the year, month, day, hour, minute, and second on the screen is valuable in data retrieval. If more than one camera image is to be combined in a "split screen" view, a "special effects" generator is needed. Equipment that can be valuable in maintaining peak performance includes waveform monitors, oscilloscopes, processing amplifiers, and time-base correctors, but these are useful only to the sophisticated technician. Video systems and their uses have been reviewed (Porter et al., 1976; Penry and Porter, 1977).

Studies characterizing the absence seizure illustrate the utility of videotape recording of epileptic seizures. Although the modern therapy of seizures is highly dependent on specific knowledge of the clinical seizure type, most patients are treated on the basis of historical information reported to the physician. The physician, in turn, develops a concept of seizures and a framework for classification. This primitive approach becomes even more ludicrous when efforts are made to study the pharmacology of antiepileptic drugs in the absence of definitive clinical data on seizure types. This is an entirely approachable problem, however, because seizures can be recorded and subsequently analyzed and categorized. This has been accomplished for the absence seizure in an analysis of 374 videotaped seizures in 48 patients (Penry et al., 1975). This seizure type is thereby relatively well-defined, and many misconceptions, such as the incidence of the various clinical manifestations, have been clarified.

SIMULTANEOUS VIDEO AND ELECTROENCEPHALOGRAPHIC RECORDING

The intensive monitoring unit is most effective if the prolonged EEG recording is teamed with the long-term video recording of the patient to yield simultaneous documentation of the clinical and EEG manifestations of the epileptic seizures. The major problem involved in accomplishing this lies in the display of the EEG on the same video screen. Three methods have been previously described (Porter et al., 1976), but only the most recent will be reviewed here; it involves the use of the analog-TV reformatter developed in the Biomedical Engineering Branch of the National Institutes of Health. In our studies at the Clinical Center, the EEGs are recorded exclusively on magnetic tape; the EEG machine is used only for playback of a specific recording. Independent of the tape recording, the analog EEG signal is displayed on the video screen by a reformatter. The signal simulates EEG and does not have the oscilloscopic appearance that is unfamiliar to many electroencephalographers. After minimal initial set-up, the system is routinely utilized for 6 hr and needs no attention other than the hourly changing of video tapes. The video display, using a special effects generator, two cameras, a time-code generator, and a reformatter, is shown in Fig. 1. Videotapes are routinely erased if no seizures are recorded. All recorded seizures are electronically transferred to master reels, and the original tapes are erased and reused.

The value of intensive monitoring, utilizing the combined system as described above, has been amply demonstrated. Twenty-three patients with intractable seizures were intensively monitored with long-term video recording and simultaneously telemetered EEG, as well as daily determinations of antiepileptic drug concentrations (Porter et al., 1977). The provisional admission diagnosis was frequent, refractory complex partial seizures. Intensive monitoring established an empirical seizure diagnosis in all but one patient, permitting the initiation of appropriate seizure-specific therapy. This therapy was instituted and delivered with maximal effectiveness through the daily determination of antiepileptic drug concentrations. Medication toxicity was eliminated in all but six patients, primarily by withdrawal of sedative antiepileptic drugs, and limited efforts were made to

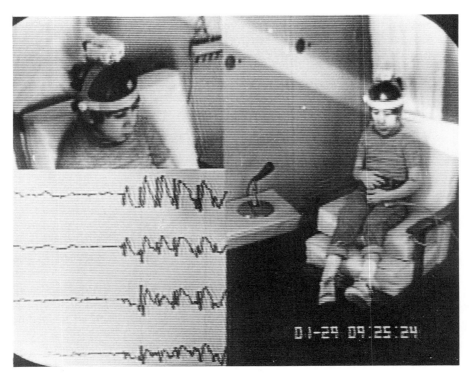

FIG. 1. Two-camera display of patient with onset of irregular, generalized spike-wave discharge with reformatted EEG in lower left quadrant.

relieve social difficulties. At 8-month follow-up, 16 patients had maintained their improvement in seizure control, 19 had sustained some decrease in medication toxicity, and 11 had preserved some social gains. Intensive monitoring has thus been shown to be of special value in the patient with seizures that are considered refractory to conventional therapeutic efforts.

Finally, some mention must be made about the location of the equipment and the type of room used for intensive monitoring. The modified hospital room, with its beds, tables, closets, curtains, and so forth, is generally used because of planning and space deficiencies. (This is the type of room utilized at the Clinical Center, in part because of severe space limitations.) The disadvantages of such a room are several. The room is likely designated for patient care, and control of its use may not be possible or may be limited by the enthusiasm of the nursing staff. If nonepileptic patients share the room, the periods of intensive monitoring may seem to be nothing but an inconvenience, and strife can arise. Further, equipment must be located so that the primary function of the room remains unchanged, i.e., the nursing function remains largely undisturbed. This limits the placement of the cameras at the Clinical Center, for example, to a rather high position on the wall so that they are not in the way of the staff, which restricts our view of the patient. Less generally available is the clinical neurophysiology laboratory solely devoted to intensive monitoring. Such a room has much greater flexibility and is obviously under more direct control of the investigative team. The single disadvantage of such a laboratory is its location with respect to a nursing unit. Nurses are available for immediate help when the unit is part of the ward; assistance may be hard to get in a remote laboratory.

In summary, intensive monitoring of the EEG and clinical manifestations of epileptic seizures is accomplished by specialized means of EEG recording, video recording, or the simultaneous application of both techniques. The usefulness of this methodology for investigators and clinicians is now generally acknowledged.

REFERENCES

Browne, T. R., Dreifuss, F. E., Dyken, P. R., Goode, D. J., Penry, J. K., Porter, R. J., White, B. G., and White, P. T. (1975): Ethosuximide (Zarontin) in the treatment of absence (petit mal) seizures. *Neurology (Minneap.)*, 25:515–524.

Browne, T. R., Penry, J. K., Porter, R. J., and Dreifuss, F. E. (1974): Responsiveness before, during and after spike-wave paroxysms. *Neurology (Minneap.)*, 24:651–665.

Goode, D. J., Penry, J. K., and Dreifuss, F. E. (1970): Effects of paroxysmal spike-wave on continuous visual-motor performance. *Epilepsia*, 11:241–254.

Ives, J. R., Thompson, C. J., and Gloor, P. (1976): Seizure monitoring: a new tool in electroencephalography. *Electroencephalogr. Clin. Neurophysiol.*, 41:422–427.

Penry, J. K., and Porter, R. J. (1977): Intensive monitoring of patients with intractable seizures. In: *Epilepsy: The Eighth International Symposium*, edited by J. K. Penry, pp. 95–101. Raven Press, New York.

Penry, J. K., Porter, R. J., and Dreifuss, F. E. (1971a): Quantitation of paroxysmal abnormal discharge in the EEGs of patients with absence (petit mal) seizures for evaluation of antiepileptic drugs. *Epilepsia*, 12:278–279.

Penry, J. K., Porter, R. J., and Dreifuss, F. E. (1971*b*): Patterns of paroxysmal discharge in 12-hour telemetered EEGs of untreated children with absence (petit mal) seizures. *Neurology (Minneap.)*, 21:392.

Penry, J. K., Porter, R. J., and Dreifuss, F. E. (1975): Simultaneous recording of absence seizures with video-tape and electroencephalography: A study of 374 seizures in 48 patients. *Brain*, 98:427–440.

Porter, R. J., Penry, J. K., and Dreifuss, F. E. (1973): Responsiveness at the onset of spike-wave bursts. *Electroencephalogr. Clin. Neurophysiol.*, 34:239–245.

Porter, R. J., Penry, J. K., and Lacy, J. R. (1977): Diagnostic and therapeutic re-evaluation of patients with intractable epilepsy. *Neurology (Minneap.)*, 27:1006–1011.

Porter, R. J., Penry, J. K., and Wolf, A. A. Jr. (1976): Simultaneous documentation of clinical and electroencephalographic manifestations of epileptic seizures. In: *Quantitative Analytic Studies in Epilepsy*, edited by P. Kellaway and I. Petersén, pp. 253–268. Raven Press, New York.

Porter, R. J., Wolf, A. A., and Penry, J. K. (1971): Human electroencephalographic telemetry: a review of systems and their applications and a new receiving system. *Am. J. EEG Technol.*, 11:145–159.

Redenbaugh, J. R., Sato, S., Dreifuss, F. E., Penry, J. K., and Kupferberg, H. J. (1977): Sodium valproate: a pilot study of pharmacokinetics and adverse reactions in patients with intractable seizures. *Neurology (Minneap.)*, 27:376.

Sato, S., Penry, J. K., Dreifuss, F. E., and Dyken, P. R. (1977): Clonazepam in the treatment of absence seizures: a double-blind clinical trial. *Neurology (Minneap.)*, 27:371.

Advances in Epileptology:
The Xth Epilepsy International Symposium,
edited by J. A. Wada and J. K. Penry.
Raven Press, New York © 1980.

Value of Intensive Monitoring

Richard H. Mattson

Epilepsy Center, Veterans' Administration Hospital, West Haven, Connecticut
06516

Diagnosis and treatment of epileptic seizures requires the accurate recognition of the specific type of attacks experienced by a patient. The distinction of epileptic seizures from other acute episodes may be difficult to determine on the basis of history alone. The ideal circumstance allows for such differentiation by the repeated observation of clinical and electrical events at the time of such attacks. Usually the physician must rely on the history of the patient or the description of untrained witnesses, since the attacks seldom occur often enough to be witnessed by a professional observer. The electroencephalographic (EEG) or polygraphic documentation of seizures is of great value in diagnosis but attacks cannot be expected to occur during the usual 1-hr EEG laboratory tracing. Making diagnosis even more difficult is the fact that in some cases attacks take place primarily or only during sleep, when observations can be expected to be even less satisfactory.

Technological advances over the past decade have led to the development of special seizure units with highly trained staff, allowing continuous intensive monitoring of clinical events with simultaneous split screen video display of EEG or other polygraphic activity over a prolonged period of time. Such display can also be tape recorded for repeated examination, which facilitates precise characterization of clinical and electrical events occurring at any time during both waking and sleeping hours. This information is of great value not only for the diagnosis of specific seizure type but also for the localization of onset of the attack. Such precise localization is especially important in the evaluation of the patient considered for surgical resection of an epileptic area of brain. At the same time, a record of events may allow the physician to distinguish between epileptic seizures and attacks of other types that may simulate epilepsy but have different causes and require alternative types of management. Prolonged recording also allows quantification of both frequency and intensity of attacks and can serve as a basis for comparison of results of treatment, which is important in evaluation of efficacy of new antiepileptic drugs.

In addition, such specially equipped and staffed units provide a capability for optimal management of acute seizures or status epilepticus. Simultaneous clinical and electrographic display provides minute-to-minute information as to the adequacy of therapy as well as the occurrence of serious side effects from the administration of potentially depressant antiepileptic drugs. The clinical/electrographic monitoring coupled with simultaneous measurement of antiepileptic drug concentration provides the physician and staff with crucial information for providing optimal medical care.

Numerous reports have appeared over this past decade describing various aspects of technological development as well as some anecdotal case reports of usefulness. Only the study by Porter et al. (1977) has carefully examined a group of patients who had been studied to assess the value of prolonged intensive monitoring. For this reason we have carried out a similar review.

METHODS

An analysis was done of the reasons for admission, the findings with intensive monitoring, and the outcome of diagnosis and treatment in a selected sample of 388 patients who entered the seizure unit of the West Haven Veterans' Administration Hospital during a 3-year period between 1975 and 1978. The unit has special videotape/polygraphic recording equipment so that two patients can be intensively monitored over 24 hr per day periods by specially trained nurses, EEG technicians, physicians, and other staff. The continuous 24-hr monitoring is facilitated by special training of the staff nurses in EEG technology so they can obtain the polygraphic recording and operate the equipment. The Seizure Unit has been operating for the past 7 years, during which time more than 1,500 patients have been admitted and intensive monitoring performed on a majority of them. More than 40,000 hr of such monitoring has been done.

The middle years were selected for detailed analysis, since the unit was fully operational during that period and accepted both veteran and nonveteran patients of all ages providing a broad spectrum of clinical epilepsy problems. Initial 21-month analysis included only nonveteran patients admitted through a "sharing agreement" with Yale New Haven Hospital but the most recent 15-month period included all admissions of both veteran and nonveteran patients. The study was accomplished through retrospective record review by three different research assistants working independently at different times, and I have reviewed the results in detail for validation and confirmation. The findings were remarkably similar among the different observers although numbers were not entirely identical and figures cited in the results should be considered very close approximations rather than absolute values.

RESULTS

During the period studied, 388 patients were admitted to the Epilepsy Unit although the number of actual admissions was greater since some patients entered more than one time. Data were not analyzed more than once for these patients since usually they were readmitted for the same reason. The numbers of reasons for admission and treatment outcome do not correspond, since some patients had more than one reason for admission or treatment given and some patients had no change made in their treatment program.

Diagnostic Evaluation

Diagnostic evaluation of seizure etiology was obtained by a thorough history, physical examination, and selected diagnostic studies, including skull X-rays, lumbar puncture, radionucleotide brain scan, computed tomography (CT) scan, and contrast studies. This etiological diagnostic evaluation had usually been completed quite adequately at other hospitals prior to referral although in recent years a number of admissions were prompted by the availability of CT scanning. The outcome of these etiological studies provided information that did not significantly differ from what would be expected in any large group of seizure patients and is not discussed further.

Diagnosis and Treatment Outcome of Epileptic Seizures

The majority of the patients were admitted for confirmation and further characterization of the specific epileptic seizure type. *Intensive videotape/ electrographic monitoring allowed us to record attacks in 194 of the 388 patients (50%).* In contrast, *seizures occurred in only 9 of 388 patients (2½%) during the routine EEG recording.* The character of the attacks was confirmed to be epileptic in type on the basis of a combination of stereotyped typical clinical events usually coupled with rhythmic electrographic ictal discharge. The recordings of attacks and/or ictal and interictal EEG epileptiform discharges characterized both the type and localization of onset of seizures. Localization of seizure onset was frequently possible and of critical importance in patients considered for surgical therapy. In most surgical candidates, however, depth electrode EEG recording was necessary for more precise localization than possible from the scalp. Determination of serum antiepileptic drug concentrations was obtained simultaneously with videotape/polygraphic monitoring to guide the medical staff in optimal selection of drug regimen.

Uncontrolled Seizures

Two hundred and sixty-seven patients were considered to have intractable or uncontrolled seizures despite standard medical therapy. Table 1 lists the types of treatment used in these patients. The largest group of patients (89) were treated by regulation of drug dosage, most often with increases to

TABLE 1. *Discharge treatment and outcome of 267 patients with uncontrolled epileptic seizures*

	Total (number)	Improved		Intractable	
		(number)	(%)	(number)	(%)
Modification of drug dose or regimen (including compliance)	89	60	67	29	33
Medication change	81	55	68	26	32
Experimental medication	47	29	62	18	38
Precipitating factors	12	8	67	4	33
Diagnosis of incorrect seizure type	10	9	90	1	10
Epilepsy surgery	12	8	67	4	33
Tumor surgery	12	10	83	2	17
Biofeedback	7	4	57	3	43
Total	270[a]	183	68	87	32

[a]Some patients had more than one type of treatment, in which case improvement was attributed to each type.

achieve high therapeutic serum concentrations short of toxicity. This category includes patients whose program needed to be modified due to non-compliance.

A trial of a different antiepileptic drug was indicated in 81 patients in whom adequate serum levels of one or more medications had been achieved without obtaining good control. Usually the total number of antiepileptic drugs was decreased and a standard drug such as carbamazepine or phenytoin started or reintroduced.

A large number of patients (47) failed to obtain control despite adequate trials of standard antiepileptic drug medications and were invited to participate in clinical trials of new antiepileptic drugs. During the years analyzed these drugs were eterobarb and valproic acid. The monitoring allowed quantitation of efficacy. For example, 6-hr EEG recordings were done before and after valproic acid therapy. In nine patients the mean number of spike wave bursts decreased from 30 to 2.

Precipitating factors played a role in seizure exacerbation in many patients and were identified as primary correctable causes of incomplete seizure control in 10 patients. Most frequently identified causes were the occasional excessive use of alcohol, sleep deprivation, and, rarely, attacks specifically triggered by music or light.

Epilepsy surgery was performed in 12 patients for removal of an atrophic lesion. Tumor surgery was carried out in another 12 patients with gliomas. These patients had been under long-term care for epilepsy for periods of up to 15 years. Although resection of the tumor was subtotal in every instance, there was a dramatic reduction in seizure frequency subsequently.

A small number of patients (7) with intractable seizures were treated with biofeedback in a controlled study and realized modest improvement.

Overall, improvement in control of seizures and severity improved in 68% and remained unimproved in 32%. The documentation of improvement of control was variable for the different categories, but was excellent in patients involved in specific experimental protocols including new antiepileptic drugs, precipitating factors, epilepsy surgery, and biofeedback. Long-term follow-up was not available for many of the patients, especially in those returned to the referring hospital.

Acute Seizure Therapy

Of the 388 patients, 88 (23%) were admitted for acute seizures or status epilepticus. Seizures usually were treated with a variety of parenteral antiepileptic drugs that were selected depending on whether the attacks seemed to be precipitated by insufficient medication, suboptimal selection of type of medication, or by factors such as withdrawal from alcohol. Many patients responded within minutes although occasional attacks persisted up to a week. No patients died or had significant residuals of the acute seizures.

Nonepileptic Attacks

Of the 388 patients, 84 (22%) proved to be having attacks that were nonepileptic in character rather than or in addition to epileptic seizures (Table 2). A large number of disorders were represented in this group of patients. The specific diagnosis was based on clinical characteristics that varied with the particular disorder. None of these nonepileptic attacks was accompanied by electrographic seizure discharge, but commonly these patients had abnormal interictal EEGs that varied with the specific disorder.

TABLE 2. *Diagnosis and treatment outcome in patients with nonepileptic attacks*

	Total (number)	Improved		Intractable	
		(number)	(%)	(number)	(%)
"Hysterical" seizures	34	25	74	9	26
Drug toxicity	15	15	100	0	0
Cerebral ischemia (syncope, TIA)	10	6	60	4	40
Vascular headache	4	2	50	2	50
Movement disorder	5	4	80	1	20
Psychiatric disorder (derealization, episodic loss of control)	9	5	56	4	44
Sleep disorders (narcolepsy, night terrors, sleep apnea)	7	6	86	1	14
Total	84[a]	63	75	21	25

[a]22% of all patients admitted.

"Hysterical" Seizures

"Hysterical" episodes were the most common type of nonepileptic attacks and this diagnosis was made in 34 patients. "Hysterical" attacks were those of histrionic character supplemented by observations such as ability of the patient to terminate an attack on command or forceful resistance to attempts by the examiner to open the eyes. Other criteria included confirmation at some later time by the patient that these attacks were not the same as their usual seizures and, indeed, were consciously produced. The fact that the EEG revealed no seizure discharge during an attack was not sufficient to constitute a diagnosis of "hysterical" seizures since a number of typical complex partial or, even more frequently, partial elementary seizures of clinically obvious epileptic type were unassociated with seizure discharge in the scalp recording. Interestingly, the recognition of the character of these attacks resulted in an improvement in 25 of the 34 (74%) patients.

Ischemic Episodes

Ischemic episodes proved to be a diagnostic problem in 10 patients, particularly those with syncopal attacks of such a severity that convulsive phenomena were present. Recording of alterations of heart rate and blood pressure concurrent with diffuse EEG slowing helped to confirm the diagnosis. Transient ischemic attacks were often difficult to separate from epileptic seizures, particularly in instances of frequent periodic dysphasia. In these cases the intensive monitoring was very helpful in distinguishing the two on the basis of slow wave activity on the one hand or rhythmic high-frequency discharge on the other.

Toxicity

Toxicity due to antiepileptic drugs or other medications was the explanation for recurrent attacks in 15 patients. The majority of these episodes correlated with peak effects from antiepileptic drug administration that occurred when carbamazepine, valproic acid, or primidone were given in high dosage once or twice daily. The signs and symptoms associated with toxicity included transient dizzy spells and complaints of confusion or epigastric disturbance but on occasion represented tonic, dystonic, or other involuntary movements simulating seizures. All of these patients improved after correction of the excessive drug dosage. The diagnoses were confirmed by clinical examination or review of videotape that revealed symmetrical incoordination or nystagmus. Characteristically the attacks developed and disappeared rather gradually and lasted longer than the usual epileptic seizures.

Other Psychiatric Disorders

A group of patients were referred for evaluation of recurrent attacks and episodic loss of control, episodes of confusion, derealization/depersonalization, hyperventilization, and acute anxiety attacks. These patients often were referred because they were found to have an abnormal interictal EEG. Nine such patients were subsequently referred for other psychiatric treatment and five were reported to have improved.

Sleep Disorders

Seven patients proved to have sleep disorders rather than seizures and included a few cases of night terrors, somnambulism, and sleep apnea. Patients with narcolepsy were also encountered although more frequently admitted for confirmation rather than because of confusion with the diagnosis of epileptic seizures. The diagnosis was made in part by recording other polygraphic variables that provide clues to sleep disorders such as eye movement, electromyogram, heart rate, and respirations.

Movement Disorders

Some movement disorders including Gilles de la Torette syndrome, dystonia, and tremors were suspected to be of possible epileptic nature at the time of admission. Four of the five patients responded to medication directed toward the movement disorder.

Atypical Headaches

Four patients were seen with attacks of severe headaches, confusion, and reports of loss of consciousness. None of these had evidence of epileptiform activity during their attacks.

Overall a specific diagnosis of these nonepileptic attacks resulted in improvement in 63 of the 84 patients (75%).

Clinical Investigation

A small number of patients were admitted for other reasons, such as clinical investigations, which utilized intensive monitoring to quantitate effect of alcohol and epilepsy, folate therapy in epilepsy, performance changes on psychometric testing during apparent subclinical seizure discharge, the effect of the menstrual cycle on epileptic seizures, and admissions designed for intensive monitoring of drug pharmacokinetics.

DISCUSSION

The analysis of the results of intensive clinical polygraphic monitoring in patients admitted to the Epilepsy Center confirmed the value of this approach in patient management. Incorrect diagnosis of seizure type was not common at the time of admission although specific seizure type was often not clear. Diagnoses often were limited to "epilepsy," "grand mal," or "seizure disorder." The recognition of specific seizure type together with monitoring of antiepileptic drug blood levels enabled an alteration of the treatment program which resulted in improvement in 183 of 267 (68%) patients having uncontrolled seizures. This figure agrees well with findings of Porter et al. (1977). Most commonly drug dosage was modified to achieve maximal nontoxic serum concentrations given in a frequency most reasonable in light of the pharmacokinetics of the drug for that particular person. The most common reason for suboptimal control proved to be an insufficient dosage of medication prescribed by the primary physician rather than noncompliance. Introduction of a different medication was often valuable in improving control and especially effective when the diagnosis of partial complex and absence seizures had been mistaken because the treatment for these two usually requires the use of quite different antiepileptic drugs. Use of new antiepileptic drugs in intractable seizure patients was often beneficial and the intensive monitoring was especially important in quantifying the effect of treatment.

The intensive monitoring was most prolonged in the surgical candidates but details are discussed elsewhere (Williamson and Mattson, *this volume*).

The intensive monitoring proved to be very valuable in treating of acute seizure or status epilepticus. The patients often demonstrated continued subclinical seizure discharge even after the acute clinical manifestations were noted. The electrographic recording at this time helped to distinguish whether earlier tonic clonic attacks were generalized or partial in onset. This was important in the selection of optimal antiepileptic medications for treatment. Similarly the finding of photosensitivity in an otherwise normal recording raised the possibility of withdrawal seizures and led to appropriate replacement therapy. The favorable outcome (no deaths or serious residuals) gives some indication of the value of intensive monitoring in the management of acute seizures or status epilepticus. It must be conceded that this unusually favorable outcome resulted in part from the fact that most of the patients had epilepsy rather than acute seizures associated with progressive neurologic disease such as meningitis or serious medical illnesses. Even in these instances, however, it is expected that availability of close monitoring capability would assist the treatment of these difficult problems.

The number of cases in which a significantly different type of seizure was diagnosed was small, which is a measure of the accuracy of diagnosis of the referring physicians, most of whom were neurologists. More surprising was the finding that 22% of the patients were having recurrent nonepileptic attacks that often presented as intractable seizures. These various disorders usually had been treated with increasing dosages of antiepileptic drugs, causing side effects that further complicated the basic underlying problem. Recognition that these attacks were of nonepileptic type allowed specific therapy and improvement in 75% of this patient group, which exceeded the favorable outcome for those patients with uncontrolled epileptic seizures. In many cases the referring neurologist and/or psychiatrist suspected the attacks were "hysterical" in type but these same patients also often had epilepsy. The precise characterization of these attacks as nonepileptic allowed the reduction of toxic doses of antiepileptic medication and more aggressive psychiatric intervention.

An attempt was made to estimate the added cost of intensive monitoring above the usual neurology service admission. Based on the added personnel and equipment it averaged $100 per day. This was considered a very reasonable cost/benefit ratio.

SUMMARY

An analysis has been performed of 388 patients admitted to the Seizure Unit over a 3-year period to determine the value of intensive clinical/polygraphic monitoring. Determination of antiepileptic blood concentrations was performed at the same time. This information allowed more precise diagnosis, with resultant improvement in 183 of 270 patients (68%) with uncontrolled seizures. Eighty-four patients were found to have attacks of nonepileptic type in addition to or rather than epileptic seizures, specific therapy of which provided improvement in 63 of the 84 cases (75%). Monitoring was especially valuable in the treatment of status epilepticus. Finally, the videotape/polygraphic recording provided a useful means of quantitating effects of clinical investigations such as introduction of new antiepileptic drugs.

ACKNOWLEDGMENTS

I wish to acknowledge the valuable assistance of Susan Trott and Gail Mattson in the collection and review of these data.

REFERENCE

Porter, R. J., Penry, J. K., and Lacy, J. R. (1977): Diagnostic and therapeutic reevaluation of patients with intractable epilepsy. *Neurology*, 11:1006–1011.

Advances in Epileptology:
The Xth Epilepsy International Symposium,
edited by J. A. Wada and J. K. Penry.
Raven Press, New York © 1980.

Intensive Monitoring of Antiepileptic Drug Serum Levels

Harold E. Booker

Department of Neurology, University of Wisconsin Medical Center
for the Health Sciences, Madison, Wisconsin 53706; currently, Neurology Service,
V.A. Central Office, Washington, D.C. 20420

Intensive monitoring in epilepsy usually refers to prolonged recording of the brainwaves derived either from the scalp or from electrodes implanted on the surface or in the depths of the brain. Telemetry and automated data reduction and analysis via a computer are often employed, as well as recording of clinical events via audio-visual taping. The main purpose of such intensive monitoring has been to gain insight into the origins and pattern of spread of the seizure process itself, and to correlate such findings with clinical events. Such studies increase our knowledge of the epileptic process in general, and can be utilized in individual patients for specific diagnostic purposes. More recently Penry and Porter (1977) reviewed the value of intensive EEG monitoring in the planning and evaluation of therapeutic response in individual patients. In recent years reliable and accurate methods for the determination of the concentration of the antiepileptic drugs and their major active metabolites in biologic fluids have been developed. These techniques have allowed the clinical pharmacology of the antiepileptic drugs to mature from empirical science to a more rational science based on a knowledge of the kinetics and metabolism of the drugs and supported by measured values in individual patients. Such efforts constitute another type of intensive monitoring in epilepsy, and are the subject of this chapter. A review of the extensive literature developed from studies in both experimental animals and man is beyond the scope of this volume, but we attempt to illustrate the kinds of knowledge that have been gained, and the potential for future application, with emphasis on practical applications.

ESTABLISHMENT OF POPULATION VALUES

Initial efforts in this area, as is usually the case in any new area, were directed toward establishing the general population values, that is, the parameters for the various drugs. With few exceptions, the relative bioavailability after various routes of dosing, the time to peak blood level after single dose, the serum half-life, and the degree of binding to serum proteins are now known for all of the major antiepileptic drugs as well as for the metabolites in those cases where major metabolites have significant antiepileptic properties themselves. In addition, a variety of drug interactions have been identified and the mechanism elaborated in some cases. These interactions can now be anticipated and thus prevented or at least controlled if simultaneous administration of the interacting drugs is necessary. These data are too extensive and too well known to need to be reviewed here. By referring to such data, however, one can quickly determine whether the results in an individual patient fall within the population values, that is, whether they are the expected results, or whether they suggest a significant individual deviation from the normal range. More detailed study of individual deviations has resulted in a number of important observations, although space will allow us to mention only a few.

It is now known that infants and young children have more rapid metabolism than adults for most of the drugs. Consequently infants and young children require different dosage schedules than adults, and dosage schedules must be adjusted during growth if one wants to maintain a constant steady-state serum level. Factors other than age also affect drug kinetics; Richens (1977) has clearly demonstrated the dose-dependent kinetics of phenytoin. Knowing that as the dose of phenytoin is increased, a point will be reached at which the serum level will rise exponentially allows one to avoid a significant degree of therapeutic "overkill" and clinical toxicity.

Recent evidence suggested that the teratologic risk of these drugs may be directly related to the serum levels during pregnancy, so that levels should be carefully monitored during pregnancy. On the other hand, occurrence of maternal convulsions also carries an obvious risk to the fetus, and since it has recently been shown (Mygind et al., 1976; Ramsay et al., 1978) that a significant degree of malabsorption of phenytoin may occur during pregnancy, intensive monitoring of serum levels during pregnancy is doubly warranted.

These few examples suffice to show that not only have general population values been established, but also that several important subgroups exist within the general population and that intensive monitoring of serum levels can be important in infants and young children and during growth, during pregnancy, and for those drugs that exhibit dose-dependent kinetics, such as phenytoin. On the other hand, the value of routine serum level determinations in individual patients has been questioned (Livingston et al., 1975), particularly in the case of patients clinically doing well without seizures and without toxicity. In these circumstances I would tend to agree, but few of us are blessed with a clinical practice composed solely of patients free of both seizures and toxicity. It is precisely in the patient who is not doing well that intensive monitoring can be important if not invaluable, and I shall give only two examples from my own experience.

VALUE OF INTENSIVE DRUG MONITORING IN INDIVIDUALS

The first case relates to unusual toxic reactions, in this case to phenytoin. The young man in question developed severe and continuous self-mutilation on two occasions, related to increased phenytoin serum levels. To our knowledge this had not been previously reported, and none of the usual clinical signs of phenytoin over dose such as nystagmus, slurred speech, and ataxia were observable in this patient on either occasion. Recognition by us at least that this was an unusual adverse reaction to phenytoin overdose was facilitated by measurement of the serum levels. It has been our experience that in cases of unusual or questionable toxicity, or when definite toxicity is present but the patient is taking more than one drug, monitoring of the serum levels has been invaluable.

The second case relates to therapeutic failure, that is, continued seizures despite generally adequate doses of antiepileptic drugs. The result in this case was attributed to very low or even absent blood levels of phenytoin and ethosuximide recorded on many occasions in the outpatient clinic or at the time of admission to the hospital. The fact that the levels of these two drugs rose to expected values while the patient was in the hospital led to the conclusion that the problem was simply that of noncompliance. However, because the family insisted this young lady indeed took her medications, and the mother's observation that seizure control had only been a problem since they moved from the city to a farm with its own water supply, we investigated the effect of water from the well on their farm on the bioavailability of phenytoin in this patient. No phenytoin was present in the serum nor were any metabolites found in urine for 48 hr after a 500-mg test dose with standard commercial capsules. Absorption was normal, however, under the same circumstances except for use of water from the city water supply. Absorption was also normal when using 500 mg of a commercial suspension preparation and water from the well on their farm. The results take on more significance when the original data are reviewed, which shows that serum levels of phenobarbital and nirvanol, active metabolites bioderived from mephobarbital and mephenytoin, were relatively high and did not change when changing from water from the well to the city water supply in the hospital. These two drugs were taken in tablet form, whereas phenytoin and ethosuximide had been taken in capsule form. Phenytoin at the same dose level was changed from the capsule form to the suspension form, and over the next several months serum levels remained high with improved seizure control. Indeed, at one point, the level was so high that clinical toxicity developed and the dose had to be lowered.

Although these two cases are interesting, they are also very unusual, but they do serve to illustrate the point that intensive monitoring of serum levels, even in individual patients, can be very productive.

Repeated serum levels when the patient should be at steady state will identify the patient who deviates significantly from the expected or population values. Absorption characteristics can be estimated by the height and the time of peak level after a test dose, and the half-life reflecting overall rate of elimination can be estimated by the tail of the curve. The more specimens obtained the more precise the results from an absorption curve, but in our experience, four samples suffice for practical purposes. Two are taken early after the dose, timed to bracket the expected time of peak level, the third is taken when the serum level would be expected to be one-half of the peak level, and the fourth when the level would be expected to be one-fourth of the peak level. Patterns of metabolism can be estimated from the ratio of parent drug to metabolite both in serum and urine, as well as the absolute amount excreted in urine over 24 hr. Binding to serum proteins can be determined by direct methods, or inferred from comparison of determinations on simultaneously collected samples of serum and saliva.

One does not need a research laboratory to accomplish these ends, as the levels can be determined by any laboratory that has the capacity to do routine determinations, if it participates in a quality control program, and such laboratories can, with only minor modifications, do urinary and salivary levels as well. Thus any practitioner who has available such a laboratory, and most now do, and who has a working knowledge of the general principles of clinical pharmacology, and all of us should, as well as a table giving the specifics for the antiepileptic drugs, should be able to work out a clinical pharmacologic profile for individual patients. The types of problems most likely to be encountered and the profile of laboratory findings in each are listed in Table 1. In our experience noncompliance has been the most common finding. This usually can be identified simply by low serum levels for dose followed by a rise in the serum levels after counseling. Often, however, as the above example illustrates, noncompliance is not the problem and an absorption curve study reveals that difficulties in absorption are the problem. The other types are far less common, but do occur and can be identified by the above described methods.

The final example, taken from the work of Rowan et al. (1975), was reserved for last for a special reason. In this case, a correlation was shown for EEG paroxysmal discharges and frank clinical seizures with fluctuations in the serum level of primidone throughout the diurnal cycle. The timing of the lower blood levels of primidone would be anticipated from the known kinetics of this drug. After adjustment of the primidone dosage schedule to provide a more smoothly plateaued serum level, improvement in the EEG and reduction of nocturnal clinical seizures were recorded. This type of study is particularly informative, as it illustrates the power of combining the two types of intensive monitoring, so that not only can we learn more about pharmacologic aspects, but also can correlate them closely with clinical and

TABLE 1. *Laboratory profile of unusual drug patterns*

	Non-compliance	Poor absorption	Rapid metabolism	Decreased protein binding	Slow metabolism (drug interactions)
Plateau value	Low	Low	Low	Low	High
Amount in urine					
Drug	Decreased	Decreased	Decreased	Variable	Increased
Metabolites	Decreased	Decreased	Increased	Variable	Decreased
Ratio					
Drug to metabolite in serum and urine	Normal	Normal	Low	Normal to low	High
Absorption curve	Normal	Flat	Normal to flat	Normal	Normal to increased
Serum half-life	Normal	Normal	Decreased	Normal to slightly decreased	Prolonged
Percent bound					
To serum protein	Normal	Normal	Normal	Low	Variable

EEG events. One hopes to see more of this combined intensive monitoring approach in the future.

SUMMARY

Although an exhaustive review was not possible, I have tried to indicate the kind of things that we have and can continue to learn by intensive monitoring of the antiepileptic drug serum levels. The general population values have been established, significant subgroups within the general population have been identified, and I have tried to illustrate the value of intensive monitoring of drug level in individual cases. I have tried to show that this approach can be practical and applied by the practitioner as well as in the major centers and research laboratories. It can be argued, however, that although it can be done, it is really not necessary, as adjustment of dosage schedules, and so forth, on the basis of clinical judgment would give equally good results in many of the cases. To this argument I can only reply that a better understanding of this process will improve the treatments we offer our patients.

REFERENCES

Livingston, S., Berman, W., and Pauli, L. L. (1975): Anticonvulsant drug blood levels. *JAMA*, 232:60–62.

Mygind, K. I., Dam, M., and Christiansen, J. (1976): Phenytoin and phenobarbitone plasma clearance during pregnancy. *Acta Neurol. Scand.*, 54:160–166.

Penry, J. K., and Porter, R. J. (1977): Intensive monitoring of patients with intractable seizures. In: *Epilepsy: The Eighth International Symposium*, edited by J. K. Penry, pp. 95–102. Raven Press, New York.

Ramsay, R. E., Strauss, R. G., Wilder, B. J., and James, L. (1978): Status epilepticus in pregnancy: Effect of phenytoin malabsorption on seizure control. *Neurology*, 28:85–89.

Richens, A. (1977): Precise adjustment of phenytoin dosage. In: *Epilepsy: The Eighth International Symposium*, edited by J. K. Penry, pp. 139–141. Raven Press, New York.

Rowan, A. J., Pippenger, C. E., McGregor, P. A., and French, J. H. (1975): Seizure activity and anticonvulsant drug concentration. *Arch. Neurol.*, 32:281–288.

Advances in Epileptology:
The Xth Epilepsy International Symposium,
edited by J. A. Wada and J. K. Penry.
Raven Press, New York © 1980.

Free-Ranging Electroencephalographic Videotelemetry in a Children's Neuropsychiatric Unit

R. D. Rafal, P. K. Garrison, K. D. Laxer,
L. Maukonen, D. S. Rushmer, and G. D. Laird

Good Samaritan Hospital and Medical Center, Portland, Oregon 97209

Telemetry has expanded the diagnostic potential of the electroencephalo-gram (EEG) by making it possible and practical to record patients for pro-longed periods to document infrequent ictal events. It has been applied clinically to the diagnosis of epilepsy, the determination of seizure type and frequency and, when used in conjunction with sphenoidal and depth re-cordings, to the localization of a seizure focus in surgical candidates (Penry et al., 1975; Porter et al., 1976; Porter et al., 1977; Belafsky et al., 1978).

In conventional practice video telemetry is conducted in a routine hospital setting. Typically, the mobility of the patient is restricted by a wall-fixed camera and there is little direct interaction between the patient and the telemetry consultant, both participating passively: the patient's time is spent *ad lib* within the confines of his/her room, while the physician waits for the data to come to him/her.

We have developed a free-ranging video telemetry technique for the dynamic study of childhood epilepsy on a special Children's Neuropsychiat-ric Unit (CNPU; see elsewhere in *this volume*). When incorporated into a comprehensive, multidisciplinary approach, free-ranging EEG video telem-etry (FRVT) provided unique opportunities for more effectively evaluating and managing children with epilepsy and related disorders.

METHODS

Telemetry was integrated into an in-depth multidisciplinary analysis of each case and was conducted in a natural milieu dynamically structured to optimize the likelihood of recording seizure-related events. Prior to telem-etry, each candidate received a complete psychosocial, neuropsychologi-cal, and neurological evaluation including routine EEG studies with con-ventional activating procedures. The Unit staff kept a seizure log recording seizure type and frequency and made detailed observations of problem behaviors. The pretelemetry work-up culminated in the formulation of the problem(s) to be addressed by telemetry and the selection of target behaviors deserving close scrutiny during the study. The telemetry consultant designed a problem-oriented, individually tailored protocol that, in addition to specifying the time of day, length of the recording, and montage to be used, also included appropriate activities or activating procedures, e.g., stressful social situations, psychometric testing, continuous performance tasks, and physical exertion.

Each study was conducted in the living area of the Unit in collaboration with its staff and the child's parents where appropriate. The patient's behavior was continuously recorded on videotape by the EEG telemetry technician, who operated a mobile camera. Four channels of EEG were displayed on the television monitor by video reformatter while eight channels of EEG were recorded intermittently on paper printout. The range of the telemetry transmitter is approximately 150 feet and it was possible to study these children in a free-ranging situation anywhere on the Unit. Thus we were able to study the interaction between environmental-behavioral events and their EEG concomitants in a wide range of structured and naturally occurring situations.

When seizures or target behaviors were observed, the time was noted from the digital clock video display and recorded for subsequent review. The records were reviewed and edited by the telemetry consultant for weekly conferences with the Unit staff. Where appropriate, the tapes were also reviewed with the patient's parents, who were instructed in the keeping of accurate seizure logs.

RESULTS

Between January, 1977 and July, 1978 we studied 50 children in one or more acute (1–6 hr), free-ranging recordings on the CNPU. Our experience is reflected in the following brief case histories, which illustrate some of the innovative applications of this free-ranging technique.

Case 1. Mary Ann was a 10-year-old girl who had had severe encephalitis at the age of 3. The sequelae were devastating and included severe mental retardation with developmental delay, a seizure disorder, and incessant, infuriating hyperactivity. It had not been possible to obtain a technically adequate EEG recording in over 5 years. At the time of her admission, she was having frequent staring spells poorly controlled on primidone.

After placement of electrodes the child was left unrestrained; she rapidly habituated to the monitoring situation and good quality records were obtained. Three absence seizures were recorded in 1 hr associated with paroxysmal, rhythmic, 3 per second spike-and-wave discharges. Two were associated with loss of postural tone. Other briefer absence spells were accompanied by frozen immobility. Telemetry helped to distinguish these from autistic reveries in which she stared vacantly as if preoccupied and continued to fiddle with her hands.

Case 2. Gigi was a 15-year-old Indian girl who had been abused as a neonate and adopted when 9 days old. Seizures began at the age of 5 years. On admission, she was having frequent absence seizures and her EEG revealed generalized 3 cycle per second spike-and-wave paroxysms. She was withdrawn and unhappy, irritable, noncompliant, and educationally crippled.

A telemetry study provided critical insight into the influence of subtle ictal events on her behavior. She was having frequent, subtle, incomplete absence spells that had been previously undetected by an experienced Unit staff. These frequent seizures were found to be principally responsible for the marked psychomotor retardation and general disorganization of her interictal behavior. Her irritability and noncompliance had previously been ascribed to psychodynamic factors and had been managed inappropriately and unsuccessfully with disciplinary action that only aggravated the child's hostility and frustration.

One prolonged episode recorded during telemetry had a focal motor component with clonic jerking of the right hand and suggested that her seizures might be focal in origin with secondary bilateral synchrony. An unsuccessful trial of ethosuximide was abandoned and carbamazepine was instituted with a gratifying improvement in seizure control.

Case 3. Rosie was a 15-year-old girl with Lennox-Gastaut syndrome who had intractable seizures from the age of 5 years. She was functioning intellectually as a 4-year-old and, at the time of admission, was having numerous major and minor motor seizures daily in spite of therapeutic doses of primidone, carbamazepine, phenytoin, and phenobarbital. Her EEG was almost continuously disorganized by irregular, slow spike and polyspike wave paroxysms. There was *no* photoconvulsive response.

Major seizures, occurring usually during sleep or on awakening, had clonic and vibratory components with occasional rhizomyelic posturing. Rhythmic blinking occurred synchronously with the slow wave component on EEG and was suppressed during bursts of high-amplitude polyspike discharge, which at times lasted as long as 4 sec.

She had been hospitalized on several occasions with status epilepticus precipitated by family stress, and academic pressure in school regularly resulted in increased seizures. It had also been noted that the slightest emotional stress caused her to blink excessively; this pathological blinking was so dramatic that she had been referred to an ophthalmologist.

Epileptiform discharges were reliably precipitated by blinking, and this linkage, although variable, was consistently demonstrated during telemetry studies over a several-day period. Frequently, isolated spike wave transients were observed to follow a single spontaneous blink. More commonly the phenomenon was associated with repetitive blinking that resulted in the recruitment of synchronous slow wave EEG activity culminating in a spike wave discharge. These blink-induced epileptiform discharges could easily be elicited by voluntary blinking on command either in the light or in the dark. They also could be elicited by reflex blinking on corneal stimulation or by psychogenic blinking triggered by social stress or cognitive effort. Usually she remained responsive during these discharges and they could be aborted simply by alerting her. However, at times they were accompanied by brief absence spells.

The introduction of sodium valproate into the regimen afforded almost complete seizure control and permitted the gradual, tapered withdrawal of her other anticonvulsants.

Case 4. Shannon was a 7-year-old girl with profound developmental delay; she did not speak and was severely autistic. A right occipital encephalocele had been repaired in infancy; repeated shunting had been required for hydrocephalus. She had had two unambiguous grand mal seizures in the 2 years prior to admission. Her EEG had a well regulated background of 11 cycle per second alpha activity, and demonstrated a right posterior slow wave focus without epileptic features.

Most of her autistic behaviors, such as rocking, repetitive head-nodding, blinking, and eye-rolling were easily distinguishable from ictal events. Others, however, included versive posturing followed by automatic, repetitive movements that were strikingly similar to psychomotor automatisms. A FRVT study permitted the confident exclusion of an ictal origin for all of these behaviors, and her anticonvulsant regimen was adjusted accordingly.

Case 5. Angie was a severely delayed 4-year-old girl who had had seizures since the age of 16 months. Her EEG revealed generalized slowing that at times was paroxysmal in character. She had generalized seizures with prolonged apneic periods that had in the past required resuscitation and emergency hospitalization. She did not speak or walk. She was severely autistic and exhibited a wide range of repetitive, ritualistic behaviors.

A curious and distressing problem studied with telemetry was the association of prolonged outbursts of terrified screaming, crying, and hand wringing, with paroxysmal, generalized, high-amplitude rhythmic, 6 cycle per second theta activity on EEG (See Fig. 1). After treatment with carbamazepine, she became more mobile and accessible. The paroxysmal screaming episodes ceased, but the other autistic behaviors changed very little.

CONCLUSIONS

To fully exploit its unique capabilities in the study of childhood epilepsy, FRVT must be carefully planned on the basis of a comprehensive, multidisciplinary approach and dynamically conducted in a natural milieu. Some of the innovative applications of this method include:

(a) For documenting seizure type, FRVT can provide good quality recordings in impulsive, hyperactive children who may not tolerate the immobilization of conventional hard-wired techniques. Most of these children will permit the placement of electrodes by a skillful technician; if then left unrestrained and are distracted for a few minutes, they rapidly habituate to the monitoring situation and forget the wires and transmitter on their backs.

(b) FRVT can provide unambiguous documentation of pseudoseizures.

(c) FRVT records are invaluable in training parents and teachers to identify, classify, and log seizures in children under their care; thus the treating physician is aided by highly reliable seizure logs on which to base management decisions.

(d) FRVT may provide critical insights into the influence of subtle ictal

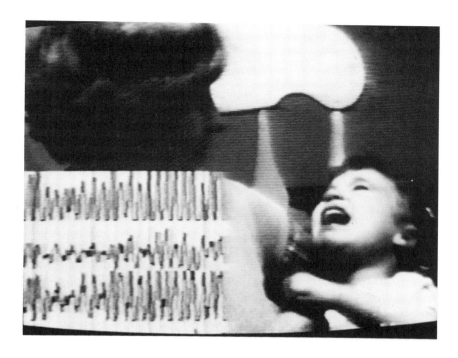

FIG. 1. Prolonged outbursts of terrified screaming and crying associated with paroxysmal theta activity in a severely autistic 7-year-old epileptic (Case 5).

events on a child's behavior by enabling *performance* to be examined in relationship to electrographic seizures.

(e) FRVT provides the flexibility and precision required for investigating patients with reflex (evoked) epilepsy or those in whom seizure frequency is heavily influenced by stress, or other environmental activators.

(f) FRVT finds its most powerful application in the study of brain-injured, autistic children where the challenge is to identify seizures against a behavioral background noise of clinically similar autisms, i.e., staring, unresponsiveness, and automatistic, repetitive, or ritualistic behaviors.

ACKNOWLEDGMENTS

This work was supported by a Comprehensive Epilepsy Program grant from NINCDS (Contract 1NS-5-2328). We are indebted to Mrs. Susan Ohlson and Ms. Jeri Janowsky for their technical assistance.

REFERENCES

Balafsky, M. A., Carwille, S., Miller, P., Waddell, G., Boxley-Johnson, J., and Delgado-Escueta, A. V. (1978): Prolonged epileptic twilight states: Continuous recordings with nasopharyngeal electrodes and videotape analysis. *Neurology (Minneap.)*, 28:239–245.

Penry, J. K., Porter, R. J., and Dreifuss, F. E. (1975): Simultaneous recording of absence seizures with videotape and electroencephalography. A study of 374 seizures in 48 patients. *Brain*, 98:400–427.

Porter, R. J., Penry, K., and Lacy, J. R. (1977): Diagnostic and therapeutic reevaluation of patients with intractable epilepsy. *Neurology (Minneap.)*, 27:1006–1011.

Porter, R. J., Penry, J. K., and Wolf, A. A., Jr. (1976): Simultaneous documentation of clinical and electroencephalographic manifestations of epileptic seizures. In: *Quantitative Analytic Studies in Epilepsy*, edited by P. Kellaway and I. Petersen, pp. 253–268. Raven Press, New York.

Advances in Epileptology:
The Xth Epilepsy International Symposium,
edited by J. A. Wada and J. K. Penry.
Raven Press, New York © 1980.

Clinical Testing During Intensive Monitoring of Ictal Events

M. L. Fay and R. H. Mattson

Epilepsy Center, Veteran's Administration Hospital, West Haven, Connecticut 06516

Intensive clinical videotape/polygraphic monitoring has been a significant advance in the diagnosis and management of epileptic seizures and related disorders. Although the electrical recordings provide important data, the information to be gained from the monitoring can be greatly increased by a clinical neurological exam during and after the attacks. Since there is rarely sufficient time to allow for detailed testing at the time of a seizure, tests need to be preselected or a screening exam planned and discussed with all potential observers. To accurately document the test results on videotape and EEG, at least two well-informed attendants should be present, one to assure proper electrical recording and one to administer the preplanned neurological exam while attending the patient (Mcfie, 1969; Strub and Black, 1977).

The exam performed during ictal events primarily involves testing for hard neurological signs (Table 1). Of primary importance is the observation of clinical events that might be out of camera range. For example, deviation of the head and eyes often takes this important clinical finding away from audio/video viewing. If there are focal contractions of the face, they may be hidden from the camera. Pupillary changes are difficult to record and should be monitored by the examiner. The clinical examination during intensive monitoring should also be used to explain findings recorded on the polygraph. Fine tremors or rhythmic contractions of various body parts out of camera view frequently give the EEG an artifact having an epileptiform appearance. Report of these observations by the examiner can be verbally presented for recording on tape.

Second, during the ictal exam, it is essential to determine the patient's level of consciousness, his ability to communicate, and the degree of orientation thereof. The significance of the more in-depth testing to follow is colored by the mental status of the patient. Frequently, patients are alert and can articulate but have no idea of where they are or what is happening. Typical answers to the question, "Where are you?" have been, "On a boat, I guess" and, "On the wall." Because of social pressures, many patients have learned to skillfully conceal the degree of confusion they are actually experiencing.

TABLE 1. *Ictal examination*

Exam	Lateralization/ localization	Supplementary information Documentation of events not recorded due to camera limitations
Supplementary clinical observation	Variable	
Level of consciousness	Generalization	Spread
Communication	Nonspecific	Confusion versus aphasia
Orientation	Nonspecific	Confusion versus aphasia
Strength (drift, grip)	Contralateral	
Eye deviation	Contralateral	
Visual fields	Contralateral	
Verbal memory (auditory)	Left temporal	Global amnesia
Nonverbal memory (visual)	Right temporal	
Nonverbal memory (auditory)	Nonspecific	
Other		Special tests for suspected nonepileptic episodes

The examiner should check for visual field deficits by confrontation and reading. Tests for verbal and nonverbal memory are given by administering a test phrase along with visual and auditory stimuli.

Finally, during the ictal period, the examiner must be prepared to administer alternate testing if the episode is suspected to be nonepileptic. Atypical toxicity requires checks for symmetrical nystagmus, ataxia, or incoordination. If the episode is due to cerebral ischemia, blood pressure and heart rate checks are essential.

"Hysterical" seizures must be tested for the typical signs such as resistance to eye opening or evidence of avoidance of harm to self. When told firmly to "cut it out," many such patients will respond by doing so.

The postictal exam is intended to add as much lateralization and localizing information as possible. Each exam is planned to cover the individual deficits suspected from baseline formal neurological testing; in particular, the area of the brain that may be surgically resected is tested. Of importance is the fact that the exam is focused also on the ability of the opposite hemisphere to function during the ictal and postictal periods. Typically the postictal examination includes the same tests but carried out in greater depth and detail as time and patient cooperation allow. These tests examine for aphasia, dysnomia, dyspraxia, alexia, dysarthria, rapid alternating movements, visual inattention, simularities, acalculia, left/right orientation, perceptual motor function, stereognosis, double simultaneous stimulation, and abstractions. Experience has shown that the exam can be administered in 10 to 15 min. Deficient areas are repeated until no longer apparent or return to baseline.

CASE HISTORIES

Case 1. Mrs. B, a 25-year-old right-handed married unemployed white female presented with a history of partial complex seizures with onset at age 7. Since that time she has had at least one seizure per week and at the time of hospitalization was frequently having one attack per day. Seizures were described subjectively as "flashbulbs going off in my face for 2 to 3 sec" or a "shaky" sensation followed by motor arrest and a disassociative state. Objectively, she had a staring spell followed by inappropriate conversation or wandering that had resulted in being picked up by the police for suspected drug abuse. Postictally she was lethargic and confused.

On admission to the Epilepsy Unit in January, 1978, two types of seizures were documented on audio/video and EEG: (a) The first was her habitual seizure with repeated complaint, "I'm dizzy, I'm tired, I'm all dizzy" followed by the disassociative state. (b) A second type was characterized by left facial clonic seizure without loss of consciousness. Extensive neurological and neuropsychological examinations were *not* done in the ictal and postictal state. Initially, continuous EEG recording showed a disorganized record of bilateral slowing and high-amplitude theta activity, sometimes more predominant on the right.

Extensive presurgical work-up including intensive monitoring, neuropsychological exam, ACTA scan, angiograph with WADA, visual fields, and pneumoencephalography suggested Mrs. B was an appropriate candidate for epilepsy surgery. A hospitalization for intensive monitoring with intracerebral electrodes was planned. She was readmitted to the Epilepsy Unit in March, 1978. Five clear clinical and electrical seizures were recorded; three of these were her habitual seizures; two were the less frequent left facial clonic seizures without loss of consciousness. Electrically, seizures were originating as suspected from the right temporal area. Detailed neurological testing was performed during ictal and postictal events. During the first of the less frequent seizures, the examiner entered the room and conversed with Mrs. B to determine her mental status. Clonic activity of left face and eye was apparent. As testing progressed, Mrs. B was asked to read *point to your nose*. Her first reply was "nose," then "your nose." A residual left homonymous hemianopsia was found on confrontation. This slowly cleared during the postictal state. Formal visual fields done after probe removal showed a congruous right inferior quadrantanopsia. Because of the possibility of significant visual problems if she lost all her left field secondary to surgery, the operation was not performed. Without careful testing during and after her seizures, the left homonymous hemianopsia field would have not been recognized. Testing in attacks without the focal facial seizures also revealed the left homonymous hemianopsia.

Case 2. In addition to eliminating the surgery possibility, testing more often gives supportive evidence of the suspected epileptiform focus. A 28-year-old left-handed white female with poorly controlled complex partial seizures was admitted for intensive monitoring of intracerebral electrodes, as was the patient in Case 1. Habitual seizures occurred two to four times each week with a vague aura of "not really tingling" and a seizure with turning to the left, automatisms, and 5 to 15 min of postictal lethargy. EEG recordings had shown an interictal left temporal spike wave focus.

Miss T underwent continuous audio/visual and EEG monitoring with depth electrodes. Three seizures were recorded. Electrically there was left-sided onset with low-voltage, high-frequency 20 Hz activity beginning in the left temporal electrode. The preplanned neurological/neuropsychological exam administered at this time substantiated those left-sided findings. Miss T demonstrated global aphasia. Left-right orientation was compromised. Evidence of normally functioning right brain was suggested by the lack of visual inattention or field deficit and the presence of perceptual motor abilities.

Because of the number of findings confirming a left temporal focus, the patient was considered a good candidate for left temporal lobectomy. Surgery has proven beneficial, with no seizures occurring since July, 1978.

SUMMARY

Intensive videotape/polygraphic monitoring of clinical and electrical seizure activity often gives incomplete data. Recordings should include a preplanned specific neurological and neuropsychological exam to supplement data recorded on the videotape and EEG.

REFERENCES

Mcfie, J. (1969): The diagnostic significance of disorders of higher nervous activity. HCN, Vol. 4.

Strub, R. T., and Black, F. W. (1977): *The Mental Status Examination in Neurology.* F. A. Davis, Philadelphia.

Advances in Epileptology:
The Xth Epilepsy International Symposium,
edited by J. A. Wada and J. K. Penry.
Raven Press, New York © 1980.

Electroencephalographic Monitoring in Patients with Absence Seizures

R. J. Quy, P. Fitch, R. G. Willison, and R. W. Gilliatt

Institute of Neurology, Queen Square, London, WC1N 3BG England

In the past, our group at Queen Square has been interested in using EEG telemetry, combined with closed-circuit television and videotape recording, to monitor epileptic patients (Bowden et al., 1975; Jestico et al., 1977). This does, of course, require the patient to remain in one room where he can be observed by the television cameras. We have found this approach particularly valuable when one wishes to match clinical events to EEG events in patients with unusual attacks in which epilepsy is suspected.

There are other situations, however, in which the problem is not one of diagnosis, but of how much epileptic activity is present at different times, and how it is related to the patient's drug treatment. For this we have developed monitoring techniques that enable us to obtain EEG recordings for 24 hr or more from patients whose activity is unrestricted, and who might be in the ward, in our special center for epilepsy, or even at home. In this we are following the pioneer studies of Penry and colleagues (Sato et al., 1976), and of Ives and Woods (1975). The approach is particularly appropriate for monitoring spike-and-wave activity in patients with absence seizures.

For these prolonged EEG recordings we need some form of automatic analysis of the spike-and-wave activity; this, in turn, requires a primary trace that is relatively free from artifact. Movement artifact is particularly a problem in recording the EEG from unrestrained patients, and to limit this we have developed a scalp-mounted preamplifier (Quy, 1978). The preamplifier is attached to the scalp with collodion and connected to a pair of silver/silver chloride electrodes. Since the preamplifier has a gain of 1,000 and a low output impedance (< 100 ohms), artifacts from external fields and triboelectric noise are minimized. In addition, this type of "stick-on" preamplifier, in contrast with other types mounted on the neck (Ives and Woods, 1975) or on a headcap (Sato et al., 1976), allows the electrode leads to be very short and flexible, which reduces the artifact produced by mechanical distortion of the electrode-electrolyte-scalp interface. It must be emphasized, however, that careful preparation and attachment of electrodes is essential for clean recordings from freely moving patients over prolonged periods.

The EEG signal is stored on a four-channel cassette recorder (Oxford Medical Systems Ltd., "Medilog"), to which we have added a connection system of our own design for electrical and mechanical termination of the input leads. Two EEG channels are normally recorded from sites selected according to the patient's abnormality. The other two channels are used for monitoring movement (using a miniature accelerometer mounted on the head), and either ECG or eye movement. The preamplifiers, electrodes, and accelerometer can be hidden under the hair for cosmetic purposes, and covered by a protective woollen cap at night. The cassette recorder is worn in a padded bag on a belt at the waist.

The cassette tapes, which run for 24 hr, are analyzed by an analog detection system. The slow wave component of spike-and-wave paroxysms is isolated by a 2 to 4 Hz bandpass filter, the output of which can be seen in trace 2 of Fig. 1. In our original system this output was compared with a preset voltage and anything exceeding this voltage produced a detector output (Jestico et al., 1977), but this system proved to be too sensitive to artefact such as eye blinking. To overcome this we tried several ways of making the system require two or more complexes before responding; we found that a more effective solution was to rectify and smooth the output of the filter to convert it to a varying DC voltage (trace 3 of Fig. 1). This is then compared with a preset voltage to produce a slow wave detector output

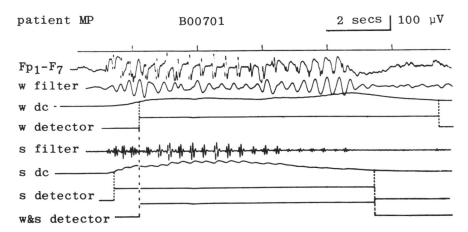

FIG. 1. Example of the operation of the spike-and-wave detection system described in the text. From **top** to **bottom**: Time marker; trace 1, primary EEG record; trace 2, output of a 2 to 4 Hz bandpass filter (24 dB per octave) used to isolate the slow-wave activity from the EEG; trace 3, the filter output after passage through a leaky integrator (time constant = 2 sec); trace 4, threshold detector operates at the points indicated by the vertical dotted lines; trace 5, spike component isolated by a 12 to 20 Hz bandpass filter (24 dB per octave); trace 6, spike DC signal (integrator time constant = 0.8 sec); trace 7, spike threshold detector operates at points indicated by *vertical dotted lines*; trace 8, combined wave-and-spike detector operates at points indicated by *vertical broken lines*.

(trace 4 of Fig. 1). The response of the detector can be modified by adjusting the time constant of the smoothing circuit and clipping the input signal.

During 24-hr recordings a further problem with this system was that the slow wave detector would sometimes register bursts of high-voltage delta activity during sleep. To avoid this we added a similar system to detect the presence of the spike component as well (traces 5–7 of Fig. 1). The spike-and-slow wave components are separately filtered from the EEG signal, converted to DC levels, and then compared with threshold voltages that are adjusted to suit the morphology of the spike-and-wave pattern for each patient. Only when both the spike and the slow wave detector outputs are present does the combined detector output shown in trace 8 of Fig. 1 operate. Note that the initial delay in the operation of the combined detector is matched by a comparable delay in switching off. This may be contrasted with the unequal on and off times of the spike and slow wave detectors themselves. This system is relatively insensitive to the shape or regularity of the spike-and-wave burst, and we have found that it will detect the degraded spike-and-wave activity that occurs during sleep. The output of the detector is coupled to a microprocessor system that sums and prints out the total number of seconds of spike-and-wave activity per 15-min intervals throughout the 24 hr. The cassette tapes are processed at 60 times real time so that a 24-hr recording can be analyzed in 24 min. A section of the primary trace can be written out automatically on paper by a Mingograf ink jet recorder whenever a spike-and-wave burst is detected, or at preset intervals, in order to check that the detection system is operating correctly (Quy et al. 1980).

The ambulatory monitoring procedure can be applied in several ways. For example, it can reveal how much spike-and-wave activity a patient is experiencing, which may not be obvious clinically. The monitoring procedure then can be repeated several times to enable the patient's response to drug treatment to be evaluated. In collaboration with Dr. Alan Richens we are at present using this method to relate drug levels and epileptic activity throughout the day in a study of the pharmacodynamics of sodium valproate. The effects of sleep and waking on spike-and-wave activity can also be assessed; in particular, we wish to study in a larger number of patients the apparent concentration of spike-and-wave activity previously observed by Jestico et al. (1977) to occur in the early morning.

Finally, not only absence seizures but also other types of epileptic activity, such as spontaneous grand mal seizures, have been successfully monitored with this technique.

In conclusion, ambulatory monitoring can provide information that would be difficult or impossible to obtain in any other way. Moreover, it should be emphasized that this approach is relatively inexpensive. The whole system, including the recording and data-analysis apparatus, could be set up for less than the cost of a conventional 16-channel EEG machine.

ACKNOWLEDGMENTS

We gratefully acknowledge support from the Medical Research Council, the Brain Research Trust, and the Mason Medical Research Foundation. A generous gift for the purchase of apparatus was provided by *The Sunday People*.
We also wish to thank Dr. W. A. Cobb for advice and encouragement.

REFERENCES

Bowden, A. N., Fitch, P., Gilliatt, R. W., and Willison, R. G. (1975): The place of EEG telemetry and closed-circuit television in the diagnosis and management of epileptic patients. *Proc. R. Soc. Med.*, 68:246–248.

Ives, J. R., and Woods, J. F. (1975): 4-channel 24 hour cassette recorder for long-term EEG monitoring of ambulatory patients. *Electroencephalogr. Clin. Neurophysiol.*, 39:88–92.

Jestico, J., Fitch, P., Gilliatt, R. W., and Willison, R. G. (1977): Automatic and rapid visual analysis of sleep stages and epileptic activity. A preliminary report. *Electroencephalogr. Clin. Neurophysiol.*, 43:438–441.

Quy, R. J. (1978): A miniature preamplifier for ambulatory monitoring of the electroencephalogram. *J. Physiol. (Lond.)*, 284:23–24 P.

Quy, R. J., Fitch, P., and Willison, R. G. (1980): High-speed automatic analysis of EEG spike and wave activity using an analogue detection and microcomputer plotting system. *Electroencephalogr. Clin. Neurophysiol.*, 49:187–189.

Sato, S., Penry, J. K., and Dreifuss, F. E. (1976): Electroencephalographic monitoring of generalised spike-wave paroxysms in the hospital and at home. In: *Quantitative Analytic Studies in Epilepsy*, edited by P. Kellaway and I. Petersen, pp. 237–251. Raven Press, New York.

Advances in Epileptology:
The Xth Epilepsy International Symposium,
edited by J. A. Wada and J. K. Penry.
Raven Press, New York © 1980.

Presurgical Intensive Monitoring Using Depth Electroencephalography in Temporal Lobe Epilepsy

P. D. Williamson, D. D. Spencer, S. S. Spencer, and R. H. Mattson

Neurology Service, Veterans Administration Medical Center, West Haven, Connecticut; and Departments of Neurology and Neurosurgery, Yale University School of Medicine, New Haven, Connecticut

Prolonged intensive monitoring of the scalp electroencephalogram (EEG) and the clinical manifestations of seizures is of proven value in patients with various types of epilepsy (Penry et al., 1969; Porter et al., 1976; Porter et al., 1977; Escueta et al., 1977). Simultaneous videotape recording of the patient and the EEG documents the presence of epilepsy and allows detailed analysis of the relationships between the electrical activity of the brain and the various clinical phases of the epileptic attack. Not all epilepsy is associated with changes in the scalp EEG. The diagnosis of epilepsy can often be established by the clinical pattern of the seizure but occasionally hysteria cannot be eliminated. Even when clear EEG changes accompany partial seizures, precise localization of the seizure onset is seldom possible.

The use of chronically implanted electrodes in the evaluation of patients being considered for epilepsy surgery is of proven value for localization of the seizure onset (Talairach and Bancaud, 1974). Most authors who have written on the subject have commented on the frequent lack of close correlation between the scalp and depth recorded paroxysmal activity both between and during seizures (Walter, 1973; Lieb et al., 1976). Since it is generally agreed that several seizures need be recorded in these patients, prolonged monitoring is usually necessary (Crandall et al., 1971).

In this chapter we present the results of prolonged depth monitoring in four patients from a group of 20 patients with complex partial epilepsy who were being evaluated for surgery. These cases illustrate findings that would not necessarily have been anticipated from the preimplant evaluation. These include "functional disorders" associated with seizure discharges, prolonged seizure discharges with no clinical manifestations, and independent right and left temporal lobe seizure onsets when scalp and interictal depth data predicted right-side disease. The electrodes are 18 contact linear probes (Ray, 1966). They are placed horizontally in the hippocampus, vertically in

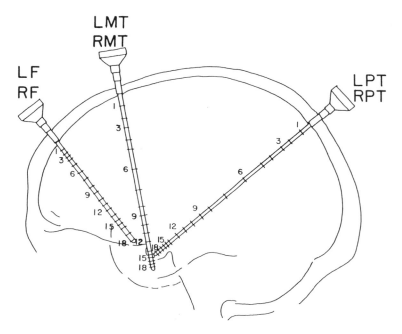

FIG. 1. Electrode placement options: hippocampal (RPT, LPT); anterior temporal (RMT, LMT); frontal (RF, LF). Eighteen contact points with number 1 near hub and number 18 at tip of electrode.

anterior temporal lobe structures, and vertically in the medial and orbital frontal structures (Fig. 1). The number and location of electrodes is determined by clinical findings in each patient.

CASE HISTORIES

Case 1. A 28-year-old male had had seizures since the age of 10. Seizures consisted of sudden motor arrest followed by some rigid posturing, automatisms, and prolonged postictal confusion. In addition, the patient was thought by some members of his family to exhibit a psychiatric disorder manifested by episodic preoccupation, talking to himself, whistling, making strange faces, and answering questions only partially and indifferently. These spells would often last for several hours, and on occasion, for a full day. Scalp recording revealed a prominent focus in the left anterior temporal frontal region with frequent secondary bilateral synchrony. Scalp recording during seizures revealed no apparent focal onset. Bilateral frontal and anterior temporal electrodes were implanted. The patient had a number of typical clinical seizures that consisted of a grimace followed by some rigid, possibly tonic posturing, lip-smacking, and a prolonged period of postictal confusion. The EEG during this period consisted primarily of high-frequency discharge from the left anterior temporal region with rapid spread to other sites, particularly the frontal lobes on both sides. On several occasions during the prolonged recording, he

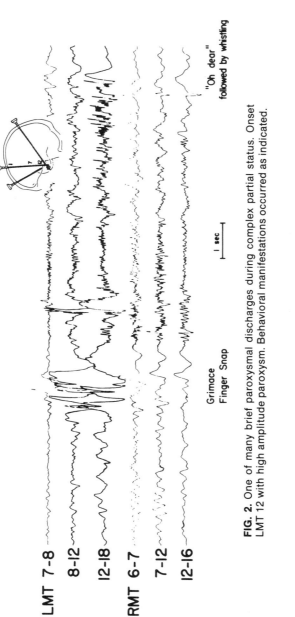

FIG. 2. One of many brief paroxysmal discharges during complex partial status. Onset LMT 12 with high amplitude paroxysm. Behavioral manifestations occurred as indicated.

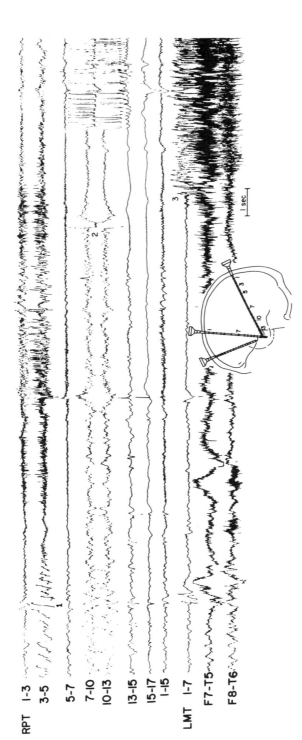

FIG. 3. Clinical seizure beginning in right occiput (1) followed by high amplitude paroxysm and desynchronization in right hippocampus (2) progressing to paroxysmal activity in left anterior temporal region (3).

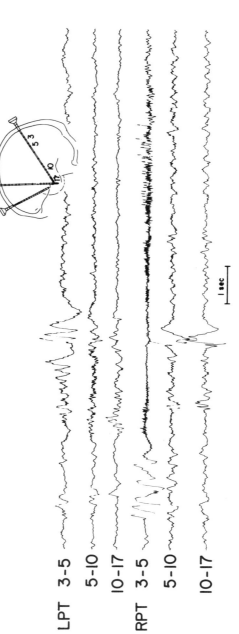

FIG. 4. Seizure discharge restricted to right occiput associated with sensation of eyes pulling.

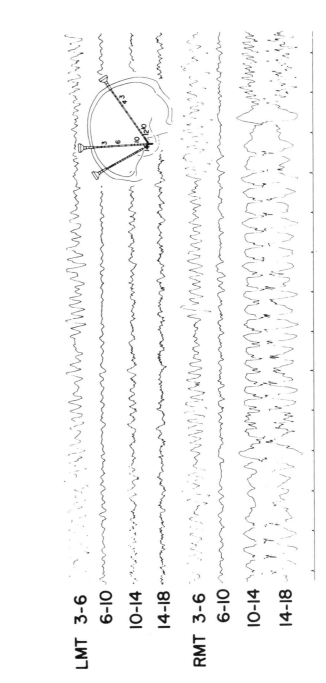

(See legend facing page.)

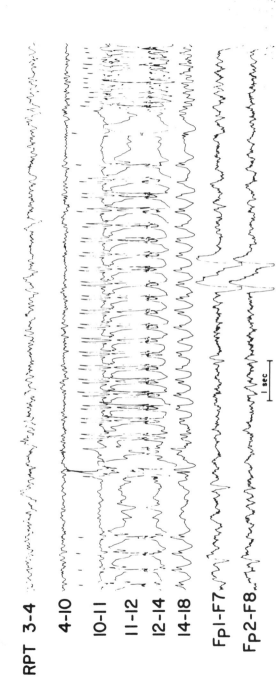

FIG. 5. A 14-sec section from subclinical seizure discharge located in right anterior hippocampus. Total duration, 80 sec. No reflection in scalp electrodes.

exhibited peculiar behavior, sometimes lasting several hours, consisting of grimacing, snapping his fingers, whistling, and repeating phrases. Depth recording revealed frequent high amplitude paroxysmal discharges followed by brief, high-frequency activity (Fig. 2). Clinical testing demonstrated disorientation to time, place, and person. It was clear that these episodes were identical to those that had previously been felt by some to have been psychiatric in nature but were actually a form of status epilepticus.

Case 2. A 34-year-old female who had had seizures since the age of 11. Her seizures occurred without warning and consisted of rigid posturing, complex turning and writhing movements, followed by a prolonged period of confusion with automatisms. She had frequent spells that she described as a sensation of pulling in her eyes. They were observed as squinting and random roving movement of the eyes. These latter attacks were thought to be clearly hysterical. Scalp EEG revealed prominent independent bitemporal spikes between seizures. Recording prior to and during clinical seizures demonstrated no focal onset or focal ictal discharge. Bilateral anterior temporal and hippocampal electrodes were implanted. Between seizures prominent independent right and left temporal paroxysmal events were noted. Typical clinical seizures began with a high-frequency discharge usually in the right occipital region but occasionally in the left occipital region as well with rapid spread to the right hippocampus, then involving the brain generally on both sides (Fig. 3). The patient did not report an aura. However, it was noted that right, and less frequently left, occipital high-frequency discharges were seen in isolation, often in flurries lasting several minutes (Fig. 4). The patient at this time would invariably complain of her "hysterical" eye-pulling sensations. There was no reflection of the electrical abnormality in the scalp recording.

Case 3. A 43-year-old male who had had seizures since the age of 29. His seizures consisted of an aura of an ill-defined epigastric sensation spreading to his head. The seizure would either end there or progress to a loss of contact with teeth clenching, automatisms, and prolonged postictal confusion. Interictal scalp recording revealed mild generalized slowing. Paroxysmal activity was only minimally apparent during drowsiness and light sleep and consisted of sharp waves predominantly in the right anterior temporal region. With use of nasopharyngeal electrodes, the sharp activity was better visualized on the right side. Several seizures were recorded and there was no clear focal onset. Bilateral anterior temporal and a right hippocampal electrode were implanted. Between seizures there was a very prominent spike focus in the right anterior hippocampus. There were numerous clear electrical seizure discharges emanating from the same area in the right hippocampus with no clinical expression (Fig. 5). Identical electrical seizure discharges would on occasion be associated with his typical aura. His usual clinical seizures with loss of contact also began with an identical right anterior hippocampal discharge. There were many more subclinical electrical discharges than either auras or full clinical seizures. At no time were the subclinical seizure discharges, the auras, or the seizure onset, observed in the simultaneous scalp recording.

Case 4. A 31-year-old male had a history of seizures since infancy. His current seizures consisted of sudden arrest of activity followed by prolonged automatisms. On occasions following the motor arrest, some left-sided clonic motor activity occurred. Scalp recording revealed bitemporal paroxysmal activity during sleep, with the abnormality being much more prominent over the right temporal region. On rare occasions bifrontal slowing was noted. Scalp recording during clinical seizures revealed either no focal onset or low-voltage fast activity in the right anterior temporal region. Depth electrodes were placed bilaterally in the frontal and anterior temporal regions. Recording from the intracranial electrodes between seizures revealed paroxysmal activity predominantly from the right anterior temporal region. During drowsiness and light sleep paroxysmal activity on occasion became more extensive, involving the frontal regions bilaterally and the left anterior temporal region as well. Seizures were recorded from the intracranial electrodes coming from the right anterior temporal region beginning with low-voltage fast activity and then rapidly spreading to involve extensive areas bilaterally. These were typical clinical seizures that on occasion were associated with some motor activity on the left side. Seizures were also recorded clearly coming from the left anterior temporal region, often remaining confined to that region for considerable periods of time with variable clinical expression and on termination were associated with prolonged postictal automatisms.

These four patients demonstrate informative and unanticipated data obtained with prolonged intracranial recording. In our series of 20 patients who have undergone intensive depth monitoring, unexpected findings were noted in 15. These findings ruled against surgical intervention or altered the surgical approach in some cases. Prolonged intensive monitoring with depth electrodes is essential in the presurgical evaluation of many cases of temporal lobe epilepsy.

REFERENCES

Crandall, P. H., Walter, R. D., and Dymond, D. (1971): The ictal electroencephalographic signal identifying limbic system seizure foci. *Proc. Am. Assoc. Neurol. Surg.*, 1:1–9.

Escueta, A. V., Kinze, U., Waddell, G., Boxley, J., Buxley, J., and Madel, A. (1977): Lapse of consciousness and automatisms in temporal lobe epilepsy: A videotape analysis. *Neurology (Minneap.)*, 27:144–155.

Lieb, J. P., Walsh, G. O., Babb, T. L., Walter, R. D., and Crandall, P. H. (1976): A comparison of EEG seizure patterns with surface and depth electrodes in patients with temporal lobe epilepsy. *Epilepsia*, 17:137–160.

Penry, J. K., and Dreifuss, F. E. (1969): Automatisms associated with the absence of petit mal epilepsy. *Arch. Neurol.*, 21:142–149.

Porter, R. J., Penry, J. K., and Lacy, J. R. (1977): The diagnostic and therapeutic reevaluation of patients with intractable epilepsy. *Neurology (Minneap.)*, 27:1006–1011.

Porter, R. J., Penry, J. K., and Wolf, A. A. Jr. (1976): Simultaneous documentation of clinical and electroencephalographic manifestations of epileptic seizures. In: *Quantitative Analytic Studies in Epilepsy*, edited by P. Kellaway and I. Petersen, pp. 253–268. Raven Press, New York.

Ray, C. C. (1966): A new multipurpose human brain depth probe. *J. Neurosurg.*, 24:911–921.

Talairach, J., and Bancaud, J. (1974): Stereotaxic exploration and therapy in epilepsy. In: *Handbook of Clinical Neurology*, Vol. 15, edited by P. J. Vinken and G. W. Bruyn, pp. 758–782. North-Holland, Amsterdam.

Walter, R. D. (1973): Tactical considerations leading to surgical treatment of limbic epilepsy. In: *Epilepsy: Its Phenomena in Man*, edited by M. A. B. Brazier, pp. 99–119. UCLA Forum in Medical Sciences, No. 17. Academic Press, New York.

Advances in Epileptology:
The Xth Epilepsy International Symposium,
edited by J. A. Wada and J. K. Penry.
Raven Press, New York © 1980.

Prolonged Seizure Monitoring with Stereotaxically Implanted Depth Electrodes in Patients with Bilateral Interictal Temporal Epileptic Foci: How Bilateral is Bitemporal Epilepsy?

P. Gloor, A. Olivier, and J. Ives

Montreal Neurological Institute, Department of Neurology and Neurosurgery,
McGill University, Montréal, Québec H3A 2B4 Canada

It is commonly assumed that temporal lobe seizures of nonneoplastic origin should only be treated neurosurgically if repeated EEG examinations disclose the presence of a unilateral or a strongly unilaterally predominant epileptogenic focus (Penfield and Flanigin, 1950; Bloom et al., 1959; Falconer and Serafetinides, 1963; Engel et al., 1975; Rasmussen, 1975; Van Buren et al., 1975).

Our recent experience in studying patients with bilateral temporal epileptogenic EEG foci by monitoring their spontaneously occurring seizures with stereotaxically implanted depth electrodes (Olivier et al., 1975) has shown that among these patients a majority can still be considered suitable candidates for a unilateral temporal lobectomy.

PATIENTS AND METHODS

This chapter deals with 18 patients with electrographic evidence of epileptogenic abnormality originating from both temporal lobes. The lateralizing evidence in repeated scalp and sphenoidal electrode EEGs of these patients was deemed insufficient for recommending surgical therapy because of the abundance of bilateral independent epileptiform abnormality showing no strong unilateral predominance. In all but one patient, at least one seizure was recorded before depth electrodes were inserted.

After a stereotaxic neuroradiological work-up, three strands of electrodes were implanted into each temporal lobe through a horizontal approach, each strand bearing 10 contacts 5 cm apart from each other. The deepest contacts of each strand were aimed at the limbic structures of the temporal lobe: the anterior at the amygdala, the intermediate at the anterior hippocampus, and the posterior strand at the parahippocampal gyrus and the body of the hippocampus. Contacts, 1, 2, and 3 were in limbic regions of the temporal lobe. The remainder of the contacts sampled activity from deep and superficial temporal neocortex. In some patients, additional depth electrodes were implanted into both frontal lobes.

The main purpose of the investigation was to record as many spontaneous seizures as possible. The patients' EEGs were monitored virtually around the clock for a period of 2 to 5 weeks. During the day, they were examined in the EEG laboratory under the direct observation of a technician. At night and over the weekends, the patients remained on the wards and their EEGs were automatically recorded by 16-channel cable telemetry (Ives et al., 1976), recently complemented by an automatic time-lapse video/audio monitoring system that, at the rate of 3.3 frames per sec, can work for 18 hrs unattended (Ives and Gloor, 1978). The automatic 16-channel cable telemetry system is designed to reduce the amount of redundant EEG data to a manageable minimum while not sacrificing any of the records of clinical seizures. This is achieved by always having the last 2 min of EEG stored on a computer disc from which it can be retrieved for permanent write-out on a 16-channel Mingograph EEG machine by pressing a pushbutton located at the patient's bedside. The button can be activated by any person witnessing a seizure (nurse, visitor, other patient) or by the patient himself. The 2-min delay on the computer disc insures that the whole seizure record, including that of the onset of the attack, is written out. The localizing information, provided by the records of repeated spontaneous seizures, provides evidence on which a decision to operate can be based.

Seizures are classified into three types: (a) clinical seizures that are socially disabling, with outward manifestations that would be obvious to a casual observer and thus would interfere with the patient's social life or cause him embarrassment; (b) clinical seizures that are not socially disabling, consisting of subjectively experienced auras or objective manifestations that are so slight that they might remain undetected by a casual observer as, e.g., change in skin color or pupillary dilatation; and (c) purely electrographic seizures with no clinical accompaniments.

At the end of the investigation, the results are tabulated and the degree of predilection of seizure onset to one side is established in quantitative terms.

RESULTS

In the 18 patients investigated in this study, a total of 555 clinical seizures were recorded, of which 142 were of the socially disabling kind and 413 of the socially nondisabling kind. In addition, more than 567 electrographic seizures were recorded. Thus, including the latter, more than 1,122 ictal events were documented. The mean number of clinical seizures per patient was 30.8 with a range from 4 to 115; the mean number of socially disabling seizures per patient was 7.8, with a range from 0 to 18.

TABLE 1. *Lateralization by depth-recorded clinical seizures*

Unilateral	7
Bilateral	11
With unilateral predominance > 90%	6
With unilateral predominance between 75 and 90%	3 (all > 80%)
With unilateral predominance between 60 and 75%	1 (64%)
No unilateral predominance	1 (50–50%)

Table 1 shows the main results regarding the lateralization of onset of the clinical seizures. In 7 patients all clinical seizures originated from one temporal lobe only. In the remaining 11 patients, some seizures arose from one, and others from the other temporal lobe. However, within this group of 11 patients, most seizures still arose from one and the same side: in 6, more than 90% of the clinical seizures originated from one lobe only, and, in an additional 3, between 80 and 90% of the clinical seizures originated from one side only. This leaves only 2 patients to be accounted for. One of them had a slight lateralizing predominance, with 64% of his clinical seizures originating from one lobe. The last patient was the only one in whom the number of clinical seizures of right and of left temporal lobe origin was equal. This patient had only 4 clinical seizures recorded. Thus, 16 of the 18 patients' clinical seizures arose from one side only or with a strong predilection for one side that exceeded 80%.

If one takes into account only the socially disabling seizures, 10 patients had evidence for unilateral onset, and seven for onset in one or the other temporal lobe, but with predilection for one side in 5, and without such predilection in two. In one patient no socially disabling seizures were recorded. Most of the socially nondisabling and electrographic seizures had the same preference for one side as the socially disabling attacks.

If one takes into account all ictal events, including the subclinical electrographic seizures, the number of cases with consistently unilateral onset of seizure discharge becomes small, amounting to only 2. However, in the additional 12 patients in whom clinical seizures showed a unilateral onset or a strong preference for one side, electrographic seizures predominated on the opposite side in only 2 individuals.

We also compared the lateralizing predominance obtained in EEGs before depth electrode implantation with that obtained through the recording of clinical seizures during depth electrode recordings. This comparison is of interest even though we are dealing with a highly selected group of patients, for intense monitoring with stereotaxically implanted electrodes was carried out precisely because the preimplantation EEGs were unable to show clear evidence for a lateralizing predominance of the epileptogenic process. Nevertheless, the interictal epileptiform abnormality in preimplantation EEGs showed some measure of lateralizing predominance in 16 of the 18 patients. In 2 patients only, no such predominance at all could be detected in preimplantation EEG records. In 12 of the 16 patients with some lateralizing predominance to one temporal lobe in preimplantation interictal EEGs, the same lobe was the exclusive or the prevailing side of onset in the seizures recorded with depth electrodes. In three patients only, the lateralization obtained through the recording of clinical seizures with depth electrodes was at variance with the side of predominance of the preimplantation interictal epileptiform EEG abnormalities. This represents 16.6% of our population. In 1 patient in whom there was a slight right-sided predominance of the preimplantation interictal EEG abnormality, the lateralization problem could not be resolved with depth electrode recordings of seizures. In 2 patients in whom the preimplantation interictal EEG abnormality showed no lateralizing predominance, the ictal recordings with depth electrodes resolved the lateralization problem in favor of one side.

The preimplantation lateralization through ictal recordings was also compared with that obtained through the recording of seizures by depth electrodes. It is not surprising that the preimplantation ictal data were unreliable or ambiguous, since the patients would not have been included in this study if the preimplantation records had resolved the lateralization problem. In only 6 of these 18 patients the preimplantation ictal records were of sufficient clarity to tentatively lateralize the onset of the seizures. In 4 of these patients, this lateralization was in agreement with that obtained with depth electrode studies; in 2 it was in disagreement. In 11 patients, the preimplantation ictal records showed no lateralizing features, or the lateralizing signs were ambiguous. In 1 patient, no seizure was recorded before depth electrode implantation.

DISCUSSION

To our surprise, the overwhelming majority of our patients showed either a consistently lateralized onset of their clinical seizures or at least a predilection for onset on one side that exceeded 80%. This strong preference for onset on one side was highly unexpected, since intensive monitoring with depth electrode recordings had been instituted precisely because the degree of bilaterality of temporal epileptiform abnormality in scalp and sphenoidal EEGs was sufficiently pronounced to suspect that seizures, at least in some patients may with equal likelihood originate at one time from one and at another from the other temporal lobe. Yet in only one patient were the number of seizures arising from one and from the other side the same. This suggests that in most patients with EEG evidence for bilateral temporal epileptogenic brain disease, a thorough search for a unilateral or unilaterally predominant focal process that could justify surgical therapy is still worthwhile. For most of these patients, this is the last remaining hope for relief from their seizures. That this hope appears justified is suggested by our preliminary follow-up results. We have operated on 15 of these 18 patients. In three patients surgical therapy was not performed for reasons that varied from case to case. One was the patient in whom no lateralizing predominance could be established on the basis of depth-recorded seizures. The second patient who was not operated upon showed a strong left-sided prevalence of seizure onset in ictal depth electrode recordings, but there were also features that suggested that the problem was more diffuse and that other lobes may also be involved. In the third patient, all seizures originated on the right side, but unfortunately he developed acute lymphoma to which he succumbed. In all other patients, a unilateral temporal lobectomy was performed. In 1 patient, the follow-up results are not available; in another the operation is too recent to allow for a reliable assessment of the surgical result. In the remaining 13 patients with follow-up periods exceeding 2 years, 46% have become seizure-free or have no more than one or two seizures per year, and 54% significantly improved (at least 50% fewer seizures than preoperatively). Social rehabilitation has been good or satisfactory in all except two patients.

The data obtained with depth electrode recordings suggest that as one progresses from socially disabling to socially nondisabling, and finally to purely electrographic seizures, the degree of unilaterality of seizure onset decreases. This suggests that the seizures representing the patient's major and often only problem, namely the socially disabling seizures, tend to have a more consistently lateralized onset than minor seizures or those that are purely electrographic.

A final point of interest is the relationship of the lateralization as established by the recorded seizures through depth electrodes with that of interictal epileptiform abnormality recorded in scalp and sphenoidal EEGS before electrodes were implanted. Even though this group of patients was highly selected and included only individuals in whom, on the basis of scalp and EEG records, a clear lateralizing diagnosis could not be made, it was found, that in most of them the seizures recorded with depth electrodes originated exclusively or with a strong predilection from that lobe in which the interictal epileptiform abnormality had predominated in EEGs taken prior to depth electrode implantation. Thus when repeated scalp and sphenoidal electrode recordings disclose a clear lateralization of the temporal epileptiform abnormality, it appears unlikely that the need to resort to the time consuming and very labor-intensive method of exploration by stereotaxically implanted depth electrodes should arise very often. It still remains true, however, that in 16.6% of this highly selected bilateral group, surgery would have been carried out on the wrong side had the decision been based on preimplantation EEG data.

REFERENCES

Bloom, D., Jasper, H., and Rasmussen, T. (1959/60): Surgical therapy in patients with temporal lobe seizures and bilateral EEG abnormality. *Epilepsia*, 1:351–365.

Engel, J., Driver, M. V., and Falconer, M. A. (1975): Electrophysiological correlates of pathology and surgical results in temporal lobe epilepsy. *Brain*, 98:129–156.

Falconer, M. A., and Serafetinides, E. A. (1963): A follow-up study of surgery in temporal lobe epilepsy. *J. Neurol. Neurosurg. Psychiatry*, 26:154–165.

Ives, J. R., and Gloor, P. (1978): A long term time-lapse video system to document the patient's spontaneous seizure synchronized with the EEG. *Electroencephalogr. Clin. Neurophysiol.*, 45:412–416.

Ives, J. R., Thompson, C. J., and Gloor, P. (1976): Seizure monitoring: a new tool in electroencephalography. *Electroencephalogr. Clin. Neurophysiol.*, 41:422–427.

Olivier, A., Gloor, P., Ives, J., Thompson, C., and Andermann, F. (1975): Chronic multiple depth electrodes in "bitemporal epilepsy." A clinical appraisal in 10 patients. *Can. J. Neurol. Sci.*, 2:339 (Abstr.).

Penfield, W., and Flanigin, H. (1950): Surgical therapy of temporal lobe seizures. *Arch. Neurol. Psychiatry*, 64:491–500.

Rasmussen, T. (1975): Surgical treatment of patients with complex partial seizures. In: *Advances in Neurology, Vol. 11: Complex Partial Seizures and Their Treatment*, edited by J. K. Penry and D. D. Daly, pp. 415–449. Raven Press, New York.

Van Buren, J. M., Ajmone Marsan, C., Mutsuga, N., and Sadowsky, D. (1975): Surgery of temporal lobe epilepsy. In: *Advances in Neurology, Vol. 8: Neurosurgical Management of the Epilepsies*, edited by D. P. Purpura et al., pp. 155–196. Raven Press, New York.

Advances in Epileptology:
The Xth Epilepsy International Symposium,
edited by J. A. Wada and J. K. Penry.
Raven Press, New York © 1980.

EEG Ambulatory Monitoring System with Visual Playback Display

*Gregory Stores, **Trevor Hennion, and R. J. Quy***

*Department of Psychiatry, Human Development Research Unit,
University of Oxford, and Park Hospital for Children, Oxford;
**Oxford Medical Systems, Abingdon, Oxford, England; and
***Institute of Neurology, Queen Square, London, England*

The National Centre for Children with Epilepsy in England is located at the Park Hospital for Children in Oxford. Referrals include children of all ages with a wide variety of problems, which are sometimes poor seizure control but often educational or other behavioral problems that may be related to their seizure disorder or its treatment. Electroencephalography, of course, is an important part of the basic investigation of these children but it is common experience that standard recording methods are of very limited value in certain clinical situations. This is particularly true where psychological or other environmental factors appear to precipitate seizures, or where episodes of altered behavior occur at home or at school that could be subtle, nonconvulsive seizures not reproducible in the standard EEG laboratory setting.

For many years ambulatory monitoring systems have been used to try to settle these diagnostic issues. Telemetry has been helpful to some extent but, in the United Kingdom, can be employed only over a limited transmission range and therefore requires hospital admission, precluding investigation in the home environment or at the child's own school. As an alternative, mini-cassette recording systems have been developed for ambulatory monitoring in recent years, notably by the groups working in the Montreal Neurological Institute (Ives, 1976) and the National Institute of Neurological and Communicative Disorders and Stroke (NINCDS) at Bethesda (Sato et al., 1976). The systems devised at both these centers have been characterized by their ability to record continuously for many hours (and even days), production of good quality EEGs recorded in various real-life situations, and high-speed playback of these long recordings for (mainly nonautomated) analysis.

However, certain modifications of these systems were needed for more effective use in centers where EEG technician time is not readily available for time-consuming analysis by hand of prolonged recordings. A joint development program, therefore, was established between the Park Hospital EEG

Department and Oxford Medical Systems Limited, who had extensive experience with the Medilog cassette recorder, for the clinical monitoring of various physiological parameters, especially ECG, for which they had developed an effective high-speed system of analysis. The display and analysis of the EEG results became a point of particular emphasis in this development program. The aim was to produce a means of rapidly scanning the prolonged EEG recordings, and assessing their content in an uncomplicated way that would easily be within the scope of an EEG technician, electroencephalographer, or clinician without any particular electronic or mathematical expertise, and without prolonged training. The system to be described meets requirements.

THE OXFORD SYSTEM

The total monitoring system consists of (a) an electrode set, (b) head-mounted EEG preamplifiers, (c) the Medilog four-channel 24-hr cassette recorder, and (d) a large-screen visual display system (the PMD 12) shown in Fig. 1.

Standard silver/silver chloride disc electrodes are used, attached with collodion glue. Electrode jelly is applied in the conventional way. The electrodes are attached by short leads to special head-mounted miniature preamplifiers (HDX-82), which greatly reduce artifact, especially from leads and mains (Quy, 1978).

The EEG is recorded onto a standard C-120 cassette tape by means of an Oxford Medilog 4–24 miniature tape recorder connected to the preamplifiers by concealed leads and worn on a belt. An event marker button, for use by an observer or the patient, is connected separately to the recorder. The electrodes, leads, and recorder can be worn unobtrusively with minimal chance of detection. This is an important feature to ensure that the child can take part in normal activities without appearing unusual.

The playback unit (the PMD 12) consists of (a) a high-speed replay deck and (b) a 12-inch visual display. Four channels are recorded. So far, the system has been used only for children known or thought likely to have a generalized form of seizure disorder. Three channels have been used for EEG (with bipolar recordings taken from approximately C4 to T6, C3 to T5, and P4 to P3) and the fourth channel has been used to mark clinical events under consideration as possible seizures.

By connecting the recorder (through a suitable coupling unit) to a conventional EEG machine, a paper trace can be obtained of the EEG signal being recorded on tape. This is used to check at the outset of the recording that the system is functioning correctly and to make any necessary adjustments.

The four channels of recorded data are shown on the visual display screen in eight second "pages" that are continually updated at a playback speed of

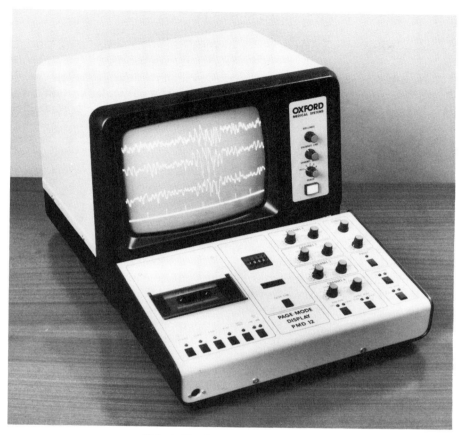

FIG. 1. The PMD 12 playback unit.

either 20 or 40 times the recording speed. The operator can compress the trace to show a 16-sec page. The uncompressed trace is very similar to a standard EEG record. The visual display also contains a calibration line that can be adjusted to appear next to any of the four channels displayed in order to measure its amplitude and frequency.

When a clinical event has been marked and the accompanying part of the tape is replayed, the event is signalled as an audible bleep and a light flashes on the replay deck. Alternatively, the replay can be made to stop automatically at the marked event.

While the tape is being replayed, the amplified EEG signal from one selected channel may be fed to a small loudspeaker on the replay deck, producing an audible tone. Seizure discharge can then be detected as a clearly defined change in the audible signal.

A control button may be used to stop the tape at any point. The visual display then holds the previous page of information in static form to allow close inspection of that part of the record. Pages can be turned back one at a time by means of another simple control on the replay deck.

The deck also contains a 24-hr clock. Providing the time at the start of the recording is noted, this clock can be used to locate a particular section of the tape in time for comparison of its contents with clinical or environmental events.

Finally, by connecting the replay deck through the headbox to the conventional EEG machine (in this case an Elema Schonander Mingograph) a paper copy of that part of the tape recording currently displayed can be obtained.

USES OF THE SYSTEM

Initial experience of the system has been in clinical circumstances similar to those described by Ives and colleagues in Montreal and the NINCDS group in Bethesda. These have included investigation of "attacks" or episodes of altered behavior in which the clinical features have made their epileptic nature certain. Teachers have used the event marker to identify such episodes in the hospital school. The appropriate section of the tape has then been located by various means, and that part of the tape examined at a slower replay speed in order to establish whether seizure activity has occurred in association with the clinical event. This procedure has been used successfully to identify the presence of particularly subtle absence seizures in a patient whose more obvious absences have been suppressed by drugs. Alternatively, more prolonged periods of behavioral change have been studied, using the replay deck's clock to locate the appropriate section of a 24-hr recording. This has revealed, in some instances, previously unsuspected episodes of minor epileptic status.

ADVANTAGES OF THE SYSTEM

In common with other miniature recording systems used for ambulatory EEG monitoring, the Oxford System offers the considerable advantage of allowing prolonged recordings to be made in real-life situations where the clinical problems in question occur. This is only possible, however, if the system is unobtrusive and does not mark out the wearer as unusual. The Oxford System requires no head or chest harness or any other real encumbrance and can be worn with minimal chance of detection by other children or adults. It is relatively lightweight (approximately 500 g) and robust and, therefore, suitable for quite small children whose natural exuberance need not be curbed during the recording period. At night, belt and recorder are easily removed and the system placed at the bedside. The system has been used for up to 24 hr continuous recording.

Apart from these practical aspects, the system offers certain technical advantages. The HDX-82 headmounted miniature preamplifiers reduce artifact significantly. A prerecording check on the integrity of the recording system is possible by means of a paper writeout. The calibration line on the visual display readily measures the amplitude and frequency of the waveforms. At the higher replay speed, a 24-hr tape can be scanned in 36 min; particular sections of the tape are scanned more carefully at 20 times the recording speed. The occurrence of clinical events can be marked on the tape and the detection of these events on replay is aided by the combined auditory and visual signal. In addition, the tape replay can be stopped automatically at the marked event. The 24-hr clock provides an additional means of relating clinical and electrographic events that take place during the recording. Seizure activity itself can also be detected by an auditory signal.

Good quality recordings have been consistently achieved that correspond closely to those obtained by conventional means. In particular, there has been very little distortion of wave morphology and signal dropouts are not seen. The large-screen visual display allows the whole record to be scanned in detail in a clinically familiar form equivalent to conventional EEG tracings, and with a minimum of expertise needed on the part of technician or clinician.

LIMITATIONS

As a four-channel system, its use is probably confined to electrographically generalized seizure disorders. Focal discharges could be missed with the limited electrode placement used. So far, no automated means of quantifying the EEG recordings have been used, although the playback lends itself to computer (or analog data reduction) techniques. This is a particularly important aspect to pursue, in order to use the Oxford System to investigate objectively and in detail the occurrence of subtle nonconvulsive seizures in relation to environmental circumstances and different treatment programs.

REFERENCES

Ives, J. R. (1976): Electroencephalogram monitoring of ambulatory epileptic patients. *Postgrad. Med. J. (Suppl. 7)*, 52:86–91.

Quy, R. J. (1978): A miniature preamplifier for ambulatory monitoring of the E.E.G. *J. Physiol. (Lond.)*, 284:23P–24P.

Sato, S., Penry, J. K., and Dreifuss, F. E. (1976): Electroencephalographic monitoring of generalised spike-wave paroxysms in the hospital and at home. In: *Quantitative Analytic Studies in Epilepsy*, edited by P. Kellaway and I. Petersén, pp. 237–251. Raven Press, New York.

Advances in Epileptology:
The Xth Epilepsy International Symposium,
edited by J. A. Wada and J. K. Penry.
Raven Press, New York © 1980.

The Advantage of Using Videotape Recording of Partial Complex Seizures

P. E. Hammerberg

Neurophysiological Department, Copenhagen County Hospital, Glostrup, Denmark

As a videotape recording is the basis for this chapter, I shall have to start with a description of the content of the videotape recording of two cases.

Case 1. A 30-year-old woman was lying in a bed. The seizure started with her pulling her left leg upward, bending her knee. There were a few slow clonic movements with an adduction of her left leg and then slow waving movements of her left arm. After a couple of minutes, her left arm was moving in more clonic jerks as she screamed, "My hand, oh my hand!" Then the seizure was over. It lasted about 4 min and she was able to talk coherently with the EEG technicians during the seizure.

Clinical comment. This patient had been of good health until 7 months earlier, when she was found—by her 5-year-old child—lying on the ground.

She was unconscious, moving arms and legs. Her husband arrived and found that she was confused, screaming, and crying for her mother and had saliva around her mouth. The observed part of the seizure—including the confusion period—lasted 30 min. Afterward she had no memory of the seizure or any possible aura.

One month later she was found on the beach unconscious with her head in the water, moving her arms and legs as if she were swimming. Otherwise the seizure was like the first one observed.

Subsequently, she started having seizures with a focal onset and with increasing frequency. She did not lose consciousness and could remember all or most of the seizures. They usually started with a peculiar feeling in her left leg followed by clonic movements of her left leg and left arm, sometimes accompanied by a blank look or a sense of unreality or a sudden fear or a feeling of heat inside her head.

Several investigations including EEG, scintigraphic studies of the brain, and a right-sided carotid angiography gave no evidence of any focal abnormality.

At the local hospital, she was regarded as a mental case and was sent to a day hospital for mental diseases.

The videotape recording compared with seizures observed during her stay at our hospital, all of the same type as recorded, convinced us of the focal pathological brain lesion, which was confirmed by a Todd paralysis of her left arm in one postictal phase and later by the neurosurgeons who extirpated a glioma at the top of her right motor area or just in front of it.

She recovered after the operation but she still had many seizures in spite of an antiepileptic treatment with phenobarbital and diphenylhydantoin.

Case 2. An 8-year-old boy was lying in a bed. He said in a frightened voice, "Now it comes." He pulled his right foot up and moved his right hand behind his head or rather tried to do so—but his father stopped his hand so as not to ruin the EEG recording. He had slight clonic movements of the facial muscles and whimpered a little.

The seizure lasted about 1 min and another seizure was shown to demonstrate that the movement of his right arm was a voluntary movement that he had learned might stop the seizure when he pressed his hand against the back of his neck. He was conscious during the seizures, scared, and made faces during tape recording.

Clinical comment. Two and a half years ago, the patient had encephalitis, which was verified by a biopsy from the brain. Two months ago, he started having the seizures for which he is currently under observation.

The seizures started with a tingling or painful sensation in his right foot ascending within seconds to his face, where clonic movements were seen either on both sides or only on his right side. He never complained of pain in his hand or arm. He felt fear but most likely it was only fear of the seizure. At the time of recording, he had several seizures a day.

All investigations were compatible with sequelae of the encephalitis.

Treatment with tegretol (carbamazepine) has had a very good effect; the patient experienced no seizures for several months.

METHOD

EEG recording was done on an 8-channel Elema Schønander electroencephalograph and mingograph writer: in Case 1 with needle electrodes and in case 2 with plate-shaped skin-scalp electrodes placed according to the 10–20 system. Through a Disa/Kaiser Telemeter system the EEG signals from 8 channels were transmitted and recorded in the sound track of a Disa Videograph system.

DISCUSSION

In both cases, the partial seizures shown on the videotape recording had a local onset and elementary symptomatology as defined by Rasmussen (1973).

Although the movements of the woman's arm (Case 1) were complicated, they had to be regarded as elementary.

The woman (Case 1) had in her earliest reported seizures some symptoms with impairment of consciousness and in later seizures a sudden sense of fear and/or unreality that may be features of "complex symptomatology" as defined by Feindel (1973).

As both cases are recorded as routine investigations, no sphenoidal or pharyngeal electrodes have been used.

At casual observation, the boy (Case 2) had seizures with the same components as the woman in Case 1, but the tape recordings demonstrated that the boy's movements of his arm were voluntary and appeared in different sequences of the seizures. The fear he demonstrated seemed to be a "normal" fear of the seizure and not a symptom in itself to be considered a part of the seizure.

The advantage of the videotape recording is apparent in the possibility of comparing several seizures in the same patient and also providing an opportunity for a better analysis of the single features of a seizure than could be obtained from the usual clinical observation, where one may even be dependent on second-hand information.

In Case 1, the movements of the woman's left arm started as waving complicated movements at times appearing almost as voluntary movements but at the end of the tape recording the clonic character of the movements was revealed, giving evidence of the focal brain lesion.

The technical possibilities might be improved by using two cameras simultaneously to enable one to see details such as eye movements or small facial myoclonic movements and prolonged videotape recordings such as those used by Escueta et al. (1977) in complex partial seizures will be of greater assistance in the diagnosis of epileptic seizures.

REFERENCES

Escueta, A., Kunze, U., Waddell, G., Boxley, J., and Nadel, A. (1977): Lapse of consciousness and automatisms in temporal lobe epilepsy: a videotape analysis. *Neurology (Minneap.)*, 27:144–155.

Feindel, W. (1973): Temporal lobe seizures. In: *The Epilepsies, Vol. 15: Handbook of Clinical Neurology*, edited by P. J. Vinken and G. W. Bruyn. North-Holland Publishing Company, Amsterdam.

Rasmussen, T. (1973): Seizures with local onset and elementary symptomatology. In: *The Epilepsies, Vol. 15: Handbook of Clinical Neurology*, edited by P. J. Vinken and G. W. Bruyn. North-Holland Publishing Company, Amsterdam.

Advances in Epileptology:
The Xth Epilepsy International Symposium,
edited by J. A. Wada and J. K. Penry.
Raven Press, New York © 1980.

Intensive Long-Term Monitoring in "Resistant" Epileptic Patients: Results of a Two-Year Study

*P. L. Morselli, **A. Baruzzi, *L. Bossi, †G. Avanzini,
†S. Franceschetti, ††R. Canger, and §F. Viani

*Laboratory of Clinical Pharmacology, Mario Negri Institute for Pharmacological Research, Milan; **Department of Neurology, University of Bologna Medical School, Bologna; †C. Besta Neurological Institute, Milan; ††University Center for the Treatment of Epilepsy, University of Milan Medical School, Milan; and §E. Corberi Children's Provincial Neuropsychiatric Hospital, Milan, Italy

The monitoring of plasma levels of antiepileptic drugs is at present, not only accepted as useful for the control of epilepsy but also considered as an essential requirement for a better and safer therapy (Morselli, 1973; Kutt and Penry, 1974; Penry, 1974; Gardner-Thorpe et al., 1977; Morselli and Baruzzi, 1978).

According to the available data, in situations where plasma levels were not monitored the efficacy of the treatment tended to be inversely related to the length of the follow-up period (Rodin, 1972): when plasma antiepileptic drug levels were monitored at regular intervals, positive results could be maintained over a prolonged period of time (Lund, 1974; Shorvon and Reynolds, 1977; Shorvon et al, 1977; Sherwin et al, 1973; Sherwin, 1977).

Most of the data supporting such evidence have been obtained in highly qualified and motivated environments. It is known, however, that a poor utilization of plasma level data by medical personnel not educated in drug disposition is not a rare event (Wilson and Wilkinson, 1974; Morselli, 1976). Furthermore, very few data are available on the significance of blood level monitoring in "difficult" epileptic patients (Porter et al., 1977; Viani et al., 1977).

On the basis of these considerations, the purpose of our study was to evaluate the significance (usefulness and limitations) of long-term monitoring of plasma antiepileptic drug concentrations in "difficult" epileptic patients in a situation very close to that encountered in everyday practice with neurologists having a very limited background in clinical pharmacology and drug disposition.

Dr. Morselli's present address is: Department of Clinical Research; Synthelabo, L.E.R.S., 58 rue de la Glacière; 75013 Paris, France

The main objectives of our study were the evaluation of the real impact of antiepileptic drug plasma levels therapeutic monitoring over a prolonged period of time in difficult epileptic patients on *drug efficacy, drug toxicity, patient's compliance,* and *physicians' prescribing habits* as well as on the *physicians' attitude toward the patients* and the *clinical pharmacologist.*

METHODS

Research Group

The initial research group consisted of three clinical pharmacologists and one chemist affiliated with the Mario Negri Institute for Pharmacological Research and one social worker and 11 neurologists affiliated with five different clinical centers. Three neurologists left the group after 3 months whereas the remaining eight continued the study up to 24 months. Contact between the physicians and the laboratory was maintained on a weekly or biweekly basis and group meetings were held once a month.

Patients

The data reported here refer to 42 patients followed for a period of at least 24 months. Two other patients underwent neurosurgery after 12 months. In 14 patients, the monitoring was continued for an additional 18 months up to a total of 42 months. Thirty-one patients were followed as outpatients, whereas the remaining 13 were hospitalized. When necessary, the ambulatory outpatients were hospitalized for periods ranging from 10 to 20 days. All the patients were known to the attending physicians for at least 1 year. Their ages ranged from 5 to 51 years (mean 16.4 ± 5.2) and there were 12 females and 32 males.

From a nosological as well as a therapeutical point of view the population was quite heterogeneous. It included 27 patients with generalized seizures (12 with atypical absences plus tonic and/or atonic seizures; five had clonic, tonic, and tonic-clonic or atonic seizures associated with complex absences; five had complex absences; two had tonic-clonic seizures plus simple absences; one had tonic-clonic seizures; one had clonic seizures; and one had simple absences). In addition, there were 15 patients with partial seizures (13 with complex symptomatology and two with elementary symptomatology). In 10 cases a secondary generalization was also present. Finally, two patients had unclassified seizures.

Operative Protocol

After an initial careful, complete physical and neurological examination the patients were monitored on a monthly basis, more frequently if necessary, as in cases of changes in therapy and control of patient compliance. Standardized forms were used for data collection. Each patient was instructed to report the frequency of the crises in a notebook. Crises were characterized by frequency and description whenever possible. During periodic controls the following examinations were performed routinely: (a) neurological examination, (b) EEG (12 leads) (at 3.00 p.m.), (c) hemotological tests, (d) performance (Gibson-Spiral and Card sorting) and psychological tests (HRS) (at 10.00 a.m.), (e) antiepileptic drug plasma levels (at 8.00 a.m. and 1.00 p.m.). On each occasion the presence of drug toxicity was evaluated by both objective neurological examination and by the spontaneous report from the patient. Clinical chemistry tests were run every 5 to 6 months unless otherwise required.

Results of antiepileptic drug plasma levels measurements were made available to the attending physicians within 24 to 72 hr together with pertinent comments, and occasionally in special cases an answer was obtained during the same day. In cases where hospitalization was made necessary, drug plasma levels were monitored daily. All drugs were measured by GLC procedures as previously indicated (Milano Collaborative Group, 1977).

Group meetings were held once a month for discussion of single cases as well as general problems.

RESULTS

Initial Assessment of the Clinical Situation

Forty-two patients included in the study were considered as "resistant" to pharmacological treatment and had a mean seizure frequency that ranged from 15 per month to several per day. Two other patients had no crisis for 6 months but suffered from severe side effects. The number of administered antiepileptic drugs to each patient ranged from one to four with a mean of 2.4 ± 0.9. Four patients were on monotherapy; 18 received two drugs; 15, three drugs; and seven, four drugs. Considering the antiepileptic drug plasma levels, 68% of the cases were within the "therapeutic range" with at least one drug but only 16% with two drugs, and none with three drugs. On the basis of plasma antiepileptic drug levels, 45% of the patients were overdosed with at least one drug and 11% were underdosed with all drugs.

Twenty patients (45%) presented disturbing side effects such as psychomotor impairment, intense drowsiness, dysarthria, ataxia, nystagmus, and gastric disturbances.

The drugs most often prescribed were phenobarbital (PB) and carbamazepine (CBZ). The most frequently (40–50%) overdosed compounds were PB and ethosuximide (ESM) whereas CBZ and phenytoin (PHT) were mostly underdosed (50–70% of the cases).

Clinical laboratory tests showed minor hematological alterations (hyper-

TABLE 1. *Effect of monitoring on drug prescribing and side effects*

	Initial	24 Months
Patients	44	42
Drug prescribed	109	91
Drug/patient	2.47	2.16
Percent patients within therapy range		
With one drug	68%	97%[b]
With two drugs	16%	86%[b]
With three drugs	0%	75%[b]
Patients overdosed	45%	7%[a]
Patients underdosed	11%	0%
Patients with side effects	45%	23%[a]

[a] $p < 0.05$.
[b] $p < 0.01$.

chromic anemia) in nine cases. Alkaline phosphatase was found elevated in 47% of the patients. A consistent reduction of IgA was observed in 13 cases, whereas skull and long bone X-rays revealed osteoporosis in four patients. These findings did not substantially change over the 24-month period.

Effects of Monitoring on Drug Prescription and Plasma Levels

As illustrated in Table 1, at the end of the 24-month period most of the patients had plasma antiepileptic drug concentrations within the "therapeutic range." Only 7% of the cases were overdosed with one drug and the mean number of prescribed drugs dropped from 2.4 to 2.1. It may be interesting to underline that changes in prescribing habit become evident only after 6 to 7 months of monitoring, being practically nonexistent for the first 5 months. The same is true for the antiepileptic drug plasma levels: Significant changes in the percentage of patients within the therapeutic range became apparent only after 5 to 6 months. Considering the drug prescribed, there was a reduction in the prescription of ESM, primidone, sodium valproate, PHT, and diazepam whereas prescriptions of PB, CBZ, and clonazepam increased.

Effects of Monitoring on Drug Toxicity and Seizure Frequency

The previously mentioned modifications in antiepileptic drug plasma levels had a clear and important effect on the incidence of side effects. As reported in Table 1, we could in fact observe a change from an initial situation where 45% of the patients suffered from severe drug toxicity to a final picture where only 23% of the cases presented less severe side effects.

More specifically, a remarkable reduction was observed for adverse reactions closely related to high antiepileptic drug plasma levels (drowsiness, psychomotor impairment, dysarthria, and ataxia) while no significant variations were present for side effects known to occur also at therapeutic antiepileptic drug levels (such as nystagmus) or not to be related to antiepileptic drug concentrations (such as hypertricosis and gingival hypertrophy) (Dam, 1977).

Again, we think it is worthwhile to stress the fact that a significant reduction in the incidence of drug toxicity phenomena was obtained only after 7 to 8 months of monitoring.

The results obtained on seizure frequency are reported in Fig. 1. A significant improvement was observed in 69% of the patients. In several instances, however, several months with antiepileptic drug plasma levels within the "therapeutic" ranges were required before any positive effect on seizure frequency could be seen.

At the end of the 24 months of monitoring, 14 patients (33% of the cases) were "free of crisis" for at least 2 months. The mean period "free of crisis" was 10.6 ± 7.8 months (range 2–24). Of these patients fully controlled, seven suffered from generalized seizures and six from partial seizures.

A reduction in seizure frequency greater than 50% was present in another 36% of the cases represented by nine patients suffering from generalized seizures [4 Lennox-Gastaut syndromes (LGS)] and six patients suffering from partial seizures.

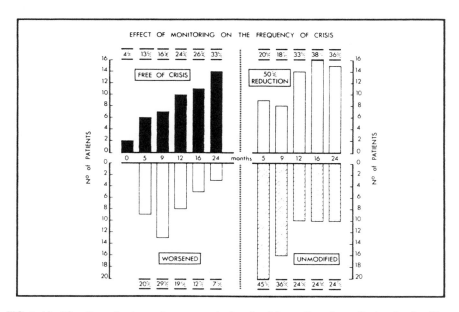

FIG. 1. Modification of seizure frequency during the 24 months of monitoring for the "free of crisis" group. The statistical significance ($p < 0.01$) was reached between the 10th and 12th months, whereas the "> 50% reduction" group's data reached the level of significance ($p < 0.01$) after 6 months.

Ten patients [six with generalized seizures (3LGS) and four with partial seizures] practically did not show any modification in their seizure frequency despite "correct" antiepileptic drug plasma levels. An evident, constant worsening was present in the three remaining cases [two generalized seizures (LGS) and one partial seizure].

The limited space available does not permit a more detailed description of the cases, but it may be worthwhile mentioning that, considering the group suffering from atypical absences with tonic-atonic seizures, in parallel with a reduction in PB plasma levels we could observe a remarkable improvement in vigilance and also a reduction in the incidence of episodes of status epilepticus (Viani et al., 1977).

In analyzing the groups "free of crisis," "> 50% improvement" and "unmodified or worsened," it was evident that they were similar with regard to age and years of disease. The only difference we could find was a trend toward a higher incidence of "brain insults" (meningitis and head trauma) in the "unmodified-worsened" group. In contrast, in nine patients in the "free of crisis" group, none of these factors could be found.

Considering the EEG data, the tracings persisted unmodified in about 50% of the cases and an improvement was present in 28%. Even if a certain relationship seemed to be present between clinical picture and EEG, a definite improvement was not always accompanied by a trend toward EEG normalization. The same holds true for the analysis of performance tests where a certain relationship could be observed between impairment of performance and antiepileptic drug plasma levels above the toxic range.

Behavior of the Group and Patients' Responses

In an analysis of the behavior of the monitoring group, four distinct phases could be observed.

(1) *A first, very brief (45–60 days) phase characterized by an enthusiastic participation:* The attitude of most of the participants was a very optimistic one mainly based on the wrong concept that antiepileptic drug plasma levels monitoring could be the "answer" to all the problems of the difficult patient.

(2) *A second phase of 4–5 months dominated by anxiety and hypercriticism:* Within 60 days the attitude described vanished and clear anxiety reactions emerged in eight neurologists and two clinical pharmacologists. The atmosphere at the meetings was very tense and there was also a more or less clear trend to reject some of the patients together with a hypercritical outlook toward the other colleagues. Laboratory data were mistrusted if not rejected and changes in therapeutic regimens continued to be done on the basis of "clinical impressions" (during this phase, three neurologists left the group).

(3) *A third, long-lasting phase (15–16 months) characterized by a positive collaborative behavior:* A common language started to develop, an-

tiepileptic drug plasma levels were considered as a useful tool, eventual "errors" were recognized, and the working atmosphere became excellent. During this phase the decision to set up laboratories for antiepileptic drug determination in the various clinical groups was also taken.

(4) *A fourth phase (lasting 2 months) where hypercritical and anxiety reactions again started to emerge, mainly with regard to worsened and unmodified patients:* The collaborative atmosphere tended to deteriorate with the appearance of individual initiatives.

If we analyze in parallel the patients' behavior, we can observe that in general most of them responded very favorably to the new situation and their demands and motivations increased considerably. Their compliance, however, improved only after 4 to 5 months of monitoring, as indicated by very stable levels between 6 and 14 to 15 months. In the final part of the study, however, their compliance tended again to deteriorate, as indicated by large fluctuations between morning and noon samples as well as between monthly samples. It may be interesting to underline that the variations in compliance parallel both the objective clinical improvement and the changes in physicians' behavior.

COMMENTS

The reported data illustrate the significance of an "integrated monitoring approach" for the epileptic patient considered either "difficult" or "resistant" to pharmacological treatment. Globally the monitoring led to: (a) a significant reduction in seizure frequency in 69% of the cases, (b) a significant reduction in occurrence of side effects and in their severity, (c) a reduction in the number of prescribed antiepileptic drugs, (d) an improved prescription concerning daily doses and dose schedules, (e) a better patient compliance, and (f) an improved patient-physician relationship.

If we consider, however, the time necessary to observe such modifications several interesting comments can be made. In general the major therapeutic difficulties were encountered with the LGS and partial seizures. Considering the antiepileptic drug plasma levels, significant improvements were attained only after 5 to 6 months, but if this was accompanied by an evident reduction in the severity of the adverse reactions, a significant improvement in seizure frequency became really evident only a few months later. Such an observation underlines on one side the "normal" retard in the utilization of pharmacokinetic data by the clinician and on the other the need of a close cooperation between the ward and the laboratory. Furthermore, it underlines also that a "therapeutic range" is not a magic threshold and its attainment does not necessarily mean "automatically" better response. In fact, in several cases "within the therapeutic range" quantitative and qualitative modification had to be performed before obtaining a positive response. These considerations also stress that among the possible causes of a poor therapeutic outcome the factor "physician" bears a remarkable role. The importance of the attitude of the attending physician is clearly stressed by the parallelism observed between the late acceptance of a collaborative dialogue and the improvement in drug toxicity and efficacy. On the other hand, the reported data demonstrate that a positive outcome is possible in a "naturalistic situation."

It may be also interesting to note that despite the very severe syndromes included in the study there was an evident trend toward a reduction in the number of administered drugs. At the end of the 2-year period, seven patients were on monotherapy and 22 on two drugs. On the other hand, any attempt at a further reduction in the number of drugs led every time to an evident deterioration of the clinical picture. This could suggest that in "severe," "old" epileptic patients, aiming at monotherapy may be not realistic.

The data obtained appear to persist. In fact, in 14 of the patients participating in the study, the follow-up has been continued for an additional 18 months with control every 2 to 5 months according to necessity. In this group, which included four patients free of crisis, five improved and six unmodified or worsened; the picture did not change concerning the unmodified and worsened cases whereas there was a trend to further reduction in crisis frequency in the "improved" group.

In conclusion, we can say that an integrated monitoring approach, such as the one we followed, seems to be valuable for the "difficult" epileptic patient also. The knowledge of antiepileptic drug plasma levels has without doubt a noticeable impact on both therapeutic decision and therapeutic efficacy even in a "naturalistic situation" provided that an adequate dialogue is established between the attending neurologist, the patient, and the clinical pharmacologist. Such a dialogue, leading to an improved knowledge of the need of each individual patient which will permit a better individualized therapy, should become an integral part of the therapeutic intervention.

ACKNOWLEDGMENTS

We wish to thank our colleagues in the Laboratory of Clinical Pharmacology of Mario Negri Institute (M. Gerna, B. Bordo and E. Soffientini) for their excellent technical help and Miss G. Pignatelli and F. Buschi, R. De Castro, C. Pruneri, S. Smirne, and P. Zagnoni for their very valuable cooperation.

A preliminary report of this study was presented at the Third WODADIBOF held in Exeter, 1976 and is reported in Gardner–Thorpe et al. (1977).

REFERENCES

Dam, M. (1977): Toxicity of antiepileptic drugs. In: *Advances in Epileptology*, edited by H. Meinardi and A. J. Rowan, pp. 330–339. Swets & Zeitlinger B. V., Amsterdam/Lisse.

Gardner-Thorpe, C., Janz, D., Meinardi, H., and Pippenger, C. E. (1977): *Antiepileptic Drug Monitoring*. Pitman Medical, Kent.

Kutt, H., and Penry, J. K. (1974): Usefulness of blood levels of antiepileptic drugs. *Arch. Neurol.*, 31:283–288.

Lund, L. (1974): Anticonvulsant effect of diphenylhydantoin relative to plasma levels. *Arch. Neurol.*, 31:289–294.

Milano Collaborative Group for Studies on Epilepsy (1977): Long-term intensive monitoring in the difficult patient. Preliminary results of 16 months of observation. Usefulness and Limitations. In: *Antiepileptic Drug Monitoring*, edited by C. Gardner-Thorpe, D. Janz, H. Meinardi, and C. E. Pippenger, pp. 197–212. Pitman Medical, Kent.

Morselli, P. L. (1973): Significato ed importanza della misura del controllo della concentrazioni plasmatiche dei farmaci uella terapia dell'epilessia. *Prospet. Pediatr.*, 12:523–538.

Morselli, P. L. (1976): Il monitoraggio dei livelli dei farmaci antiepilettici. Considerazioni critiche sulla situazione attuale. In: *La Epilessie*, edited by E. Lugaresi, P. Parraglia, and R. Canger, pp. 169–180. Aulo Gaggi Publ., Bologna.

Morselli, P. L., and Baruzzi, A. (1978): Serum levels and pharmacokinetics of anticonvulsants in the management of seizure disorders. In: *Pediatric Clinical Pharmacology and Therapeutics*, edited by B. Mirkin, pp. 89–106. Year Book Medical Publisher, Chicago.

Penry, J. K. (1974): The usefulness of serum antiepileptic drug levels in the treatment of epilepsy. In: *Drug Interactions*, edited by P. L. Morselli, S. Garattini, and S. M. Cohen, pp. 299–308. Raven Press, New York.

Porter, R. J., Penry, J. K., and Lacy, J. R. (1977): Diagnostic and therapeutic revaluation of patients with intractable epilepsy. *Neurology (Minneap.)*, 27:1006–1011.

Rodin, E. A. (1972): Medical and social prognosis in epilepsy. *Epilepsia*, 13:121–131.

Sherwin, A. L., Robb, J. P., and Lechter, M. (1973): Improved control of epilepsy by monitoring plasma ethosuximide. *Arch. Neurol.*, 28:178–181.

Sherwin, A. L. (1977): Pharmacological principles in the management of patients with epilepsy. In: *Advances in Epileptology*, edited by H. Meinardi and A. J. Rowan, pp. 211–219. Swets & Zeitlinger B. V., Amsterdam/Lisse.

Shorvon, S. D., and Reynolds, E. N. (1977): Unnecessary polypharmacy for epilepsy. *Br. Med. J*, 1:1635–1637.

Shorvon, S. D., Chadwick, D., Galbraith, A. H., and Reynolds, E. H. (1977): One drug in the treatment of epilepsy. In: *Advances in Epileptology*, edited by H. Meinardi and A. J. Rowan, pp. 300–304. Swets & Zeitlinger B. V., Amsterdam/Lisse.

Viani, F., Avanzini, G., Baruzzi, A., Bordo, B., Bossi, L., et al. (1977): Long-term monitoring of antiepileptic drugs in patients with the Lennox Gastaut Syndrome. In: *Epilepsy*, edited by J. K. Penry, pp. 131–138. Raven Press, New York.

Wilson, J. T., and Wilkinson, G. R. (1974): Delivery of anticonvulsant drug therapy in epileptic patients assessed by plasma level analysis. *Neurology (Minneap.)* 24:614–623.

Advances in Epileptology:
The Xth Epilepsy International Symposium,
edited by J. A. Wada and J. K. Penry.
Raven Press, New York © 1980.

Sodium Valproate, Correlation Between Serum Level and Clinical Effect: A Controlled Study

*Lennart Gram, **Helga Flachs, **Annelise Würtz-Jørgensen,
and *Josef Parnas

*Epilepsy Department and **Laboratory, The Filadelfia Colony,
Dianalund, Denmark*

The antiepileptic effect of sodium valproate (VPA) has been established in several controlled trials (Meinardi, 1971; Suzuki et al., 1972; Richens and Ahmad, 1975; Gram et al., 1977; Vasella et al., 1978).

Serum levels of the drug have been reported in a number of studies, but only few and uncontrolled data concerning correlation between serum level and clinical efficacy have been published.

Accordingly we performed a controlled study in which patients were randomized to different preestablished serum levels of VPA.

PATIENTS AND METHODS

The design of the trial was double-blind with an open therapeutic control with multiple crossovers in randomized blocks.

Patients with clinical effect from VPA, but who in spite of continued treatment with the drug still suffered from at least two seizures per month, were considered for admission. Patients entered the trial regardless of seizure type, sex, and age, but the seizure type(s) of the individual patient was classified according to the International Classification of Epileptic Seizures (Gastaut, 1970). Thirteen inpatients, eight males and five females, entered the trial. The age ranged from 15 to 67 years, median 28 years. Informed consent was obtained from all patients or their legal guardian.

All patients were in concomitant antiepileptic treatment. For all administered antiepileptic drugs, i.e., diphenylhydantoin, phenobarbital, carbamazepine, clonazepam, primidone, sulthiame, ethosuximide, acetazolamide, and dimethadione, serum levels were kept constant by dose adjustments throughout the trial. Other drugs were administered in fixed doses during the trial.

Seizure frequency and possible side effects in each patient were recorded on three different serum levels of VPA. The applied VPA levels were: A level, 110 to 140 μmoles/liter; B level, 206 to 244 μmoles/liter; and C level, 300 to 350 μmoles/liter.

The observation periods were 8 weeks on each level with intermittent crossover periods of varying duration. Patients entered the observation period the first time the serum level was within the interval.

Throughout the trial blood samples were drawn *at least* once a week. Blood sampling was always done before the morning dose.

VPA was administered as Deprakine® 100 mg and 300 mg tablets together with placebo tablets. Each patient received the same total number of tablets throughout the trial.

Patients were excluded during the trial if an unwarranted aggravation of seizures or side effects occurred and the condition could not be improved by a premature crossover. Two patients were excluded. One patient died, an event bearing no relationship to the study. One patient was excluded because of somnolence already on the lowest VPA level, which he had tolerated well at an earlier stage.

RESULTS

Eleven patients completed the trial. No significant period or carryover effect as to seizure frequency or serum levels was observed ($p > 0.10$, nonparametric analysis of variance).

Table 1 shows the main results of the trial. The difference between number of seizures on the three VPA levels was statistically significant ($p < 0.005$, Friedman test). No significant differences between proposed and achieved serum levels were demonstrated ($p > 0.10$, Sign test). All patients had a few serum concentrations outside the stipulated intervals. The difference between the number of these at the three levels was not significant ($p > 0.10$, Friedman test). The relationship between dose and obtained serum concentrations was found to be curvilinear. Ratio between dose and serum level showed a significant increase with increasing serum concentration ($p < 0.01$, Friedman test). No significant differences in serum levels or doses of diphenylhydantoin, phenobarbital, and carbamazepine during the three periods were found ($p > 0.10$, Friedman test).

The number of patients in concomitant treatment with other antiepileptic

TABLE 1. *Sodium valproate: relationship between dose, serum level, and number of seizures*

Period	Serum level (μmoles/liter)		Dose (mg/day)		Number of seizures		
	Median	Range	Median	Range	Total	Median	Range
A	128	113–149	700	300–800	482	24	0–218
B	230	200–238	1,400	950–2,400	345	35	3–141
C	312	271–344	3,050	2,000–4,000	151	6	0–46

drugs was too small to allow statistical evaluation of data. Except for trimethadione and dimethadione no systematic or consistent change could be seen.

Increasing serum levels of VPA seems to inhibit the demethylation of trimethadione to dimethadione, causing a decrease in the serum concentration of dimethadione and an increase in trimethadione serum concentration.

Except for patients with absences the number of patients with a single seizure type was too limited to permit statistical evaluation of correlation between seizure type, clinical effect, and serum concentration. For the absences the result was consistent with the main result.

Eight patients experienced side effects during the trial. Anorexia, hypersalivation, and drowsiness occurred without obvious dependence of VPA serum concentration. Vomiting, diarrhea, and vertigo occurred most frequently at the C level.

DISCUSSION

Controlled clinical trials are the only scientifically valid comparisons between different treatment. In our opinion the comparison between clinical effect of different serum levels of a certain drug corresponds methodologically to a comparison between different drugs and therefore requires a similar scientific approach.

In the majority of studies on the relationship between serum levels and clinical response, patients have not been randomized to specified levels. As a consequence, the observed levels may be influenced by factors that simultaneously influence response.

Our study shows an evident correlation between serum levels of VPA and reduction of seizures. Increasing serum levels reduce seizure frequency.

The only conclusion that can be drawn from this study is that a serum level of 300 to 350 μmoles/liter has a superior clinical effect compared with that of lower serum concentrations. It is still an open question whether serum levels above 350 μmoles/liter may render even better clinical results.

The application of *therapeutic serum levels* for antiepileptic drugs is complicated by the hypothesis advanced by Kutt and Penry (1974) that increasing serum concentrations are required to control an epileptic process of increasing severity. This hypothesis seems obvious, but has never been confirmed by controlled prospective studies.

All patients in our study suffer from severe epilepsies. Possibly patients with mild epilepsies can be controlled at a lower VPA serum level.

ACKNOWLEDGMENTS

Our statistical adviser was chief surgeon Bjørn Andersen, M.D.

Deprakine® was placed at our disposal by Orion OY, who also supported the study financially. We wish to express our gratitude.

REFERENCES

Gastaut, H. (1970): Clinical and electroencephalographical classification of epileptic seizures. *Epilepsia*, 11:102–113.

Gram, L., Wulff, K., Rasmussen, K. E., Flachs, H., Würtz–Jørgensen, A., Sommerbeck, K. W., and Løhren, V. (1977): Valproate sodium: A controlled clinical trial including monitoring of drug levels. *Epilepsia*, 18:141–148.

Kutt, H., and Penry, J. K. (1974): Usefulness of blood levels of antiepileptic drugs. *Arch. Neurol.*, 31:283–289.

Meinardi, H. (1971): Clinical trials of anti-epileptic drugs. *Psychiatr. Neurol. Neurochir.*, 74:141–151.

Richens, A., and Ahmad, S. (1975): Controlled trial of sodium valproate in severe epilepsy. *Br. Med. J.*, 4:255–256.

Suzuki, M., Maruyama, H., Ishibashi, Y., Ogawa, S., Seki, T., Hoshino, M., Maekawa, K., Yo. T., and Sato, Y. (1972): A double-blind comparative trial of sodium dipropylacetate and ethosuximide in epilepsy in children, with special emphasis on pure petit mal seizures. *Med. Progr. (Japan)*, 82:470–488.

Vasella, F., Rudeberg, A., da Silva, V., and Pavlincova, E. (1978): Double-blind study on the anti-convulsive effect of phenobarbital and valproate in the Lennox syndrome. *Schweiz Med. Wochenschr.*, 108:713–716.

Advances in Epileptology:
The Xth Epilepsy International Symposium,
edited by J. A. Wada and J. K. Penry.
Raven Press, New York © 1980.

Anticonvulsant Drugs and Cognitive Function

Michael Trimble and **John Corbett

*Department of Psychological Medicine, The National Hospitals for Nervous Diseases, Maida Vale and Queen Square, London; and **Department of Psychiatry, The Bethlem Royal and the Maudsley Hospitals, Denmark Hill, London, England*

Although it has been suspected for a long time that anticonvulsant drugs have an adverse effect on the mental state of epileptic patients, review of the literature reveals only few studies that have been carried out to assess the situation in an experimental way (Trimble and Reynolds, 1976). Many anecdotes are recorded, but it is often unclear exactly what aspect of the mental state is thought to be affected by drugs, and little attempt has been made to quantify the actual changes observed. Only a few of the drugs available for the management of epilepsy have been assessed, and most studies were carried out prior to the introduction of serum anticonvulsant estimations. It is nevertheless suggested that some drugs have more adverse effects on patients than others, and that changes in the mental state may be observed at serum levels of anticonvulsants regarded as "therapeutic" (Reynolds and Travers, 1974). In this study an attempt has been made to evaluate such effects more comprehensively, using as far as possible serum anticonvulsant estimations. In order to gather as complete information as possible it was decided to study residents at a hospital school for epileptic children. The effects of anticonvulsant drugs on cognitive abilities have been assessed separately from their possible effects on other aspects of behavior such as conduct disorder and depression. The results of the latter will be reported elsewhere (Trimble and Corbett, 1980). In view of the suggestion that folic acid abnormalities may be related to changes in the mental state in patients on anticonvulsant drugs (Reynolds, 1975), serum folic acid levels have also been assessed.

PATIENTS AND METHODS

Of 314 children resident at Lingfield Hospital School, 312 were examined. Information was gathered from case notes on their age, sex, seizure onset, seizure type, and drugs prescribed. An estimate of seizure frequency was obtained by examination of the number of seizures the children had in the month prior to the examination, and they were divided into three groups: those having more than ten seizures a month, those having one to nine seizures a month, and those having no seizures a month. A clinical neuro-psychiatric examination was performed to look for gross neurological abnormalities above the brainstem, and the presence of psychomotor slowing. The latter was assessed on a four-point scale depending on the clinical findings, and in the analysis of the results a score of 0 or 1 (i.e., absent or minimal) was regarded as negative and a score of 2 or 3 (i.e., moderate or severe abnormality) was regarded as positive. Prior to the examination a small sample of children was examined to assess the interobserver reliability of this measure, and it was found to be 79.5% between two observers.

Results of psychological testing were provided by the school psychologist. Not only was there an estimate of full-scale I.Q., but also where possible verbal and performance scales were documented. It was the intention of the study to examine children with cognitive deterioration, and therefore from those children who had received two or more estimates of their I.Q. while at the Hospital School, a group whose I.Q. had actually deteriorated were detected. The criteria for "I.Q. fall" were a drop of more than 10 points on two tests (WISC or equivalent) assessed more than 1 year apart. These data were provided "blind" and knowledge of the I.Q. status was not available during the clinical examination. Blood was taken for measurement of serum phenytoin, phenobarbitone, primidone, folic acid, and in some children, carbamazepine. Blood samples were taken as near as possible to the clinical examination, and were taken in the early morning in the fasting condition. A pilot study had indicated that blood levels of phenobarbitone, primidone, and phenytoin remained constant for those children who received the same dose of the drug over a period of 12 months.

Results

Of 312 children, 219 were males and 267 were older than 10 years of age. The drug most commonly prescribed was phenytoin (67.6%), followed by carbamazepine (42.3%) and sodium valproate (42.0%), then primidone (28.0%), sulthiame (18.3%), and phenobarbitone (15.1%). Other drugs that were prescribed to a smaller percentage of the children have not been assessed in this study. Of all the children, 10.5% had a gross neurological disorder above the brainstem, and psychomotor slowing was found in 19.2%. A fall in I.Q. was found in 15.2% of 204 children who had two or more I.Q. estimates. The mean I.Q. of the total population of children was 66.2 (± 18.8) and verbal and performance I.Q. estimates were available in 244 children. The means were 71.7 (± 15.6) and 73.6 (± 20.4), respectively. For those with a fall in I.Q. the majority had a fall that was greater than 15 points, and in some the fall was considerable (range, 10–48 points).

Table 1 shows the mean serum levels and the folate estimations of the anticonvulsant drugs that have been measured. Comparison is made between the mean levels of groups of children with abnormalities and the rest

TABLE 1. Mean serum levels (± SD) in μmoles/liter in children with and without neuropsychiatric abnormalities

	Slowing		Fall in I.Q.	
	Present	Absent	Present	Absent
Phenobarbitone	73.8 ± 35.0(23)	68.9 ± 40.1(100)	80.5 ± 40.9(13)	68.8 ± 38.3(97)
Phenytoin	33.6 ± 21.9(41)	30.3 ± 25.6(171)	39.2 ± 28.5(19)[a]	28.4 ± 22.2(166)
Primidone	25.9 ± 17.1(16)	19.9 ± 12.5(63)	23.4 ± 3.8(10)[a]	19.5 ± 13.8(63)
Carbamazepine	17.4 ± 9.6(15)	16.0 ± 6.4(38)	15.5 ± 2.6(3)	16.7 ± 7.6(48)
Serum folic acid	4.6 ± 5.8(59)	3.5 ± 3.3(235)	3.0 ± 1.3(29)[a]	3.9 ± 4.4(227)

[a] $p < 0.05$, present versus absent.
n Values indicated in parentheses.

of the population. Statistical analysis used was t-test between the means and p values of significance are given. Table 1 shows that children with a fall in I.Q. have significantly higher mean levels of phenytoin and primidone than the rest of the population, and a significantly lower serum folic acid level. Although mean levels of phenytoin and primidone are higher in the children with slowing this does not reach statistical significance.

Table 2 shows the number of children with a fall in I.Q. and slowing who have high levels of serum anticonvulsants compared with the number of children with the abnormality who have lower serum levels. It can be seen that there is a significantly higher incidence of fall in I.Q. in children with high levels of phenytoin and primidone as opposed to phenobarbitone and carbamazepine.

Pearson Correlation Coefficients were estimated for children with an I.Q. greater than 70 between the actual serum anticonvulsant levels measured and the I.Q. estimates. By omitting children with low I.Q. it was hoped to eliminate some of the difficulties of measurement of I.Q. at the lower end of the scale and to minimize effects of gross brain damage. These data indicated significant negative correlations between phenobarbitone and phenytoin and the performance I.Q. ($p < 0.05$) and a trend toward significance with primidone ($p < 0.1$). No relationship to the verbal scale of the I.Q. was noted.

In order to rule out some of the other factors such as seizure frequency and brain damage, which may be influencing these results, the mean serum levels of the anticonvulsants were reassessed in a group of patients who were having infrequent seizures, leaving from the analysis those having more than 10 seizures a month. These results again indicated significantly greater levels of phenytoin and lower levels of serum folate in the population with a fall in I.Q.

In addition, analysis revealed no significant differences in the distribution of age, sex, site of EEG abnormality, length of time of epilepsy, or neurological disorder above the brainstem between the children receiving the various drugs under study. No relationship was found between the seizure frequency and the fall in I.Q., although psychomotor slowing was related to seizure frequency, there being a significantly larger number of children with slowing in association with a greater number of seizures ($p < 0.05$). Although there was no statistical difference between the seizure frequency of the children receiving the various anticonvulsants it was noted that there were more children with greater than 10 seizures a month on sodium valproate.

DISCUSSION

These results suggest that anticonvulsant drugs are related to impairment of cognitive function in epileptic patients, and that some drugs are more involved in this process than others. It is acknowledged that the population

TABLE 2. Numbers and percentages of children on high and lower levels of anticonvulsants with abnormalities

	Slowing			Fall in I.Q.		
	Absent	Present	Percent	Absent	Present	Percent
Phenytoin <60 μmoles/liter	234	57	19.6	228	26	10.2
>60 μmoles/liter	16	3	15.8	11	5	31.2[a]
Primidone <20 μmoles/liter	207	46	18.1	199	21	9.5
>20 μmoles/liter	43	14	24.6	41	10	19.6[a]
Phenobarbitone <80 μmoles/liter	214	48	18.3	203	24	10.5
>80 μmoles/liter	36	12	25.0	37	7	15.9
Carbamazepine <24 μmoles/liter	6	2	25.0	8	0	0
>24 μmoles/liter	33	11	25.0	42	2	4.5

[a] $p < 0.05$
X^2 analysis.

under study is highly selective. Nevertheless, in order to collect such information it was necessary to define a population where abnormalities were likely to be frequent, and in any case it is often patients such as the ones we have studied who present with problems that are therapeutically the most difficult to manage. It is recognized that few of the children were on a single drug and it has not been possible to assess interactional effects that in themselves may be important. The interpretation of these results therefore depends to some extent on whether or not they find support from other studies.

The design of the study initially intended to separate out varieties of behavior that could be effected by the drugs, and thus changes in cognitive abilities have been assessed separately. Three possibly different aspects have been examined. First, a group of children has been identified whose intellectual abilities have actually deteriorated, in some cases markedly, while at a hospital school with special educational facilities. Second, correlation between actual I.Q. scores and anticonvulsant levels on a much larger number of children have been calculated in order to explore a possible direct relationship. Third, psychomotor slowing has been assessed. With regard to the actual deterioration of ability it is suggested that phenytoin and primidone are related to this process in that the mean levels of the drugs are higher in the populations with this abnormality than in the rest of the children, and that this difference is still noted when, for example, children with a large number of seizures are left out of the analysis. The mean values for the children with these abnormalities are well within the so-called therapeutic range for these drugs. In addition, patients with a deterioration are over-represented in the groups with high serum levels of these two drugs. There have been several studies in the literature supporting these results indicating, for example, that phenytoin may be associated with a subacute encephalopathy (Rosen, 1968; Logan and Freeman, 1969). Some authors suggest that such a clinical picture of deterioration may occur at serum levels regarded as therapeutic (Glaser, 1972; Reynolds and Travers, 1974). This is consistent with other information indicating that phenytoin may induce irreversible neuronal damage, for example, cerebellar damage (Reynolds, 1975), and that after intoxication experimentally electron microscopic changes equivalent to those seen in the lipoidoses are seen (del Cerro and Snider, 1967). Clearly not all patients on phenytoin develop such problems, but some, for reasons not yet established, do seem susceptible, and the possibility that a drug effect may be involved when there is decline in intellectual function must always be considered.

The situation with regard to primidone is much less clear as there are no other studies that have looked at this drug and, because it breaks down to phenobarbitone, there are problems with interpretation of results. Nevertheless the possibility that it too is implicated in a process similar to that suggested for phenytoin requires consideration. The two drugs least implicated in this process from these studies would appear to be phenobarbitone and carbamazepine. Again, this is in keeping with the literature which, for the former, is rather inconclusive regarding its effect on cognitive abilities, and for carbamazepine suggests psychotropic properties (Trimble, 1978).

The negative correlation between performance I.Q. scores and phenytoin, phenobarbitone, and primidone levels are again in accord with other reports that indicate a direct interference by anticonvulsant drugs on the abilities of patients to perform I.Q. tests, in particular those tests of spatio-temporal and motor competence (Trimble and Reynolds, 1976). This is particularly true with regard to phenytoin and phenobarbitone, although again results with primidone have not been replicated elsewhere. The lack of a relationship with carbamazepine on this measure is further support for the contention that this drug is less implicated in cognitive disabilities than some of the other anticonvulsants.

Psychomotor slowing seems to be related more to seizure frequency than to anticonvulsant levels, unlike the deterioration in I.Q. It is suggested that two different clinical abnormalities have been assessed and the failure of other studies to distinguish in this way has led to some of the confusion in the literature regarding the effect of seizure frequency on cognitive function (Bagley, 1971).

The actual mechanisms whereby anticonvulsant drugs could produce an effect on cognitive processes has not been adequately explored. There are several possibilities, including a direct effect of the drugs themselves on neuronal activity; a secondary effect due to disturbances of conduct provoked by the drugs leading to a deterioration of abilities; and secondary metabolic effects of the drugs. Work published elsewhere suggests that influences on other aspects of behavior are not responsible (Trimble and Corbett, 1980). One of the metabolic effects that has been studied here has been the role of folic acid. There have been several suggestions that abnormalities of folic acid metabolism may be related to abnormalities of the mental state both in epileptic and nonepileptic adult populations (Reynolds, 1976). The results of this study suggest that children with epilepsy and cognitive deterioration also have serum folic acid abnormalities. The effects of many years of folate deficiency as the children grow older are unknown and need assessment in view of the possibly important role of folic acid in central nervous system (CNS) metabolism (Reynolds, 1976). In that recent evidence has suggested that abnormalities of central monoamine metabolism are a consequence of anticonvulsant therapy, and in particular that patients with anticonvulsant intoxication have greater abnormalities than those that do not (Chadwick et al., 1977), and the fact that folic itself may be involved in the metabolism of the monoamines (Reynolds, 1976) provides a link that deserves further investigation.

SUMMARY

Of 312 epileptic children resident at a hospital school a group of 31 were identified whose I.Q. had actually deteriorated over a period of time. In addition, clinical assessment was made of the whole population for psychomotor slowing and data was provided on I.Q. assessments. Serum anticonvulsant levels were measured for phenytoin, primidone, phenobarbitone, and carbamazepine as well as serum folate levels. Analysis of the results showed significantly greater mean phenytoin and primidone levels in the children with I.Q. deterioration, and a significantly higher number of children with such deterioration having high serum levels of these two drugs. In addition, negative correlation coefficients were obtained between the performance I.Q. and serum levels of phenytoin, primidone, and phenobarbitone. Children whose I.Q. scores had deteriorated had significantly lower serum folate levels than the rest of the population. The implications of these findings are discussed and possible mechanisms whereby anticonvulsant drugs could affect the mental state suggested.

ACKNOWLEDGMENTS

The authors wish to thank Drs. P. Dupré, T. C. Nicol, E. M. Bayliss, D. Donaldson, and Miss M. Wiseman for their help in collecting and providing information without which the study could not have been undertaken.

REFERENCES

Bagley, C. (1971): *The Social Psychology of the Child with Epilepsy*. Routledge-Kegan Paul, London.

Chadwick, D., Jenner, P., and Reynolds, E. H. (1977): Serotonin metabolism in human epilepsy, the effect of anticonvulsant drugs. Ann. Neurol., 1:218–224.

del Cerro, M. P., and Snider, R. S. (1967): Studies on dilantin intoxication. *Neurology (Minneap.)* 17:452–466.

Glaser, G. H. (1972): Diphenylhydantoin toxicity. In: *Antiepileptic Drugs*, edited by D. M. Woodbury, J. K. Penry, and R. P. Schmidt. Raven Press, New York.

Logan, W. J., and Freeman, J. M. (1969): Pseudodegenerative disease due to diphenylhydantoin intoxication. *Arch. Neurol.*, 21:631–637.

Reynolds, E. H. (1975): Chronic antiepileptic toxicity: A review. *Epilepsia*, 16:319–353.

Reynolds, E. H. (1976): Neurological aspects of folate and B12 metabolism. *Clin. Haematol.*, 5:661–694.

Reynolds, E. H., and Travers, R. (1974): Serum anticonvulsant concentrations in epileptic patients with mental symptoms. *Br. J. Psychiatry*, 124:440–445.

Richens, A. (1976): *Drug Treatment of Epilepsy*. Henry Kimpton, London.

Rosen, J. S. (1968): Dilantin dementia. *Trans. Am. Neurol. Assoc.*, 93:273.

Trimble, M. (1978): Anticonvulsant drugs, behaviour and cognitive abilities. In *Current Developments in Psychopharmacology*, edited by W. B. Essman and L. Valzelli. Spectrum Publications, New York. (*in press*).

Trimble, M. R., and Corbett, J. (1980): The effects of anticonvulsant drugs on behaviour. *J. Irish Med. Assoc.* (*in press*).

Trimble, M. R., and Reynolds, E. H. (1976): Anticonvulsant drugs and mental symptoms: A review. *Psychol. Med.*, 6:169–178.

Advances in Epileptology:
The Xth Epilepsy International Symposium,
edited by J. A. Wada and J. K. Penry.
Raven Press, New York © 1980.

Very Accurate Computer Recognition of Three-per-Second Generalized Spike-and-Wave Discharges

* **A. Gevins, **J. Blackburn, and **M. Dedon

EEG Systems Laboratory, University of California School of Medicine,
*San Francisco 94143; and **Neuro-Analysis Computing Systems,*
San Francisco, California 94143

If computer analysis is to replace tedious manual scoring of very long (12 hr) polygraph tracings in the evaluation of the effectiveness of anticonvulsant control of absence seizures, high recognition accuracy of generalized 3/sec spike-and-wave discharges (GSWDs) is mandatory (Penry et al., 1975; Sato et al., 1976).

Only a few of the many previously published quantitative EEG studies have specifically been concerned with the detection of GSWDs. Ehrenberg and Penry (1976) implemented a system based on the comparison, with a fixed threshold, of a running sum of the integrated, weighted amplitudes of four EEG channels. In order to increase sensitivity to slow waves and spikes, ad-hoc procedures were applied that attenuated EEG components above 5 Hz, but did not attenuate activity in the 14 to 20 Hz band (which potentially contained spikes). During a comprehensive evaluation of the detection accuracy of this system, 12-hr, telemetered, daytime EEG recordings from seven patients with absence seizures were analyzed. Of 609 discharges found by all three scorers, the computer system detected 85%. Approximately as many isolated detections were made by the computer as by any of the three scorers. The performance of this system was not deemed adequate for routine use.

Carrie and Frost (1972; 1977) implemented a GSWD detection system in which separate detectors searched for spikes, muscle action potentials (EMG), and slow waves. Several ad-hoc criteria were then applied to the individual detections in order to reach a final decision that a GSWD was actually present. Ten- to twelve-hour, one-channel waking recordings from each of five patients with absence seizures were analyzed. Ninety-five percent of those seizures rated by two electroencephalographers as lasting longer than 3 sec were detected, but only 30% of those seizures lasting between 1 and 3 sec were picked up. The authors concluded that implementation of multi-channel processing would be required to attain a clinically acceptable level of performance. In our previous work on this problem (Gevins et al., 1975; 1976), we devised simple computer algorithms for the detection of randomly occurring sharp and slow transient waveforms. We estimated their accuracy in detecting 3/sec GSWDs to be in the 80 to 90% range, with a number of false detections of variant abnormal patterns and artifacts.

In understanding why these systems did not attain adequate levels of detection accuracy, one must consider the distinction between the rather infrequently occurring "ideal" 3/sec GSWD (which consists of clearly defined sequences of alternating, well-formed spikes and waves appearing suddenly in the context of a low-amplitude background EEG (e.g., Gibbs, and Gibbs, 1952, p. 66), and the more commonly occurring type of GSWD in which there is considerable morphological and temporal variation in the spike and slow wave components (Fig. 1, top). (Slow waves may be rounded and smooth, or relatively sharp and jagged. Spikes may be of large amplitude and clearly demarcated from the slow waves, of low amplitude and superimposed on the slow waves, or they may even be entirely obscured on the polygraph recording.) To complicate matters, 3/sec GSWDs may arise in the context of an abnormal background EEG (i.e., one that is of high amplitude and diffusely slow), and the EEG may itself be contaminated with EMG, movement, and other physiologic and instrumental artifact. Furthermore, relatively "minor" variations from the ideal pattern (i.e., multiple spikes between slow waves, 2 slow waves per second instead of 3, etc.) may be the accompaniment of clinically distinct types of seizure activity.

In order to cope with these problems, it is clear that considerably more complex and flexible computer procedures would be required than have been applied previously. In this chapter, we present a second generation of computer algorithms specifically designed with these considerations in mind. Overall, these algorithms are similar to first-generation algorithms in that multi-channel EEGs are digitally filtered and searched for the occurrence of slow waves, spikes, and EMG. The decision that an EEG sample containing slow waves and spikes is a 3/sec GSWD is then made by applying criteria modeled on the traditional visual interpretation of polygraphs, including the obvious requirement that slow waves occur at roughly 3/sec and that nearly simultaneous detections of a criterion percentage of both slow waves and spikes occur on homologous channels. The major improvements incorporated in these second-generation algorithms are found in the increased sophistication of the digital filtering, primary waveform detectors for slow waves and spikes, and in the flexibility of the criteria used to assemble GSWDs from the primary detections. The algorithms described below are implemented in an on-line, interactive computing system that is detailed elsewhere. The output of this system consists of histograms of the number of seizures versus time of day and versus seizure length, and computer reconstructed EEG excerpts corresponding to each detected GSWD (Fig. 1).

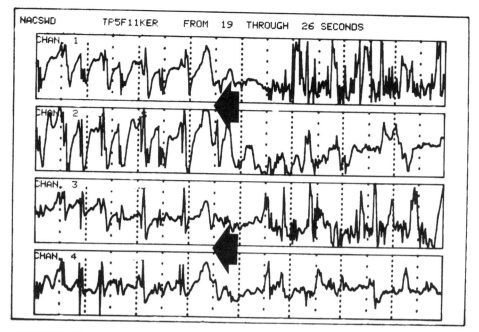

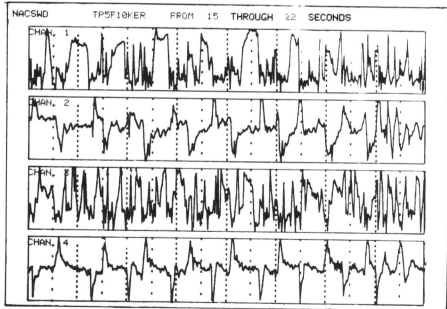

FIG. 1. Top: Computer reconstructed four-channel, 8 sec EEG excerpt from a patient (W.A.) with absence seizures. The *large arrow* points to the end (time 22.48 sec) of a computer-detected 3/sec generalized spike and wave discharge (GSWD) that began at time = 7.18 sec. The high-amplitude, irregular activity, consisting of spikes, EMG artifact, and slow waves (beginning at time 23.5 sec and extending to the end of the excerpt) was not considered part of the GSWD by the computer algorithm. Channel 1, F3C3; Channel 2, F4C4; Channel 3, T3T5; Channel 4, T4T6. *Vertical dotted lines* are at 0.5 sec intervals. Amplitude scale is in arbitrary units. **Bottom:** A different EEG excerpt from the same patient. Since there were not approximately 3 spike waves per second, and since spikes and slow waves on homologous channels were not approximately synchronous, the computer algorithm did not consider the activity to constitute a GSWD.

METHODS

Definitions of Waveforms

Each channel of EEG is transformed into a time series of digitized values with 0.01 sec between samples. y_{ij} represents the time series value for channel j at time i samples after the beginning of the analysis, and $y(i)$ represents the value for an unspecified channel at time i.

A segment $S(i_1, i_2)$ of a time series $y(i)$ is said to be monotonic over the domain (i_1, i_2) if and only if the first differences are all of the same sign:

$$[y(i + 1) - y(i)] * [y(j + 1) - y(j)] \geq 0$$

for all $i_1 \leq i, j \leq i_2$. A segment is monotonic increasing (decreasing) if all first differences are either positive (negative) or zero. A simple wave $\omega(i_1, i_2)$ consists of a monotonic increasing segment $s(i_1, i_3)$ and a monotonic decreasing segment $s(i_3, i_2)$. A wave complex $c(i_1, i_n)$ is composed of $n - 1$ contiguous simple waves:

$$\omega(i_1, i_2), \omega(i_2, i_3), \ldots, \omega(i_{n-2}, i_{n-1}), \omega(i_{n-1}, i_n).$$

The peak over the time domain (i_1, i_2) is the relative maximum of $y(i)$: $P(i_1, i_2) \geq y(i)$ for all $i_1 \leq i \leq i_2$. There is a distinction between maximal segments and less-than-maximal segments. In general, a simple wave is composed of nonmaximal segments and therefore is a nonmaximal wave. By definition, the "interior" simple waves of a wave complex (all but the first and last) are all maximal in order to meet the "contiguous" requirement. Both simple waves and wave complexes may or may not be maximal depending on whether the first and last segments of the wave are both maximal. The geometrical interpretations of these definitions are obvious and correspond to the common meaning of the terms.

Primary Wave Detectors

Three types of patterns are detected in the time series.

Spikes

A wave complex $C(i_1, i_2)$ is declared to be a spike at time i_2 if:
(a) $i_2 - i_1 \leq 100$ msec; that is, the apparent frequency of the wave complex is at least 10 Hz.

(b)
$$P(i_1, i_2) - y(i_1) \geq \text{SPKAMP}$$

$$\text{and } P(i_1, i_2) - y(i_2) \geq \text{SPKAMP}$$

where $P(i_1, i_2)$ is the peak and SPKAMP is the minimum spike amplitude.

(c) There is a "peak region" defined by i_3 and i_4 where:

$$i_1 \leqslant i_3 \leqslant i_4 \leqslant i_2$$
$$P(i_3, i_4) = P(i_1, i_2)$$
$$i_4 - i_3 \leqslant 20 \text{ msec}$$
$$y(i_3 + 1) - y(i_3) \geqslant \text{SPKCRV}$$
$$y(i_4) - y(i_4 + 1) \geqslant \text{SPKCRV}$$

That is, there is a peak region not wider than 20 msec that passes a curvature test.

(d) If $\text{SPK}(i)$ is a spike detection on the same channel as SPK (i_1), and if $i < i_1$, then $i_1 - i \geqslant 90$ msec, the minimum time between successive SPs.

EMG

An EMG event is declared at time i_1 if:

(a) There are at least three contiguous maximal simple waves the last of which ends at time i_1.

(b) The absolute value of each wave segment in this wave train $\geqslant$ EMGAMP—a minimum EMG amplitude.

(c) The period of each simple wave $\leqslant 50$ msec.

(d) The number of simple waves necessary to declare an EMG event is incremented each time an event is found (on a channel). At the end of each 0.25 sec epoch, this number is reset to 3. This limits the number of EMG detections in "noisy" data. An EMG detection turns off subsequent SP detections on the EMG-contaminated channel(s) for the remainder of the 0.25 epoch.

Slow Waves

In order to attenuate unwanted high frequency signals, the original time series are filtered using a 15-wide symmetric, FIR numerical filter, F15. Since the filter was designed to cut off above 16 Hz, the filtered data is decimated by a factor of $3:1$ in order to reduce computational load. Slow waves are then detected in the filtered data:

$$y^*(i) = \omega_0 y(i) + \sum_{k=1}^{7} \omega_k [y(i + k) + y(i - k)]$$

where $\omega_0, \omega_1, \ldots \omega_7$ are the normalized F15 filter weights. A slow wave in the raw data is defined as a maximal wave complex (that is, all segments are maximal and so the complex is "geometrically isolated" from the surrounding time series) that meets several conditions:

(a) The period of the wave is between 250 and 500 msec.

(b) The leading and trailing edges of the wave exceed an amplitude threshold, WAVAMP.

(c) There is no pair of adjacent simple waves, both contained in the composite wave, where the first simple wave has a "significant fall" and the next simple wave has a "significant rise." A wave is defined as having "significant rise/fall" if (1) the period of the wave exceeds 210 msec and (2) the amplitude of the wave exceeds a minimum value, EPSLON.

This requirement imposes a condition of "geometrical isolation" on a slow wave. This means that the first simple wave does not have a "significant fall." If the second simple wave in the wave complex has a "significant fall" then it marks the end of this complex (the next complex is started by the next simple wave having a "significant rise"), and so on. This allows individual wave complexes to be properly separated from each other at the appropriate places.

(d) The amount of energy in the wave complex due to frequency components between 4 and 16 Hz is less than a maximal fraction of the integrated amplitude of the wave, ALIASA. This requirement rejects slow waves with excessive, superimposed high-frequency activity.

GSWD Assembly

The primary slow wave, spike, and EMG detections are evaluated by a "seizure assembly" program that examines the temporal arrangement of the detections and determines whether or not a 3/sec GSWD is present. If a GSWD is found, the time of its onset and offset are determined.

For each 2 sec interval (which overlaps the previous interval by 1.5 sec) the following requirements must be met for a GSWD detection to occur: (a) between three and eight slow waves on at least three out of four channels; (b) no more than 80 msec difference in the time of slow wave peaks on homologous channels (a slow wave "match"); (c) one or more spike detections for at least three out of four channels; (d) no more than 30 msec difference between time of spike peaks on homologous channels (a spike "match"); and (e) a sufficient number of slow wave and spike matches determined as a nonlinear function of the GSWD length. In the presence of a large number of EMG detections, the requirement for spike detections is waived, but more rigid criteria are applied to the slow wave detections (five or more slow waves on four out of four channels, and four or more slow wave matches on both homologous channel pairs).

In order to accurately determine the start and ending times of a GSWD occurring in the context of a background EEG containing high-amplitude delta waves, a simple algorithm searches inward from the initially determined ends of the GSWD for slow waves whose amplitudes (expressed as Z scores) exceed a threshold of -0.07 standard deviations. (This algorithm is not applied to those GSWDs whose slow wave components have very low amplitude variance.) If the length of a potential GSWD is less than 2 sec, more rigid criteria are applied to make the final determination (spike and slow wave matches are required on four out of four channels). When a GSWD is longer than 6 sec, criteria 1 to 5 above are slightly relaxed. Finally, simple algorithms allow for gaps of up to 2 sec to occur during long GSWDs.

RESULTS

As of September, 1978, the algorithms have not yet been formally evaluated on an independent set of data (that is, data that were not used in development). On a preliminary evaluation of their performance on the training data, 27 of 27 GSWDs were detected during 900 sec of four-channel EEG excerpts from eight patients with absence seizures. There were no misses or false detections. Figure 1 shows two computer-reconstructed EEG excerpts from a difficult case in which the background was highly abnormal and in which the EEG was contaminated with physiologic and instrumental artifact. The arrow in the upper half of the figure shows the end of a seizure (time = 22.48 sec) found by the computer (the start occurred 15.3 sec earlier). Note that the high-amplitude, irregular activity beginning at time 23.5 sec and extending to the end of the excerpt is not considered to be part of the GSWD. In the lower half of Fig. 1 is shown another 8 sec excerpt from the same patient. Although there were many detections of slow waves and spikes, the activity shown was not considered to be a part of a GSWD (there were not approximately three slow waves per second, and slow waves and spikes on homologous channels were not approximately synchronous.)

ACKNOWLEDGMENTS

The research and development reported here was supported by the Epilepsy Branch of the National Institutes of Neurologic and Communicative Diseases and Strokes, J. K. Penry, Director. We are grateful to H. Moore and B. G. White of the Epilepsy Branch for technical and logistical assistance and to S. Sato of the Epilepsy Branch for polygraph evaluations.

REFERENCES

Carrie, J. R. G. (1972): A hybrid computer system for detecting and quantifying spike and wave EEG patterns. *Electroencephalogr. Clin. Neurophysiol.*, 33:339–341.

Carrie, J. R. G., and Frost, J. D., Jr. (1977): Clinical evaluation of a method for quantification of generalized spike-wave EEG patterns by computer during prolonged recordings. *Comput. Biomed. Res.*, 10:449–457.

Ehrenberg, B. L., and Penry, J. K. (1976): Computer recognition of generalized spike-wave discharges. *Electroencephalogr. Clin. Neurophysiol.*, 41:25–36.

Gevins, A. S., Yeager, C. L., Diamond, S. L., Spire, J., Zeitlin, G. M., and Gevins, A. H. (1975): Automated analysis of the electrical activity of the human brain (EEG): A progress report. *Proceedings of the Institute of Electrical and Electronics Engineers*, 63:1382–1399.

Gevins, A. S., Yeager, C. L., Diamond, S. L., Zeitlin, G. M., Spire, J. P., and Gevins, A. H. (1976): Sharp-transient analysis and thresholded linear coherence spectra of paroxysmal EEGs. In: *Quantitative Analytic Studies in Epilepsy*, edited by P. Kellaway and I. Petersen. Raven Press, New York.

Gibbs, F. A., and Gibbs, E. L. (1952): *Atlas of Electroencephalography, Vol. 2, Epilepsy.* Addison-Wesley, Reading, Massachusetts.

Kooi, K. A. (1971): *Fundamentals of Electroencephalography.* Harper & Row, New York.

Penry, J. K., Porter, R. J., and Dreifuss, F. E. (1975): Simultaneous recording of absence seizures with video tape and electroencephalography. *Brain*, 98:427–440.

Sato, S., Penry, J. K., and Dreifuss, F. E. (1976): Electroencephalographic monitoring of generalized spike-wave paroxysms in the hospital and at home. In: *Quantitative Analytic Studies in Epilepsy*, edited by P. Kellaway and I. Petersen, pp. 237–251. Raven Press, New York.

Abstracts

AED CONCENTRATIONS IN DISCRETE BRAIN AREAS OF EPILEPTIC PATIENTS UNDERGOING SURGICAL INTERVENTION — PRELIMINARY OBSERVATIONS

C. Munari, V. Rovei, J. Talairach, E. Sanjuan, J. Bancaud and P. L. Morselli

Paris

Plasma and brain levels of PB, DPH, CBZ and its epoxide were monitored in 11 epileptic patients who underwent surgical intervention (after acute or chronic stereo EEG recording) because of severe seizures resistant to pharmacological treatment. Monitored cortical brain samples included: epileptogenic focus and "lesional" and "irritative" areas. Normal brain tissue was obtained on a few occasions when its ablation was considered necessary. Results indicate that AED brain concentrations were frequently lower than the plasma ones in most of the cases. Furthermore a remarkable variability (PB 3 fold, DPH and CZB 2 fold) was observed for different brain specimens within the same patient, without any evident relationships with either topography or type of tissues. Such a variability in AED brain concentrations within the same patient appears somehow in contrast with current knowledge on the AED brain/plasma relationship. The clinical bearing of this data will be discussed together with the questions relevant to a better understanding of the "resistant" patient. The data underline the need for more observations and for more experimental work on AED concentrations in discrete brain areas in animal models for epilepsy.

24-HOUR 8-CHANNEL EEG DIGITAL CASSETTE RECORDING IN PATIENTS WITH COMPLEX PARTIAL SEIZURES

S. Sato and J. K. Penry

Bethesda

Previously, we described an 8-channel EEG digital cassette recorder and playback system, and proposed its usefulness in patients with partial seizures (Academic Press 1978, in press). Subsequently, we have used this system to define distribution and quantification of epileptiform discharges continuously during wakefulness and sleep.

Eight patients (5 males and 3 females, 16-43 years of age) with complex partial seizures underwent 24-hour EEG monitoring with the 8-channel digital cassette recorder, which was preceded by routine EEG examination. The latter showed left temporal epileptiform discharges in two patients, right tem-poral discharges in three, bitemporal, bilateral, or independent discharges with bilateral irregular spike-wave paroxysms in two, and sharp waves in the left parietal-posterior temporal area in one patient.

The discharge rates (number of discharges/min) were 0.002-1.112 during wakefulness, 0-6.592 during REM sleep, 0.097-6.615 during stage I, 0.035-9.067 during stage II, 0.198-17.244 during stage III, and 0.285;9.970 during stage IV. Epileptiform discharges increased as non-REM sleep deepened, regardless of their origin — left or right temporal or bilateral. There was no significant difference in the distribution of the epileptiform discharges of left and right temporal origin during a 24 hour period.

Therefore, the 8-channel EEG digital cassette recorder is very useful in recording and localizing epileptiform discharges for the purpose of quantification.

LONG-TERM MONITORING OF INTERICTAL EPILEPTIC EEG ACTIVITY

J. Gotman, J. R. Ives and P. Gloor

Montreal

A method of automatic recognition and quantification of interictal epileptic activity in the human EEG had previously been developed and tested using short recordings from awake subjects. This method has been adapted for the monitoring of interictal activity in free-moving, unattended patients.

EEGs were recorded overnight from scalp and sphenoidal electrodes, using cable telemetry and a PDP-12 computer. Simultaneous on-line pattern recognition analysis of 16 channels allowed to detect waveforms having the morphology of epileptic spikes and sharp waves. Sections including one second before and one second after each detected spike were saved on magnetic tape. Upon completion of the monitoring session the spike sections were played back on the EEG machine. This gave a highly concentrated view of the epileptic activity, on a traditional paper tracing. Spike sections were further analyzed by computer to determine the spatial and temporal distributions of the epileptic activity, providing a complete synopsis of the recording session.

Thirty 6-hour monitoring sessions were performed. The proportion of false detections was very variable, depending mostly on the presence of technical artefacts. Even with high false detection rates however, data reduction can be considerable, when comparing to a continuous recording. Examples will be shown and possible improvements discussed.

INTENSIVE ALL-NIGHT MONITORING OF PATIENTS WITH COMPLEX SEIZURE DISORDERS

C. T. Lombroso, G. Erba
Boston

Some ictal patterns, such as tonic seizures, are known to be activated by drowsiness and slow-wave sleep. All-night sleep studies, therefore, became necessary to quantify such "activation" and to assess its consequences. Examples of the value of this monitoring is shown in patients in whom sleep deprivation from unrecognized activation of clinical or subclinical ictal discharges triggers certain types of status epilepticus or aggravates periodically some epileptic syndromes. The validity of such cause-effect in these patients is indirectly suggested by the use of hypnotic drugs. Observations in our laboratories utilizing continuous EEG monitoring during specific neuropsychological evaluation have shown an "increased vigilance" state during the initial part of the "beta-like" discharge accompanying minor tonic attacks.

The hypothesis is advanced that such "arousal" effects may explain the disruptive influence by this type of discharge on sleep organization. Illustrative cases will be presented.

A STUDY OF NOCTURNAL SEIZURES OF THE LENNOX-GASTAUT SYNDROME BY ALL-NIGHT EEG AND VIDEO RECORDINGS

K. Yagi, T. Morikawa, M. Miyakoshi, N. Kekegawa, T. Fujiwara, O. Ishihara, T. Osawa
Shizuoka

In an attempt to elucidate the versatile nature of nocturnal seizures which are observable among patients with the Lennox-Gastaut syndrome, all-night sleep polygraphic recordings of EEG were carried out with intensive monitoring devices on 22 intractable cases aged 7-29 years to assess 1264 seizures in total.

They were: axial to global tonic seizures accompanying runs of rapid spikes, and periocular to massive myoclonic twitching accompanying bursts of slow (poly-) spike and wave discharges associated with tachy- and/or brady-pnea and -cardia.

Notwithstanding that each sleep stage was rather undistinguishable on the EEG background activities, the presence of REM sleep was unmistakably distinct since REM was witnessed on the video-minitor along with the polygraph throughout.

The average percentage ratio of REM to all the sleeping time was as low as 11.0% : 56 ± 37 min. (min. 0, max. 122) to 528 ± 54 min. (min. 394, max. 624).

It was exemplified that not only seizure discharges but also clinical seizures took place quite exceptionally during REM sleep; namely, 1249 seizures — 1

seizure per 8.3 min. — occurred during NON-REM sleep, while only 15 seizures — 1 seizure per 84.3 min. — occurred during REM sleep.

Judging from paroxysmal discharges of generalized nature augmented during light sleep, these nocturnal seizure phenomena, though so subtle and mild, appeared to prevent the patients from falling asleep and resulted in a vicious circle of seizure and hyposomnic state.

INTENSIVE EEG MONITORING BY MEANS OF PATTERN RECOGNITION IN THE TREATMENT OF SOME FORMS OF EPILEPSY

L. O. Ferrer-Vidal, J. Sabater, A. Maya
M. A. Lagunas, L. Oller-Daurella
Barcelona

An intensive EEG monitoring is the basis of the work. The correlations between the interical EEG activity and drug plasma levels are the purpose of the work, in order to know the efficacy of one drug introduced in the treatment of some forms of Epilepsy.

The monitoring is carried out along a period of 12 hours with the patient continuously connected to the EEG system and every hour the EEG was recorded for a period of 15 minutes. The total number of paroxysms and their characteristics (spikes, sharp waves, high voltage slow waves, polispikes, 3 Hz spike-waves, slow spike and wave) being evaluated by means of a computerized system. The software was original from the authors based on Pattern Recognition by means eigenfonctional digital filters and the hardware was a PdP8, Lab 8/E, with 28K words of core. The drug under testing (Carbamazepine, Sodium Valproate or Ethosuximide) was administered orally every two hours and at the same time blood was sampled for the drug plasma level determination, carried out by gas chromatography. The patients were followed up weekly for a period of six months. The correlations between drug plasma level and interictal EEG activity, was evaluated any way it related with the frequency of seizures. The results of some cases will be discussed.

STANDARDIZED METHODS OF VIDEODOCU-MENTATION IN INTENSIVE MONITORING

H. Stefan, H. Penin, Bonn

Videodocumentation takes substantial part in objective seizure management and in evaluation of drug therapy. The intensive monitoring of patients with intractable seizures led to a more exact observation of the course. We see in the area of videodocumentation supplementary possibilities to gain more exact and detailed information of ictal behaviour. The combination of several methods, leading to a more standardized documentation of ictal phenomena, provides more qualitatively and quantitatively positive evidence. These simultaneously used methods are:

1) Polygraphic recordings of EEG, poly-EMG, EKG,

respiration, etc. in split screen videodocumentation.

2) Transmission of biosignals with telemetry.
3) Videometric analysis of videotapes including slow motion play-back.

The difficulties of comparison of videodocumentation made by different investigatiors require more standardized methods. Based on our experience, the standardization should include:

1) Standardized view of the cameras (frontal *and* side).
2) Standard position of the patient, i.e., documentation of seizures in a *defined* (sitting, standing, and lying) position.
3) *Simultaneous* videorecording of each seizure from frontal and side view.
4) Use of *standard leads* in telemetered biosignals.
5) *Constant sequence* of investigation during videodocumentation: at first exploration including the subjective perception of ictal phenomena, then recording of spontaneous seizures (first without interaction, then with psychopathometry) and after all defined provocation.

Different syndromes of seizures demand variations in derivation technique, examples are demonstrated, inspiring discussion aimed at reaching agreement on standardization among different investigators.

SEIZURE MONITORING: ITS COST-EFFECTIVENESS

J. W. Whisler, W. J. ReMine, R. J. Gumnit
Minneapolis

Intensive seizure monitoring of hospitalized patients usually includes periodic determination of blood anti-convulsant concentrations and prolonged EEG recordings. Data will be presented regarding its cost-effectiveness based on experience with over 90 patients in over 800 hours of monitoring. The analysis revealed the following central problem: Prolonged EEG or EEG/video recordings permit much more accurate seizure classification and quantification than otherwise possible. This is especially useful in surgical cases and patients with mixed seizure types. However, the cost of such recordings is relatively high in relation to the information obtained for some patients. The time-consuming task of identifying clinical and EEG seizures in the long records accounts for most of the cost. Relying on patient reporting or on machine seizure detection substantially reduces the cost but severly limits the range of applicability in the patient population.

A revised monitoring system is presented combining patient and nurse reporting, machine seizure detection, and constant observation to maximize reliability of the system while minimizing costs. A time code system and paper printer produce a list of reported seizures including time of day, source of report, and a patient identifier. Initial experience with the system is encouraging and preliminary cost-effectiveness data will be presented.

This work was supported by NINDS contract number Nol-NS-5-2327.

PSYCHOSIS OR EPILEPSY

S. Gladwell, K. Kaufman, M. Driver
Pittsburgh, Pennsylvania, U.S.A.

It is often extremely difficult to differentiate between "psychotic" and "epileptic" phenomenology. This becomes an even greater problem when the seizure pattern is variable and episodes of minor epileptic status or complex partial seizures occur. We report a complex case where the symptomatology had several possible explanations and in which evaluation was difficult.

A 15-year-old patient was hospitalized with a 12-year history of idiopathic epilepsy and abnormal behavior. The patient presented in an acute psychotic state. Clonic, tonic, tonic-clonic, and automatistic seizures were noted clinically in addition to incoherent speech, hallucinations, and psychotic posturing. This complex pattern had led previous physicians to diagnose this patient as hysterical with psychogenic psychosis. Serial split-screen videotaped EEGs revealed a clear association among the psychotic features, clinical seizure activity, and paroxysmal spike-wave EEG rhythms during which the patient was undergoing status epilepticus. Multiple anticonvulsants were tried, but only sodium valproate has recently resulted in remission.

The authors conclude that in order to differentiate conditions directly related to ictal activity from those in which psychological symptoms are primary, it may be necessary to carry out simultaneous observations of clinical and electroencephalographic features — specifically by split-screen videotaped recordings.

HYSTERICAL SEIZURES IN EPILEPTIC PATIENTS

S. V. Ramani, D. Olson, R. J. Gumnit
Minneapolis, Minnesota, U.S.A.

The coexistence of real and hysterical seizures in the same patient is not rare and creates problems in diagnosis and management. Prompt recognition of hysterical seizures is important to prevent overtreatment with anticonvulsant drugs. The diagnosis of hysterical seizures is difficult to make on clinical grounds alone. Simultaneous video EEG monitoring techniques were used in the diagnosis of hysterical seizures in ten epileptic patients. Diagnostic monitoring and intensive psychotherapy were carried out during four to nine weeks of hospitalization period. During an average follow-up period of 13 months, five patients demonstrated marked improvement in seizure control as well as psychosocial status. Significant reduction in hysterical seizures with some psychosocial improvement was noted in four. One patient did not respond at all. The implications of our findings pertaining to the nature of hysterical seizures will be briefly considered.

PRIMIDONE WITHDRAWAL IN PATIENTS WITH INTRACTABLE EPILEPSY

D. Schmidt, H. J. Kupferberg
Berlin
R. J. Porter, J. K. Penry
Bethesda

Primidone was withdrawn in three patients with complex partial seizures uncontrolled by phenytoin-primidone combination treatment. After a temporary increase the number of complex partial seizures fell below the pre-withdrawal frequency in two patients and was unchanged in one patient. The paroxysmal abnormal discharges disappeared in one patient who became seizure-free after withdrawal. Video-EEG-analysis of 77 complex partial seizures demonstrated modification of ictal signs during withdrawal. Generalized tonic-clonic seizures occurred in two patients dispite phenytoin plasma levels between 12 and 20 μg/ml. The plasma half-lives of primidone, phenobarbital and PEMA were followed.

It is concluded that the withdrawal of primidone may be beneficial for selected patients with intractable epilepsy. Phenytoin does not prevent primidone withdrawal seizures.

THE EFFECT OF VALPROIC ACID ON THE EEG BACKGROUND

J. C. Sackellares, S. Sato, F. E. Dreifuss,
Charlottesville
J. K. Penry
Bethesda

Electroencephalograms of patients receiving valproic acid (VPA) in a double blind study were computer analyzed as to the influence of VPA on the background frequency distribution. In each patient, the EEG frequency distribution before and after VPA therapy was compared. Group I received no drug prior to initiation of VPA. Group II received ethosuximide before crossing over to VPA. Group III received a barbiturate before and during VPA therapy.

In Group I there was a trend toward increase in the 0-4 and 12-24 cps bands and reduction in 4-8 and 8-12 cps bands. These changes were more prominent during the first week than during the sixth week of treatment. In Group II there was also a shift toward the 0-4 cps band and reduction in the 8-12 cps band during the first week, but these changes were not evident by the sixth week when the 12-24 cps frequencies were more prominent. Group III showed similar shifts toward slower frequencies during the first week which persisted to a lesser degree after six weeks, but there was little change in the 12-24 cps band. Thus, VPA may initially induce slowing of the EEG background and later accentuate beta frequencies. These changes will be discussed in relation to clinical alertness and serum levels.

THE EFFECT OF PLASMA LEVEL MONITORING ON THERAPEUTIC OUTCOME IN EPILEPTIC OUTPATIENTS.

W. Froscher, H. Penin, M. Eichelbaum, R. Gugler,
G. Hildenbrand, Bonn

127 epileptic outpatients (seizure type: grand mal, grand mal and psychomotor epilepsy, grand mal and absences) were randomly assigned to two groups. During one year of follow-up plasma levels were determined in either group by means of gas-chromatography and high-pressure-liquid-chromatography (the following compounds were determined: carbamazepine, ethosuximide, phenobarbital, primidone, phenytoin, valproic acid). Of group B (controls) the treating physician was not informed on the results of plasma level determinations. Drug dosage was adjusted in the traditional way by using history, clinical and EEG-findings. Plasma levels of group A were reported to the treating physician who should attempt to have the plasma levels in the "therapeutic range" (the therapeutic concentrations were as defined by Kutt and Penry (Arch. Neurol. 31,283, 1974) and by Meinardi and Magnus (In: Vinken and Bruyn, The Epilepsies 1974) as to valproic acid. In either group number of seizures and frequency of side effects were compared to a control period. The results of group A were compared to group B. From a total of 127 patients 105 could be evaluated at the end of the study year. Therapeutic results of group A and group B were not significantly different at the end of one year. The number of seizures decreased to a similar extent in both groups during the observation period. The reduction in seizure frequency was accompanied by an increase in plasma concentrations of the antiepileptic drugs. The type of the treatment as well as the number of drugs prescribed were identical in both groups. No change was observed in the type and the number of drugs during the year of observation. The frequency of side effects was identical in both groups.

NATURAL HISTORY AND
PROGNOSIS OF EPILEPSY

Advances in Epileptology:
The Xth Epilepsy International Symposium,
edited by J. A. Wada and J. K. Penry.
Raven Press, New York © 1980.

Natural History and Prognosis of Epilepsy

*Teruo Okuma and **Hisashi Kumashiro

*Group for the Study of the Prognosis of Epilepsy in Japan,
Department of Psychiatry, Tohoku University School of Medicine, Sendai;
and **Department of Psychiatry, Fukushima Prefectural Medical College,
Fukushima, Japan*

The continuous acquisition of new knowledge regarding the causes, courses, and consequences of epilepsy is essential to achieve the goal of primary and secondary prevention of epilepsies. Significant insight into the natural history and prognosis of epilepsy may be gained by comparing the outcome of epileptic symptoms before the development of advanced drug treatment with those under a modern treatment approach.

In studies performed some 70 years ago, before development of antiepileptic drug therapy, the percentage of complete remission of epileptic seizures as a whole was reported to be 10% (Habermaas, 1901) and 32% (Turner, 1907). Introduction of potent antiepileptic drugs such as phenobarbital (1912), diphenylhydantoin (1938), and other new drugs between 1940 and 1970, however, could not elevate the remission rate of seizures as much as expected, and the remission rate remained at 20 to 40%. In Japan, reliable data on the outcome of epileptic seizures before the era of modern drug treatment are not available. The remission rate of seizures reported in the literature was 27% (Akimoto and Okamoto, 1940), 22% (Uchimura et al., 1952) and, more recently, 41% (Wada, 1963) and 46% (Fukushima, 1969).

To obtain reliable information on the outcome of epileptic patients under a modern treatment approach, a multi-institutional investigation, which included 20 institutions, was performed in Japan from 1975 to 1977 (Okuma, 1977) by using the International Classification of Epileptic Seizures (Gastaut, 1970). The investigation team consisted of 12 psychiatric, four pediatric, and three neurosurgical clinics, and one neurological clinic, as listed at the end of this chapter.

PATIENTS AND METHODS

The outcome of epilepsy 10, 5, and 3 years after the onset of the illness was investigated in three groups of patients who fulfilled the following criteria. The subjects of the study on outcome 10 years after onset were selected as follows. As the first step, epileptic patients who had visited a given institution as new patients 10 to 13 years before the present investigation (September 1976 or September 1977) were listed. Next, among these patients, only those whose onset of seizure had occurred within 5 years of the first visit were selected as the "original group of patients" to be followed up. In this way, an outcome of at least 10 years after the onset of the illness was investigated. The subjects of the studies on outcome 5 and 3 years after onset were selected in a similar way to those of the 10-year outcome study. Patients who were not attending the clinic at the time of the investigation were surveyed by a mail questionnaire or by telephone.

Twenty-four variables were evaluated at the time of the initial examination (Table 1). Variables evaluated at the time of follow-up were: state of seizures, personality disturbances, psychotic disturbances, state of social ad-

TABLE 1. *Relationships among variables at initial examination and outcome of seizures—analysis of variance*

Variables	F
Intellectual deficits	30.2[a]
Frequency of seizures	20.4[a]
Time of occurrence of seizures	19.5[a]
Neurological symptoms	15.1[a]
Personality disturbances	14.4[a]
Age of onset of seizures	14.0[a]
EEG background activity (grade)	7.4[a]
Lennox's classification	5.8[a]
Institution	3.3[a]
International classification	3.2[a]
EEG background activity (general)	5.5[b]
Idiopathic, symptomatic	5.0[b]
Period of follow-up	2.7[b]
Precipitating factors	2.7[b]
Pretreatment period	4.5[c]
Psychotic disturbances	3.3[c]
EEG general findings (topography)	2.8[c]
Age at investigation	2.7[c]
EEG background activity (topography)	2.7[c]
EEG paroxysmal activity (topography)	2.5[c]
EEG background activity (grade-topography)	2.3[c]
Surgical treatment	3.7[d]
Exogenous etiology	1.7[d]
EEG general findings (general-1)	1.9[d]
EEG general findings (general-topography)	1.8[d]
Marital status	1.7[e]
Infantile convulsion (febrile)	1.1[e]
Aura	1.1[e]
EEG paroxysmal activity (laterality)	1.1[e]
EEG general findings (general-2)	0.8[e]
Heredity	0.6[e]
Sex	0.5[e]
Method of investigation	0.0[e]

Significance level (%): [a]$p < 0.001$; [b]$p < 0.01$; [c]$p < 0.05$; [d]$p < 0.1$; [e]NS.

justment, antiepileptic medication, EEG findings, and clinico-EEG correlations.

The data from the 10-year, 5-year, and 3-year outcome groups were summed up and analyzed together to obtain a general information picture, and the subjects were subdivided into 10-year, 5-year, and 3-year outcome groups or into child (onset before 10 years of age) and adult groups, when necessary. In order to find those factors having a close relation to the outcome of seizure or social adjustment, and also to find interactions between variables, analysis of variance was chiefly used, and both F test and χ^2 tests were utilized.

RESULTS

Outcome of Seizure Control and Social Adjustment

The total number of epileptic patients successfully followed up was 1,868, i.e., 795 in the 10-year outcome group, 665 in the 5-year outcome group, and 409 in the 3-year outcome group. The rate of follow-up in all institutions averaged 42%. The rate of complete remission of seizures in all of the 1868 patients irrespective of seizure type, age, and period of follow-up was 58.3%. The rate of normal social adjustment was 62.6%, and that of moderate to severe maladjustment was approximately 12%.

Relationships Between Variables at Initial Examination and Outcome of Seizure Control

Result of Analysis of Variance

As shown in Table 1, the type of seizure, frequency of seizures, state during occurrence of seizure such as sleep, waking, and diffuse, precipitating factors, age at onset of seizures, and period prior to the first treatment, showed a significant relationship to the outcome of seizures. Regarding etiology, idiopathic epilepsy and patients without any exogenous etiology showed a favorable outcome. Presence or absence of intellectual deficits, personality disturbances, psychotic disturbances, and neurological symptoms showed a close relationship to the outcome of seizure. With regard to the EEG findings at the time of initial examination, the abnormality of background activity, particularly the grade of abnormality, showed high F value.

Relationship of Each Variable to the Outcome of Seizures

No statistically significant difference was found among the remission rates of seizures in the three groups of patients with different follow-up periods. This finding is inconsistent with those in the literature, where the longer the follow-up period the lower the remission rate. The remission rate was significantly higher in the group with onset before 10 years of age (66%) than in those of the other two groups (10–19 years, 54%; over 20 years, 51%). The remission rate in cases with onset before 1 year, however, was 51% and was significantly lower than that of patients with onset between 1 and 4 years (73%) and between 5 and 9 years (69%). It has been reported in the literature (Rodin, 1968) that the younger the patient at the time of onset of the illness, the less likelihood there is of complete control being achieved, but this notion applies only to patients with onset before 1 year of age as far as the present study is concerned.

Patients diagnosed as having idiopathic or cryptogenic epilepsy showed a significantly higher remission rate (62%) than residual (52%) or symptomatic (50%) epilepsies. It was shown, in general, that the lower the frequency of seizure, the better the outcome of seizure control. In patients with simple absences, however, no significant relationship was observed between the frequency and outcome of seizure. With regard to the time of occurrence of seizures, the remission rate was highest in sleep epilepsy (69%), and lowest in diffuse epilepsy (50%), with waking epilepsy in the middle (62%). As for the relationship between the variables such as neurological symptoms, intellectual deficits, personality disturbances, and psychotic disturbances, and the outcome of seizures, very similar relationships were found between each of these variables and the outcome of seizures. The remission rate was highest in patients without such disturbances (60–65%), middling in those with mild disturbances (33–44%), and lowest in those with severe disturbances (31–38%).

Insofar as the type of seizure was concerned, the remission rate for partial seizure with elementary symptomatology was 60% and for partial seizure with complex symptomatology, 61%. The outcome of seizure was rather favorable in those patients with single-type seizure but the remission rates in combined types (partial seizures with generalized tonic-clonic seizures) were significantly lower than those of the single types, i.e., 42% and 30%, respectively. The remission rate of 61% for partial seizure with complex symptomatology in the present study seems to be higher than those rates reported in the literature (Currie et al., 1971). It should be remembered, however, that the 61% rate was for single type cases, and when the combined types were included, the remission rate was lowered to 46%, coming closer to those rates reported by other authors. The remission rate of the Lennox syndrome (this category was added to the International Classification in the present study) was only 37%, and that of infantile spasms (West syndrome), 51%.

The remission rate in tonic-clonic seizure in total was 69%, and no significant difference was found between those with and without exogenous etiology. The remission rate of tonic-clonic seizure in the present study is higher than those reported for grand mal seizures by other authors. This is because the so-called grand mal seizure includes partial seizure secondarily generalized and combined types that show very low remission rates, i.e., 39% and 37% in the present study. If tonic-clonic seizures, partial seizure secondarily generalized and combined types were grouped together in our study, the remission rate would be 59%. One of the merits of the International Classification is that we can distinguish generalized convulsions of different origin and also of different prognosis.

The remission rate of simple absence was 68% and was almost the same as that of tonic-clonic seizures, whereas the remission rate of simple absence combined with generalized convulsion was 50% and was significantly lower than that of the single type. The result of the present study seems to be close to those reported in the literature (Livingston et al., 1965; Dalby, 1969).

Relationships Between Variables at Initial Examination and Outcome of Social Adjustment

The variables that showed significant relationship to the outcome of social adjustment in analysis of variance were almost the same as those of seizure control, and the F values were generally larger for social adjustment than for seizure control. Neurological symptoms, intellectual deficits, personality disturbance, and psychotic disturbance showed very close relationship to the outcome of social adjustment, and those patients with such disturbances showed a much lower rate of normal social adjustment (5–40%) than those without any disturbances (75–87%). Patients who had neither intellectual nor personality disturbance showed a very high rate of normal adjustment, 92%. The rate of normal social adjustment of patients with only personality disturbance was 52%, whereas that of patients with intellectual deficits only was 21%. This fact suggests that intellectual deficits play a more important role toward social adjustment than does personality disturbance.

With regard to the seizure type and outcome of social adjustment, the rate of normal social adjustment in simple absence was 87%—the highest among all seizure types, with that of tonic-clonic seizure without exogenous etiology (85%) following it. The rate was very low in the West (30%) and Lennox (22%) syndromes. The rate of normal social adjustment was usually higher than that of seizure control in each seizure type, but the tonic-clonic seizure with exogenous etiology, West syndrome, and Lennox syndrome showed poorer outcome of social adjustment as compared with that of seizure control.

DISCUSSION

The main object of the present study was not to detect any new findings relating to the prognosis of epilepsy, but to obtain reliable information on the prognosis of epilepsy based on a large number of patients, in which the follow-up rates as well as drop-out rates are clearly demonstrated. I would say that these objectives have been almost attained in the present study. Many of the previous findings reported in the literature have been confirmed statistically in our study.

The remission rate in our patients, 58%, seemed to be high as compared with those rates reported in the literature. There may be several factors that have made the remission rate in our study relatively high. One possibility might be that the subjects of our study were outpatients of university hospitals. In Japan, however, the majority of epileptic patients, not only severe cases but also mild cases, visit university hospitals and are treated there as outpatients. The assumption that we are dealing with only mild cases, therefore, does not apply to the present study. The next factor might be that the follow-up rate, 42%, was not sufficiently high. However, the correlation coefficient between the rate of follow-up and remission rate in our study was 0.55 ($p < 0.05$). This means that the remission rate tended to be higher as the follow-up rate became higher. Therefore, the remission rate of seizure would not become lower if the follow-up rate had been higher.

Another and most desirable possibility would be that the remission rate of seizures has been elevated by the recent progress in pharmacological treatment. The fact that most of our patients were still under medication at the time of follow-up may also be a factor that made the remission rate higher.

To predict a prognosis of seizure control and social adjustment more accurately and systematically from the information obtained at initial examination, we should have a certain formula or argolism based on these statistical data, thus making it possible to calculate a coefficient for prognosis by using these variables. Rodin reported this kind of trial that employed a technique of discriminant function analysis. We are now trying to make an argolism based on the technique of multicontingency table.

It has been demonstrated in the present study that many different factors exert influence on the prognosis of epilepsy. The study suggests that, in order to improve the prognosis of epilepsy, not only medical treatment but also comprehensive care is urgently needed.

ACKNOWLEDGMENTS

The author would like to express his gratitude to Yukio Takahashi of Nippon Roche Company for his cooperation in the statistical analysis of the data.

This study was carried out by the Group for the Study of the Prognosis of Epilepsy in Japan chaired by T. Okuma and H. Kumashiro. Investigators collaborating in this study were: Y. Hirabayashi and I. Yamashita (Psychiatry, Hokkaido University); T. Sato and H. Fukushima (Psychiatry, Hirosaki University); T. Okuma (Psychiatry, Tohoku University); H. Kumashiro, K. Maruko, Y. Takahashi, and T. Ono (Psychiatry, Fukushima Medical College); Y. Fukuyama, and M. Hara (Pediatrics, Tokyo Women's

Medical College); T. Seki, Y. Kawahara, and H. Yamawaki (Pediatrics, Keio University); K. Sano, S. Manaka, and H. Shimizu (Neurosurgery, Tokyo, University); R. Inoue, K. Seki, M. Nakamura, K. Tomita, M. Inagaki, T. Yamazaki, and T. Sato (Psychiatry, Juntendo University); N. Yamaguchi, J. Sano, H. Kawada (Psychiatry, Kanazawa University); S. Okamoto, S. Kamiya, K. Minami, S. Kita (Psychiatry, Kansai Medical College); H. Hori, S. Miyamoto, H. Terada, T. Naito, K. Kinugawa, S. Utsumi (Neurosurgery, Nara University); S. Ohtahara, Y. Yamatogi, Y. Ohtsuka (Pediatrics, Okayama University); K. Hosokawa, T. Kugoh (Psychiatry, Okayama University); H. Hazama, R. Kawahara (Psychiatry, Tottori University); H. Yamada, H. Yoshida, H. Ninomiya, Y. Kato (Pediatrics, Kyushu University); K. Inanaga, Y. Nakazawa, M. Kotorii, M. Ohoshima, T. Kotorii, H. Hasuzawa, T. Ohokawa, H. Sakurada, K. Nonaka (Psychiatry, Kurume University); K. Sarai, H. Kodama, T. Nakahara, K. Nakagawa, M. Tamazaki (Psychiatry, Hiroshima University); K. Sumi (Pediatrics, Osaka University); J. Mukawa (Neurosurgery, Osaka University); and T. Kitagawa (Neurology, Tottori University).

REFERENCES

Akimoto, H., and Okamoto, T. (1940): Prognosis of epilepsy. *Psychiatr. Neurol. Jpn.*, 44:471 (*Jap.*).

Currie, S., Healthfield, K. W. G., Henson, R. A., and Scott, D. F. (1971): Clinical course and prognosis of temporal lobe epilepsy. A survey of 666 patients. *Brain*, 60:13.

Dalby, M. A. (1969): Epilepsy and 3 per second spike and wave rhythms. *Acta Neurol. Scand.* (*Suppl.* 40), 45:1–183.

Fukushima, Y. (1969): Prognosis and EEG of epilepsy with special reference to the focal spike abnormality. *Clinical EEG*, 11:287–290 (*Jap.*).

Gastaut, H. (1970): Clinical and electroencephalographic classifications of epileptic seizures (ILAE). *Epilepsia*, (*Amst.*), 11:102–113.

Habermaas, S. (1901): Ueber die Prognose der Epilepsie. *Z. Psychiatr.*, 58:243–253.

Livingston, S., Torres, I., Pauli, L. L., and Rider, R. V. (1965): Petit mal epilepsy: results of a prolonged follow-up study of 117 patients. *JAMA*, 194:227–232.

Okuma, T. (1977): Prognosis of epilepsy: a preliminary report of a multi-institutional study in Japan. *Folia Psychiatr. Neurol. Jpn.*, 31:291–299.

Rodin, E. A. (1968): *The Prognosis of Patients with Epilepsy*. Charles C Thomas, Springfield, Illinois.

Turner, W. A. (1907): *Epilepsy. A Study of the Idiopathic Disease*. Macmillan, London.

Uchimura, Y., Taen, S., Shimazono, Y., and Kawada, H. (1952): Prognosis and classification of epileptic seizures. In: *The Study of Epilepsy*, edited by Y. Uchimura, pp. 218–229. Igaku-Shoin, Tokyo (in Japanese).

Wada, T. (1962): Present state of anti-epileptic drug treatment in Japan. *Rihsho-to-Kenkyu*, 40:914 (*Jap.*).

Advances in Epileptology:
The Xth Epilepsy International Symposium,
edited by J. A. Wada and J. K. Penry.
Raven Press, New York © 1980.

Remission and Relapse of Seizures in Epilepsy

*J. F. Annegers, **W. A. Hauser,
*L. R. Elveback, and *L. T. Kurland

*Department of Medical Statistics and Epidemiology,
Mayo Clinic, Rochester, Minnesota 55901; and
*Department of Neurology, College of Physicians
and Surgeons, Columbia University,
New York, New York 10032

Our study is concerned with several key questions: (a) What are the chances that patients with epilepsy will have remissions of their seizures? (b) Does the likelihood of a remission vary by seizure type, sex, age of onset, or predisposing cause? (c) What are the prospects for discontinuing anticonvulsant medication, as well as being seizure-free sometime in the future?

We have attempted to answer these questions by a follow-up study of a cohort of patients with epilepsy.

METHODS

The medical records linkage system of the Mayo Clinic has been utilized to identify all diagnosed cases of epilepsy in the population of Rochester, Minnesota. A total of 618 patients had their initial diagnosis of epilepsy while residents of Rochester between 1935 and 1974. All have had at least two seizures that did not appear to be provoked by an acute cause. Thus, this series excludes over 1,000 Rochester residents who had febrile convulsions or other symptomatic convulsions and 159 patients who had one seizure without an apparent cause. The patients we have included were followed through the medical records and by follow-up inquiries from the date of diagnosis of epilepsy, usually the time of their second seizure.

For purposes of this discussion, remission of epilepsy is defined as a seizure-free period of 5 years. A relapse is one or more seizures after a remission. We also consider the prospect for successfully discontinuing anticonvulsant medication after the patient has been without seizures or medication for at least 5 years.

Of the 618 Rochester patients with epilepsy, 475 have been followed at least 5 years from diagnosis. Among the others, 93 died within 5 years of diagnosis and 50 have been followed less than 5 years. Of those followed at least 5 years, our information concerning subsequent seizures and anticonvulsant medication was judged inadequate for 18, and these were deleted from this analysis. Thus, our study is concerned with 457 patients, of which 328 were followed at least 10 years and 141 at least 20 years.

The net probabilities of remission have been determined by actuarial methods, with the risk of death set at zero. The results at each time interval after diagnosis apply to the survivors to that time.

RESULTS

The prognosis in all patients is presented in three ways in Fig. 1. The time scale begins at 5 years and the probabilities refer to completion of 5 seizure-free years. Another and convenient interpretation involves subtracting 5 years from each point on the time scale, in which case the ordinate corresponds to the probability of entering a 5-year period free of seizures. For example, at 1 year after diagnosis, 42% of the patients have entered this 5-year remission state and at 2 years, 51%. The longer patients continue to have seizures after the date of initial diagnosis, the lower the probability of a subsequent remission. The estimates of prognosis, therefore, apply only from diagnosis.

The top curve is the probability of ever being in remission (i.e., 5 years seizure-free from the 6th through the 20th years after diagnosis). The probability of ever achieving remission is 65% by 10 years and 76% by 20 years. The second curve is the net probability of being in remission a given point in

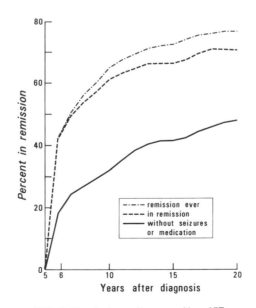

FIG. 1. Remission, all cases; *N* = 457.

time. The fact that some patients have a relapse of seizures after being in remission accounts for the difference in these two curves. The net probability of being seizure-free at 10 years after diagnosis for all cases is 61%, and this slowly rises to 70% at 20 years. You will note that both curves become rather stable 10 to 15 years after diagnosis. The percent in remission did not change between 20 and 30 years.

The bottom curve presents the probability of being without seizures for 5 years and not taking anticonvulsant medication. As we would expect, the initial slope of this curve is much less than the slope for remission but it continues to rise throughout the 20 years. Ten years after diagnosis, almost one-third of the patients have been without seizures or medication for 5 years, and by 20 years after diagnosis this figure approaches 50%. Thus, 20 years after the initial diagnosis, about 30% continue to have seizures, 20% are using anticonvulsant medications but have been without recent seizures, and one-half have been without seizures or anticonvulsant medication for at least 5 years.

When one reviews the literature, it is apparent that these rates of remission are greater than those that have usually been reported. In most reports about one-third of all patients achieve remission of epilepsy, usually using a 2-year seizure-free definition (Rodin, 1972). In our cohort, 76% of all patients achieve remission within 20 years of diagnosis. However, our data and that of the others cannot be readily compared. First, the duration of follow-up is usually less than in our material. The chance of remission increases with the period of follow-up, although we have found that 15 years after diagnosis, there is little likelihood of remission. More important, our cases are derived from the total population and not from a selected specialty clinic or institution. Thus, it includes the entire spectrum of cases of epilepsy in the community from the mildest to the most severe. Another major difference is that the prognostic assessment begins at the time of diagnosis, frequently the second seizure. If a series consists of patients who have had seizures for longer periods of time, their follow-up would begin after the annual rates of remission have diminished considerably. For example, the net probability of all patients achieving remission within 10 years after diagnosis is 65%. However, patients who still have seizures 5 years after the diagnosis have only a 21% chance of going into remission during the next 10 years.

The prospects for remission are not the same for all subgroups of the epilepsy cohort. We have classified the patients into three groups according to presumed etiology: first, idiopathic, or those without a known predisposing cause; second, those with secondary epilepsy, or those with central nervous system (CNS) lesions acquired postnatally from trauma, brain tumor, cerebrovascular disease, infection, or chronic degeneration; and third, patients with major neurological dysfunction present or presumed to have been present at birth, manifested by cerebral palsy, mental retardation, i.e., I.Q. under 70, or a CNS malformation.

The idiopathic group has 335 patients, and for this group the net probability of being in remission after 20 years is 74%. The 73 patients with secondary epilepsy have slightly lower rates of remission in the earlier years, but eventually the prospects for remission among the survivors are quite good. The 49 patients with major neurological dysfunction from birth have only a 46% net probability of a remission by 20 years.

The idiopathic cases tend to discontinue anticonvulsant medication much more rapidly than the secondary or the congenital neuro-dysfunction group. Ten years after diagnosis, 36% of the idiopathic group, but less than 20% of the secondary group, have been without seizures or medication for at least 5 years.

The remission rates in idiopathic epilepsy are higher for patients with generalized onset seizures than those whose seizures are focal at onset. By 20 years after diagnosis, 85% of those with generalized tonic clonic seizures and 80% with absence seizures are in remission, whereas the rate for partial complex seizures is 65%. There are also large differences in treatment. By 20 years after diagnosis, over one-half of those with generalized onset seizures have been seizure-free and have discontinued medication whereas only 35% of those with partial complex seizures achieve this status.

Among those with idiopathic epilepsy, younger patients have a more favorable prognosis. Ten years after diagnosis, the probability of being in remission is 75% in those whose epilepsy was diagnosed under age ten, 68% among those diagnosed from age 10 to 19 years, and 63% among those diagnosed between 20 to 59 years of age. If we consider medication as well, the age differentiation is even greater. At 10 years after diagnosis, 51% of those with diagnosis under 10 years of age have had no seizures or medication for 5 years; 40% of those age 10 to 19 years, 28% of those age 20 to 59 years, and only 6% of those age 60 years or more.

Relapse

In our cohort, 45 of the 305 patients with a remission (followed a total of 2,750 person-years) had subsequent seizures. Since we would expect only about one new case of epilepsy to occur during this follow up, it is apparent that virtually all represent relapses. The average annual rate of relapse is 1.6%. Most relapses occurred in the first 10 years, and all in the first 20 years after remission. Among all patients, the net probability of a relapse the first 5 years after a remission is 8%, to 10 years after remission is 15%, and 24% through 20 years. The net probabilities of relapse vary greatly by seizure type. The net probabilities for relapse 20 years after remission are 6% for those with absence seizures, 21% for those with generalized tonic clonic seizures, and 32% for partial complex seizures. The chances for relapse are lowest among those under age 9 at diagnosis, 13% by 20 years after remission. Among those age 10 to 19 years, it is 22% and in those age 20 to 59 years, 32%.

CONCLUSIONS

In our longitudinal study of patients with epilepsy from Rochester, Minnesota, we find that the net probability of being in remission is 70% 20 years after diagnosis. The rates of remission in this series are generally higher than those reported previously. Three major factors apparently account for this difference: first, the long follow-up in this series; second, the cases of epilepsy include all that occurred in a defined population; and third, the prognosis for follow-up begins with the initial diagnosis of epilepsy.

The prognosis is poor for epilepsy associated with congenital neurological dysfunctions. The survivors of postnatally acquired epilepsy, as well as those with idiopathic seizures have good prospects for eventual remission. The prospects for remission are best in patients with generalized onset seizures and epilepsy diagnosed under 10 years of age. The prognosis is less favorable for partial complex seizures and adult onset epilepsy.

ACKNOWLEDGMENT

This study was supported in part by NIH contract NO1–NS–5–2327.

REFERENCE

Rodin, E. A. (1972): Medical and social prognosis in epilepsy. *Epilepsia (Amst.)*, 13:121–131.

Advances in Epileptology:
The Xth Epilepsy International Symposium,
edited by J. A. Wada and J. K. Penry.
Raven Press, New York © 1980.

Prognosis of West Syndrome with Special Reference to Lennox Syndrome: A Developmental Study

Shunsuke Ohtahara, Yasuko Yamatogi,
Yoko Ohtsuka, Eiji Oka, and Takashi Ishida

Department of Pediatrics, Okayama University,
Medical School, Shikata-Cho, Okayama 700, Japan

It is generally known that epilepsy in childhood is characterized by specific clinical and electroencephalographic (EEG) features that undergo changes as the child ages. This fact must be taken into consideration in the long-term prognosis of epilepsy in childhood.

West and Lennox syndromes have the typical characteristic of displaying developmental disorders, and, therefore, emphasis on the developmental aspect is especially important in the study of their prognosis.

CONCEPT AND CATEGORIZATION OF AGE-DEPENDENT EPILEPTIC ENCEPHALOPATHY

The authors would like to apply the term "age-dependent epileptic encephalopathy" to a group of epileptic disorders comprising the aforesaid syndromes and the "early-infantile epileptic encephalopathy with suppression-burst (EIEE)" (Ohtahara et al., 1976, *a* and *b*).

These encephalopathies share the following common characteristics: (a) age dependency, (b) characteristic minor seizures, (c) outstanding epileptic EEG abnormality, (d) heterogenous etiology, (e) frequent association of mental defect, and (f) refractoriness to treatment and grave prognosis.

It is important to note that a mutual transition occurred among these three encephalopathies. There was a considerable number of cases whose clinical course developed with age from EIEE to West syndrome and then from West to Lennox syndrome (Ohtahara, 1978).

Underlying pathologies in cases of these encephalopathies are quite heterogenous, and there is no particular difference among the three groups. If a common polyetiology underlies all the characteristic clinico-electroencephalographic patterns in each syndrome, specific ages must act as the only conjugate factor associated with their pathogenesis.

In other words, these encephalopathies can be regarded as an age-specific form of epileptic reaction against diverse, nonspecific exogenous causes that occur at specific developmental stages of brain maturation. This hypothesis is supported by the fact that evolution from one to another of these three encephalopathies occurs with age.

MUTUAL RELATIONSHIP AMONG THE ENCEPHALOPATHIES AND THEIR SEQUENTIAL TRANSITION

A long-term follow-up study was made for elucidation of age dependency, prognosis, and mutual relationship between these three types of encephalopathies.

In 10 cases of EIEE, suppression-burst was confirmed until 6 months after birth in one case, but in the others it became indistinct after almost 3 months and gradually disappeared. Interestingly, in six of nine cases, hypsarhythmia developed in the EEG between 3 to 10 months of age. In four of these six cases, moreover, evolution to West syndrome was observed clinically. It is clear from the above findings that EIEE is closely correlated with West syndrome. It has to be pointed out that, because of the limited cases and period of the follow-up study, the question of whether West syndrome, when evolved from EIEE, displays any specific features has not yet been made clear in the present study.

West syndrome was seen to evolve to Lennox syndrome with progress of age in 51 (54.3%) of 94 cases in our series, whereas history of West syndrome was found in 42 (36.2%) of 116 cases of Lennox syndrome.

LONG-TERM PROGNOSIS OF WEST SYNDROME

The above-mentioned findings clearly suggest that prognosis of these epileptic encephalopathies should be studied from the developmental point of view with due regard to the mutual relationship among them. This is the point the authors would like to emphasize. However, no studies on the long-term prognosis of these encephalopathies seem to have been conducted from this standpoint.

In the present chapter, the prognosis of West syndrome is mainly discussed with respect to its relationship with Lennox syndrome.

The subject studied includes 108 cases with West syndrome.

The long-term follow-up study of these cases was conducted for a period of 3 to 17 years, with the average period being 7 years and 8 months.

Table 1 indicates the results. Since a high incidence of mental defect is an important characteristic of West syndrome, its prognosis should be discussed with special reference to mentality as well as to seizure control. As many as 92 cases (85.2%) had accompanying mental defects whereas only 16 cases (14.8%) remained intact.

TABLE 1. *Clinical state on follow-up in patients with West syndrome*

No gross mental defect (I.Q. > 75)		16 (14.8%)
Persistence of Lennox syndrome	1 (6.3%)	
Transition to other seizure types	1 (6.3%)	
Free from seizure	14 (87.5%)	
With gross mental defect (I.Q. < 75)		92 (85.2%)
Persistence of Lennox syndrome	54 (58.7%)	
Transition to other seizure types	8 (8.7%)	
Free from seizure	30 (32.6%)	
Total		108 cases

Of 108 cases, 64 (59.3%) had persistent seizure whereas 44 cases (40.7%) had controlled seizure. It was noteworthy that, of the persistent cases, as many as 55 (85.9%) showed the evolution to Lennox syndrome that remained persistent. It was also noted that, of the controlled 44 cases, 35 cases (79.6%) were affected only with West syndrome that was controlled without shifting to any other seizure type.

The findings in Table 1 suggest that the presence of mental defects noted at the time of follow-up resulted in a great difference in the distribution of intractable cases: A large number of mentally defective cases were intractable and persistently affected with the Lennox syndrome. This indicates the refractoriness of this syndrome. In the prognosis of West syndrome, therefore, the Lennox syndrome occupies an important place.

On the other hand, the results of follow-up on 116 cases of Lennox syndrome, persistent seizure was found in 71 (61.2%). Of these, 70 remained as Lennox syndrome, which testifies to the refractoriness of Lennox syndrome in spite of the progress in antiepileptic treatment.

It is noteworthy that mental defect was present in 40 of 42 cases of Lennox syndrome that had evolved from West syndrome, and seizure remained in 31 of these 40 cases.

The aforementioned facts indicate that prognosis for the Lennox syndrome is especially unsatisfactory in cases evolved from West syndrome and that persistent seizure in patients with West syndrome are mostly those of Lennox syndrome.

The authors should like to stress, therefore, that prognosis for both West and Lennox syndromes should be studied with special attention to a mutual relationship.

Generally the factors affecting the prognosis for West syndrome are enumerated as follows: (a) underlying disease, (b) age at onset of seizures, (c) treatment lag, (d) EEG, (e) radiological signs of cerebral atrophy, and (f) neurological abnormalities (Yamatogi et al., 1977).

We will mention briefly the important items in our own study.

With respect to the relationship between the age of onset and prognosis, the cases with onset from 3 to 9 months after birth apparently took a favorable course, whereas those with onset earlier or later than the above period showed an unfavorable prognosis.

Regarding the relationship between EEG pattern and prognosis, those cases with asymmetric hypsarrhythmia showed a markedly poor prognosis in seizure control and mentality. Treatment lag also affects the prognosis: the shorter the treatment lag the better the prognosis and vice versa. The authors presume that the problem of transition to Lennox syndrome is above all the major factor determining the prognosis of West syndrome.

For the clinician, the greatest concern should be whether or not seizures can be controlled in the stage of West syndrome. It is almost certain that there must be other factors than that of age involved in the mechanism for evolution of West syndrome to that of Lennox. Elucidation of such a mechanism is an important task for the future, and could lead to the clarification of the pathogenesis of Lennox syndrome.

MENTAL DETERIORATION IN PATIENTS WITH WEST SYNDROME

One of the important characteristics of epileptic encephalopathies is a high incidence of the complication of mental defect. It is also an important fact that the seizures observed in epileptic encephalopathies are "minor seizures" but they give rise to progressive mental deterioration.

In order to study this matter, the authors followed up for more than 3 years 28 idiopathic cases of West syndrome who had been free from developmental retardation prior to the initial seizure. Even in this group a large number of cases were found to have deterioration after seizure, including five cases of idiots. Furthermore, the severity of deterioration was correlated with the duration of seizures.

The minor seizures are presumed to have provoked mental deterioration. This fact also suggests the importance of controlling seizures at the earliest possible stage.

The authors presume that the subcortical structures, especially of the thalamus and its surrounding structures, are largely involved in the pathophysiology of both syndromes (Ohtahara, 1977).

In order to follow this question further from a neurophysiological viewpoint, the authors studied it from the aspect of visual evoked potential (VEP). The authors previously reported that VEP can be a useful indication from the dynamic aspect for the functional development of the brain (Ohtahara, 1974). From this point of view, VEPs of 56 patients with West syndrome were measured and follow-up study was done for chronological changes.

As compared with the mean value of normal children (Ban, 1974), increased latency was apparently observed in a majority of these cases. The relationship between the state of psychomotor development and VEP latency at the time of first consultation was investigated. The latencies of all eight cases having normal development were within normal range. In the retarded cases, however, as many as 16 of 25 cases showed increased latency.

A follow-up study of the five cases who displayed mentally normal development at the time of first consultation revealed that in three cases of mental deterioration with aging, a gradual increase of latency was observed, whereas in the remaining two cases who have been intact thereafter such a tendency was not seen.

CONCLUSIONS

The authors have pointed out that age-dependent epileptic encephalopathies (EIEE, West, and Lennox syndromes) develop in the course of brain maturation during childhood and the three syndromes are mutually transferred with aging. Therefore, their prognosis should be studied with special attention to mutual relation.

This chapter has dealt with the findings of a long-term follow-up study on 108 cases of West syndrome observed for more than 3 to 17 years while the patients were receiving treatment from the author's group.

Ninety-two cases (85.2%) had mental defects. Persistent seizure was found in 64 cases (59.3%), and was observed in a high percentage among the mentally defective cases. It was noted that the persistent seizure type was found in as many as 55 cases (85.9%) of Lennox syndrome. It was pointed out that this means a majority of refractory cases in West syndrome are taking a converted course to Lennox syndrome. It is still unknown, however, what types of West syndrome will evolve to Lennox syndrome.

The suggested factors affecting the prognosis of West syndrome include age of onset, EEG pattern, and treatment lag. The transition to Lennox syndrome is, however, the primary clinical problem in the prognosis of West syndrome. Therefore, the utmost effort should be given in the future to probe any factors involving this phenomenon. It has been pointed out, finally, that minor seizures in West syndrome can be a causative factor for mental deterioration. The results of a VEP study for the purpose of elucidating the underlying mechanisms of this phenomenon are also discussed. The authors are of the opinion that these findings will provide a new insight and standpoint for neurophysiological research on mental deterioration.

REFERENCES

Ban, T. (1974): A study on development of visual evoked potential during infancy and childhood. *Acta Paediatr. Jpn.*, 78:548–558 (*Jap.*).

Ohtahara, S. (1974): Developmental aspects of electroencephalography. *Pediatr. Rev.*, 7:372–408 (*Jap.*).

Ohtahara, S., Ishida, T., Oka, E., et al. (1976a): On the specific age-dependent epileptic syndrome: The early-infantile epileptic encephalopathy with suppression-burst. *Brain Develop.*, 8:270–280 (*Jap.*).

Ohtahara, S., Yamatogi, Y. and Ohtsuka, Y. (1976*b*): Prognosis of the Lennox syndrome. *Folia Psychiatr. Neurol. Jpn.*, 30:275–287.

Ohtahara, S. (1977): A study on the age-dependent epileptic encephalopathy, *Brain Develop.*, 9:2–21 (*Jap.*).

Ohtahara, S., Yamatogi, Y., Ohtsuka, Y., et al. (1977): Prognosis in childhood epilepsy: A prospective follow-up study. *Folia Psychiatr. Neurol. Jpn.*, 31:301–313.

Ohtahara, S. (1978): Clinico-electrical delineation of epileptic encephalopathies in childhood. *Asian Med. J.*, 21:499–509.

Yamatogi, Y., Ohtsuka, Y., and Ohtahara, S. (1977): Prognosis of West and Lennox syndrome: An electroencephalographic study. *Clin. EEG*, 19:456–465 (in Japanese).

Advances in Epileptology:
The Xth Epilepsy International Symposium,
edited by J. A. Wada and J. K. Penry.
Raven Press, New York © 1980.

Outcomes of Infants with Neonatal Seizures

*,**Kenton R. Holden, *,**John M. Freeman,
and **,†E. David Mellits

*Departments of *Neurology, **Pediatrics, and †Biostatistics,
Johns Hopkins University School of Medicine,
Baltimore, Maryland 21205*

The NIH Collaborative Perinatal Project prospectively registered a population of approximately 54,000 randomly selected pregnant women for the purpose of studying the mothers throughout pregnancy and the infants from birth through 7 years of age. Two hundred seventy-seven infants (0.5%) had documented neonatal seizures.

The neonatal seizure population (NSP) was compared with the general collaborative study population (CSP). A number of parameters were examined to determine what relationship, if any, existed between each parameter and the eventual outcome of the child who had experienced neonatal seizures.

DESCRIPTION OF POPULATION

The 277 neonates with seizure activity were classified as to seizure type, onset, duration, number, treatment, and laboratory data. Excluded were neonates who were only jittery, hyper- or hypotonic, had myoclonic jerks, or had apnea spells unaccompanied by definite seizure activity. The NSP included 130 whites, 124 blacks, and 23 infants of other races. There were 157 males and 120 females. While the socioeconomic index of the NSP was similar to that of the CSP, the percentage of mothers greater than 30 years of age exceeded that of the CSP. There were fewer primiparas and more mothers who had had more than five pregnancies in the NSP than in the CSP as well as a greater percentage of women in the NSP who had experienced prior perinatal losses.

The mean birth weight of the NSP was 2,849 g, with an excess as compared with the CSP of infants less than 2,500 g and greater than 4,000 g. The mean Apgar score was 5.3 at 1 min and 6.8 at 5 min for the NSP. At 5 min 34.8% had an Apgar score of ≤ 6 and 17.2% had a score ≤ 3.

The onset of the initial neonatal seizure occurred during the first 24 hr of life in 37.9% of the NSP, during the second 24 hr in 24.9%, and during the third 24 hr in 14.4%. In 86.3% of cases seizures had begun by the end of the first week of life.

RESULTS

Death

Of the 277 infants comprising the NSP, 96 (34.7%) died. Of the 96 deaths, 29.2% occurred in the first 36 hr. Two-thirds of the deaths occurred in the neonatal period. Significant positive correlations were found between death and: (a) birth weight ($p < 0.001$), (b) gestational age ($p < 0.05$), (c) a 5-min Apgar score of < 7 ($p < 0.001$), (d) number of days of seizures ($p < 0.001$), and (e) duration of seizure, i.e., less than or greater than 30 min ($p < 0.01$).

When apnea spells were present in addition to seizures, only 40% of the infants survived; without apnea spells, there was a 77% survival rate ($p < 0.001$). The time of onset of the first seizure was significantly related both to the percent of infants who died ($p < 0.001$) and to the time of death ($p < 0.001$).

Autopsy results were available in 77 of the 96 deaths. Fifty-three of the 77 autopsies revealed CNS involvement. These 53 included 14 with congenital CNS anomalies, 13 with CNS infection, and 26 with evidence of significant intracranial bleeding.

Cerebral Palsy

Of the 181 survivors in the NSP, 21 (11.6%) had moderate or severe cerebral palsy (CP) at 7 years of age, and 4 (2.2%) had mild, nonhandicapping CP. Eleven additional infants with CP are not included in the 7-year data due to death before the age of 7.

Although the NSP survivors comprised less than 1% of the entire CSP survivors, NSP survivors accounted for 21% of the moderate or severe CP cases found among the entire CSP. Cerebral palsy types included six with hemiparesis, nine with diplegia (of whom four died), and 18 with quadriplegia (of whom seven died). There were three "pure" ataxias/dyskinesias and 10 "mixed" with other palsies. An infant from the NSP who survived was 30 to 40 times more likely to have CP at age 7 years than an infant from the CSP and was 55 to 75 times more likely to have moderate or severe CP. It should be noted, however, that 88.4% of the NSP survivors did not have handicapping CP.

Mental Retardation

Mental retardation (full-scale I.Q. < 70) was present in 31 NSP survivors (18.8%). Twenty-five (15.2%) had a full-scale I.Q. of 70 to 79.

NSP survivors with a normal full scale I.Q. had had a mean 5-min Apgar score of 7.8, which was significantly different ($p < 0.0005$) from the mean Apgar of 5.3 for those who were retarded.

Of the various types of neonatal seizures, tonic stiffening and myoclonic correlated with mental retardation ($p < 0.05$). There was also a significant difference ($p < 0.001$) between the number of days of seizures for those who had a normal I.Q. (2.3 days) and those who were retarded (4.5 days). Neonates who had had any seizure lasting longer than 30 min were more likely ($p < 0.001$) to be retarded at 7 years of age.

Mental retardation correlated significantly ($p < 0.001$) with moderate and severe CP and later epilepsy.

Subsequent Seizures

The NSP included 47 children (22.0%) who had at least one afebrile seizure after the neonatal period. Of these, 9 had multiple types of seizures. Twenty-three (12.7%) had at least one afebrile seizure after 3 years of age and were considered cases of active epilepsy. The types of subsequent seizures included generalized tonic-clonic (23); focal motor (13), minor motor (16), and temporal lobe (1). Fifteen had subsequent febrile convulsions. Epilepsy, mental retardation, and cerebral palsy commonly coexisted.

SUMMARY

An infant who experienced neonatal seizures had a 34.7% chance of dying, with two-thirds of the deaths occurring during the neonatal period. One hundred twenty-eight (70.7%) of the 181 survivors had no major neurological deficit. The major neurological outcomes of infants who experienced neo-

TABLE 1. *Outcome at age 7 Years of children from neonatal seizure population*

Race	*n*	Dead	Survived age 7	CP	MR	Seiz.	Survived Age 7 with no CP, MR, or seiz.
White	130	39	91	15	15	9	67
Percent survived				16.5	16.5	9.9	73.6
Black	124	51	73	5	12	11	51
Percent survived				6.8	16.4	15.1	69.9
Other	23	6	17	1	4	3	10
Percent survived				5.9	23.5	17.6	58.8
Total	277	96	181	21	31	23	128
Percent survived				11.6	18.8	12.7	70.7

Abbreviations: CP, moderate or severe cerebral palsy; MR, I.Q. < 70; 165 of 181 were tested; Seiz, afebrile seizures after age 3 years.

A number of children had a combination of CP, MR, and/or seiz.

natal seizures are summarized in Table 1. The infant who survived had an 11.6% chance of having moderate or severe CP, an 18.8% chance of having mental retardation, a 22.0% chance of having subsequent afebrile seizures, and a 12.7% chance of having active epilepsy. There were a significant number of patients with a combination of neurological deficits. Low birth weight, Apgar less than 7, a neonatal seizure lasting longer than 30 min, an early onset time, a greater number of days of seizures, and seizures with accompanying apnea spells all had a significant adverse effect on the outcome.

ACKNOWLEDGMENT

Supported in part by NIH grant 03-11-000-143-06.

Advances in Epileptology:
The Xth Epilepsy International Symposium,
edited by J. A. Wada and J. K. Penry.
Raven Press, New York © 1980.

Course and Prognosis of Certain Childhood Epilepsies with Predominantly Myoclonic Seizures

Jean Aicardi

Institut National de la Sante et de la Recherche Medicale,
INSERM, U 154, 75674, Paris, Cedex 14, France

Childhood epilepsies featuring predominantly myoclonic phenomena still raise unsolved nosological and clinical problems (Harper, 1968; Aicardi and Chevrie, 1971; Loiseau, 1971, Jeavons, 1977). Since myoclonic seizures often present as falls or head-noddings, the myoclonic epilepsies are often confused with infantile spasms or with Lennox-Gastaut syndrome, depending on the age of affected children. Moreover, myoclonic phenomena are a common feature of widely different types of epilepsy. Some of them belong to progressive encephalopathies of a metabolic origin (Tassinari et al., 1976). Others are associated with static encephalopathies, especially postanoxic ones (Aicardi and Chevrie, 1971). Myoclonic seizures unassociated with diffuse cerebral lesions may belong to epilepsies already well defined, such as those of the generalized epilepsies of adolescence or early adulthood (Janz and Christian, 1957; Janz, 1976), photosensitive epilepsies (Jeavons, 1977), or certain forms of petit mal (Tassinari et al., 1969).

RESULTS

Patients

This chapter reports on 55 cases of epilepsy characterized by prominent myoclonic seizures, selected among a series of 141 children with various myoclonic phenomena, according to the following criteria: (a) massive myoclonias of brief duration (less than 3 sec), frequently repeated, as the main seizure type; (b) bilateral synchronous bursts of spike waves or polyspike waves at a rhythm of 3 per sec or more, generally arrhythmical, lasting less than 5 sec, ictal or interictal; (c) no evidence of a static or a progressive encephalopathy; and (d) lack of associated tonic seizures. Patients in whom petit mal absences were present in association with the myoclonias, as defined above, were excluded.

Thirty-three patients were boys and 22 were girls. Mean age at the time of the first seizure was 23 months, and 31 months at the time of the first myoclonia (range: 3 months–9 years, 5 months). Age of onset of myoclonic seizures was before 1 year in 10 patients (18%), before 2 years in 20 patients (36%), and before 3 years in 37 children (67%). The mean follow-up was 75 months (6 years, 3 months) ± 49.5 months (SD). The range was from 8 months to 22 years.

Clinical Features

The myoclonic seizures belonged to the bilaterally symmetrical or massive type in 48 children (87%). Head and trunk were most commonly affected but myoclonias of the lower limbs were responsible for repeated falls in 30 children (55%). In several patients, an atonic component was associated with the myoclonus, affecting predominantly the posterior neck muscles. In these patients a saccadic fall of the head forward was observed in association with active myoclonias of the upper limbs in the sitting position, whereas only the latter was apparent when the patient was lying down.

Ocular and facial myoclonias were recorded in 27 children (47%), almost always associated with massive myoclonias. Segmental and/or erratic myoclonias were rarely observed (7 patients or 13%). Myoclonic status occurred once or several times in 4 children (7%).

The myoclonic seizures occurred frequently each day in all patients.

Electroencephalographic Features

The clinical myoclonias were accompanied by bursts of polyspikes or polyspike wave complexes lasting less than 5 sec, with a rhythm of 3 per sec or more. These were always irregular and arrhythmic. They were recorded on the whole scalp but usually predominated in the fronto-central areas and were generally symmetrical (Fig. 1). In 8 patients, these bursts were associated with paroxysmal discharges of a different type, especially with polyspike waves at a rhythm of 2 per sec. All myoclonias occurring during the recording of EEG were accompanied by bursts of paroxysmal activity. Numerous bursts in the EEG remained without clinical expression. The paroxysmal EEG activity was activated by intermittent photic stimulation in 58% of the cases, and by hyperventilation in 40% of the 30 patients in whom it could be performed. The initial stages of sleep also increased the frequency of the discharges in 25% of the patients.

The first tracings displaying 3 per sec spike wave discharges were often recorded in very young patients. In 6 patients (11%) they were recorded before the age of 1 year, in 14 children before the age of 2 years (25%), and in 19 patients (35%) before 3 years. Mean age of the first EEG containing paroxysmal bursts was 40 months (range 4 months–13 years). As a rule, the occurrence of fast spike waves or polyspike waves under the age of 2 years is

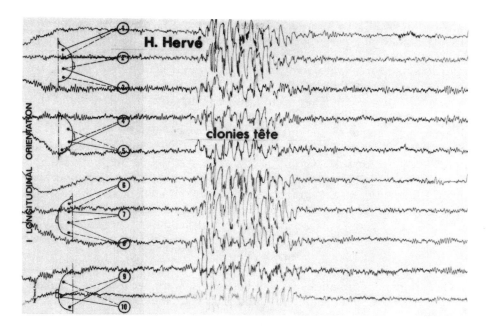

FIG. 1. Polyspike wave complexes (*see text*).

accompanied or announces epilepsies with a marked myoclonic component (Aicardi and Chevrie, 1973).

Associated Seizures

Thirty-one patients (56%) had seizures other than myoclonias, either prior to, or in association with their myoclonic seizures. These seizures were, most commonly, generalized ones, often exclusively clonic in nature. Unilateral seizures were known to have occurred in four children.

Course and Prognosis

At the end of follow-up, 27 patients (49%) had been seizure-free for a minimum of 1 year. Most of them were still on medication at that time and late recurrences have been observed in a few patients; thus our figures cannot be considered as a "cure-rate."

At the same time, 20 patients (36%) had a normal or borderline intellectual level (I.Q. ≥ 80). Thirty-five children (64%) had some degree of mental impairment. However, only six patients (11%) had an I.Q. of less than 51 and a majority were only slightly retarded.

We searched for factors influencing the prognosis. An early age of onset was not significantly associated with the persistence of seizures or with a low intellectual level at end of follow-up. Epileptic seizures occurring prior to the myoclonic seizures were significantly less frequent in those children who were seizure-free at the end of follow-up than in those who still had fits (29% versus 51%, $p < 0.02$). They were also less common in those without intellectual deficit at the end of follow-up. A suspect or abnormal mental development antecedent to the myoclonias was significantly linked with the persistence of seizures (11% versus 46%, $p < 0.005$) and with mental subnormality (15% versus 51%, $p < 0.01$).

The effect of treatment was difficult to assess as the course was spontaneously a fluctuating one. Nitrazepam, clonazepam, and sodium dipropylacetate seemed at least partly effective. Ethosuximide appeared dramatically effective in six patients who had never experienced any other seizure type.

Etiologic Factors

Gestational abnormalities or a difficult birth were recorded in 8 patients but were not of a severe nature, making their etiologic role difficult to assess. The distribution of birthweights was not different from that in the general population, and only one infant weighed less than 2,500 g at birth.

A family history of epilepsy and/or of febrile convulsions in first or second degree relatives was found in 21 cases (38%). This proportion is as high or higher than in a series of febrile convulsions (Chevrie and Aicardi, 1975) and suggests that genetic factors play a significant role in this type of myoclonic epilepsy.

DISCUSSION

On the basis of the criteria outlined above, it seems possible to tentatively isolate, among the many types of epilepsy of infancy and childhood featuring prominent myoclonic phenomena, a group of patients with a distinctive EEG and clinical picture and a relatively good prognosis. Such patients are often misdiagnosed as cases of Lennox-Gastaut syndrome, or of infantile spasms when the onset is before 1 year of age. The prognosis for children fulfilling the criteria for "cryptogenic myoclonic epilepsy" is, however, much less unfavorable than that in Lennox syndrome or infantile spasms, and the clinical and EEG picture is different. Tonic and atonic seizures and atypical absences are lacking or inconspicuous and the slow spike wave pattern is not commonly encountered, whereas fast polyspike wave complexes are predominant. Clinical and EEG diagnosis of "cryptogenic myoclonic epilepsy" is thus feasible and makes it possible to avoid grave errors in prognosis.

The exact limits of the syndrome are difficult to delineate and the present series may well be a heterogeneous one. Transitional forms exist and similar patients have been reported as having a myoclonic variant of the Lennox syndrome (Erba and Lombroso, 1973) or as myoclonic astatic petit mal (Doose, 1964; Kruse, 1968: Doose et al., 1970) of the "centrencephalic" type.

We feel that the use of terms suggestive of the most severe types of childhood epilepsy is best avoided even though a definitive nosological classification of the myoclonic epilepsies is not yet available.

REFERENCES

Aicardi, J., and Chevrie, J. J. (1971): Myoclonic epilepsies of childhood. *Neuropädiatrie*, 3:177–190.

Aicardi, J., and Chevrie, J. J. (1973): The significance of electroencephalographic paroxysms in children less than three years of age. *Epilepsia*, 14:47–55.

Chevrie, J. J., and Aicardi, J. (1972): Childhood epileptic encephalopathy with slow spike-wave. A statistical study of 80 cases. *Epilepsia*, 13:259–271.

Chevrie, J. J., and Aicardi, J. (1975): Duration and lateralization of febrile convulsions. Etiological factors. *Epilepsia*, 16:787–789.

Doose, H. (1964): Das akinetische Petit Mal. I das klinische und elektroencephalographische Bild der akinetischen Anfälle. *Arch. Psychiatr. Nervenkr.*, 205:625–631.

Doose, H., Gerken, H., Leonhardt, R., Völzke, E., and Volz, C. (1970): Centrencephalic myoclonic-astatic petit mal. Clinical and genetic investigations. *Neuropädiatrie*, 2:59–78.

Erba, G., and Lombroso, C. T. (1973): La sindrome di Lennox-Gastaut. *Prospettive in Pediatria*, 3:145–165.

Harper, J. R. (1968): True myoclonic epilepsy in childhood. *Arch. Dis. Child.*, 43:28–35.

Janz, D., and Christian, W. (1957): Impulsive Petit Mal. *Dtsch. Z. Nervenheilk.*, 176:346–386.

Janz, D. (1976): The natural history of primary generalized epilepsies with sporadic myoclonias of the "impulsive Petit Mal" type. In: *Evolution and Prognosis of Epilepsies*, edited by E. Lugaresi, P. Pazzaglia, and C. A. Tassinari, pp. 55–61. Aulo Gaggi, Bologna.

Jeavons, P. M. (1977): Nosological problems of myoclonic epilepsies in childhood and adolescence. *Dev. Med. Child Neurol.*, 19:3–8.

Kruse, R. (1968): *Das myoklonisch-astatische Petit Mal*, p. 131. Springer, Berlin.

Loiseau, P. (1971): Epilepsies myocloniques. *Encephale*, 60:245–264.

Tassinari, C. A., Coccagna, G., and Dalla Bernardina, B. (1976): Dissinergia cerebellare mioclonica di Ramsay-Hunt, epilessia mioclonica progressiva di Unverricht-Lundborg con corpi di Lafora, neurolipidosi. In: *"L'Epilessie,"* edited by E. Lugaresi, P. Pazzaglia, and R. Canger. Aulo Gaggi, Bologna.

Tassinari, C. A., Lyagoubi, S., Santos, T., Gambarelli, G., Roger, J., Dravet, C., and Gastaut, H. (1969): Etude des decharges de pointes-ondes chez l'homme. Les aspects cliniques et électro-encephalographiques des absences myocloniques. *Rev. Neurol.*, 121:379–383.

Advances in Epileptology:
The Xth Epilepsy International Symposium,
edited by J. A. Wada and J. K. Penry.
Raven Press, New York © 1980.

Seizure History in Families: Factors Affecting Sibling Risk for Seizures

*W. A. Hauser, **Myra M. Chern, †V. E. Anderson,
and ††Asa Mayersdorf

*Departments of *Neurology, **Health Computer Sciences, †Genetics and Dight
Institute, University of Minnesota, and ††Veterans Administration Hospital,
Minneapolis, Minnesota*

Epilepsy has long been recognized as a common disorder caused by heterogeneous genetic and environmental mechanisms. The mode of inheritance, however, has been in question. It is our feeling, based on our own studies and those of others, that the inheritance of epilepsy is multifactorial. Given the correctness of this hypothesis, siblings of most patients with epilepsy will have an increased risk for seizures. Depending on the degree of genetic and common environmental effects, the risk for seizures in each sibship varies. The present analysis represents an attempt to evaluate individual variables as well as combinations of medical, demographic, and family history information in seizure probands to better assess the level of liability for seizures in their siblings.

Whereas previous studies have looked at the effect of single variables such as age at onset of epilepsy or specific EEG traits (i.e., spike wave patterns) on sibling risk for seizures, the present analysis represents a multivariate evaluation of numerous variables, utilizing a stepwise regression technique to select the more important combinations of variables that are associated with an increased sibling risk for seizures.

PATIENTS AND METHODS

The present study was performed as part of the Comprehensive Epilepsy Program for the State of Minnesota. The probands are 559 individuals with a new diagnosis of seizures or epilepsy at the University of Minnesota affiliated hospitals. Patients with diagnosis and treatment for convulsive disorder more than 3 months prior to their initial visit to the hospitals or

---

*Present address: Sergievsky Center, College of Physicians and Surgeons, Columbia University, New York, New York.

clinics and/or patients with the diagnosis of epilepsy prior to January 1, 1976 were excluded from this analysis.

The 559 probands have 2,282 siblings, 60 of whom (2.6%) have had seizures. Of the siblings, an additional 24 have had migraine headaches and 42 have had seizure-like symptoms, i.e., syncope.

Variables considered for the multivariate analysis were divided into three subcategories. The first category was family history data. In this, we included as potential risk factors a maternal or paternal history of seizures, and a maternal sibling or paternal sibling with history of seizures.

Clinical data analyzed included proband's age at onset of seizures, proband's seizure type (utilizing a modification of the international classification of epileptic seizures), presumed etiology of the proband's seizures, and selected EEG variables (photoconvulsive responses, generalized spike-and-wave discharges, 6 per second spike-and-wave, focal spikes and/or focal EEG slowing and rolandic spike discharges).

Demographic data analyzed included proband's sex, sibling's sex, sibling's age, paternal age at the sibling's birth, maternal age at sibling's birth, and sibship size.

The analysis was further modified by the seizure categorization of the proband. This included three separate subsets: first, a comparison between those probands with single seizures or acute symptomatic seizures with those experiencing more than one seizure episode (recurrent); second, a comparison between individuals with convulsions following an identified insult to the central nervous system (CNS) (remote symptomatic episodes), with those probands with seizures only occurring in association with acute CNS insults such as meningitis, stroke, or acute head trauma (acute symptomatic seizures) and those individuals with no discernible antecedent cause for the epilepsies (idiopathic cases). We then subdivided the idiopathic group according to presence or absence of CNS pathology (generally based on the findings at time of neurologic examination) and the presence or absence of specific EEG abnormalities, including focal abnormalities and generalized spike-and-waves.

A statistical procedure designed for analyzing categorical data at a multivariate level was programmed to handle the stepwise analysis (Higgins and Koch, 1977). At each step, the differences in the rate of seizures in the siblings were compared among the different groups of individuals representing different combinations of the variables.

RESULTS

The Pearson χ^2 calculated for cross-tabulations for seizures in siblings and each individual variable have been ranked in order of decreasing significance based on p-values of the χ^2. The variable most highly correlated with seizures in siblings was the proband's age at onset of seizures. This rate was significantly higher ($p = 0.00008$) for siblings of probands under age 20 at first seizure compared with siblings of probands with onset after age 20. Myoclonic seizures in the proband was the next most important single variable ($p = 0.002$). One or both parents affected ($p = 0.01$), presence of generalized spike-and-wave ($p = 0.07$) or a photoconvulsive response in the proband ($p = 0.04$) or maternal sibling history of seizures ($p = 0.15$) were all associated with an increased sibling risk for epilepsy. Risk was somewhat higher for siblings of probands with recurrent seizures (4%) when compared with those with single seizures (3%), and for siblings of female probands (3% versus 2%).

When we evaluated two-way combinations of the influencing variables, the probands with onset of epilepsy prior to age 20 and maternal sibling history of seizures demonstrated the highest risk for seizures ($p = 0.008$). This is followed by the following combinations: onset prior to age 20 and either generalized spike-and-wave ($p = 0.009$) or a focal EEG abnormality ($p = 0.01$). Risk to siblings of probands with onset of partial complex seizure prior to age 20 was also increased ($p = 0.01$).

The step-wise strategy was carried out for three more rounds. The collection of variables was terminated at a point where there were too few cases in individual cells to allow a meaningful χ^2 analysis. An additional three variables were included in the model. The 32 combinations of the five selected variables and their respective observed sibling risks for seizures are summarized in Table 1.

When examining the five-factor model, we found the highest seizure risk for siblings of female patients with seizures starting prior to age 20 with nonfocal EEGs and both a maternal and paternal sibling with seizures. The last three factors (presence or absence of focal EEG, proband's sex, and positive paternal family history of epilepsy) each provided little additive information.

On evaluating the risk for seizures among siblings with probands with "idiopathic seizures," the highest rate was among siblings of patients with both focal and generalized spike wave abnormalities (based on a small number of cases). Risk to siblings of probands with generalized spike waves alone was 4.8%. The risk for siblings of probands with focal EEG abnormalities was somewhat less than that for siblings of probands with normal EEGs or EEGs with nonspecific findings (2.4% versus 3.3%), although differences are not significant.

DISCUSSION

The importance of proband's age at onset of seizures for sibling risk has been documented by Eisner et al. (1959), who reported an increased risk for seizures among siblings of probands with idiopathic major motor epilepsy and first seizure occurring before age 16. Members of this study team previ-

TABLE 1. *Risk of seizure in siblings for a five-factor model*

Proband's onset age	Number of mother's siblings having seizures	Proband with focal EEG abnormality	Proband's sex	Number of father's siblings having seizures	
				No	Yes
≤19 0.055 (23/419)	0 0.049 (19/385)	No 0.031 (4/131)	M 0.029 (2/70)	0.031 (2/65)	0 (0/5)
			F 0.033 (2/61)	0.034 (2/59)	0 (0/2)
		Yes 0.069 (12/173)	M 0.048 (5/105)	0.043 (4/92)	0.077 (1/13)
			F 0.103 (7/68)	0.091 (6/66)	0.500 (1/2)
	1+ 0.118 (4/34)	No 0.190 (4/21)	M 0.500 (3/6)	0.400 (2/5)	1.00 (1/1)
			F 0.067 (1/15)	0.071 (1/14)	0 (0/0)
		Yes 0 (0/5)	M 0 (0/2)	0 (0/2)	0 (0/0)
			F 0 (0/3)	0 (0/3)	0 (0/0)
20+ 0.020 (37/1821)	0 0.021 (36/1754)	No 0.023 (20/886)	M 0.017 (12/691)	0.018 (12/681)	0 (0/0)
			F 0.041 (8/195)	0.041 (8/195)	0 (0/0)
		Yes 0.015 (10/654)	M 0.015 (7/476)	0.015 (7/458)	0 (0/18)
			F 0.017 (3/178)	0.018 (3/169)	0 (0/9)
	1+ 0.015 (1/67)	No 0.042 (1/24)	M 0.053 (1/19)	0.053 (1/19)	0 (0/0)
			F 0 (0/5)	0 (0/5)	0 (0/0)
		Yes 0 (0/33)	M 0 (0/16)	0 (0/16)	0 (0/0)
			F 0 (0/17)	0 (0/17)	0 (0/0)

ously reported an increased frequency of seizures among the offspring of epileptic females when compared with the population rates, whereas the offspring of epileptic males demonstrated no increased risk for seizures (Annegers et al., 1976). This, along with the observation that the average annual incidence rate for epilepsy is lower in females, led us to suggest a genetic loading hypothesis with a higher genetic threshold for seizure trait in females. The important effect of maternal sibling history of epilepsy and the effect of proband sex would seem to support this hypothesis. Paternal history of epilepsy seems to be important in our study, although up to this point it has the lower level of predictive value for sibling risk.

The observed lower risk for siblings of our probands with focal EEG abnormalities would seem to support the interpretations of studies in which seizure risk has been lower for relatives of neurologically handicapped patients compared to those without (Alstrom, 1950), and studies in which increased sibling risk has been associated with a spike wave trait in probands (Metrakos and Metrakos, 1960).

While most of the significant factors have been associated with increased sibling risk for seizures in previous reports, the relative importance of these variables has not been analyzed in combination. The relative level of importance of these predictors may be modified as our sample size increases. This statistical procedure seems promising for the development of a model of sibling risk for epilepsy. Predictive information derived will be of considerable value to the clinician for genetic counseling and, in addition, will be useful in understanding the underlying heterogenicity.

ACKNOWLEDGMENTS

This study was supported in part by NIH contract NO1-NS-5-2327.

REFERENCES

Alstrom, C. H. (1950): A study of epilepsy in its clinical, social, and genetic aspects. *Acta Psychiatr. Neurol. Scand. (Suppl.)*, 63:5–276.

Annegers, J. F., Elveback, L. R., Hauser, W. A., Anderson, V. E., and Kurland, L. T. (1976): Seizures in the offspring of patients with a history of seizures. *Epilepsia*, 17:1–9.

Eisner, V., Pauli, L. L., and Livingston, S. (1959): Hereditary aspects of epilepsy. *Johns Hopkins Hospital Bull.*, 108:245–271.

Higgins, J. E., and Koch, G. G. (1977): Variable selection and generalized Chi-square analysis of categorical data applied to a large cross-sectional occupational health survey. *Int. Statistic. Rev.*, 45:51–62.

Metrakos, J. D., and Metrakos, K. (1969): Genetic studies in clinical epilepsy. In: *Basic Mechanism of the Epilepsies*, edited by H. H. Jasper, A. A. Ward, Jr., and A. Pope. pp. 700–708. Little, Brown and Company, Boston.

Advances in Epileptology:
The Xth Epilepsy International Symposium,
edited by J. A. Wada and J. K. Penry.
Raven Press, New York © 1980.

Three Pairs of Monozygotic Twins with Rolandic Discharges

Takashi Kajitani, Makoto Nakamura, Kiyotaka Ueoka, and Seiko Kobuchi

Department of Pediatrics, Kawasaki Hospital, Kawasaki Medical School, Okayama, Japan

In recent years, a prognostically benign childhood epilepsy has been reported and called "benign epilepsy of children with rolandic discharge." It features rolandic (central-midtemporal) spikes on the EEG, generalized convulsions or simple partial motor seizures, usually nocturnal, onset of seizures between 3 and 8 years of age, absence of evidence of brain damage, good response to anticonvulsant therapy, and the disappearance of seizures and EEG abnormalities before 15 years of age. It is suggested that this epilepsy is inherited as a single autosomal dominant trait with age-dependent penetrance (Bray and Wiser, 1964; Bray et al., 1965; Heijbel et al., 1975).

We recently studied three pairs of identical twins, all of whom showed rolandic discharges on the EEG. We report their clinical manifestations and EEG findings, and comment on the genetics of rolandic discharges.

The definition of rolandic discharge is based on the following EEG findings: spikes and sharp waves of maximal amplitude in centrotemporal regions, the individual potentials appearing on normal background activity with an almost identical appearance and amplitude in each recording. They are often followed by a small slow wave, usually sporadic but occasionally pseudorhythmic, activated by sleep and not affected by hyperventilation, photic stimulation, or by opening the eyes.

CASE REPORTS

Case 1. Y. A., an 8-year-old boy, is one of the first pair of twins. His chief complaint was generalized convulsions. At birth he weighed 2,540 g. His growth through the neonatal and infantile stages was normal. He had two febrile convulsions at the age of 2 and 3, both with 39°C fever. Convulsions were generalized, tonic and clonic in nature, and lasted 2 to 3 min each. At 3½ years he had an episode of generalized seizures without fever with increased oral secretion while he was taking a nap, lasting 1 to 2 min. He was examined with EEG at 6 years and 5 months, and his parents were told that he had abnormal epileptic discharges in the right hemisphere. Anticonvulsants have been administered since that time and he had no recurrence of seizure. At the age of 6 years and 11 months EEG was taken in the spindle stage of sleep and showed a few pseudorhythmic focal spikes on the right rolandic region. All spikes shared similar appearances and amplitude.

Case 2. M.A., an 8-year-old boy, is the second twin of the first pair. His chief complaint was left hemifacial seizures during sleep. His birthweight was 2,900 g. He had no medical problems during infancy. At 8 years and 1 month he experienced a focal convulsive seizure on the left half of his face during sleep, with salivation and clonic twitches of the jaw. Duration of the seizure was only a minute or so. He was conscious throughout, but he could not talk during the seizure. Characteristics of his seizure correspond to the description of a typical benign focal epilepsy in children. EEG was taken at the age of 8 years and 3 months. Background activities were normal, but there were focal spikes at the right central-midtemporal region (near the sulcus rolandi). At 9 years and 3 months of age his EEG showed diffuse HVS bursts as well as right rolandic spikes.

This pair of twins share very similar features—hair color, skin color, shape of nose, ears, and lips—and are diagnosed as monozygotic by detailed blood typings (type A, Rh(+), CCDee).

Their mother is one of identical twins and experienced a febrile convulsion during infancy but has been free from seizures since. Her EEG at 36 years of age was not normal, however, and showed generalized, episodical abnormal activities. It showed bursts of 3 c/sec high-voltage slow wave during hyperventilation, but did not have any rolandic discharge. EEGs of the twins' father and elder brother were normal (Fig. 1).

Case 3. M.I., a 5-year-old boy, one of the second pair of twins, weighed 3,950 g at birth and had no sign of asphyxia. His neonatal and infantile period was uneventful, as was his psychomotor development. He had two episodes of febrile convulsions at 1 year and 5 months, and an EEG was interpreted as normal. He had the third episode of febrile convulsions at 5 years and 7 months and a second EEG was taken. It showed left central-midtemporal focal spikes (left rolandic discharges).

Case 4. T.I. is the second twin of the second pair. His pre-, peri-, and postnatal history were uneventful. His birthweight was 3,300 g. His psychomotor development was normal. He also had two episodes of febrile convulsions at 1 year of age, but had not experienced any seizures since that time. His EEG had similar left central-midtemporal focal spikes.

These twins shared similar features and were diagnosed as identical twins by blood typings (type A, Rh(+), DccE). They have a cousin who experienced episodes of febrile convulsion.

Case 5. Y.T., an 11-year-old boy, is one of the third pair of identical twins. He was born prematurely in the 32nd week and at birth weighed 1,700 g. He had no medical problems during infancy, but had at least 20 febrile convulsions between 2 and 4 years of age. He has been treated with anticonvulsants since age 4. He had a grand mal seizure without fever during sleep at 10 years and 11 months of age. EEG was taken when we was 11 years and 5 months. It showed right rolandic spikes.

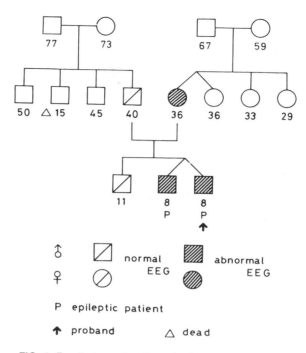

FIG. 1. Family tree of patients in Case 1 and Case 2.

Case 6. T.T., the second twin of the third set of twins, weighed 1,700 g at birth. He also had several febrile convulsions between 2 and 5 years of age, and has been treated with anticonvulsants. He did not experience any other convulsive seizures. He had focal spikes on the left rolandic area, in contrast with his brother.

These twins were diagnosed as identical twins because of similar physical features and blood typings (type A, Rh(+), CċDEe).

The father of these twins and a cousin on the father's side have histories of febrile convulsions.

DISCUSSION

The clinical and EEG findings of the first pair of twins and their mother are suggestive of the possibility that rolandic discharges may disappear before 15 years of age, but that diffuse HVS burst may remain into the adult years, as in the case of their mother. Thus, the history of the mother and of the twin brothers should be interpreted as an autosomal dominant trait of rolandic discharge with multiple clinical manifestations rather than three different unrelated convulsive disorders, i.e., simple febrile convulsion, generalized seizure without fever, and focal motor seizure during sleep.

Lennox-Buchthal (1971) studied 24 pairs of monozygotic twins (19 pairs in whom one or both had febrile convulsions, and five pairs in whom one or both had nocturnal convulsions). She concluded that susceptibility to febrile convulsions is transmitted by a single dominant gene with incomplete penetrance and the specific trait, susceptibility to febrile convulsions, is related to susceptibility to nocturnal convulsions. She did not refer to the EEG findings, but these nocturnal convulsions may belong to benign epilepsy of children with rolandic discharge.

Bray and Wiser (1964, 1965), in describing the genetics of rolandic discharge, noted that the occurrence of the temporal central focal spikes is inherited as an autosomal dominant gene, but that penetrance is low and clinical and EEG manifestations are age-dependent. Their cases include not only epilepsies with the rolandic discharge but also psychomotor seizures with anterior temporal focus.

Heijbel, Blom, and Rasmuson (1975) studied genetically 19 probands with benign epilepsy of children with rolandic discharges, 36 full parents, and 34 full siblings and concluded that an autosomal dominant gene with age-dependent penetrance is most probably responsible for the EEG changes in benign epilepsy of children with rolandic (centrotemporal) EEG foci. Among 32 siblings who were examined by EEG, five had rolandic discharges with clinical seizures, and six had rolandic discharges without clinical seizures. We agree with their opinion from the observations of our twins and several other cases. The rolandic discharges are considered as a functional, hereditary abnormality of EEG originating probably from the subcortical structures, mainly due to functional disturbance in cortico-subcortical networks, and they usually disappear with the maturing of the brain at adolescence, or approximately 15 years of age.

These findings strongly suggest that a certain genetic factor is concerned with the appearance of a rolandic discharge in the EEG. This factor seems to be autosomally dominant in its mode of inheritance and probably has age-dependent penetrance, being maximal between 3 and 13 years and decreasing thereafter almost to zero. The extreme variability of the clinical manifestations of rolandic discharge is worth mention. Thus, in some cases there is lifelong freedom from attack, whereas in others simple febrile convulsion is the only manifestation, and in extreme cases there is partial motor seizure, generalized seizure or partial motor, secondarily generalized seizure that occurs during sleep, i.e., benign epilepsy of children with rolandic discharge (Fig. 2).

SUMMARY AND CONCLUSIONS

Three pairs of monozygotic twins all of whom showed rolandic discharges on the EEG were presented. Clinical seizure patterns were not always concordant in these twins. They showed simple febrile convulsion, generalized

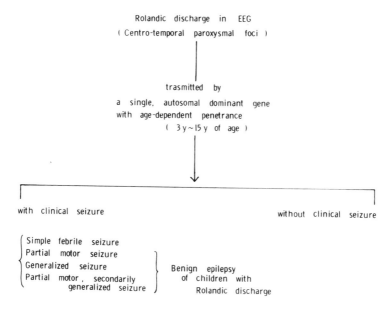

FIG. 2. Inheritance of rolandic discharge in EEG

seizure without fever or partial motor seizure (hemifacial seizure) during sleep. It can be said that an autosomal dominant gene with age-dependent penetrance is most probably responsible for the rolandic discharges, but the clinical manifestations of the rolandic discharges have an extreme variability.

REFERENCES

Bray, P. F., and Wiser, W. C. (1964): Evidence for a genetic etiology of temporal-central abnormalities in focal epilepsy. *N. Engl. J. Med.*, 271:926–933.

Bray, P. F., Wiser, W. C., Wood, M. C., and Pusey, S. B. (1965): Hereditary characteristics of familial temporal-central focal epilepsy. *Pediatrics*, 36:207–211.

Heijbel, J., Blom, S., and Rasmuson, M. (1975): Benign epilepsy of childhood with centrotemporal EEG foci: a genetic study. *Epilepsia*, 16:285–293.

Lennox-Buchthal, M. (1971): Febrile and nocturnal convulsions in monozygotic twins. *Epilepsia*, 12:147–156.

Advances in Epileptology:
The Xth Epilepsy International Symposium,
edited by J. A. Wada and J. K. Penry.
Raven Press, New York © 1980.

Natural History of Posttraumatic Epilepsy

*William F. Caveness, **Arnold M. Meirowsky,
†Berkley L. Rish, ††Jay P. Mohr, †††J. Philip Kistler,
§J. Daniel Dillon, and ‖George H. Weiss

*Laboratory of Experimental Neurology, NINCDS, National Institutes of Health,
Bethesda, Maryland 20205; **Department of Neurosurgery, Vanderbilt University,
Nashville, Tennessee 37240; †Department of Neurosurgery, Eastern Virginia Medical
School, Norfolk, Virginia 23508; ††Department of Neurology, University of South
Alabama Medical School, Mobile, Alabama 36617; †††Department of Neurology,
Harvard Medical School, Boston, Massachusetts 02115; §Department of
Neurosurgery, U.S. Naval Hospital, Portsmouth, Virginia 23708; and ‖Laboratory of
Clinical Sciences, DCRT, National Institutes of Health, Bethesda, Maryland 20205

The relationship of craniocerebral trauma to convulsive seizures was clearly recognized by Hippocrates (460–357 B.C.) in his treatise *Injuries of the Head*, for he noted that a wound of the left temporal region would cause convulsions on the right side of the body, and vice versa. John Hughlings Jackson in the 19th century added precise details for the association between wound location and attack pattern. Penfield and associates extended Jackson's concepts and provided a scholarly appraisal of the meningocerebral cicatrix as the cause of the discharging lesion (Penfield and Jasper, 1954). In addition, a host of astute physicians and surgeons have recognized a variability in the head injured toward the development of fits. For an understanding of the natural course of the disorder a relatively large cohort of head-injured subjects who can be followed for a least a decade are needed. The use of animal models is hampered by a difference in craniocerebral configuration, which results in a difference in response characteristics to physical impact when compared with man, and by the extreme difficulty in producing seizures in lower animals by physical trauma. Posttraumatic epilepsy is an affliction of man and as a clinical entity must be studied in man. Investigations from the civilian sector have been remarkably sparse over the past decades, with the exception of the detailed studies by Jennett (1975) and colleagues.

PATIENTS AND METHODS

The military experience offers the advantage of similarity in age and general health of the subjects at the time of injury and the relative ease with which they can be followed in subsequent years. This opportunity was exploited following World War I, World War II, and the Korean Campaign. During a period in the Vietnam war, 1967–1970, a roster of 1,250 head-injured men was developed by military surgeons. The injured received definitive care within an average of 6 hr after injury. Through the completion of registry forms, by those trained in neurological surgery, subjects were selected for future study. This provided a uniformity in the initial neuro-logical status, particularly regarding level of consciousness, and in location and extent of craniocerebral damage, not previously recorded in military or civilian populations of the head injured. After the identified men returned to the United States, their military and veterans administration hospital records were assembled by the medical follow-up agency of the National Research Council. These records, along with the registry forms, were then reviewed by a team of neurologists and neurological surgeons, the pertinent data being stored on magnetic tape. This activity began in July 1976 with the support of NINCDS, NIH, and to date, July 1978, there are 1,030 cases on tape, and their analyses have begun. The mean age at time of injury was 21 years, and the agents of injury were missile fragments in 76%, gunshot wound (bullets) in 16%, and vehicular and those attributable to other accidents in 8%. The severity of injury adjudged by loss in consciousness and depth of penetration varied from the apparently trivial to an amount of brain destruction barely compatible with life. At the time of initial examination, within 6 hr of injury, 55% were fully alert, 25% were unresponsive, or responded only to pain, and the remaining 20% responded inappropriately to the environment. Seven-teen percent received injuries to the scalp and skull, without penetration of the dura, 41% had penetration of at least two lobes of the brain, and the remaining 42% had penetration of a single lobe.

With the availability of sequelae of these injuries, consistent findings have been abstracted from these and previous data to provide an outline of the phenomena of posttraumatic epilepsy as they are known today.

RESULTS

Characteristics of the Injury

A highly significant relationship exists between the degree of focal brain destruction and the liability to fits. This has been noted by Credner (1930), Ascroft (1941), Russell and Whitty (1952), Walker and Jablon (1961), Cave-ness (1963), and Jennett (1975) regarding both penetrating injuries and in the focal damage or "areal density," in closed injuries. The same holds true for the Vietnam series: 27.9% developed fits after penetration limited to a single lobe; 43.7%, when the penetration involved multiple lobes. Within the latter, the through and through injuries had a fit incidence of 58.6%. It has been the general experience that when focal damage is associated with prolonged loss in consciousness the liability to seizures is enhanced. Injury to any part of the brain may result in fits, but the incidence is greater when the damage is in the regions adjacent to the central sulcus than at either pole. Russell and Whitty (1952) in a study of penetrating injuries of limited depth stressed the importance of injury to the parietal lobe.

Characteristics of the Fit

Latency in onset: Attacks may occur within moments of injury or be delayed for 20 years or longer. This distribution in time is not random, but follows a consistent pattern. The curve of new fit cases is at first steep, leveling off at 1 or 2 years. Reports from military experience indicate that 40 to 50% of the new cases occur by 6 months, 70% by 1 year, and 80% by 2 years. The steepness of this curve is influenced by the severity of the injury and by the duration of follow-up. When stated more precisely as monthly rate of new fit cases, 7 to 9% of the injured have their first fit within the first month, with the rate falling to 2 to 3% for the next 6 months and 1% or less thereafter. Within this distribution, another division is now clearly recognized (Jennett, 1975), that is "early," meaning within the first week and "late," meaning all those cases having their first fit beyond 7 days. Those within the first week are less precisely related to local brain destruction than to diffuse damage as indicated by loss in consciousness.

Frequency: The number of attacks varies within a wide, but graded range. There may be but a single seizure, or two or three. There may be 20 to 30 scattered over a 10-year period, or there may be so many attacks that they defy an accurate count. In the Korean series each of these groups comprised about one-third of those who developed seizures (Caveness, 1963).

Duration: As some men are developing their first attack, others are experiencing their last. Cessation, like onset of fits, is a dynamic process. When the cumulative onset was correlated with the cumulative cessation in the series from the Korean campaign, the increase in onset was at first greater than that for cessation, but after a period of $1\frac{1}{2}$ years, these trends were reversed to a modest degree. From the fifth year the onset and cessation remained approximately parallel. The difference at any given period represented the prevalence of active cases at that time after injury. Based on a 10-year follow-up, attacks ceased in terms of abatement for 2 years from the first day to the eighth year after injury. In this sense, attacks ceased in just over one-half of the men. This is consistent with that reported for other series (Russell and Whitty, 1952; Walker and Jablon, 1961).

Attack pattern: Irrespective of time of onset or frequency, any of the seizure patterns may be seen. Focal attacks alone appear in approximately one-quarter; focal attacks progressing to or occurring in conjunction with general attacks in about one-half, and general attacks alone in about one-quarter of those that develop seizures (Caveness, 1963).

Although there is a clear correlation between severity of injury and onset of fits, there is no correlation between severity of injury and cessation of attacks. However, there is a correlation between the attack frequency and persistence of fits, as demonstrated by Weiss and Caveness (1972).

Characteristics of the Individual

Multifactorial Genetic Traits: Although predisposing factors have been assumed to be significant additions to the severity of injury in the causation of posttraumatic epilepsy, the attempts to demonstrate a genetic influence have been inconclusive. It now seems clear that there are multifactorial traits that must be considered in judging an individual's susceptibility to seizures in general. Moreover, these genetic traits are thought to be interacting with multiple environmental factors. The principles for this were set forth by Carter (1973) and Nova and Fraser (1974) in their consideration of developmental anomalies, e.g., cleft palate and spina bifida, and metabolic disorders, e.g., diabetes and rheumatic fever. Metrakos (1975) has put this succinctly, with regard to seizures, and has provided a schematic representation of the theoretical distribution of liability in the general population. If we include craniocerebral trauma as a significant environmental factor interacting with the existing genetic traits, we can visualize the effect in an elaboration of Metrakos' schema (Fig. 1).

This attractive but still unproven hypothesis is supported by inference from clinical experience. Evidence for the graded distribution of the genetic trait in the population at risk is afforded by: (a) The occurrence of fits over a 10-year period ranges from none in 70% to a few in 10%, many in 10%, and to a number that defy an accurate count in 10% (Caveness, 1963). (b) Of those fits that occur, one-half stop, one-quarter may be controlled, and one-quarter are intractable (Caveness, 1963). (c) Cessation or persistence is not related to the amount of brain damage; nor is latency in onset (Caveness, 1963). The single highest correlation with persistence is frequent attacks (Weiss and Caveness, 1972).

Evidence for the strength of the genetic factors is the similarity in overall fit incidence after World War I, 32%, World War II, 34%, the Korean campaign, 30% (Caveness et al., 1962), and the Vietnam war, 33%, in spite of the rather profound advance in wound handling and overall patient care from 1914 to 1970. Further, a concerted prophylactic anticonvulsant regime carried out for the first time in Vietnam yielded no demonstrable benefit. The institution of the regimen was incorporated within the postoperative orders, 84% of the men receiving their anticonvulsants, intramuscularly if unconscious, within 24 hr of injury. There were no blood levels determined, but the amount of medication, dilantin 300 to 400 mg/day in 75%, accompanied by phenobarbital 96 mg/day in an additional 20% was consistent with the best medical practice of 1967–1970. In 453 cases, the medical records indi-

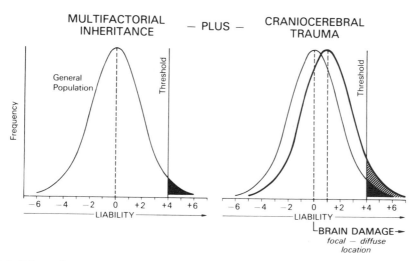

FIG. 1. Schematic representation of the distribution of genetic traits toward epilepsy in the general population, shown on the **left**. Subjects at the far **right** of the bell-shaped curve are the most susceptible and may exhibit "spontaneous" seizures. Subjects at the far left are least susceptible to any influence. When the environmental factor of craniocerebral trauma is added, as indicated on the **right**, a large number cross the threshold and exhibit attacks. Of pertinence is the fact that beyond the threshold, there remain different degrees of susceptibility.

cated continuous medication through successive hospital admissions for periods ranging from 3 months to 9 years. Three hundred and thirty-five men were thus monitored for at least 1 year. During that year, 113 of these men developed one or more fits. In 524, the medication was interrupted at varying periods after injury, and in 53 men, there was no anticonvulsant medication. The incidence of posttraumatic epilepsy in those with a continuous medical regime was somewhat greater than the incidence in those with an interrupted or no medical regimen.

Even more surprising is the comparability of fit data from the Vietnam injuries, 93% of which resulted from missiles, to fit data from two sets of civilian, non-missile injuries, with varying ages, reported by Jennett (1975). Early fits, within 7 days, were similar in incidence for the 1,030 cases from Vietnam and the Oxford series of 1,000 relatively mild injuries, 4.4% and 4.6%, respectively. Cumulative incidence for the first 5 years, excluding the first 7 days, were similar for the Vietnam casualties and the Glasgow-Rotterdam series of 1,005 depressed fractures plus 420 intracranial haematomas, 27.9% and 28.6%, respectively.

COMMENT

From the preceding, two principal determinants are evident: the constitutional tendency toward fits, probably a multifactorial genetic trait; and the brain damage. In onset of fits, both play a part, the constitutional factor apparently determining severity of attacks. In cessation or persistence of fits, the constitutional factor plays the dominant role.

REFERENCES

Ascroft, P. B. (1941): Traumatic epilepsy after gunshot wounds of the head. *Br. Med. J.*, 1:739–744.

Carter, C. O. (1973): Multifactorial genetic disease. In: *Medical Genetics*, edited by V. A. McKusick and R. Clairborne, pp. 199–208. H. P. Publishing Co., New York.

Caveness, W. F. (1963): Onset and cessation of fits following craniocerebral trauma. *J. Neurosurg.*, 20:570–583.

Caveness, W. F., Walker, A. E., and Ascroft, P. B. (1962): Incidence of posttraumatic epilepsy in Korean veterans as compared with those from World War I and World War II. *J. Neurosurg.*, 19:122–129.

Credner, L. (1930): Klinische und soziale Auswirkungen von Hirnschadigungen. *Z. Ges Neurol. Psychiatr.*, 126:721–757.

Jennett, W. B. (1975): *Epilepsy after Non-Missile Head Injuries.* Year Book Publishers, Chicago.

Metrakos, J. D. (1975): *Genetics of Epilepsy, The Lennox Lecture.* In: *American Epilepsy Society Meeting*, Dec. 3–4, 1975.

Nova, J. J., and Fraser, F. C., editors (1974): Multifactorial inheritance. In: *Medical Genetics: Principles and Practice*, pp. 221–230. Lea and Febiger, Philadelphia.

Penfield, W., and Jasper, H. H. (1954): *Epilepsy and the Functional Anatomy of the Human Brain.* Little, Brown and Co., Boston.

Russell, W. R., and Whitty, C. W. M. (1952): Studies in traumatic epilepsy; factors influencing the incidence of epilepsy after brain wounds. *J. Neurol. Neurosurg. Psychiatry*, 15:93–98.

Walker, A. E., and Jablon, S. (1961): *A Follow-up Study of Head Wounds in World War II*, p. 202. U.S. Government Printing Office, Washington, D.C.

Weiss, G. H., and Caveness, W. F. (1972): Prognostic factors in the persistence of posttraumatic epilepsy. *J. Neurosurg.*, 37:164–169.

Advances in Epileptology:
The Xth Epilepsy International Symposium,
edited by J. A. Wada and J. K. Penry.
Raven Press, New York © 1980.

Withdrawal of Anticonvulsant Medications in Successfully Treated Patients with Epilepsy

*,**E. A. Rodin and **G. John

*Department of Neurology, Wayne State University, Department of Neurology and Electroencephalography, Lafayette Clinic; and **Epilepsy Center of Michigan, Detroit, Michigan 48202*

The literature dealing with the results of discontinuation of anticonvulsant medication in successfully treated epileptic patients shows considerable discrepancies (Yahr et al., 1952; Zenker et al., 1957; Strobos, 1959; Juul-Jensen, 1964; Juul-Jensen, 1968; Holowach et al., 1972; Janz and Sommer-Burkhardt, 1976; Oller-Daurella et al., 1976; Rodin et al., 1977). This is demonstrated in Table 1, which lists the most prominent studies to which are added our current results. The range of recurrences, between a high of 80% and a low of 6%, is so startling that it can only be explained on the basis of the type of patient population served and, to some extent, how the anticonvulsant medication withdrawal was achieved.

The literature is in agreement that better results are accomplished in children than in adults when only primary generalized seizures—either of the tonic-clonic type or absence variety—or febrile convulsions are present. The results are also better when there was only one seizure type rather than two or three different ones, and when the patients had responded relatively rapidly to anticonvulsant therapy that was continued for a minimum of 2 to 3 years. The value of the EEG in prognosis for seizure recurrence after anticonvulsant discontinuation remains controversial.

Keeping this relative consensus from the literature in mind, anticonvulsant medications were discontinued in 44 children during the past 5 years. Of these, only 32 could be followed for a 2-year period after anticonvulsants had been withdrawn. The others were either lost to follow-up or have not yet reached the 2-year period since medications were completely stopped. Inasmuch as both Juul-Jensen (1968) and Janz and Sommer-Burkhardt (1976) agreed that approximately 88% of patients who experience a recurrence of seizures will do so in the first 2 years, this follow-up period appears reasonable and although some recurrences will still occur in the future, they are not likely to be of major proportions. This report will concentrate, therefore, only on those patients who have been followed for 2 years after attempted or completed withdrawal.

TABLE 1. *Anticonvulsant therapy discontinued*

N	Recurrence rate (%)	Population	Length of follow-up	Reference
26	81	—	—	Yahr et al. (1952)
117	21	Children	At least 1 Year	Zenker et al. (1957)
25	76	—	—	Strobos et al. (1959)
200	35	Mostly adolescents and adults	2 Years	Juul-Jensen (1964)
196	40		5 Years	Juul-Jensen (1968)
148	24	Children	5–12 Years	Holowach et al. (1972)
138	21	—	—	Oller-Daurella et al. (1976)
	34	—	6 Months–21 years (average 5 years)	Janz et al. (1976)
32	6	Children	2–5 Years	Rodin and John (1978)

As far as description of the sample is concerned, there were 10 males and 22 females. Mean age at first seizure was 4.4 years (range between birth and 17 years), age at time of last seizure was 7.3 years (range, 4 months–23 years), and the mean interval from the last seizure to discontinuation of medication was 5.6 years (range, 21 months–13 years). As far as seizure types are concerned, 23 patients suffered from grand mal seizures; five, febrile convulsions; two, petit mal absences; and one, minor focal motor seizure. One was difficult to classify. All patients had had one seizure type only.

Since this report is in part retrospective and different physicians were involved in the withdrawal process, there is a certain amount of variability in the time over which withdrawal was achieved. Some pediatricians followed the conservative route of using up to 4 years for the process (15%), others 2 to 6 months (18%), but 30% of the patients were discontinued over a period of 1 to 6 weeks. In 31%, the information contained in the chart was inconclusive because parents had already begun to decrease or even discontinue medications on their own without medical authorization. Our findings agreed with those of Juul-Jensen (1964) that the time taken for discontinuation of anticonvulsants was irrelevant in regard to recurrence of seizures. As a matter of fact, there were only two patients who experienced recurrences. One occurred 1 year after dilantin and phenobarbital had been discontinued; the other while phenobarbital was being reduced over a 2-year period.

The 21 patients whose anticonvulsant program was personally discontinued by the authors have fulfilled the following criteria: (a) complete seizure freedom for at least 3, preferably 5 years, and (b) normal or only slightly nonspecifically disorganized EEG. The withdrawal process itself was initiated after an anticonvulsant blood level determination was done and an EEG obtained. If the patient was on only one drug, which was most commonly phenobarbital, diphenylhydantoin, or ethosuximide and the anticonvulsant level was in the therapeutic range, the dose was reduced to half over a 2-week period. The patient was then returned for another EEG and anticonvulsant blood level. If the EEG remained normal, elimination of the rest of the compound was achieved over the next 2 to 3 weeks and the patient returned for another EEG and medical follow-up at that time. If there were no complications, the patient was then advised to return in 1 month for another EEG and medical follow-up, thereafter in 3 months, 6 months, and subsequently at yearly intervals. In addition, the patient and parents were strongly encouraged to call us immediately if they noted any adverse change in the behavior of the child, even if the symptoms were as mild as dizzy spells or headaches.

If the patient was on two drugs, one drug was initially reduced and eliminated and if this was well tolerated, the same was done with the second one thereafter. This tended to increase the duration of the withdrawal process to about 6 weeks. Although there were, as mentioned, only two patients in the series who had clinical seizures after withdrawal—which were promptly controlled by re-institution of the anticonvulsant program—there were another two in whom the discontinuation process was abandoned and the patients were returned to their previous anticonvulsant regimens because the EEG had shown definite deterioration in the form of spike wave discharges. Under the circumstances, it was felt that we were potentially jeopardizing the future of the child by continued reduction of medications. Adding these two patients to the previously mentioned ones in whom overt seizures had recurred, one can say that successful withdrawal of anticonvulsants could be achieved in 88% of this population. Although this figure may decay in time, as has been mentioned, it is sufficiently high to recommend adoption of the above mentioned schedule for patients who fit the criteria listed.

Nevertheless, it is essential that anticonvulsant withdrawal is done not only with full consent, but also in concordance with the wishes of patients and family. Since a recurrence of a grand mal seizure or a first occurrence of a grand mal seizure after the patient had previously been successfully treated for petit mal absences is a very real threat, the following additional precautions should be taken: (a) To prevent embarrassment to the child in school, anticonvulsant withdrawal should be attempted during summer vacations, when there is also time available for the frequent EEG studies. (b) The risk has to be fully explained to patient and parent and if there is any hesitation on either part, the attempt to discontinue anticonvulsants should be postponed for at least another year. (c) The physician should document in the chart that the risks were explained to the patient as well as parents and that they were desirous of following the regimen as outlined. The latter recommendation is especially important for physicians in practice in the United States where litigation has assumed epidemic proportions. Keeping these precautions in mind, it is clear that a certain, but unfortunately fairly small, proportion of patients can safely discontinue their anticonvulsant program.

REFERENCES

Holowach, J., Thurston, D. L., and O'Leary, J. (1972): Prognosis in childhood epilepsy. *N. Engl. J. Med.*, 286:169–174.

Janz, D., and Sommer-Burkhardt, E. -M. (1976): Discontinuation of antiepileptic drugs in patients with epilepsy who have been seizure free for more than two years. In: *Epileptology*, edited by D. Janz, pp. 228–234. Georg Thieme, Germany.

Juul-Jensen, P. (1964): Frequency of recurrence after discontinuance of anticonvulsant therapy in patients with epileptic seizures. *Epilepsia*, 5:352–363.

Juul-Jensen, P. (1968): Frequency of recurrence after discontinuance of anticonvulsant therapy in patients with epileptic seizures: A new follow-up study after 5 years. *Epilepsia*, 9:11–16.

Oller-Daurella, L., Pamies, R., and Oller F. V., L. (1976): Reduction or discontinuance of antiepileptic drugs in patients seizure-free for more than 5 years. In: *Epileptology*, edited by D. Janz, pp. 218–227. Georg Thieme, Germany.

Rodin, E. A., John, G., Kobiljak, J., and Green, M. A. (1977): Discontinuation of anticonvulsant medications in remitted epileptic patients. *Electroencephalogr. Clin. Neurophysiol.*, 43:905.

Strobos, R. R. J. (1959): Prognosis in convulsive disorders. *Arch. Neurol.*, 1:216–225.

Yahr, M. D., Sciarra, D., and Carter, S. (1952): Evaluation of standard anticonvulsant therapy in three hundred nineteen patients. *JAMA*, 150:663–667.

Zenker, C., Groh, C., and Roth, G. (1957): Probleme und Erfahrungen beim Absetzen antikonvulsiver Therapie. *Neue Oest. Z. Kinderheilk.*, 2:152–163.

Abstracts

NEUROLOGIC, NEUROPSYCHOLOGICAL, AND GENETIC INTERACTIONS IN EPILEPSY

R. S. Thomas, W. A. Hauser, M. M. Chern,
A. Mayersdorf, S. E. Strauman, V. E. Anderson
Minneapolis

A battery of neuropsychological assessment instruments was utilized to evaluate 63 probands and 42 relatives of three patient groups selected on the basis of: (1) recent diagnosis of epilepsy, (2) seizures in one or more first degree relatives of the proband, (3) EEG manifestations of generalized spike and wave, photoconvulsive response, and/or rolandic spikes. A similar battery was used to evaluate a group of 90 patients in whom seizures were refractory under routine medical management.

The neuropsychological patterns in the probands are presented as a function of seizure type, presumed etiology of seizures, nature and location of EEG abnormality, and years since diagnosis of epilepsy. The neuropsychological patterns for affected and unaffected siblings are also compared with the profiles for the probands.

On many tests, (particularly those assessing memory, judgment, and sustained vigilance), patients with chronic refractory seizures showed the greatest deviation from norms. Probands with better seizure control were less abnormal. On some tests, unaffected siblings were found to lie between affected siblings and population norms.

Supported in part by N.I.H. contract number N01-NS-5-2327.

CONTRIBUTION OF THE EEG TO PROGNOSIS IN LATE ONSET EPILEPSY

S. Kawaguchi, M. Shimoyama
Sapporo, Hokkaido, Japan
T. Moriyama, Y. Fukushima
Hirosaki, Aomaori, Japan

The relationship between the EEG findings at the time of initial examination and the clinical outcome of seizure was studied in 248 patients who developed their first seizure at the age of 20 or older. The average follow-up period was 4.6 years, the shortest period being at least 2 years.

Seizures were completely or almost completely controlled in 169 patients (68%). Seizures were decreased in frequency but were not sufficiently controlled in 61 cases (25%). No change or aggravation of seizures was seen in 18 cases (7%).

The following conclusions were obtained.

1) The relationship between EEG and prognosis of seizure control appeared to be influenced by age of onset, type of seizure and presence of exogenic factors.

2) In patients with the onset of seizure in the 3rd decade or with grandmal seizures, a normal initial EEG related to good seizure control.

3) The presence of temporal spikes on the initial EEG led to poor prognosis in patients with onset in the 3rd and 4th decades, or with grandmal seizures.

4) These correlations between EEG and prognosis are significant in cases with "idiopathic" seizures, whereas these correlations were not significant in 80 cases with presumable organic causes.

NATURAL HISTORY OF 1000 PATIENTS WITH EPILEPSY

H. Sugiyama, S. Manaka, N. Basugi, K. Sano
Tokyo

One thousand patients with epileptic seizures at our out-patient clinic from April 1976 to March 1977 were statistically analyzed. Their average ages were 34 ± 13 (SD) years. They had been under constant observation in our clinic for 12.5 ± 7.5 years. 14% of them were patients with intractable epilepsy and 48% were seizure free for more than 2 years. Of those intractable epileptic patients, 51% had primary generalized epilepsy, 32% partial complex seizures and 14% partial elementary seizures. The partial complex seizure was found with statistical significance among intractable epileptic patients ($p < 0.001$). The age of onset did not differ significantly with each group. Patients with intractable epilepsy secondary to organic lesions, such as head injury or encephalitis, were 29%. Plasma levels of anticonvulsant drugs of the intractable epilepsy were 13.4 ± 9.3 μg/ml for Diphenylhydantoin (DPH) and 18.8 ± 12.1 for Phenobarbital (PB). These high plasma levels of DPH and PB in the intractable epilepsy were statistically significant ($p < 0.001$, $p < 0.001$, respectively).

A STUDY ON THE LONG-TERM PROGNOSIS OF PSYCHOMOTOR SEIZURES

T. Ohtaka, M. Miyasaka
Tochigi
H. Fukuzawa, K. Sugano
Tokyo

We believe that clinico-electroencephalographically, psychomotor seizures consist of four successive phasic structures: subjective seizure, psychomotor lapse, oral automatism and behavioral automatism phases. From this point of view, the long-term prognosis was studied on 43 patients aged 17-69 years (average 37.0 years). The observation period was 8-22 years (average 13.3 years).

On the frequency change, the most intractable was the aura phase and the most controllable was the oral automatism phase. Of the total 43 patients, 19 (44.2%) were seizure-free for 3 years or more and 17 (39.5%) for 5 years or more. Recurrence occurred in 3 cases (15.8%) in the former and 2 cases (11.8%) in the latter. Those cases with a favourable course were compared to the others, and the factors relating to the good prognosis were studied. The results were as follows:

1. Psychomotor seizures without aura.
2. Low frequency of seizures before the onset of treatment.
3. Onset of psychomotor seizures in school age or puberty.
4. Patients without apparent etiology.
5. Patients with psychomotor seizures only.

A SYNDROME OF "SPIKE-WAVE STUPOR"

K. Hosokawa, T. Kugo, J. Hirata, S. Otsuki
Okayama

Since the original description of "petit mal status" by Lennox in 1945, many workers have described prolonged stupor associated with bilateral synchronous spike and wave discharges seen on the electroencephalogram. The more descriptive term "spike-wave stupor" suggested by Niedermeyer and Khalifeh in 1965 is now widely used. We encountered ten patients with spike-wave stupor during the years from 1966-78. These ten were separated into three groups; 1) typical cases of petit mal status as reported in the literature, 2) recurrent episodes of spike-wave stupor as the only manifestation with no history of epileptic seizure, 3) cases in which the stupor occurred in association with an acquired disease of the central nervous system. We considered such to be a syndrome in which a variety of mechanisms may be involved. Thus we use the term "spike-wave status syndrome". A summary of our patients is compared with other patients reported in the literature of Japan during the same period. Also discussed is one case of hepatic encephalopathy in which there were stupor episodes lasting almost an entire day. These recurrent episodes were not "comatose" in disturbed consciousness, but "stupor" with spike-wave continuity. Furthermore, the prognostic aspect in ten cases, and particularly the mode of onset and problem of epileptic classification of the second group is discussed.

EPILEPTIFORM ACTIVITY, ACUTE SEIZURES AND EPILEPSY WITH ACUTE CEREBRAL VASCULAR DISEASE

M. Ramirez-Lassepas, W. A. Hauser, S. R. Bundlie, and B. B. Cleeremans
St. Paul

The interrelationship between epileptiform activity, acute seizures (occurring within the first 48 hours of insult) and subsequent recurrent seizures has been evaluated in 102 consecutive patients with the diagnosis of acute cerebral infarct admitted to the cerebral vascular intensive care unit at St. Paul-Ramsey Hospital in 1975 and 1976. All patients had EEG examinations within the first 48 hours and 22 (22%) demonstrated epileptiform activity (spikes, sharp waves or continuous rhythmic slow waves of a focal nature). Six of the patients, all with epileptiform activity, also had seizures occurring during this acute stroke period.

Followup in this group ranged from 4 to 22 months. Ten patients, including three with acute seizures, developed recurrent seizures while two patients in the group with recurrent seizures had a prior history of epilepsy. Neither had been on medication or experienced seizures for at least a ten year period prior to the acute cerebral vascular insult and their seizure type was different. Of the surviving patients 12% had developed recurrent seizures within one year following the onset of their stroke.

A higher proportion of females and a higher proportion of individuals with vascular lesions in the posterior quadrant demonstrated epileptiform activity in the acute stroke and mortality tended to be slightly, but not significantly, greater in patients with epileptiform activity when this group was compared to the remainder of the patients. An additional 200 patients admitted between 1973 and 1975 with acute cerebral vascular disease are in the process of evaluation and followup. The significance of epileptiform activity as well as the frequency of acute seizures and epilepsy in this larger group will be discussed.

PREDICTION OF OUTCOME IN GENERALIZED TONIC-CLONIC SEIZURES IN CHILDHOOD

P. Camfield, C. Camfield, A. How, J. Tibbles
Halifax

This study examined whether any features at the onset of pure generalized tonic-clonic epilepsy (G.T.C.E.) in children predicted subsequent seizure control. One neurologist examined 30 children with only G.T.C.E. without structural or metabolic cause within one year of their first seizure (age of onset 1-14 yrs., average 6.6 yrs.). Treatment was diphenylhydantoin, phenobarbital, and primidone alone or in combination. Outcome was assessed 5-11 yrs. after onset (average 8.5 yrs.) by chart review, interview or mail.

Features evaluated for predictability included age of onset, stress factors at onset, previous febrile seizures, family and perinatal history, developmental and physical examination and EEG. Outcome was scored, whether or not they still received medication, as excellent (17), good (3), fair (6) or poor (4), defined by length of terminal remission or continuing seizure frequency. Multivariant analysis showed no significant relationships between these features and outcome. It was impossible at the time of initial diagnosis to identify children with G.T.C.E. whose seizures would not be controlled. Clustering of features that were anticipated to be risk factors for poor seizure control did not influence prognosis.

OUTCOME OF EARLY TRAUMATIC EPILEPSY IN INFANCY AND CHILDHOOD

J. Okada, M. Ogashiwa, and K. Takeuchi
Tokyo

Post-traumatic epilepsy, particularly immediate and early epilepsy as described by Jennet, was studied in a series of 14 cases among 2,300 children with head injuries aged 15 or less. The 14 cases consisted of 10 cases of immediate epilepsy demonstrating convulsive seizure within six hours of receiving head injuries and four cases of early epilepsy in the narrow sense demonstrating seizures within seven days. There were concentrations of patients under one and between 12 and 15. EEGs of 13 children recorded in the first seven days showed abnormal findings in eight cases were persistent localized spikes indicated subclinical epilepsy.

Early epilepsy in the broad sense requires clinical and EEG follow-up, and its relation to "once and for all" seizure, subclinical epilepsy, late traumatic epilepsy and serious head injuries should not be ignored even though early traumatic epilepsy has been given little attention to date. Throughout the series, a spike followed by a wave suggested a worse prognosis than a spike alone. Answers sought from the medicolegal field are increasing, and therefore conclusive information concerning post-traumatic epilepsy and EEG abnormalities is required.

LONGITUDINAL OBSERVATION OF ROLANDIC DISCHARGES WITH AND WITHOUT EPILEPSY

N. Nishiura, T. Miyazaki
Osaka

Concerning Rolandic (centro-temporal) discharge, Gastaut reported in 1952 that there were many patients without epileptic symptoms showing biphasic spikes around the central areas. As for the prognosis of mid-temporal spikes, Gibbs and Gibbs studied 739 children with epilepsy and mid-temporal spikes, and noted that these EEG abnormalities appeared at eight years of age, and disappeared after 15 years of age. The present investigation deals with an analysis of the characteristic differences of Rolandic discharge with and without epilepsy, with respect to the cerebral maturation.

The patients selected out by symptoms and features of EEG's, consisted of 30 children with Rolandic discharges and epilepsy, and 20 without epilepsy. The latter were from post traumatic sequelae. Rolandic discharge with epilepsy showed a clear age dependency in rate and also of its amplitude, which manifested remarkably between the age of four and nine. However, Rolandic discharge without epilepsy appeared less frequent even during sleep activation than in the EEGs with epilepsy and was usually localized to the ipsilateral side of the brain. Finally, the combination of Rolandic discharge with other paroxysmal discharges was common in the patient with epilepsy, but this combination was rare in non-epileptics.

CLINICAL AND GENETIC ASPECTS OF SEIZURE DISORDERS PREVALENT IN AN ISOLATED AFRICAN POPULATION

L. Jilek-Aall, W. Jilek, J. R. Miller
Vancouver

In an isolated Bantu population in the interior of Tanzania the authors found that about 200 of the 10,000 tribesmen presented at the bush clinic with *kifafa*, a convulsive seizure disorder which often led to severe burns in the so afflicted. Many of these cases showed definite Parkinsonian symptoms and/or other neurological abnormalities, mental deterioration, and high mortality. A frequent variant of the disease in children involved "nodding of the head" which was often a precursor of later grand mal. Transient psychotic episodes were seen in about 23% of the cases. The clinic patients were followed up to ten years. The necessarily simple anticonvulsive treatment with phenobarbitone reduced the seizure frequency and intensity in the majority of cases and also ameliorated the Parkinsonian features.

The authors discuss possible reasons for the high prevalence of seizure disorders in this population, indicating infective processes, birth trauma, malnutrition, and inbreeding.

Genetic factors appear to be of major importance for the development of the suspected systemic disease of the central nervous system and are reflected in the demonstrated high family incidence of *kifafa*. A genetical analysis of the data will be presented and discussed by the geneticist-author. Slide illustrations of typical cases and of pedigrees will be shown.

MARRIAGE AND FERTILITY IN EPILEPTIC PATIENTS

L. Dansky, E. Andermann, F. Andermann
Montreal

We compared the marriage and fertility rates of 100 male and 100 female epileptics to those for a matched normal cohort. The marital rates for females and males respectively were 83.2% and 59.6% of expected. Only female patients showed a significant improvement in their marital opportunities over the past 30 years. Males with onset of seizures at 0-9 years had the poorest chance of marriage (32.2% of expected), followed by males with onset at 10-19 years (46.9%) and females with onset at 0-9 years (58.4%). Patients of both sexes whose seizures began at 20 years or over fulfilled their marital expectations. Married males attained their expected liveborn fertility, irrespective of the age at which their epilepsy began, whereas married females had only 70% of the expected number of liveborn children. The lower fertility of female patients was particularly evident for those who married prior to 1950 and for those with very early onset of seizures. However, females who married during recent years showed a fertility approaching that of the general population.

In summary, the present study indicates that the marital and reproductive performance of epileptic patients is strongly influenced by sex, age at onset of seizures, and year of marriage.

THE SIGNIFICANCE OF DATA SELECTION IN DIAGNOSIS AND TREATMENT OF EPILEPSY

F. Hajnsek
Zagreb

The treatment of epilepsy is characterized by the permanent trends of replacement of the clinical empiricism with more complex information. This tendency exhibits by the introduction of more sophisticated diagnostic techniques (monitoring, CEAN), by the precise determination of drug serum level (EMIT, GC-MS-COM), and by obtaining a better insight into biotransformation of antiepileptics. Computer analyses manipulates with a large number of data, using them successfully in research, but scarcely in everyday practice. Therefore, there is a growing need for a reasonable data selection of that pertinent information which will enable us to answer properly the following simple questions: is there an epilepsy or not, if so, where lies the cause, what is the nature of it, and what should be the optimal treatment?

Following several thousands of patients for more than twenty years, the fundamental information that should be collected by using the modern neurophysiological and biochemical diagnostic tools, is discussed in this paper. Some practical suggestions are proposed.

DRUG REGIME IN EPILEPSY

A. Das-Gupta
Calcutta

Despite plentiful knowledge about Epilepsy, exact guidelines regarding drug regime to follow have remained relatively poor. This paper is based on observation of 25,000 patients in a busy neurology outpatient clinic over a period of 15 years. After establishing an effective dose on an individual patient, it is continued without interruption for two years. When there is no recurrence, the dose is reduced a little and continued for a further period of one year at the end of which EEG is repeated. Drug is stopped only when EEG becomes completely normal. Following this regime, it has been possible to stop completely the drugs without recurrence of fits after 3 to 5 years of continuous treatment in about 85% of patients. In the remaining 15%, however, fits recurred after 1 to 10 years of drug stoppage. Prognosis is poor where: 1) fits continue in spite of regular drugging, or 2) with dose reduction after 2 years of freedom, or 3) in those 15% of patients where fits recur after 1 to 10 years of drug stoppage, or 4) when EEG remains abnormal throughout in spite of clinical absence of fits. In these situations, drug is continued for the rest of the patient's life.

A STUDY OF THE CORRELATION BETWEEN CLINICAL PROGNOSIS AND EEG CHANGES OF EPILEPTIC PATIENTS

J. Sano, H. Kawada, Y. Wada
Kanazawa

The purpose of the present study was to examine the long-term correlation between the alterations of the frequency of seizures and EEG findings in epileptic patients. The material consisted of 53 outpatients who had been followed for more than 10 years and examined by EEG more than five times each patient. A large number of epileptic patients with primary generalized tonic clonic convulsive seizures showed rapid improvement, while many patients with partial seizures repeatedly showed some improvements and aggravations in the frequency of seizures and also in EEG findings. EEG findings generally improved later in one-third and the frequency of seizure improved earlier in two-thirds of the patients. Only one half of the patients showed close correlation between changes in the clinical course and EEG but in particular this was evident in a few cases with elementary partial seizure. The fact that there is considerable dissociation between clinical prognosis and EEG changes is very important for the comprehensive care of epileptic patients.

STUDY OF LONG TERM FOLLOW UP OF EPILEPTIC PATIENTS

V. Virmani and M. Behari
New Delhi

This is a long term follow up study of 2000 epileptic patients. A small number of patients discontinued medication on their own after a fit free period of 2 to 7 years. They have remained free of fits from 1 to 5 years after stopping all medication. Another group of patients had a relapse after a fit-free period varying from 4 to 8 years. This occurred within 1½ to 4 years of stopping medication. A large majority of patients remained free of fits while taking prescribed anticonvulsants regularly. There was another group of patients who continued getting attacks in spite of adequate dosage of various combinations of anticonvulsants. The common factors in the first and second group appears to be early onset of epilepsy and occurrence of 1 to 4 fits before medication was started. There was no correlation between the type of epilepsy, EEG abnormality and freedom from fits in the first 3 groups. The groups of patients whose fits were intractable, showed intellectual and personality disintegration which was not necessarily progressive. The results of the trial of an indigenous drug in these intractable cases will also be presented. Analysis of various factors in the 4 groups of patients will be discussed.

CHILDHOOD EPILEPSY WITH ROLANDIC DISCHARGES AND AGE DEPENDENCY, WITH SPECIAL REFERENCE TO BENIGN EPILEPSY WITH CENTRO-TEMPORAL EEG FOCI

T. Miyazaki, N. Nishiura
Takatsuki

Childhood epilepsy with nocturnal seizure and Rolandic (centro-temporal) discharge on EEG have recently been reported. These types of epilepsy usually appear in middle childhood and show a favorable response to anticonvulsant therapy. The present investigation deals with an analysis of seizure patterns and of some characteristics of Rolandic discharge, particularly with respect to the cerebral maturational process.

The patients, consisting of 30 children in total, were selected according to their symptoms of epilepsy and the EEG features. Twenty-two patients showed somatomotor attacks and eight showed somatosensory as well as somatomotor attacks. As for the duration of seizure, those who had seizures before three and after 10 years of age, had attacks for relatively short periods, whereas those who had attacks from four to nine years of age, usually had longer duration. The amplitude of Rolandic (centro-temporal) discharge remained lower than 50 microvolts up to three years of age, reached as high as 200 microvolts up to nine years, particularly during sleep, but became lower after the age of 10. It was concluded that, between the ages of four to nine, there is an age dependency to the occurrence of seizures and Rolandic discharges.

A COMPARISON OF FOLLOW-UP STUDIES OF EPILEPTICS — A FIVE YEAR AND TEN YEAR PROGNOSIS OF EPILEPSY

H. Yamada, H. Yoshida, N. Ninomiya, Y. Kato
Fukuoka, Japan

A 10 year follow-up study of 97 epileptics was carried out and compared with the five year follow-up study previously reported. The types of seizures of 97 patients were as follows: five partial elementary seizures; seven partial complex seizures; 37 partial seizures secondarily generalized; four absences; and 44 tonic clonic seizures. The clinical states of the patients at 10 years from onset of seizures were as follows: 42 (43.3%) of 97 patients were controlled (no seizures had occurred for at least three years); 33 (34.3%) were improved; 15 (15.5%) were unchanged; and seven (7.2%) became worse.

As compared to the five year follow-up study, seizure controlled patients were increased from 22.7% to 43.3% and unchanged patients decreased from 30.3% to 15.5%. The predictability of follow-up studies at five years and at 10 years on the same subjects is discussed.

It is concluded that the time of improvement of epileptic seizures differs with seizure type. The prognosis for generalized seizures, especially tonic clonic seizures, is predictable at the first five year period, but the prognosis for partial seizures is not predictable at an early stage.

NEW SURGICAL TREATMENT
THROUGH EXPERIMENTAL MODELS

Advances in Epileptology:
The Xth Epilepsy International Symposium,
edited by J. A. Wada and J. K. Penry.
Raven Press, New York © 1980.

New Surgical Treatment Through Experimental Models

Juhn A. Wada

Electroencephalography Department, University of British Columbia Health Sciences Center Hospital, Vancouver, British Columbia, Canada V6T 1W5

The future outlook for the treatment of epilepsy with drugs is becoming brighter as we acquire new antiepileptic drugs, an increasing knowledge of their respective actions, and a greater capability of more precise diagnostic assessment. Excluding patients whose seizures are a manifestation of a primarily neurosurgical concern such as neoplasm or vascular malformation, it can be safely estimated that medical treatment affords the majority of patients with epilepsy the opportunity to become seizure-free, or nearly seizure-free, so that they can live comfortably as contributing members of our society. However, some patients do not respond to available medication, or to a combination of medications. Among those medically intractable patients, a percentage can be helped by surgical means, which are based on a century-old Hughlings Jackson concept that "epilepsy is the name for occasional, sudden and excessive, rapid and local discharges of grey matter" that can then spread to the rest of the brain. It follows, therefore, that a surgical approach can be directed to removal of the source of local discharge or to interruption of the route of discharge propagation.

CLASSIC OPEN SURGERY

Classic open surgery is a method elaborated by the late Penfield and associates patterned after that of Foerster of Breslau. Classic open surgery can be applied to patients (a) with frequent and severe seizures that cannot be controlled by medication over a reasonable trial period under competent medical supervision, (b) with significant psychosocial handicap secondary to uncontrolled seizures and/or often due to the large amount of medication or combination of medications, and (c) whose site of origin of habitual seizure can be traced to a localized and accessible area on one side of the brain, and where removal of that area is likely to benefit the patient, making the seizure condition more amenable to available drug treatment without producing an additional handicap, such as disturbance of speech, memory or sensory-motor functions.

In Canada, a large number of patients with focal epilepsy have undergone this remedial surgery at the Montreal Neurological Institute. Long-term follow-up of the Montreal series indicates that more than three-fifths of operated patients become completely seizure-free or nearly so. The majority of the remainder of the patients benefited to varying degrees with significant reduction in seizure tendency (Rasmussen, 1975). In the Montreal series, patients who had undergone temporal lobe excision represented, according to the primary brain area involved, the largest group and consisted of more than 50% of the total surgical population. When this particular group is examined, the success rate is somewhat higher (71%) than that of the total series (64%). Since seizures originating from temporal lobe structures are the most prevalent among the focal epilepsies and since they are also known to be generally resistant to drug treatment, this success rate with medically intractable seizure of temporal lobe origin is quite encouraging. Follow-up study of surgical resection of the temporal lobe in 2,282 patients who were medically intractable indicates that two-thirds of the patients were free or almost free from seizures, and if one adds those patients whose seizure frequency was reduced by at least 50%, almost four-fifths of the patients appear to have benefited (Jensen, 1975). The operative risks have always been low and complications after the operation are few and not serious. Thus, it can be concluded with confidence that classic open excisional surgery has a very definite place in the treatment of medically intractable seizure disorder of focal origin.

WHY THIS SURGERY IS NOT PERFORMED MORE FREQUENTLY

At this point one might examine the rate with which such surgery is performed in Canada. We have a population of about 23 million and approximately 1 to 2% of this general population is estimated to be affected by epilepsy. If we take the smaller figure, this represents 230,000 patients. Since about 80% of these patients can benefit significantly from appropriate medication, the remaining 20%, that is, 46,000 patients, remain resistant to drug treatment. Among this large number of medically intractable patients, about 10%, that is, about 4,600 patients, can be estimated to be appropriate candidates for open excisional surgery. Yet, during 1977, the total number of patients in Canada who underwent this operation was less than 80. There are possibly multiple reasons for this discrepancy between the large number of potential surgical candidates and the actual number of patients who undergo surgery (Ojemann, 1978). One of the most probable and important reasons why open excisional surgery is not performed more often is a lack of awareness, on the part of the treating physician and the public alike, of the availability of alternative surgical treatment of proven effectiveness. It must be noted that if this situation exists in Canada, where surgical treatment of epilepsy is, in general, more actively pursued following the tradition established by the late Wilder Penfield, one can only assume that a much smaller proportion of medically intractable patients undergo surgery in many other nations. There is an abundance of clinical and experimental evidence to suggest that recurrent seizure states are a progressive and malignant process (Scheibel et al., 1974; Harris, 1972; Brown, 1973). Therefore, an early attempt to determine whether the patients can benefit from excisional surgery when reasonable medical trial has failed is imperative, and cannot be overemphasized, in order to minimize potential neurobiological risks and to prevent sociopsychological disabilities stemming from uncontrolled seizures from becoming permanent.

NEW SURGICAL TREATMENT FOR 90% OF MEDICALLY INTRACTABLE PATIENTS WHO DO NOT QUALIFY FOR EXCISIONAL SURGERY

The above discussion of classic excisional surgery is concerned with 10%—a very definite majority—of drug-resistant patients. Therefore, even if all candidates were operated on, 90% (that is, 44,400 in Canada) will continue to have uncontrolled seizures in spite of heavy medication in many cases. These individuals are almost entirely dependent on our society. What can we do about this problem? There are some technical approaches one may consider for relief of this "medically hopeless" group of patients who do not qualify for excisional surgery due to, for example, multifocal or diffuse epileptogenic abnormalities or the superimposition of nondispensable cortex on the epileptogenic area. The surgical strategy for such a group would be to interrupt seizure propagation pathways or to suppress the mechanisms that tend to initiate seizures. Alternatively, the enhancement of mechanisms that tend to suppress seizure by selective stimulation or destruction of certain target structures is possible. Many procedures have been described and the results have been reported with varying degrees of success. Since the criteria for surgery are not as clearly established as in the case of selecting candidates for classic open surgery, it is often difficult to assess objectively the results of these procedures. Therefore, the effectiveness of some of the procedures with reported promising results was evaluated experimentally and the results are summarized below.

EXPERIMENTAL OBSERVATIONS[1]

The effect of surgical procedures on kindling (seizure development) and/or kindled (developed) seizures was examined in a kindling model of epilepsy involving epileptic baboons (*Papio papio*) and nonepileptic rhesus monkeys.

[1]Supported by grants from the Medical Research Council of Canada and the National Institutes of Health to Juhn A. Wada.

They were kindled by daily threshold electrical stimulation lasting for 1 sec at the amygdala (Wada and Osawa, 1976; Wada et al., 1978) or mesial frontal cortex (Wada et al., 1975). Although both baboons and monkeys will respond to kindling procedures with a sequential development of epileptic seizure having distinct clinical stages over a period of time, the speed of seizure development, as well as the final pattern of developed seizure, differs significantly between these two species. With amygdaloid kindling, stage 3 partial motor seizure can develop in an average of 11 days in *Papio papio*, in contrast with 196 days in monkeys and primary generalized convulsions develop in 72 days in *Papio papio*, in contrast with a failure to progress beyond secondary generalized convulsion in Rhesus monkeys in spite of more than 400 daily stimulations. These differences are most likely related to the presence (*Papio*) and absence (Rhesus) of an epileptogenic predisposition. Therefore, use of these species was expected to provide us with information that is required for extrapolation of experimental results to the problems of human epilepsies.

Forel-H-Lesion

Forel-H-tomy, based on extensive animal studies defining the pathway of convulsive seizure of neocortical (frontocentral) origin (Jinnai, 1966) is claimed to be highly effective with more than three-fourths of the cases remaining seizure-free postoperatively for 1 year or more (Mukawa and Jinnai, 1975).

In our animals, neither unilateral nor bilateral electrolytic lesion placement showed any effect on amygdaloid kindled convulsions. On the other hand, all the frontally kindled animals showed regression of primary generalized convulsion to asymmetrical generalized seizure in *Papio papio* whereas secondary generalized convulsion became incomplete in Rhesus monkeys. However, the effect in Papio papio was transient with reemergence of primary generalized convulsion in about 4 months, whereas Rhesus monkeys showed a persistent minor "beneficial" effect at 12 months postoperatively. Since these animals are still being used for other studies, we do not possess the exact histological information. However, it should be noted that it had no effect on amygdaloid kindled seizure, an aspect already emphasized by Jinnai.

Cerebellar Stimulation

Results of central stimulation on various epileptiform activity have been reviewed (Ajmone-Marsan and Gumnit, 1974). Among the structures so studied, the cerebellum appears to have been examined most intensively. Although effects of cerebellar stimulation vary considerably, according to experimental models and conditions, it appears predominatingly suppressive so far as cortical ictal activity is concerned. This is in contrast with a tendency to enhance such manifestations by lesioning or cooling of the cerebellum. Since favorable effects of chronic cerebellar surface stimulation on some intractable seizure patients have been reported (Cooper, 1973; Cooper et al., 1976), it became the subject of intensive experimental reevaluation.

Through the courtesy of Dr. Cooper, we were able to use one of his original stimulators and electrode systems for our primate study, using the kindling preparation. No observable suppressive or beneficial electroclinical effect was noted with photosensitivity or kindled convulsion in *Papio papio*. Concurrent cerebellar stimulation from the outset of amygdaloid kindling was also disappointing, although there was an intriguing tendency to accelerate amygdaloid seizure development in Rhesus monkeys (Wada, 1974–1975).

Forebrain Commissurotomy

The possible role played by the commissural and/or subcortical mechanisms in generalization of epileptic seizures has been the subject of many investigations. Among the forebrain commissures, the corpus callosum plays a major role in transmission of seizure activity (Erickson, 1940; Wada, 1951; Marcus and Watson, 1966; Marcus and Watson, 1968). Considerable variation of experimental results in this regard appears to be related to species difference; that is, the higher the animal in the phylogenic scale, the more likelihood there is that the corpus callosum will play the dominant role for seizure generalization than will the subcortical mechanisms. An additional difficulty in evaluating the experimental data is that, in spite of their undeniable and significant contributions made to our knowledge of pathophysiology, uncertainty remains as to the relevance of the observations made in acute or semi-acute "normal" animal preparations for the problem of human epilepsy with chronic epileptogenic brain processes that are often associated with predisposed seizure susceptibility. With the realization that the only genuine model of human epilepsy is human epilepsy, therefore, use of animal models with (*Papio papio*) and without (Rhesus monkeys) natural epileptogenic predisposition should help us to gain better insight into the intriguing controversies generated by investigations using different animal species.

Based on the assumption that the corpus callosum is preferentially used for bilateralization of seizure, Van Wagenen and Herren (1940) performed bisection of various portions of the corpus callosum and other forebrain commissures in medically intractable seizure cases. Although results were inconclusive, long-term follow-up of some of the operated cases indicated very definite beneficial effects with minimal or no obvious postoperative deficits (Goldstein and Joynt, 1969). Encouraging results have since emerged in a highly selected group of medically intractable seizure patients who did not qualify for cortical excision (Bogen and Vogel, 1975; Luessenhop, 1970; Luessenhop et al., 1970; Wilson et al., 1975; Wilson et al., 1977; Wilson et al., 1978).

Although our current understanding of seizure generalization and the possible role played by individual commissural pathways is not clear, it is highly conceivable that the corpus callosum is the predominant structure, since the beneficial effects were reported with sections of corpus callosum with or without additional commissural bisections. In spite of the promising results so far reported, commissurotomy has not been readily adopted, possibly due to uncertainty as to the precise criteria with which to select candidates for this procedure and also fear of the disconnection syndrome as a result of the procedure.

Our experiments were designed to investigate: (a) the effect of prior bisection on convulsive seizure development from one hemisphere (Wada et al., 1977), (b) the effect of bisection on generalized convulsion triggered from one hemisphere, and (c) the extent of commissural bisection required to achieve an optimal result.

Effect of Prior Bisection

In Papio papio: Despite the fact that more than twice the number of daily stimulations required for the development of primary generalized seizure in intact animals was applied, seizure development was arrested at stage 3 hemiconvulsion, with a minimal tendency to partial bilateralization. An identical suppressive effect in terms of seizure generalization was noted at the secondary site amygdala despite a large number of stimulations.

In Rhesus monkeys: The result after 8 months of daily stimulation was, at the primary site amygdala, the development of hemiconvulsion. This is in contrast with the approximately 7 months of daily stimulation required for the development of secondary generalized convulsion in this species with intact commissure. At the secondary site, seizure development was similarly arrested at the hemiconvulsion stage.

Effect of Bisection after the Development of Kindled Primary Generalized Convulsion in *Papio papio*

The animals were subjected to forebrain commissural bisection after the completion of amygdaloid kindling with the development of stable stage 5 primary generalized convulsive seizures. After the surgery, all the animals showed immediate and persistent regression to stage 3 hemiconvulsion with minimal evidence of impairment of the conscious state. There was no further development despite repeated stimulation at the primary amygdaloid site. When the animals were subjected to secondary site amygdaloid kindling, the results were essentially identical to those of prior bisection (Wada and Komai, *in preparation*).

The above observations clearly indicate that in both the epileptic baboon and Rhesus monkeys the presence of the forebrain commissure is essential for the generalization of convulsive seizures of amygdaloid origin. It is particularly interesting to note that a tightly organized low-amplitude fast discharge in the brainstem so characteristic of the onset of stage 5 primary generalized convulsion of the epileptic *Papio papio* was recognized bilaterally and yet the clinical seizure remained lateralized. This finding suggests that ictal involvement of the bilateral and probably the neocortical structure is essential for the development of primary generalized convulsion.

In spite of the general similarity of the effect of forebrain bisection on the clinical seizure pattern in *Papio papio* and Rhesus monkeys, several distinct differences were noted.

The speed of both the longitudinal seizure development and the clinical ictal march within individual seizures was much faster and the intensity of clinical seizure appears to have been enhanced in Rhesus monkeys. An entirely opposite effect was noted in *Papio papio*. This finding suggests that forebrain commissures play "suppressive" and "facilitating" effects in nonepileptic Rhesus monkeys and epileptic baboons, respectively.

Extent of Commissural Bisection

Although we do not yet possess information on the precise extent of bisection in all the animals the clinical results obtained were identical regardless of whether the corpus callosum alone was bisected in its anterior two-thirds only or in its entirety (including the hippocampal commissure). Similarly, additional bisection of the anterior commissure did not appear to influence the surgical outcome. Therefore, bisection of the anterior two-thirds of the corpus callosum alone appears sufficient for the purpose of containing and lateralizing a seizure discharge of amygdaloid origin to one hemisphere.

DISCUSSION

The percentage of patients who are refractory to medical treatment will hopefully diminish in the future with the availability of a new generation of antiepileptic drugs, improved technical diagnostic assessment, and increased knowledge of drug action. In the meantime, we must deal with those patients who can be helped by alternative surgical treatment. We must increase our awareness of these alternatives, since the development of more precise assessment technology, such as positron emission tomography, will undoubtedly increase the percentage of candidates for open excisional surgery in the near future. However, as such, candidates will most likely remain a minority among medically intractable patients, a concerted effort must be made to develop surgical strategy to help those patients who do not qualify for standard cortical excision.

In an attempt to achieve this goal, reevaluation of some of those procedures that have been reported to have some beneficial effect was made in the kindling model of epilepsy, using both epileptic and nonepileptic primates.

While the effect of cerebellar stimulation was disappointing, Forel-H-lesion produced some beneficial results in animals with frontal but not amygdaloid stimulation, suggesting the necessity of further investigation.

Examination of the results of forebrain bisection indicates striking and contrasting differences between baboons and monkeys. It appears that the role played by the forebrain commissure is significantly different in epileptic animals in that its presence seems to support and facilitate the development of seizure generalization. This finding further supports the concept that forebrain commissurotomy might be helpful not only in preventing the generalization of partial seizures, but also in exerting a beneficial effect in patients with a predisposition to primary generalized seizures. Although our commissurotomy study is limited to observations involving amygdaloid kindling, results obtained are sufficiently encouraging to support its rationale and the previously reported favorable results of forebrain commissurotomy. Our results also suggest that complete bisection of all the commissures may not be necessary and that the actual extent and location of bisection could vary, depending on the individual clinical situation. It appears that in order to prevent bilateralization of convulsive seizure of amygdaloid origin, bisection of the anterior two-thirds of the corpus callosum is sufficient. Whether this would apply to patients with generalized seizures of a nonconvulsive nature must await further evaluation.

Encouraged by our experimental findings, two patients with medically intractable seizures having multifocal EEG abnormalities underwent commissurotomy here in Vancouver. One of these patients had severe behavior problems in addition to frequent automatism with or without convulsive seizure, whereas the other patient had up to eight atonic seizures with loss of consciousness. Both cases have been seizure-free since the surgery, that is, 18 months for the first case and 8 months for the second. Their EEG abnormalities remain unchanged but both are being rehabilitated. For the first time in their lives they are attending schools and learning social skills. The first case underwent bisection of the anterior commissure and anterior two-thirds of the corpus callosum and had a rather stormy course postoperatively, lasting for several months.

In our animal studies, saving of the ventricular lining has significantly reduced postoperative morbidity. The animals are able to be up and about as soon as they recover from anesthesia, in contrast with the prolonged nursing care required after opening of the ventricle. Based on our animal experience, the second case underwent bisection of the anterior two-thirds of the corpus callosum, leaving the ventricular lining intact. Her recovery was swift and uneventful and this finding is entirely consistent with an earlier suggestion made from clinical experience with commissurotomy (Wilson et al., 1977).

CONCLUSION

(a) When a patient fails to respond to medication or to a combination of medications supervised by a competent physician, in-depth evaluation should be undertaken to see whether the patient qualifies for classical open excisional surgery.

(b) Surgical excision of localized epileptogenic brain tissue is quite effective in helping patients who are drug resistant and whose origin or seizure can be traced to an accessible, dispensable, and circumscribed brain area. One can expect two-thirds of patients who undergo this operation to become completely or almost completely free of seizures. In spite of the proven value of this surgery, it is not used as extensively as it should be.

(c) When the patient does not qualify for open excisional surgery due to widespread areas of epileptic activity, or for other reasons, the possibility of an alternative surgical strategy must be entertained. Division of the corpus callosum (commissurotomy) appears to be one of the most promising approaches, with substantial support from animal investigation and some extremely encouraging clinical results in a limited number of patients. Elaboration of clinical criteria for case selection remains a challenge for the future.

(d) Increased awareness by the public, as well as by treating physicians, of the availability of such an alternative must be the first step toward rescuing the small percentage, but large number of "hopeless" patients before medically abandoning them.

REFERENCES

Ajmone-Marsan C., and Gumnit, R. J. (1974): Neurophysiological aspects of epilepsy. In: *Handbook of Clinical Neurology, Vol. 15: The Epilepsies*, edited by R. P. J. Vinken and G. W. Bruyn, pp. 30–59. American Elsevier, New York.

Bogen, J. E., and Vogel, P. J. (1975): Neurologic status in the long term following complete cerebral commissurotomy. In: *Les Syndromes de Disconnexion Calleuse Chez l'Homme*, edited by F. Michel and B. Schott, p. 227. *Hop. Neurol.*, Lyon.

Bogen, J. E., Sperry, R. W., and Vogel, P. J. (1969): Commissural section and the propagation of seizures. In: *Basic Mechanisms of the Epilepsies*, edited by H. Jasper, A. A. Ward, and A. Pope, p. 439. Little, Brown and Company, Boston.

Brown, J. W. (1973): Structural substrates of seizure foci in the human temporal lobe. In: *Epilepsy, Its Phenomena in Man*, edited by M.A.D. Brazier, pp. 341–374. Academic Press, New York.

Cooper, I. S. (1973): Chronic stimulation of paleocerebellar cortex in man. *Lancet*, i:306.

Cooper, I. S., Amin, I., Riklan, M., Waltz, J., and Poon, T. (1976): Chronic cerebellar stimulation in epilepsy. *Arch. Neurol.*, 33:559–570.

Erickson, T. C. (1940): Spread of the epileptic discharge. *Arch. Neurol. Psychiatry.*, 32:429–452.

Goldstein, M. N., and Joynt, R. J. (1969): Long-term follow-up of a collossal-sectioned patient. *Arch. Neurol.*, 20:96.

Harris, A. (1972): Degeneration in experimental epileptic foci. *Arch. Neurol.*, 26:434–449.

Jackson, J. H. (1958): In: *Selected Writings of John Hughlings Jackson, Vol. 1: On Epilepsy and Epileptiform Convulsions*, edited by James Taylor. Basic Books Incorporated, New York. Original in London 1931, Hodder and Stoughton.

Jensen, I. (1975): Temporal lobe surgery around the world: Results, complications and morality. *Acta Neurol. Scand.*, 52:354–373.

Jinnai, D. (1966): Clinical results and the significance of Forel-H-tomy in the treatment of epilepsy. *Conf. Neurol.*, 27:219–236.

Luessenhop, A. J. (1970): Interhemispheric commissurotomy as an alternate to hemispherectomy for control of intractable seizures. *Am. Surg.*, 36:265.

Luessenhop, A. J., De la Cruz, T. C., and Fenichel, G. M. (1970): Surgical disconnection of the cerebral hemispheres for intractable seizures. *JAMA*, 213:1630.

Marcus, E. M., and Watson, C. W. (1966): Bilateral synchronous spike wave electrographic patterns in the cat: Interaction of bilateral cortical foci in the intact, the bilateral cortical-callosal and adiencephalic preparation. *Arch. Neurol.*, 14:601–610.

Marcus, E. M., and Watson, C. W. (1968): Bilateral symmetrical epileptogenic foci in monkey cerebral cortex. *Arch. Neurol.*, 19:99–116.

Mukawa, J., and Jinnai, D. (1975): Forel-H-tomy for the treatment of intractable epilepsy. Special reference to postoperative electroencephalographic changes. *Conf. Neurol.*, 37:302–307.

Ojemann, G. A. (1978): The future role of surgery in the treatment of epilepsy. In: *Modern Perspectives in Epilepsy*, edited by J. A. Wada, pp. 209–226. Eden Press, Montreal.

Rasmussen, T. (1975): Cortical resection in the treatment of focal epilepsy. In: *Advances in Neurology, Vol. 8: Neurosurgical Management of the Epilepsies*, edited by D. P. Purpura, J. K. Penry, and R. D. Walter, pp. 139–154. Raven Press, New York.

Scheibel, M. E., Crandall, P. H., and Scheibel, A. B. (1974): The hippocampal-dentate complex in temporal lobe epilepsy. A Golgi study. *Epilepsia*, 15:55–80.

Van Wagenen, W. P., and Herren, R. Y. (1940): Surgical division of commissural pathways in the corpus callosum. *Arch. Neurol. Psychiatr.*, 44:740–759.

Wada, J. A. (1951): An experimental study on the neural mechanism of the spread of epileptic impulse. *Folia. Psychiatr. Neurol. Jpn.*, 3:27–33.

Wada, J. A. (1974–1975): Progressive seizure recurring in subhuman primate and effect of cerebellar stimulation upon developed versus developing amygdaloid seizure. In: *10th Anniversary Symposium of Mexican National Institute of Neurology*, edited by A. Escobar. *Bol. Estud. Med. Biol.*, 8–10:285–301.

Wada, J. A., Osawa, T., and Mizoguchi, T. (1975): Recurrent spontaneous seizure state induced by prefrontal kindling in Senegalese baboons *Papio papio*. *Can. J. Neurol. Sci.*, 2:477–492.

Wada, J. A., and Osawa, T. (1976): Spontaneous recurrent seizure state induced by daily electric amygdaloid stimulation in Senegalese baboons. (*Papio papio*). *Neurology (Minneap.)*, 26:273–286.

Wada, J. A., Mizoguchi, T., and Komai, S. (1977): Effect of prior forebrain bisection on amygdaloid seizure development in subhuman primates. In: *American Epilepsy Society Meeting*, New York, November 30, 1977 (Abstr. 7).

Wada, J. A., Mizoguchi, T., and Osawa, T. (1978): Secondarily generalized convulsive seizure induced by daily electrical stimulation in rhesus monkeys. *Neurology (Minneap.)*, 28:1026–1036.

Wilson, D. H., Culver, C., Waddington, M., and Gazzaniga, M. (1975): Disconnection of the cerebral hemisphere: An alternative to hemispherectomy for the control of intractable seizures. *Neurology (Minneap.)*, 25:1149–1153.

Wilson, D. H., Reeves, A. G., Gazzaniga, M., and Culver, C. (1977): Cerebral commissurotomy for control of intractable seizures. *Neurology (Minneap.)*, 27:708–715.

Wilson, D. H., Reeves, A. and Gazzaniga, M. (1978): Division of the corpus callosum for uncontrollable epilepsy. *Neurology (Minneap.)*, 28:649–653.

Advances in Epileptology:
The Xth Epilepsy International Symposium,
edited by J. A. Wada and J. K. Penry.
Raven Press, New York © 1980.

Corpus Callosotomy for Control of Intractable Seizures

Donald H. Wilson, Alexander Reeves, and Michael Gazzaniga

*Departments of Neurosurgery and Neurology, Dartmouth-Hitchcock Medical Center
Hanover, New Hampshire 03755*

Cerebral commissurotomy, or the "split-brain procedure," is defined as the surgical division of one or more forebrain commissures for the control of intractable seizures. The corpus callosum (including the underlying, adherent, hippocampal commissure), fornices, anterior commissure, and massa intermedia of the thalamus comprise the commissures that have been divided in man.

There is persuasive evidence that these neocommissures, especially the corpus callosum, are the preferred pathways for seizure discharges passing from one hemisphere to another, whereas subcortical routes play a secondary role. When they are divided, discharges should be confined to the abnormal hemisphere, thereby converting a generalized seizure to a partial one. Furthermore, an overall reduction in the number of discharging neurons should raise the threshold for partial seizures, allowing them to be controlled by moderate doses of anticonvulsant drugs. These are the theoretical bases for commissurotomy, which seem to be confirmed in the small number of patients who have undergone the operation.

This chapter describes the evolution of commissurotomy with particular reference to the most recent experience in a series of 13 consecutive cases.

HISTORICAL BACKGROUND

In 1940, Erickson described the results of his research in the monkey on the spread of epileptic discharges from one cerebral hemisphere to the other. He stated that "this spread occurs largely or entirely via the corpus callosum" and "with the cerebral cortex intact, subcortical centers play a secondary role. . . ." He made another important observation that was overlooked when the animal experiments were transferred to man: "Partial division of the corpus callosum, even of all the fibers responding to electrical stimulation, does not abolish the spread of epileptic discharge from one hemisphere to the other, although it may cause delay."

In the same year, Van Wagenen reported his experience with the first cerebral commissurotomies performed on humans. It was a remarkable example of synchronicity if Van Wagenen were unaware of Erickson's experiments. He made no reference to them, claiming that the idea for commissurotomy came from his observations on epileptics who subsequently developed tumors or infarcts of the corpus callosum; as their new diseases became manifest their seizures diminished. Although he operated on 26 people, Van Wagenen discussed only the first 10 in his paper. Most of them underwent partial division of the corpus callosum, usually completed at a second operation. He also divided the left fornix in four, and the anterior commissure in one. He did not discuss his reasons for fornicotomy or anterior commissurotomy. His results appeared to be good: All 10 patients recovered from surgery with few ill effects and seizures appeared to be improved. But the longest follow-up, in his paper, was only 5 months. In 1944, Akelaitis performed psychological tests on some of Van Wagenen's patients and concluded that commissurotomy had no obvious effect on cognition, affect, memory, or behavior. However, he had little interest in the effect of the operations on epilepsy and only mentioned that seizures seemed to be improved.

Commissurotomy was revived by Bogen in 1962. He and Vogel had operated on 15 or more patients by 1970 but the results of their series as a whole remain unreported. Bogen's papers on selected patients, and his last one in 1975 on 10 patients, showed that the operation had powerful potential for relieving intractable seizures (Bogen and Vogel, 1965, 1975). Bogen performed two kinds of commissurotomy—"complete" and "frontal." The "frontal" operation (Bogen et al., 1971) was reserved for multifocal seizures that involved only the frontal or anterior temporal areas of the brain, where the anterior commissure and the anterior part of the corpus callosum (to the splenium) were divided. Sometimes one fornix was included. In his "complete" commissurotomy, Bogen divided the anterior commissure, the whole corpus callosum, one fornix, and at times, the massa intermedia of the thalamus (primarily to gain access to the anterior commissure through the third ventricle). Those patients whom Bogen discussed recovered from surgery without undue difficulty and many had dramatic relief of their seizures, which was sustained by moderate doses of anticonvulsants.

While Bogen and Vogel were performing these operations, Sperry and Gazzaniga were studying the subtle effects of the "split-brain procedure" (as they called it) on monkeys. They discovered that the forebrain commissures, especially the corpus callosum, conveyed sensory information from one hemisphere to the other that allowed the hemispheres to work as an integrated unit. When the commissures were divided, each hemisphere became independent of the other. At Bogen's invitation, Gazzaniga and Sperry (1962) adapted their neuropsychological tests to humans and tested his patients. Until this time the normal functions of the commissures were unknown. These subtle tests showed that humans, like monkeys, became "disconnected"; two minds dwelled in one brain. Information processed by one hemisphere was no longer available to the other. When Akelaitis said that Van Wagenen's patients seemed to show no defects in cognition, memory, or affect after commissurotomy, he was also right, for in everyday life each hemisphere received the same information from the environment at the same time. The "split-brain" became such a fine tool for extracting information on the normal functions of the brain that it overshadowed its ability to alter seizures.

In 1970, Luessenhop et al. reported the results of "complete" commissurotomy on four children. They were excellent when brain damage was clearly limited to one hemisphere, and he believed that commissurotomy was a better alternative to hemispherectomy for the control of incapacitating seizures.

THE DARTMOUTH SERIES

The Dartmouth series of commissurotomies began in 1972 after a review of the available literature, consultation with Luessenhop, and a visit to Bogen. We believed that the operations could be made safer by using microsurgical techniques, and that the proposed series should be carefully organized. A neurologist (Reeves) chose the candidate from his service after performing the following tests: physical examination, skull X-rays, CT scan (which has largely replaced pneumoencephalography and angiography), blood levels of anticonvulsants, serial EEGs, careful recording of seizures, and further manipulations of drugs if appropriate. Seizures had to be intractable; i.e., at least four daytime generalized seizures each month, uncontrollable on a supervised regimen of anticonvulsants for 4 years and not amenable to standard methods of surgery; intelligence adequate to lead a reasonably independent life; and relatives who cared enough to see the patient through a long convalescence. A determined effort was made to localize the areas of brain damage but patients who lacked definitive signs of unilateral damage were not excluded. Tores and French (1973) demonstrated that it was often impossible to distinguish a primary from a propagated seizure, and Goldring (1972) believed that the EEG was limited in its ability to localize multiple discharges. An experimental neuropsychologist (Gazzaniga) conducted special preoperative and postoperative "split-brain" tests. A clinical psychologist (Culver) performed a battery of standard psychological tests before and after surgery to determine intelligence and the extent of brain damage (Reitan and Davison, 1974). The operations were performed by one surgeon (Wilson) who returned patients to the Neurology Service after they had recovered from the effects of surgery. Every patient was followed at regular intervals by the team.

The first series of eight patients consisted of three "complete" commissurotomies and then five "frontal" commissurotomies (Wilson et al. 1977).

The first patient, a 9-year-old boy, was a candidate for hemispherectomy (Wilson et al., 1975). He had a left hemiparesis and was experiencing so many seizures each day that he lived on a mattress on the floor. By mistake, no anticonvulsants were given after "complete" commissurotomy. He has had no seizures since his operation 6 years ago. The fifth patient underwent a "frontal" commissurotomy in 1973 and has been without seizures for 5 years. He was on phenytoin 300 mg daily until this treatment was stopped 1 year ago. These two cases seemed to reflect the full potential of commissurotomy for relieving uncontrollable epilepsy.

In the others, it was difficult to define improvement of seizures since postoperative complications often obscured the effect of commissurotomy. In spite of the change to microsurgical technique and to smaller craniotomies, ventriculitis (sterile and bacterial) was frequent and disabling; morbidity was not reported by others. The eighth patient died suddenly from a hemorrhagic infarct in her right frontal lobe, probably from the excessive traction required in getting around the genu of the corpus callosum to divide the anterior commissure from the outside: The attempt to resect all the recommended commissures, while trying to respect the integrity of the ventricular system, had failed. The risk : benefit ratio was too high.

No further operations were performed for 18 months, during which time the series was carefully analyzed. It was finally concluded that commissurotomy did, indeed, alter seizures for the better but the technical aspects of the operation had to be improved. A review of all available clinical and laboratory data on the subject provided the clue: The corpus callosum seemed to be the problem. Because of its large size and outstanding function in conveying sensory data from one hemisphere to the other, it was probable that this was also the major pathway for seizure discharges, and that the other commissures together with the brainstem played a secondary role. Even if these smaller commissures did play a larger role in conducting discharges it was clear that seizures still utilized the largest and most accessible commissural system to the greatest degree. It appeared to be quite feasible to divide the entire corpus callosum down to (but not through) the ependymal lining of the ventricles. Also, by restricting the operation to one commissure, it would be possible to glean more precise information on its role in seizures and in health, and to perhaps indirectly discover what role the other commissures played in epilepsy.

In 1975, beginning with case 9, a second series of operations began. Five patients underwent total extraventricular division of the corpus callosum (Wilson et al., 1978). All had a smooth recovery from surgery; and with one exception, all had a decided improvement in their seizures. The exception, case 11, deserves discussion.

Case Report

A 24-year-old man had a cystic astrocytoma removed from his left frontal lobe at age 14, followed by irradiation. Generalized tonic-clonic seizures then occurred as well as partial conscious adversive seizures to the right. These became incapacitating and unresponsive to anticonvulsants. The cause of his seizures was found to be an area of scar tissue in the left frontal lobe, close to Broca's area, a residual from previous surgery and irradiation. The risk of motor aphasia was considered to be too high for a focal resection to be performed. Since this was a unique problem of partial and generalized seizures beginning at a known site, it was decided that the corpus callosotomy be performed in two stages. EEGs showed bilateral symmetrical spike discharges in the frontal lobes. If Bogen was right, then division of the anterior part of the corpus callosum back to the splenium would relieve seizures, prevent the "acute disconnection syndrome" of the "complete" commissurotomy, and maintain some integration of the partially isolated hemispheres. In April, 1976, the rostrum, splenium, and body of the corpus callosum back to the splenium were divided. All other commissures were spared and the ventricles were not opened. Recovery from surgery was prompt and uncomplicated. For 5 months, the patient had no seizures and EEGs showed disappearance of the epileptic activity in his right frontal lobe. This suggested that the anterior commissure was not being used by the discharges. Then convulsions recurred, at first partial (but not adversive) and then generalized. EEGs underwent a striking change: Spike discharges spread from the primary locus in the left frontal lobe to the right parietooccipital lobe, but *not* to the right frontal lobe, suggesting that they had eventually found their way across the intact part of the corpus callosum.

Erickson was probably right when he predicted that partial division of the corpus callosum would delay, but not abolish, the spread of discharges from one hemisphere to the other. In February, 1977, the splenium was divided. Once more recovery was swift and uneventful. Seizures diminished but did not stop and Gazzaniga showed by his special "split-brain" tests that a bridge of intact callosum remained. This was confirmed by the EEGs, which showed spread to the right temporal area this time. At the second operation, we had been unable to insure that the corpus callosum had been completely divided by our usual patty-retrieval method. Since the patient's seizures were under reasonable control, a third operation could not be justified. But his case was a striking demonstration of the importance of the corpus callosum in conducting seizure discharges

Since postoperative recovery was smooth in the five cases of series two, the results of neuropsychological tests were not obscured by operative trauma to the brain, and they showed the effects of dividing only one commissure. Much information on the normal function of the brain was gleaned (Gazzaniga et al., 1975; Gazzaniga et al., 1977; Gazzaniga and LeDoux, 1978; Greenwood et al., 1977; LeDoux et al., 1977; LeDoux et al., 1978; Risse et al., 1978).

TECHNIQUE OF CORPUS CALLOSOTOMY (FIG. 1)

Under endotracheal anesthesia, the patient was in a semi-sitting position with his head fixed in a skull clamp. While the scalp was clipped and cleansed, an infusion of mannitol (0.5 g per minute per kilogram) was begun. First a posterior craniotomy was performed with the head well flexed. A 9-cm linear incision was made in the right parietal area and separated by

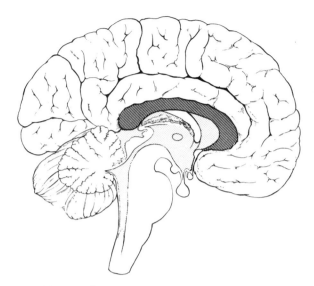

FIG. 1. The corpus callosum (*shaded area*), was the only commissure divided in series 2.

self-retaining retractors (Fig. 2). A D'Erico trephine (with guard), 2 inches in diameter, attached to the Hudson adapter in the arc craniotome, was used to remove a bone disc whose medial edge crossed the sagittal sinus while the anterior edge lay 1 inch behind the midpoint of nasion and inion; i.e., just behind the motor cortex (Wilson, 1971). The dura was opened and the medial edge of the right parietal lobe was retracted away from the falx (Fig. 3). A 3× loupe was worn. When the white splenium came into view, a self-retaining

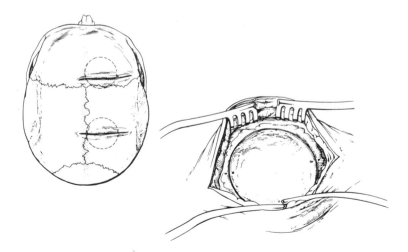

FIG. 2. Incision must cross midline for adequate exposure of sagittal sinus.

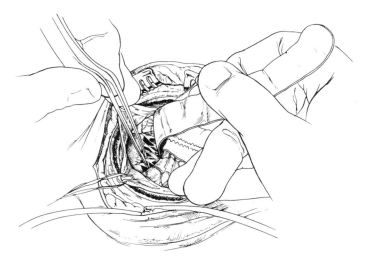

FIG. 3. Adhesions between brain and falx coagulated with bipolar forceps.

retractor maintained gentle traction on the brain and the operating microscope was brought into play. Under 16 power (with a 300-mm focal length), a central portion of the callosum was cleared of vessels with bipolar cautery forceps. A thin sucker transected the fibers down to the fairly tough ependymal lining of the ventricular roof (Fig. 4). This lining was not penetrated. Callosal fibers were divided posteriorly until the arachnoid over the tentorial notch was reached, and then anteriorly as far as possible. A cottonoid patty was left behind at the anterior limit of the resection, to be

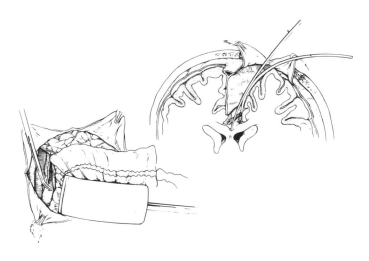

FIG. 4. Sucker divides callosum in an avascular area.

retrieved later through the anterior craniotomy. This insured that the callosum was divided between the wounds. The dura was closed, the bone disc replaced, and the scalp apposed.

The head was extended for an anterior craniotomy. An incision was made 9 cm behind the nasion. The medial aspect of the bone disc was again over the sagittal sinus and the posterior edge on the coronal suture. The callosum was divided around the genu until it trailed off in the rostrum, and posteriorly to the patty which was retrieved. The wound was closed.

Dexamethasone 10 mg i.v. was given during surgery, and thereafter 4 mg every 6 hr. The dosage was gradually tapered over 7 days. The patient's usual anticonvulsant medication was continued, and then lowered and simplified as seizures and blood levels dictated.

CONCLUSIONS

Extraventricular microsurgical division of the corpus callosum was safer than multiple intraventricular commissurotomies and appeared to be equally effective in controlling seizures.

Surgery was not a substitute for continued use of anticonvulsants; seizure discharges still utilized other pathways, but these could usually be blocked with moderate doses of anticonvulsants.

If brain damage was found to be limited to one hemisphere before *or* after surgery, a good outcome could be predicted. Frequently, primary discharges lateralized only after surgery.

ACKNOWLEDGMENTS

The authors are grateful to the editor of *Neurology* for permitting them to reproduce some of the figures and part of the text from their article, "Division of the Corpus Callosum for Uncontrollable Epilepsy" which appeared in the July, 1978 issue.

REFERENCES

Akelaitis, A. J. (1944): A study of gnosis, praxia, and language following section of the corpus callosum and anterior commissure. *J. Neurosurg.*, 1:94.

Bogen, J. E., Gordon, H. W., and Sperry, R. W. (1971): Absence of deconnexion syndrome in two patients with partial section of the neocommissures. *Brain*, 94:327.

Bogen, J. E., and Vogel, P. J. (1965): Cerebral commissurotomy in man. *Bull. Los Angeles Neurol. Soc.*, 27:169.

Bogen, J. E., and Vogel, P. J. (1975): Neurologic status in the long term following complete cerebral commissurotomy. In: *Les Syndromes de Disconnexion Calleuse Chez L'homme*, edited by F. Michel and B. Schott, p. 227. *Hop. Neurol. Lyon.*

Erickson, T. C. (1940): Spread of the epileptic discharge. *Arch. Neurol.*, 43:429.

Gazzaniga, M. S., Bogen, J. E., and Sperry, R. W. (1962): Some functional effects of sectioning the cerebral commissures in man. *Proc. Natl. Acad. Sci. USA*, 48:1765.

Gazzaniga, M. S., and LeDoux, J. E. (1978): *The Integrated Mind.* Plenum Press, New York.

Gazzaniga, M. S., Risse, G. L., Springer, S. P., et al. (1975): Psychologic and neurologic consequences of partial and complete cerebral commissurotomy. *Neurology (Minneap.)*, 25:10.

Gazzaniga, M. S., Wilson, D. H., and LeDoux, J. D. (1977): Language, praxis and the right hemisphere: Clues to some mechanisms of consciousness. *Neurology (Minneap.)*, 27:1144.

Goldring, S. (1972): The role of prefrontal cortex in grand mal convulsion. *Arch. Neurol.*, 26:190.

Greenwood, P., Wilson, D. H., and Gazzaniga, M. S. (1977): Dream report following commissurotomy. *Cortex*, 13:311.

LeDoux, J. E., Risse, G. L., Springer, S. P., et al. (1977): Cognition and commissurotomy. *Brain*, 100:87.

LeDoux, J. E., Wilson, D. H., and Gazzaniga, M. S. (1978): A divided mind: Observations of the conscious properties of the separated hemispheres. *Ann. Neurol.*, *(in press)*.

Lussenhop, A. J., Delacruz, T. C., and Fenichel, G. M. (1970): Surgical disconnection of the cerebral hemispheres for intractable seizures. *JAMA*, 213:1630.

Reitan, R. M., and Davison, L. A. (editors) (1974): *Clinical Neuropsychology: Current Status and Applications*. John Wiley and Sons, New York.

Risse, G. L., LeDoux, J. E., Springer, S. P., et al. (1978): The anterior commissure in man: Functional variation in a multisensory system. *Neuropsychologia*, 16:23.

Tores, F., and French, L. A. (1973): Acute effect of section of the corpus callosum upon "independent" epileptiform activity. *Acta Neurol. Scand.*, 49:47.

Van Wagenen, W. P., and Herren, R. Y. (1949): Surgical division of commissural pathways in the corpus callosum. *Arch. Neurol.*, 44:740.

Wilson, D. H. (1971): Limited exposure in cerebral surgery. *J. Neurosurg.*, 34:102.

Wilson, D. H., Culver, C., Waddington, M., et al. (1975): Disconnection of the cerebral hemispheres: An alternative to hemispherectomy for the control of intractable seizures. *Neurology (Minneap.)*, 24:1149.

Wilson, D. H., Reeves, A., Gazzaniga, M. S., et al. (1977): Cerebral commissurotomy for the control of intractable seizures. *Neurology (Minneap.)*, 27:708.

Wilson, D. H., Reeves, A., and Gazzaniga, M. S. (1978): Division of the corpus callosum for uncontrollable epilepsy. *Neurology (Minneap.)*, 28:649.

Advances in Epileptology:
The Xth Epilepsy International Symposium,
edited by J. A. Wada and J. K. Penry.
Raven Press, New York © 1980.

Some Effects of Chronic Cerebellar Stimulation on EEG and Epilepsy in Man

*I. S. Cooper, **A. R. M. Upton, and *I. Amin

*Center for Physiologic Neurosurgery, Westchester County Medical Center,
Valhalla, New York 10595; and **Department of Neurology,
McMaster University Medical Center, Hamilton, Ontario, Canada*

Chronic cerebellar stimulation (CCS) was conceived as a method of prosthetically activating inhibitory mechanisms in the nervous system in order to ameliorate symptoms resulting from neuronal hyperactivity (Cooper, 1973a,b). It has been investigated on our service during the past 6 years in several syndromes that we consider to be disorders of sensory communication or disinhibition (Cooper and Upton, 1978).

Of 375 patients who have undergone CCS on our service, the majority had suffered primarily from spasticity or cerebral palsy. We investigated the effect of inhibitory mechanisms on seizures in 36 cases (Cooper et al., 1976). Sufficient time has elapsed to permit us to evaluate the rationale, safety, and efficacy of neurosomatory activation of inhibitory mechanisms on seizures.

METHODS OF INVESTIGATION

The population consisted of 36 patients suffering from intractable epilepsy. Each patient in this group had proved unresponsive to a prolonged period of treatment with commonly used anticonvulsant drugs in therapeutic doses. In each instance, the epilepsy was of long duration, in some cases almost lifelong, without any reasonable likelihood of spontaneous remission. The mean age was 28.0 years. The mean length of illness was 17.6 years. The time since surgery ranged from 12 to 65 months. Among the specific selection criteria, in addition to an intractability to previous therapy, were definitive electroencephalographic (EEG) abnormalities, an I.Q. score of at least 70 on standardized intelligence tests, and the absence of any demonstrable mass lesion.

Each patient was clinically evaluated with reference to frequency, severity, and type of seizures before and after treatment with CCS. Seizure evaluation was based on pre- and postoperative records maintained by the patient's family, on inpatient hospital records maintained by the patient's family, on inpatient hospital records, and on detailed interviews with patients and their families. The psychological status of the patients was assessed by standard psychological tests, including the Wechsler Adult Intelligence Scale (WAIS), the Wechsler Memory Scale (WMS), and the Bender Gestalt (BG) administered before and after surgery. Standardized psychological interviews were also undertaken to evaluate emotional status and behavioral functions.

In 13 of the epileptic patients, in addition to EEG, special neurophysiologic studies were carried out (Upton and Cooper, 1976). These included the acute effects of cerebellar stimulation on H reflexes, V_1, and V_2 late reflexes, blink reflexes, subcortical and cortical somatosensory evoked potentials (SSEP) after median nerve stimulation, visual evoked responses, and subcortical auditory evoked responses. More recently, we have employed split-screen videomonitoring of the EEG and the patient before, during, and after cerebellar stimulation. Biopsy material from the posterior lobe of the cerebellum prior to implantation of electrodes was obtained in 12 patients. These biopsies were stained with hematoxylin and eosin and examined to determine the presence or absence of Purkinje cell loss or other signs of cerebellar cortical atrophy (Urich et al., 1978).

SURGICAL TECHNIQUES

Results

The electrode-bearing pads are placed on the anterior or the posterior cerebellar cortex or both and the lead from each electrode configuration is carried subcutaneously to a receiver placed inferior to the clavicles or some other subcutaneous position preselected by the surgeon (Fig. 1). Bilateral anterior and posterior electrode placement is currently considered the configuration of choice. Stimulation is achieved by transcutaneous induction of a radio-frequency signal from a power pack carried by the patient.

We have employed bipolar electrodes with a capacitively coupled monophasic pulse (Avery, Medtronic) as well as electrodes with a modified biphasic pulse (Avery). Each is capable of inducing neurophysiological evidence of CNS inhibition. There are some indications that the monopolar, biphasic, capacitively coupled wave may be effective at lower levels of current than the bipolar, monophasic, capacitively coupled pulse wave.

Of the 36 patients, 20 were considered to demonstrate a good clinical response to CCS. In these patients, seizures were reduced at least 50%, with other significant signs of clinical improvement as well. One patient died postoperatively due to a posterior fossa hematoma.

There have been no observable undesirable neurological sequelae of CCS. Thus far CCS has not resulted in abnormal neurological signs in any patient from among either the epilepsy or cerebral palsy group.

Detailed clinical evaluation of our experience with epilepsy has been pre-

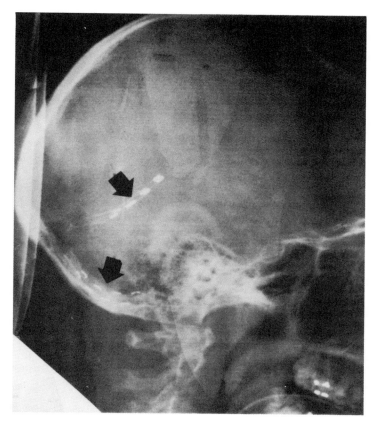

FIG. 1. Lateral X-ray showing location of anterior and posterior arrays of 8 platinum electrodes on right anterior and posterior cerebellar cortex.

viously reported. One case will be presented to illustrate the potential of neurostimulatory inhibition as a therapeutic approach to seizures.

Case Report

J. D., a 28-year-old man, developed seizures at the age of 6 years, which continued despite regular medical treatment. For 3 years prior to admission frequent episodes of status epilepticus had occurred. There were multiple daily seizures, and the patient was bedridden and totally incapacitated. The seizures were typically grand mal in type, without aura, the frequency varying up to 200 daily. On January 24, 1974, the patient underwent placement of cerebellar electrodes over the left anterior and posterior cerebellum. An initial improvement occurred after cerebellar stimulation, with frequency of seizures reduced to one attack every 3 to 4 weeks. However, 3 months after the onset of stimulation, frequent grand mal attacks in status epilepticus recurred. The patient returned to the hospital, and on June 24, 1974, electrodes were implanted over the right anterior cerebellum. Stimulation then led to marked alleviation of the seizures, with reduction in frequency and severity of attacks. The frequency of major seizures decreased from as many as 100 daily to one every 2 to 3 weeks. When the patient was seen on August 4, 1976, 31 months after initiation of cerebellar stimulation, he reported marked improvement of his seizures, with the frequency reduced from a preoperative level of approximately 100 daily to five to six a day. At the present time, the seizures he does experience are much shorter in duration, with a faster recovery and much less postictal drowsiness. The patient is now working part-time in his father's store and is functionally independent.

In the majority of epileptic patients, we have not observed an effect on seizure activity in the EEG (Fig. 2). This is similar to the findings of others who have confirmed significant seizure reduction during cerebellar stimulation in the absence of EEG changes (Fenton et al., 1977). However, in three of six cases in our series, subjected by Upton and McLellan to statistical analysis of paroxysmal discharges before, during, and after cerebellar stimulation, a comparison of epochs with stimulator on and off shows statistically significant ($p < 0.0001$) reduction in duration of discharges during stimulation (Upton, 1978).

Figure 3 demonstrates the effect of cerebellar stimulation on paroxysmal discharges in the EEG of the 26-year-old male described above (patient J.D.). Duration of paroxysmal discharges per 10-sec page is shown for periods when the stimulator was on by the black columns and off by the white columns. The recording reads continuously. In this case, the marked decrease in paroxysmal discharges was in conformity with the marked decrease in seizures during CCS.

A rebound increase in paroxysmal discharges frequently followed cessation of stimulation (Upton and Cooper, 1976; Upton and Cooper, 1977; Cooper and Upton, 1978) (Fig. 3B).

Figure 4 illustrates the computation of paroxysmal discharges in EEG for 270 sec (27 pages) of recording in the case of C. W., a 22-year-old epileptic patient. During cerebellar stimulation clinical seizures and abnormal EEG discharges were markedly reduced. There was a sharp increase in number and duration of paroxysmal discharges after the stimulator was switched off. Statistical analysis revealed significant ($p = < 0.0005$) increase in both number and duration of paroxysmal discharges following CCS.

Additional neurophysiologic evidence of inhibition followed by a rebound is observed at the spinal level.

Figure 5 demonstrates the effect of cerebellar stimulation on H responses in a 17-year-old epileptic female patient. Each frame represents five superimposed H reflex responses. The response is decreased during and after 1 min of cerebellar stimulation. There is a larger rebound amplitude of the H response 7 minutes after cessation of cerebellar stimulation.

A study of brainstem somatosensory and auditory click evoked responses generally reveals a suppression of the "thalamic response" (Fig. 6) and we have been able to confirm this observation with direct recordings from the

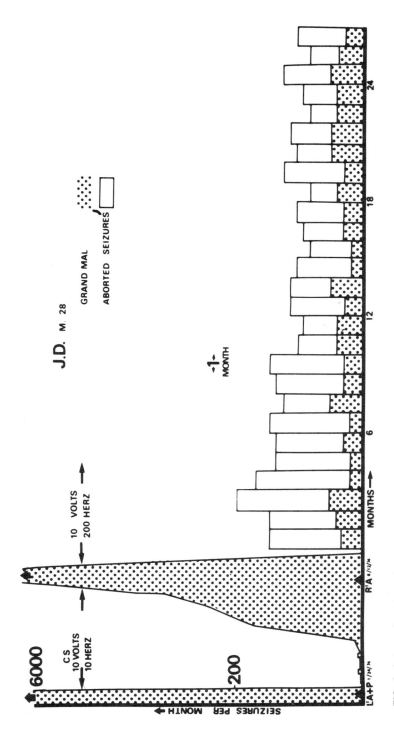

FIG. 2. Seizure frequency is displayed for each month and for 27 months after CCS in patient J. D. There was initial improvement after stimulation of left anterior and posterior cerebellar electrodes (Lt A + P) but seizures recurred and right anterior electrodes (Rt A) were inserted 6 months later.

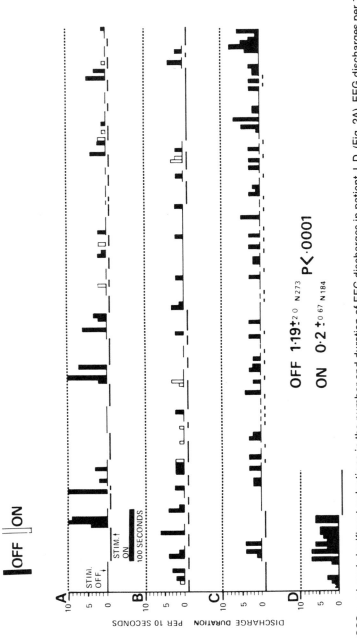

FIG. 3. CCS produced significant reductions in the number and duration of EEG discharges in patient J. D. (Fig. 2A). EEG discharges per 10 sec have been quantified during epochs when the cerebellar stimulator was ON (white columns) or OFF (black columns) (from Upton, 1978).

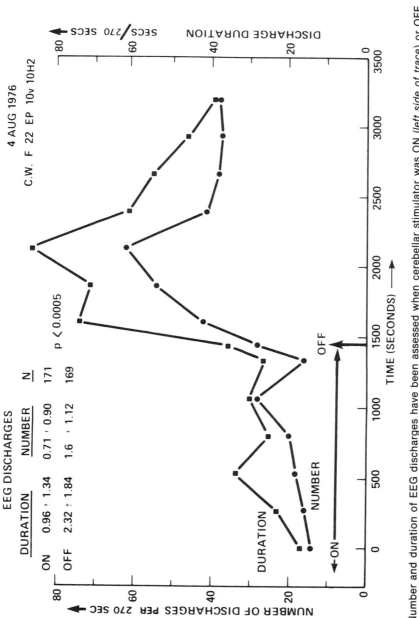

FIG. 4. Number and duration of EEG discharges have been assessed when cerebellar stimulator was ON (*left side of trace*) or OFF. The number of discharges per 270 sec showed significant increase (*p* < 0.0005) after cessation of CCS, and such *rebound* effects may well complicate interpretation of the results of double-blind studies of the effects of CCS (from Upton, 1978).

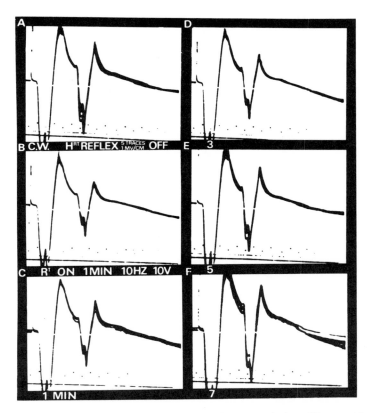

FIG. 5. H reflexes were recorded from the right soleus muscle in a 17-year-old epileptic girl. Each trace represents five superimposed traces on a Tektronix RM64 oscilloscope. Right sided CCS produced a reduction in amplitude of the H reflex response (B) with increasing amplitudes over the next 1(C), 3(D), 5(F) min periods. The response was larger (F) than control values (A) 7 min after 1 min CCS at 200 Hz and 10 V (from Upton, 1978).

thalamus during CCS. Often there is an augmentation of the midbrain response, which we believe represents an increase in reticular inhibitory activity.

These physiological studies conducted in our laboratory in the Westchester County Medical Center and at McMaster University Medical Centre illustrate the need for individual biocalibration of stimulation parameters in each case (Upton et al., 1977). The point is emphasized by the following examples.

Figure 7 demonstrates the fact that subthreshold stimulation fails to elicit an inhibitory effect on SSEP. Threshold stimulation (3V, 4V) inhibits various elements of the evoked response, whereas supramaximal (6V, 8V) stimulation results in no effect or a paradoxical increase in the response. Repeated biocalibration of each instrument and each patient should be an integral part of all neurostimulatory procedures, although clinical effects may be

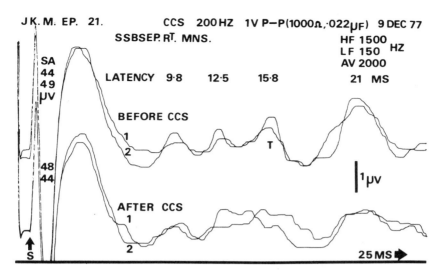

FIG. 6. Brainstem somatosensory-evoked responses were obtained after electrical stimulation of the right median nerve (Rt MNS). Each trace represents an average of 2,000 potentials after stimulation at 9.8 shocks/sec using a Nicolet CA 1000 averager with artifact rejection. An upward deflection on the trace represents a positive response at the CZ (vertex) electrode in comparison with a supraclavicular electrode contralateral to the stimulus. It can be seen that CCS produces a marked reduction in amplitude of responses at peak positive latencies of 12.5, 15.8, and 21 msec after the stimulus to the median nerve.

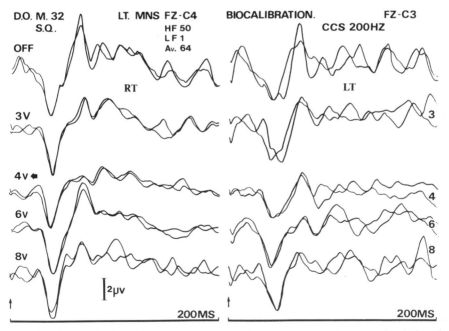

FIG. 7. Cortical somatosensory-evoked responses after left median nerve stimulation (Lt MNS) have been recorded over the right (RT) and left (LT) hemispheres between FZ and C4 or C3 electrodes. CCS produces a reduction in amplitude of responses at settings of 4 V, but responses are larger in amplitude at lower (subthreshold) and higher voltages. Excessive charge levels may produce *paradoxical* increases in the amplitude of evoked responses or in the number of paroxysmal EEG discharges. Such results may well explain the results of Van Buren et al. (1978).

seen at lower settings of the stimulator than those required to produce acute changes in evoked responses.

BEHAVIORAL STUDIES

Among patients undergoing CCS for periods of 1 to 5 years, none demonstrated any pattern of impairment in any measurable area of behavior or intellectual function. There is some evidence that tests of memory and/or cognitive functions show improvement over the longer term, which appears to be a manifestation of impairment in behavioral changes (Cooper et al., 1978*a,b*).

PATHOLOGICAL STUDIES

Urich and colleagues at the University of London studied biopsies from cerebellum prior to stimulation in 30 of our patients, 12 of whom had intractable epilepsy. They also studied the brains of four patients, two of whom were epileptic, who underwent cerebellar stimulation from 3 to 26 months.

They concluded that all of the epileptic patients had moderate to severe

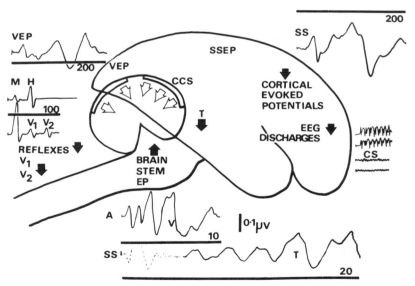

FIG. 8. Summary of effects of CCS (*white arrows*) on neurophysiological responses. *Upward arrows* indicate increased amplitudes and *downward arrows* indicate decreased amplitudes of cortical evoked responses (VEP = visual evoked responses after pattern stimulation; SSEP = somatosensory evoked responses after electrical stimulation of the median nerves), subcortical responses (A = Brainstem auditory evoked responses after biphasic click stimulation; SS = subcortical somatosensory-evoked responses after median nerve stimulation) thalamic potentials (T) and brainstem responses (Brainstem EP). Reflexes are generally reduced in amplitude after CCS (H = H reflex. V_1, V_2 = late responses) (Upton, 1978).

cerebellar pathology prior to electrode placement. It was also evident that placement of the electrodes can produce localized lesions subjacent to them due to mechanical, possibly unavoidable, factors. They concluded further that electrical stimulation, within the parameters we have employed, does not produce widespread or diffuse cerebellar damage.

The pathological changes produced in cerebellum by repeated seizures or long term phenylhydantoin therapy, are more severe and diffuse than the localized changes subjacent to the surface cerebellar electrodes (Urich et al., 1978).

MECHANISM OF ACTION OF CCS

In view of the striking loss of Purkinje cells in cerebellar cortex of epileptics, we believe that the inhibition produced at spinal, brainstem, and cortical levels by CCS is provoked by antidromic stimulation of deep cerebellar nuclei, inferior olivary nucleus, and brainstem reticular substance.

A REVIEW OF OTHER STUDIES OF CCS

The results of animal studies are conflicting. Human studies have been few and anecdotal. Fenton et al. (1977) reported encouraging results of CCS in one epileptic patient and Dow et al. (1977) found some improvement in three cases. Levy and Auchterlonie (1979) have published the results of CCS in six patients with intractable epilepsy. Two patients were greatly improved after CCS and were able to hold employment. One patient felt better despite no change in frequency of seizures, and another patient denied improvement despite 50% reduction in seizures.

Correll (1977) reported disappointing results of CCS in patients with psychomotor and generalized convulsive seizures, and only two of seven patients showed any improvement. Van Buren et al. (1978) attempted a double-blind controlled study of CCS in five patients. They chose to avoid any form of biocalibration, and set the stimulators at charge levels that were just below those required to produce headaches, despite good evidence that such stimulating levels are well above those required for therapeutic effects and paradoxical effects might be expected (Upton and Cooper, 1976; Upton, 1978; Cooper and Upton, 1978). Van Buren et al. (1978) reported no decrease in seizure frequency with CCS even though four patients reported improvement in seizure frequency and were enthusiastic about the treatment.

CONCLUSION

It is our conclusion that this study has demonstrated clinical and physiological evidence of CNS inhibition and suppression of seizure activity by CCS in some patients. Further definition of proper patient selection, improved stimulation equipment, and perfection of biocalibration techniques should potentiate the usefulness of this particular procedure. More important perhaps is the support that this study lends to the concept and rationale of the safety and efficacy of prosthetically mobilizing CNS inhibitory mechanisms (Cooper and Upton, 1978) as a primary or ancillary means of suppressing seizure activity.

REFERENCES

Cooper, I. S. (1973a): Chronic stimulation of palaeocerebellar cortex in man. *Lancet*, i:306.

Cooper, I. S. (1973b): Effect of chronic stimulation of anterior cerebellum on neurological disease. *Lancet*, i:1321.

Cooper, I. S., Amin, I., Riklan, M., Waltz, J. M., and Poon, T. P. (1976): Chronic cerebellar stimulation in epilepsy. *Arch. Neurol.*, 33:559–570.

Cooper, I. S., and Upton, A. R. M. (1978): Use of chronic cerebellar stimulation for disorders of disinhibition. *Lancet*, i:595–600.

Cooper, I. S., Riklan, M., Amin, I., and Cullinan, T. (1978a): A long-term follow-up study of cerebellar stimulation for the control of epilepsy. In: *Cerebellar Stimulation in Man*, edited by I. S. Cooper, pp. 19–38. Raven Press, New York.

Cooper, I. S., Riklan, M., Tabaddor, K., Cullinan, T., Amin, I., and Watkins, E. S. (1978b): A long-term follow-up study of chronic cerebellar stimulation for cerebral palsy. In: *Cerebellar Stimulation in Man*, edited by I. S. Cooper, pp. 59–99. Raven Press, New York.

Correll, J. (1977): Cerebellar stimulation. *Panel Presentation to the American Association of Neurological Surgeons*. Toronto, April 24–28.

Dow, R. S., Smith, W., and Mankonen, L. (1977): Proc. Western EEG Society, *Electroencephalogr. Clin. Neurophysiol.*, 43:906.

Fenton, G. W., Fenwick, P. B. C., Brindley, G. S., Falconer, M. A., Polkey, C. H., and Rushton, D. N. (1977): Chronic cerebellar stimulation in the treatment of epilepsy: A preliminary report. In: *Epilepsy: The Eighth International Symposium*, edited by J. K. Penry. Raven Press, New York.

Levy, L. F., and Auchterlonie, W. C. (1979): Chronic cerebellar stimulation in the treatment of epilepsy. *Epilepsia (Amst.)*, 20:235–245.

Upton, A. R. M. (1978): Neurophysiological mechanisms in modification of seizures. In: *Cerebellar Stimulation in Man*, edited by I. S. Cooper, pp. 39–57. Raven Press, New York.

Upton, A. R. M., and Cooper, I. S. (1976): Some neurophysiological effects of cerebellar stimulation in man. *Can. J. Neurol. Sci.*, 3:237–254.

Upton, A. R. M., and Cooper, I. S. (1977): Prolonged neurophysiological effects of cerebellar stimulation in man. *Electroencephalogr. Clin. Neurophysiol.*, 43:906.

Upton, A. R. M., Dunn, J., McLellan, D. L., and Cooper, I. S. (1977): Biocalibration of cerebellar stimulators in man. In: *American Association of Neurological Surgeons (Cushing Meeting)*, Toronto, Ontario, April 25.

Urich, H., Watkins, E. S., Amin, I., and Cooper, I. S. (1978): Neuropathologic observations on cerebellar cortical lesions in patients with epilepsy and motor disorders. In: *Cerebellar Stimulation in Man*, edited by I. S. Cooper, pp. 145–159. Raven Press, New York.

Van Buren, J. M., Wood, J. H., Oakley, J., and Hambrecht, F. (1978): Preliminary evaluation of cerebellar stimulation by double blind stimulation and biological criteria in the treatment of epilepsy. *J. Neurosurgery*, 48:407–416.

Advances in Epileptology:
The Xth Epilepsy International Symposium,
edited by J. A. Wada and J. K. Penry.
Raven Press, New York © 1980.

Forel-H-tomy for the Treatment of Intractable Epilepsy

*D. Jinnai, **J. Mukawa, **Y. Iwata, and †K. Kobayashi

*Department of Surgery, Kinki University Hospital, Osaka;
**Department of Neurosurgery, Osaka University, Osaka; and
†Institute for Neurobiology, Okayama University, Okayama, Japan

The long-term follow-up results of Forel-H-tomy (Jinnai and Nishimoto, 1966; Jinnai, 1966; Jinnai and Mukawa, 1970; Jinnai and Mukawa, 1973; Jinnai et al., 1976; Mukawa et al., 1975) for the treatment of epilepsy are summarized in this chapter.

PATIENTS AND METHODS

Sixty-eight patients with intractable epilepsy, 12 of whom were idiopathic and 56 symptomatic, were treated by Forel-H-tomy. There were 40 male and 28 female patients ages 2 to 33 years at the time of operation. The follow-up period was over 3 years, with a maximum period of 14 years and 4 months.

Bilateral operations were initially performed with an interval of 0 to 2 weeks, but in recent years the interval has routinely been over 6 months, which seems to be long enough to evaluate the postoperative course of the first operation. The target point is located 2 mm posterior to the midpoint of the AC-PC line, 4 mm ventral to the line, and 4.5 to 5 mm lateral to the third ventricle wall (Schaltenbrand and Bailey, 1959; Spiegel and Wycis, 1952; Van Buren and Borke, 1972). The criteria of clinical evaluation and location of lesion are the same as already reported (Jinnai and Mukawa, 1970). Cryogenic lesions were made at the beginning and later by a radiofrequency electrocoagulation method.

CLINICAL RESULTS

Clinical Seizures

As summarized in Table 1, strategically placed lesions produced better results both in the idiopathic and symptomatic groups. If the lesion missed the target point, the effectiveness was decreased. It is to be noted that some of the cases of unilateral surgery have remained under observation awaiting

Effect on Clinical Seizures

(idiopathic epilepsy)

	Lesions	Excellent	Good	Poor or no effect
Bilateral surgery (6)	Bilaterally complete	2	1	
	Others	3		
Unilateral surgery (6)	Complete	2	1	1
	Incomplete or out of target			2

TABLE 1A.

Effect on Clinical Seizures

(symptomatic epilepsy)

	Lesions	Excellent	Good	Poor or no effect
Bilateral surgery (21)	Bilaterally complete	3	6	4
	Others	1	2	5
Unilateral surgery (35)	Complete	11	14	7
	Incomplete or out of target			3

TABLE 1B.

surgery on the opposite side, especially in the symptomatic group, for example, cases with Lennox syndrome.

Seizure Types

In three idiopathic cases with well-placed lesions, grand mal seizures were abolished in three patients and myoclonic seizures were abolished in one case and diminished in one case.

In 13 symptomatic cases with well-placed bilateral lesions, generalized and focal convulsions and Lennox syndrome were controlled, but psychomotor seizures were not (Table 2).

In 32 symptomatic cases with well-placed unilateral lesions (Table 3), generalized, hemi-, and focal convulsions were controlled. Psychomotor seizures were not controlled. Lennox syndrome was slightly controlled by a

Effect on Clinical Seizure Types

(13 symptomatic cases with bilaterally
complete lesions)

	abolished	diminished	unchanged
general. convul.	7	1	
focal convul.	2	1	
Lennox	2	2	1
reflex epilepsy		·1	
psychomotor			4

21 in total

TABLE 2.

unilateral lesion. One patient of status petit mal who was operated on unilaterally had an excellent result, but the seizures, although controllable, recurred 1 year later but the patient was without status epilepticus for 6 years.

Electroencephalographic Changes

As reported in a previous paper (Mukawa and Jinnai, 1975), an increase of background activity and improvement of abnormal discharges, especially of spike-and-wave complex type, were found after Forel-H-tomy, although there was no direct correlation with the clinical course. There was no evidence to indicate epileptogenicity produced by the lesion of Forel's H field.

Other Symptoms

Unstable behavior, especially aggression, was markedly improved in three cases. Motivation was improved in nine cases, including six cases of Lennox

Effect on Clinical Seizure Types

(32 symptomatic cases with unilaterally
complete lesion)

	abolished	diminished	unchanged
general. convul.	17	6	
hemiconvul.	2	1	
focal convul.	8	6	
akinetic		2	
petit mal		1	
Lennox		4	3
psychomotor			3

53 in total

TABLE 3.

syndrome, together with seizure improvement. Cerebellar signs were completely abolished in one patient, enabling him to stand and walk without disturbance of balance after operation. Stridor, one of the most controllable symptoms often causing respiratory infection in severely debilitated children, was cleared up in two cases of postmeningitic epilepsy.

Social Evaluation

Social evaluation was carried out on the basis of prognosis (Table 4). Out of 12 patients in the idiopathic group, seven were employed, three were institutionalized, and two died. Out of 56 cases in the symptomatic group, 36 were employed or in school, 17 were institutionalized, and 3 died.

One idiopathic and four symptomatic patients have remained well without any necessity of anticonvulsant medication.

Social Evaluation in Idiopathic Epilepsy
(follow-up: over 3 years)

	Lesions	Employ.	Institut.	Dead
Bilateral surgery (6)	Bilaterally complete	2 (1 without anticonvul.)	0	1 (myoclonus)
	Others	1	2	0
Unilateral surgery (6)	Complete	4	0	0
	Incomplete or out of target	0	1	1

TABLE 4A.

Social Evaluation in Symptomatic Epilepsy
(follow-up: over 3 years)

	Lesions	Employ. or school.	Institut.	Dead
Bilateral surgery (21)	Bilaterally complete	7 (2 without anticonvul.)	4	2 (heart failure)
	Others	3	4	1 (heart failure)
Unilateral surgery (35)	Complete	15 (2 without anticonvul.)	7	0
	Incomplete or out of target	1	2	0

TABLE 4B.

Side Effects

Side effects were observed in four cases (Table 5). An akinetic type of motor disturbance was found in two and speech and swallowing disturbances in four cases. These four patients were operated on by bilateral Forel-H-tomy. Psychometric tests (Table 6) revealed no intellectual deficit after operation. The deficits appear, therefore, to be due to extrapyramidal lesions.

DISCUSSION

Forel-H-tomy was originally designed to interrupt the pathway of epileptic discharges at the level of Forel's H field between the lenticular nucleus and substantia nigra as summarized in a previous paper (Mukawa and Jinnai, 1971). However, the control of seizures was found to be due not only to interrupting the descending convulsive impulses but also to elevating the seizure threshold, possibly by interrupting the cortico-subcortical reverberating circuit (Iwata, 1967; Kobayashi, 1972; Mukawa, 1964a,b).

Clinically, this is explained by the improvement of EEG abnormalities, especially of seizure discharges (Mukawa and Jinnai, 1975). As mentioned above, the improvement of "other symptoms" such as aggression and lack of motivation was found after operation irrespective of drug dosage. Stridor was also cleared up by the operation. These behavioral and respiratory abnormalities are often found in severe epileptic patients, and the improvements coincide with the clinical course of the seizures.

There have been many reports describing psychoneurological abnormalities in epilepsy, but correlation as to whether these abnormalities are primary or secondary to the seizures is difficult from a clinical point of view. It is reasonable to postulate, from our surgical experiences, that some of them are directly associated with seizures and some with clinically latent seizure episodes, and the improvement in these psychoneurological abnormalities immediately after operation indicates the improvement of epileptic disturbance of the nervous system.

The problem is how to determine the stereotaxic coordinates in epileptic patients. As summarized in Table 7, most of our patients have dilatation of the lateral and third ventricles. A normal range of the VC-index (less than 0.25) is found only in 12 out of 50 cases (minimum 0.22). The same number of patients have definite dilatation (over 0.3 based on Evans criteria: maximum 0.57). On the other hand, a normal range of the width of the third ventricle (less than 5 mm) is found in only four patients (minimum 4 mm) out of 50 based on Taveras criteria. Marked dilatation (over 10 mm) is found in 11 patients (maximum 17 mm). The lateral distance between the target point and the lateral ventricle wall is, therefore, usually set at 4.5 to 5 mm in the adult so as not to involve the hypothalamus and internal capsule. It is to be

TABLE 5. Side effects (four cases of bilateral surgery)

Patient	Diagnosis	Lesions	Follow-up	Motor disturbance (akinetic type)	Speech and swallowing disturbance
Nob. Miz. (11-year-old male)	Reflex ep. CP Idiocy Left: spastic paralysis	Bilaterally complete (left and right)	Institutionalized	+	+
Chih. Yuz. (12-year-old female)	General and psychomotor Aggressive Idiocy (WISC: 39)	Bilaterally complete (right and left)	4 Years, 6 months, school		+
Kok. Chin (13-year-old male)	General CP Idiocy	Left: complete Right: out of target	6 Years, 9 months Died after institutionalization	+ Left: hemiparesis	+
Kyok. Kos. (18-year-old female)	Myoclonic	Bilaterally complete (left and right)	9 Years, 11 months Employed		+

Takeshi Shima 6y male

Date	Binet (Tanaka)	WISC V	P	F
8.10.'72	82	99	74	84
1.31.'73	88	86	72	75
7.23.'74	(r-Forel-H-tomy)			
6. 6.'75	82	79	92	84

Hiroko Shin 7y female

Date	Binet (Suzuki)	WISC V	P	F
4.21.'70	unable			
12. 7.'70	(r-Forel-H-tomy)			
8.25.'71	62			
3.10.'72	67	61	50	49
3.11.'74		53	50	45
4. 8.'75		54	46	46

Chihiro Yuza 10y female

Date	Binet (Tanaka)	WISC V	P	F
10. 6.'69	45			
7. 7.'71	(r-Forel-H-tomy)			
10.21.'71	45	47	46	46
11.30.'73		48	45	47

Yumi Koba 11y female

Date	WISC V	P	F
11. 9.'73	45	40	under 36
11.13.'73	(r-Forel-H-tomy)		
2. 1.'77	58	46	46
3. 8.'77	60	50	49

Atsushi Usu 11y male

Date	WISC V	P	F
4.22.'70	88	72	77
5. 4.'71	(r-Forel-H-tomy)		
6.18.'71	100	104	102
11.12.'71	93	88	90

Bunji Matsu 30y male

Date	WB V	P	F	WAIS V	P	F
12. 8.'71	65	85	72			
12.22.'71	(r-Forel-H-tomy)					
4.11.'72	80	85	82			
6. 4.'73	86	97	90			
5.17.'75				79	73	76

Keiko Kon 10y female

Date	Binet (Tanaka)	WAIS V	P	F
5.21.'73	51	57	72	59
7. 2.'73	(l-Forel-H-tomy)			
5.21.'75	84	70	77	70

Kazunori Muka 23y male

Date	WB V	P	F
10.29.'71	79	87	79
11.10.'71	(l-Forel-H-tomy)		
3.14.'72	81	89	83

Minoru Naka 27y male

Date	WB V	P	F	WAIS V	P	F
10. 2.'71	82	105	91			
10. 5.'71	(l-Forel-H-tomy)					
5.11.'72	92	98	94			
8.23.'73				73	74	73

TABLE 6.

VENTRICULAR DILATATION

—— 50 CASES ——

I) LATERAL VENTRICLE

VC-INDEX (0.22~0.57)

0.2~	12 CASES
0.25~	26
0.3~	12

SIDE / INDEX	LT (0.16~0.61)	RT (0.20~0.63)
0.15~	2 CASES	0 CASES
0.2~	18	25
0.25~	18	17
0.3~	12	8

2) ⅢRD VENTRICLE (4~17mm)

2.5mm~	4 CASES
5 ~	24
7.5 ~	11
10 ~	8
12.5 ~	3

TABLE 7.

noted that there is no direct correlation between the surgical effect and ventricular dilatation, and ventricular dilatation is not a contraindication to surgery.

Side effects were found in four cases of bilateral surgery, although there were no discouraging complications in unilateral surgery. The symptoms were akinetic motor disturbance and disturbances of speech and swallowing. As previously mentioned, the evidence of no postoperative intellectual deficit shows that these disturbances are due to extrapyramidal lesions. Two of them were cases of cerebral palsy with idiocy, whose preoperative motor deficit including speech and swallowing difficulty might aggravate the disturbances after surgery.

With regard to age distribution, 29 cases were 2 to 10 years of age at the time of operation. Among them, 12 patients had intractable epilepsy with Lennox syndrome showing diffuse slow spike and wave (Gastaut et al., 1966). Forel-H-tomy showed excellent results in two out of five bilateral operations. These data encourage us to carry out this type of stereotaxic surgery before epileptic brain damage and personality changes have been widely and uncontrollably built up in these children.

CONCLUSIONS

Sixty-eight cases of intractable epilepsy were operated on by Forel-H-tomy and analyzed from a clinical point of view.

Lesions should be made accurately at the target point, 2 mm posterior to the midpoint of the AC-PC line, 4 mm ventral to the line, and 4.5 to 5 mm lateral to the third ventricle wall.

Forel-H-tomy resulted not only in seizure control, but also in improvement of EEG abnormality and associated psychoneurological abnormalities.

Side effects are found in four cases of bilateral surgery—akinetic motor disorder and disturbance of speech and swallowing, which are due to extrapyramidal lesions.

When surgery is indicated, it is considered essential to carry out stereotaxic surgery before epileptic brain damage and personality changes have become irreversible.

REFERENCES

Gastaut, H., Roger, J., Soulayrol, R., Tassinari, C. A., Regis, H., Dravet, C., Bernard, R., Pinsard, N., and Saint-Jean, M. (1966): Childhood epileptic encephalopathy with diffuse slow spike-waves (otherwise known as "petit mal variant") or Lennox syndrome. *Epilepsia*, 7:139–179.

Iwata, Y. (1967): Experimental study of epileptic excitability—its intracerebral facilitation and inhibition. I. On pentetrazol induced seizure. II. On electrically induced major seizures. *Osaka Daigaku Igakuzashi*, 19:295–312 (in Japanese).

Jinnai, D. (1966): Clinical results and the significance of Forel-H-tomy in the treatment of epilepsy. *Conf. Neurol.*, 27:129–136.

Jinnai, D., and Mukawa, J. (1970): Forel-H-tomy for the treatment of epilepsy. *Conf. Neurol.*, 32:307–315.

Jinnai, D., and Mukawa, J. (1973): Surgery for epilepsy. In: *Progress in Neurological Surgery Vol. 5*, edited by H. Krayenbühl, P. E. Maspes, W. H. Sweet. S. Karger, Basel/Munchen/Paris/London/New York/Sidney.

Jinnai, D., Mukawa, J., and Kobayashi, K. (1976): Forel-H-tomy for the treatment of intractable epilepsy. *Acta Neurochir. (Suppl.)*, 23:159–165.

Jinnai, D., and Nishimoto, A. (1966): Stereotaxic destruction of Forel-H for the treatment of epilepsy. *Neurochirurgia*, 6:164–175.

Kobayashi, K. (1972): Effects of brain-stem stimulation on seizure discharges of neo-, archi- and paleocortex with special reference to the subthalamus. *Psychiatr. Neurol. Jpn.*, 74:124–150 (in Japanese).

Mukawa, J. (1964a): Effect of brain stem and subcortical lesions on corticogenic epileptic convulsion with special reference to Forel-H-field. *Acta Med. Okayama*, 18:153–171.

Mukawa, J. (1946b): Fiber connections of the Forel-H-field as seen in Marchi preparations. *Acta Med. Okayama*, 18:207–220.

Mukawa, J., and Jinnai, D. (1971): The propagation of focal cortical epilepsies and its modes. *Acta Neurol. Latinoamer*, 17:613–643.

Mukawa, J., et al. (1975): Forel-H-tomy for the treatment of intractable epilepsy. Special reference to postoperative electroencephalographic changes. *Conf. Neurol.*, 37:302–307.

Schaltenbrand, G., and Bailey, P. (1959): *Introduction to Stereotaxis with an Atlas of the Human Brain*. Georg Thieme, Stuttgart.

Spiegal, E. A., and Wycis, H. T. (1952): *Stereoencephalotomy*. Grune & Stratton, New York.

Van Buren, J. M., and Borke, R. C. (1972): *Variations and Connections of the Human Thalamus*. Springer-Verlag, New York/Heidelberg/Berlin.

Advances in Epileptology:
The Xth Epilepsy International Symposium,
edited by J. A. Wada and J. K. Penry.
Raven Press, New York © 1980.

Effect of Stimulation of the Caudate and Ventral Anterior Thalamus on Seizure Frequency in the Chronic Primate Model of Epilepsy

George Ojemann and John C. Oakley

Department of Neurological Surgery, University of Washington,
Seattle, Washington 98195

The evaluation of new drug treatments for epilepsy is now fairly standardized throughout the world. After initial identification of a potentially effective agent in animal screening tests, systematic evaluation for efficacy and safety is undertaken in animal models and then in clinical trials, culminating in "double blind" evaluations. Evaluation of surgical treatments for epilepsy has been much less standardized. Often experimental hints that surgical manipulation of a particular brain site might alter seizure frequency have been directly applied to patients, bypassing systematic animal evaluation for efficacy and safety. Evaluation of efficacy in patients with complex intractable seizure disorders is difficult. As a result, clear efficacy of many newer surgical procedures has not yet been demonstrated. Because of this, systematic evaluation in animal models is needed. This chapter reports such systematic evaluations of efficacy for several newer or potential surgical treatments.

The animal model for epilepsy produced by the injection of alumina cream into one sensory motor cortex of Rhesus monkeys, as developed by Kopeloff et al. (1955) and modified by Ward and associates (1972) has a number of advantages for this type of study. Almost alone among experimental models of epilepsy, these animals develop persisting chronic spontaneous seizures of both partial elementary motor and secondarily generalized types. These spontaneous seizures appear 60 to 90 days after injection of the alumina and persist indefinitely, at frequencies of 2 to 20 per week. A number of parallels have been established between the physiologic and biochemical changes in the epileptic foci of these animals and human epilepsy (Calvin et al., 1973; Rapport et al., 1978). When this animal model of chronic spontaneous recurring seizures is combined with a technique for continuous measurement of seizure frequency, an accurate assessment of efficacy of a treatment can be obtained. Continuous 24-hr assessment is essential, however, since only then can seizure counts be obtained that are independent of factors known to influence seizure frequency such as sleep or other circadian cycles, and feeding. Such a technique for continuously measuring seizure frequencies has been developed by Lockard and Barensten (1967). It involves placing animals in activity chairs instrumented so that patterns of movement are recorded on a polygraph. Seizures produce relatively unique envelopes on these records, which trigger a videotape recording of the animals' movement during that time, allowing confirmation that the movement actually represents seizure activity. This technique has been used for the evaluation of efficacy of anticonvulsants (Lockard et al., 1975, 1977) and in assessing the effects of behavioral manipulation on seizure frequency (Lockard et al., 1972). In this chapter, studies of the effects of several surgical manipulations on seizure frequency measured with this technique of continuous monitoring in the alumina monkey model of chronic recurrent spontaneous seizures are reviewed.

The surgical manipulations to be considered are placement of lesions in one ventral anterior thalamus and head of the caudate nucleus ipsilateral to the focus, and electrical stimulation of the midline anterior cerebellar surface, ipsilateral ventral anterior thalamus and caudate head, at a number of stimulation parameters. Additional advantages of studying efficacy in animal models, besides accurate counts of seizures, are the ability to perform "sham" operations as controls for the placement of lesions, and to obtain histologic verification of the location of the lesion or stimulating electrode. Occasionally these are not in the site where the surgeon thought he had placed them, and these animals then provide "double blind" controls for the effects obtained with lesions or stimulation of the chosen target.

VENTRAL ANTERIOR THALAMIC LESIONS

With John Kusske and Arthur Ward, I have previously reported on the effects of stereotaxic lesions at the rostral pole of the thalamus in the medial side of the ventral anterior nucleus on seizure frequency, in the 4- to 8-week period after placement of these lesions compared with a 4-week period immediately prior to lesioning, in five chronically epileptic monkeys (Kusske et al., 1973). In four of these animals the lesions were confirmed histologically in the ventral anterior nucleus. These animals showed a 74.4% mean *decrease* in seizure frequency after placement of the lesions (range, 52.1– 85.8% decrease). In a fifth animal, the lesion was displaced posterio-laterally into the ventral lateral nucleus. This animal demonstrated only a 6.2% decrease in seizure frequency. Sham operations in three animals did not change seizure frequency. Three animals had transient motor deficits after these lesions, which cleared in all within 3 weeks. Alertness, desire for food, and motor activity in the chair were not otherwise changed by these lesions. Ventral anterior lesions seem to be effective in decreasing frequency of seizures in this model of epilepsy.

CAUDATE LESIONS

A second study undertaken with Kusske, previously unreported, evaluated effects of stereotaxic lesions in the head of the caudate nucleus in four chronically epileptic monkeys. Seizure frequency was unchanged in three animals and increased in the fourth, from 10.2 seizures per week to 38.5, comparing a 4- to 9-week period after the lesion to a 4-week preoperative control period. Seizure duration was not altered in any animal by the caudate head lesions, but amplitude of movements during both focal and generalized seizures was significantly increased in three monkeys; nonseizure activity levels of these animals were also noted to be increased postoperatively. A fifth monkey with a lesion in the caudate body showed no effects, nor did an animal with a sham lesion in the white matter dorsal to the caudate head. Caudate head lesions do not change seizure frequency or duration, but increase the magnitude of movements during seizures.

CEREBELLAR STIMULATION

The efficacy of cerebellar surface stimulation was next determined in this chronic primate model. A preliminary study with John Oakley involved four animals with strip electrodes on the anterior midline cerebellar surface. These animals received bipolar stimulation with 1 msec unidirectional pulses at 10 Hz applied 10 min on, 10 min off, using current levels below those evoking behavioral changes (2 to 7 mA). Comparisons were made between control periods and periods of stimulation of the same duration, varying from 1 to 10 weeks, followed by a poststimulation period of the same duration. Seven pairs of comparisons between prestimulation and stimulation periods are available in these four animals. Four showed increased seizure frequency during stimulation (mean increase, 33%); three showed decrease (mean decrease, 20%) (Ojemann and Oakley, 1977; Ojemann, 1978).

Although this pilot study failed to show effectiveness of cerebellar stimulation in reducing seizure frequency, a more comprehensive study was undertaken with Joan Lockard, and is reported in this volume. In a dozen monkeys with 6 weeks of cerebellar stimulation, a significant increase in seizure frequency could be demonstrated, and a further rebound increase was encountered in the several weeks after terminating stimulation.

STIMULATION OF VENTRAL ANTERIOR THALAMUS AND CAUDATE

Oakley and I are now studying the effects of stimulating the ventral anterior thalamus and head of the caudate nucleus in this chronic primate model of partial elementary and secondary generalized epilepsy. Concentric electrodes with 2 mm between tips were stereotaxically implanted into each of these target sites in four animals. Then protocols for stimulation for each animal were instituted, alternating 1 month of control measures with a month of stimulation of either ventral anterior thalamic or caudate head at either low (10 Hz) or high (100 Hz) frequency, using bipolar stimulation with 1 msec unidirectional pulses at constant currents (0.3–6 mA), in each case a current just below the threshold for overt behavioral manifestation. The order of these conditions varies between animals. Initial plans were to carry out all stimulations in an intermittent mode, 10 min of stimulation alternating with 10 min without stimulation.

Ventral anterior thalamic stimulation at 10 Hz was evaluated in two animals. In each case seizure frequency *increased,* 16% in one animal, 72% in the other. The animal with the larger increase in seizure frequency had an electrode high in medial ventral anterior thalamus, the other low. The other two animals received ventral anterior thalamic 100 Hz stimulation. In each case seizures decreased (23%, 33%). Again the animal with the larger effect had an electrode located relatively high in the medial ventral anterior thalamus. In both these animals the seizure frequency during the poststimulation month showed a further decline, but increased toward the end of this control period, suggesting that this was a persisting effect of stimulation rather than one of the periodic fluctuations in seizure frequency that can complicate evaluation of efficacy even under the control conditions obtained in chronic animal models. Thus high-frequency VA stimulation may be effective in decreasing seizure frequency. This deserves further evaluation.

In each of these same four monkeys, another electrode had been directed toward the head of the caudate nucleus. Histologic examination after the termination of stimulation demonstrated that the electrodes were in the head of the caudate nucleus in only two animals. In a third the electrode was deep to the caudate nucleus in internal capsule (IC), and in the fourth had bent posteriorly on insertion, passing into medial globus pallidus (GP). These latter two animals thus represent "double blind" controls for the effects of caudate stimulation. In both of the animals with electrodes in the caudate nucleus, 10 Hz intermittent stimulation produced a moderate decrease in seizure frequency (of 28 and 50%). In one of the animals seizure frequency returns to baseline, in the other it remains reduced in the month after termination of stimulation.

Intermittent stimulation of 100 Hz had a most dramatic effect in these animals. In both animals status epilepticus was precipitated, after 16 and 17 days of stimulation, respectively. Seizures then recurred at exactly 20-min intervals, occurring at the termination of each period of stimulation. In one animal, status was aborted both by turning off the stimulating current, and by turning on the current continuously. The other animal tolerated the frequent seizures well enough that intermittent 100 Hz stimulation was continued for the full month, seizure frequency gradually declining after 2 days of status, returning to baseline by day 25 of stimulation. The marked increase in seizures was not observed with stimulation of the two animals whose electrodes were not in the head of the caudate nucleus at the same parameters.

In view of the relationship of the seizures to the termination of stimulation and the apparent ability to control status by continuous high-frequency caudate stimulation, we added another control and stimulation period to each of the animals with caudate electrodes, in which 100 Hz stimulation would be carried out continuously for a 1-month period. It was possible to accomplish this in three or four animals; illness terminated the experiment prematurely in the animal with an electrode in GP. In both animals with caudate electrodes, high-frequency continuous stimulation decreased seizure frequency, slightly (3%) in one, and substantially (54%) in the other. In both cases termination of stimulation was followed by a rebound increase in seizure frequency to levels higher than the initial control period. The animal with the IC electrode showed minimal changes and no rebound after continuous high-frequency stimulation.

This effect of continuous high-frequency caudate stimulation is now being further evaluated in an additional four monkeys. Nearly complete data are available for two, two still have 10 days remaining on stimulation and no histologic data for these animals are presently available. Stimulation now uses biphasic pulses, 1 msec total duration 100 Hz continuously at 1 to 6 mA. Seizure frequency during stimulation has *decreased* in three of the four animals (51%, 29%, and 87%), and increased in one (46%), compared with the previous month's period after implantation but without stimulation. One animal has had only a single seizure while on stimulation. Rebound increases in seizure frequency have followed termination of stimulation in both animals with poststimulation data. No overt behavioral changes have been noted during the continuous stimulation. Continuous high-frequency stimulation of the caudate head is often an effective method for reducing seizure frequency in this animal model, to date showing an average 45% reduction in five of six animals with confirmed or presumed caudate electrodes.

DISCUSSION

In this chronic primate model of epilepsy, two surgical approaches seem to be effective in reducing seizure frequency: lesions of the medial portion of the ventral anterior nucleus and continuous high-frequency stimulation of the caudate head. Two other approaches show promise, but need further evaluation: intermittent high-frequency stimulation of ventral anterior nucleus, and intermittent low-frequency stimulation of the caudate head. Several approaches were either ineffective or increased seizure frequency: anterior cerebellar surface stimulation, lesions of the caudate head, and intermittent high-frequency caudate stimulation. Note that effects vary both by target site (internal capsule and globus pallidus near to the caudate head have little of the effects of stimulating that target) and by stimulation parameter (only frequency and train duration have been manipulated to date, current levels have been held constant in each animal at levels just below any overt behavioral manifestations). The applicability of these findings to patients with epilepsy depends on how well the alumina monkey models human partial elementary motor and secondarily generalized seizures. Drug therapies effective in reducing seizures in the model are effective in patients (Lockard et al., 1975, 1977). Based on that parallel, medial ventral anterior lesions, and especially continuous caudate head stimulation, seem ready for carefully designed clinical trials in patients with similar types of intractable epilepsy.

ACKNOWLEDGMENTS

This study was supported by NIH grant NSO4053. George Ojemann is an affiliate of the Center for Child Development and Mental Retardation, University of Washington.

REFERENCES

Calvin, W., Ojemann, G., and Ward, A., Jr. (1973): Human cortical neurons in epileptogenic foci: comparison of inter-ictal firing patterns to those of "epileptic" neurons in animals. *EEG Clin. Neurophysiol.*, 34:337–351.

Kopeloff, L., Chusid, J., and Kopeloff, N. (1955): Epilepsy in *Macaca Mulatta* after cortical or intracerebral alumina. *Arch. Neurol. Psychiatr.*, 74:523–526.

Kusske, J., Ojemann, G., and Ward, A. Jr. (1973): Effects of lesions in ventral anterior thalamus on experimental focal epilepsy. *Exp. Neurol.*, 34:279–290.

Lockard, J., and Barensten, R. (1967): Behavioral experimental epilepsy in monkeys. I. Clinical seizure recording apparatus and initial data. *EEG Clin. Neurophysiol.*, 22:482–486.

Lockard, J., Levy, R., Congdon, W., DuCharme, L., and Patel, I. (1977): Efficacy testing of valproic acid compared to ethosuximide in monkey model: II. Seizure, EEG, and diurnal variations. *Epilepsia*, 18:205–224.

Lockard, J., Uhlir, V., DuCharme, L., Farguhar, J., and Huntsman, B. (1975): Efficacy of standard anticonvulsants in monkey model with spontaneous motor seizures. *Epilepsia*, 16:301–317.

Lockard, J., Wilson, W., and Uhlir, V. (1972). Spontaneous seizure frequency and avoidance conditioning in monkeys. *Epilepsia*, 13:437–444.

Ojemann, G. (1978): The future role of surgery in the treatment of epilepsy. In: *Modern Perspectives in Epilepsy*, edited by J. Wada. Eden Press, Montreal.

Ojemann, G., and Oakley, J. (1977): Effect of chronic cerebellar stimulation on seizure frequency in alumina monkey model of epilepsy. In: *American Association of Neurological Surgeons*, Toronto, April 25, 1977.

Rapport, R., Harris, A., Lockard, J. and Clark, A. (1978): Na, K. ATPase in serially excised segments of epileptic monkey cortex.

Ward, A., Jr. (1972): Topical convulsant metals. In: *Experimental Models of Epilepsy*, edited by D. Purpura, J. Penry, D. Tower, D. Woodbury, and R. Walter, Raven, New York.

Advances in Epileptology:
The Xth Epilepsy International Symposium,
edited by J. A. Wada and J. K. Penry.
Raven Press, New York © 1980.

Cerebellar Stimulation in Alumina-Gel Monkey Model: Differential Effects on Clinical Seizures and EEG Interictal Bursts

Joan S. Lockard, George A. Ojemann, John C. Oakley, and Leonard D. Salonen

Department of Neurological Surgery, University of Washington, Seattle, Washington 90195

After a demonstration of a decrease in seizures in several acute animal models of epilepsy (reviewed by Dow, 1974) with electrical stimulation of the surface of the anterior vermis of the cerebellum, Cooper et al. (1973, 1974, 1978) reported a reduction in seizure frequency with similar stimulation in man. However, other series have not achieved similar results (Correll, 1977; Van Buren et al., 1977). The findings of preliminary studies utilizing alumina-gel monkeys have also been unclear. Black et al. (1976) reported for one of six monkeys a reduction in spontaneous epileptic activity, but not in precipitated seizures. Ojemann and Oakley (1977) showed no dramatic effects of cerebellar stimulation in four monkeys and only in one of the animals did a detectable change occur.

The present study addresses the question of efficacy of cerebellum stimulation in a comprehensive manner in the alumina-gel model. Using techniques (e.g., Lockard et al., 1976b) allowing round-the-clock monitoring of clinical seizures and periodic sampling of EEG paroxysms in 12 epileptic monkeys, the anterior cerebellar vermis was stimulated, employing the same parameters used in man. Six weeks of stimulation were compared with before and after baseline periods of the same length.

METHODS

Animals and Epileptic Preparation

Two years prior to the commencement of the study, 12 subadult Rhesus monkeys *(Macaca mulatta)*, weighing 4 to 6 kg, were injected (under sterile craniotomy) with aluminum-hydroxide (approximately 0.3 cc total) in the left pre- and postcentral gyrus, sensory hand and motor areas (confirmed by physiological stimulation). The animals were also instrumented with an EEG plug (e.g., Lockard et al., 1976*b*). Several weeks preceding the study, three monkeys (Nos. 4, 5, and 6) were administered 6 mg/kg phenobarbital i.m. b.i.d. and were maintained on the drug at that dose throughout the study, including baseline periods, as a consequence of their predilection for excessive seizures. Plasma drug levels for each animal were obtained periodically.

EEG and Seizure Recording

The monkeys were manifesting stable daily seizure frequencies and EEG paroxysms at the onset of the study. Twenty-four hour monitoring of clinical seizures was accomplished by a closed-circuit television system (the cameras had infrared vidicons for night coverage) with videotape recorders activated by accelerometers on the primate chairs. Diurnal EEG samples of half an hour twice a week per monkey and one all-night EEG (12 hr) per monkey every 3 weeks were gathered. The recordings were readable only during the 10-min *off* periods between the alternating 10-min *on* stimulation periods. Diurnal samples were scored for EEG bursting and the night records for EEG bursting and sleep stage (0–4, REM).

Cerebellar Electrode Implants

Two weeks prior to the onset of the study, the animals were implanted with platinum electrodes over anterior superior cerebellum by a posterior fossa craniotomy under halothane anesthesia. Each monkey received three electrodes, 2 mm × 3.8 mm × 0.1 mm platinum strips spaced 2 mm apart and imbedded in silastic; therefore, each electrode pair was a square approximately 4 × 4 mm. Electrode placement was confirmed by X-ray. Electrode leads were connected to an external stimulator when the animals were returned to their primate chairs.

Experimental Design

Cerebellum stimulation was instituted after a 2-week postsurgical period and a 6-week baseline period and was followed by a 6-week (9 weeks in some animals) poststimulation baseline period. Stimulation was bipolar, utilizing a Grass PSIU 6 at 10 hz, with 1 msec pulses, 10 min on, 10 min off, providing an average current of 2.0 mA. The current was checked daily for each monkey during the stimulation weeks. The animals were sacrificed for histological follow-up within one month after the completion of the study, with the exception of one monkey which died earlier from unrelated causes.

RESULTS

Seizure Frequency

As shown in Fig. 1 for the no-drug animals, there were appreciable differences in seizure frequency between baseline and the first 5 weeks of the post-baseline period ($t = 4.37$, $p < 0.05$). In the last post-baseline week, the number of seizures returned to baseline levels and remained at a low level [as indicated by those animals that were monitored for 9 weeks (not shown) after stimulation]. There was a significant increase in seizure frequency during stimulation as compared with baseline ($t = 3.71, p < 0.05$) and the increase was even greater in the post-baseline period, relative to the weeks of stimulation ($t = 5.41, p < 0.05$). The results for the three phenobarbital monkeys were similar to the other monkeys.

Seizure Envelopes

If the seizure envelopes from the polygraph readout of activity are classified as to partial or secondarily generalized seizures, the increase in seizure frequency during weeks of cerebellar stimulation is attributable to an increase in long-duration ($t = 7.41, p < 0.05$) partial seizures. However, the elevated seizure frequency in the post-baseline period was a function of shorter duration, low-amplitude ($t = 16.64, p < 0.005$) secondarily generalized tonic-clonic seizures. The implications of these findings will be discussed.

EEG and Sleep Data

The diurnal EEG samples that were scored for mean number of interictal spikes per 10-sec page revealed a trend ($t = 1.90, 0.20 > p > 0.05$) toward *decreased* bursting during weeks of stimulation. An analysis of variance of the all-night EEG records for each monkey every 3 weeks supported this outcome, showing a significant attenuation of bursting during the stimulation period ($F = 2.69, p < 0.05$), as a function of sleep stage. The reduction in EEG bursting during weeks of cerebellar stimulation was *not* a function of the animals' sleeping less during those periods, as there were no significant differences between mean minutes of sleep for any of the five stages of sleep (1–4, REM) throughout the study (e.g., $t = 0.16, p > 0.05$).

Histological Findings

Cellular damage of the cerebellum in the vicinity of the electrode placement was evident to varying degrees in 9 of the 12 monkeys. Granulation

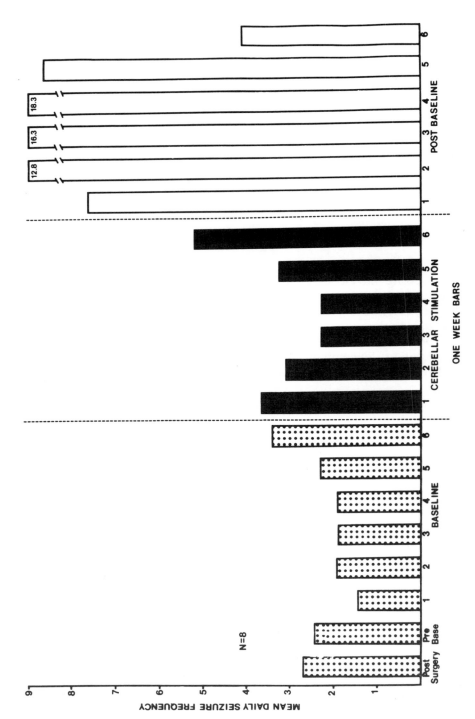

FIG. 1. Mean seizure frequency before (baseline), during, and after (post-baseline) cerebellar stimulation in eight monkeys.

tissue encapsulated abscesses, the extent of which (as quantified by relative weight) for each of the affected animals did *not* correlate significantly with seizure frequency (e.g., $t = 0.61, p > 0.05$) or EEG bursts (e.g., $t = 0.96, p > 0.05$) during either baseline, stimulation, or post-baseline weeks. Therefore, it is assumed that the differences in the paroxysms evident during and after cerebellar stimulation are not attributable in any direct way to the tissue damage itself. Moreover, the seizure and EEG activity of the three animals (Nos. 5, 10, and 11) not exhibiting abscesses was similar to those of the other animals.

DISCUSSION

Cerebellar stimulation in patients has been most consistently effective in movement disorders (Cooper, 1978) and *not* epilepsy (Correll, 1977; Van Buren, 1977). It may well be that this conclusion has been obscured by the seemingly favorable outcome of some studies utilizing animal models of epilepsy. Our results in monkeys indicate that although interictal EEG bursting does decrease with cerebellar stimulation, seizure frequency increases during, and especially after, weeks of stimulation. In fact, when cerebellar stimulation has been efficacious in other animal models, its influence has been most obviously manifested on EEG concomitants of epilepsy other than ictal events (e.g., Boone et al., 1974; Dow, 1974; Meyers and Bickford, 1974; Soper et al. 1977). Either minimal effects to no changes (Babb et al., 1977; Black et al., 1976; Strain et al., 1977), or an increase in frequency (Bantli et al., 1978) has been reported for animals with overt seizures.

In the evaluation of anticonvulsant drugs (e.g., Lockard et al., 1975, 1976 *a, b*; Lockard and Levy, 1977*a*) and EEG biofeedback (Lockard et al., 1977*b*; Wyler et al., 1977) in our primate model, mean interictal EEG spikes and clinical seizures have correlated directly with one another. The present study was the first instance in this model when the correlation was inverse. Whereas in previous studies, desynchronization of neuronal bursting was suggested to result in fewer ictal as well as interictal events, this explanation is not appropriate when the frequency of seizures is augmented rather than attenuated. Rather, in this case, it is hypothesized that cerebellar stimulation through cellular projections from the cerebellum differentially affects group I and II epileptic neurons (e.g., Wyler et al., 1975; Wyler et al., 1978) such that its influence on ictal and interictal events are separable. It is suggested that those neurons responsible for interictal spikes are cells that may fire in either a normal or epileptic mode, i.e., group II neurons, which are cells at the periphery of the epileptogenic focus still having considerable afferent input. These neurons may be inhibited from firing in either mode by cerebellar stimulation via brain circuitry as would be involved with the activation of Purkinje cells (Julien, 1974) or, more probably, by way of the reticular formation (Bantli et al., 1976). On the other hand, group I neurons (i.e., cells central to the epileptogenic focus that are largely deafferented and fire exclusively in an epileptic mode) may be bursting more frequently. Their limited afferent input may be diminished still further by cerebellar stimulation inhibiting cells that project to the focus. If this were true, then a decrease in interictal spikes and fewer secondarily generalized seizures but considerably more partial seizures would be manifested during weeks of cerebellar stimulation, as was observed in the present study. In other words, inhibited group II cells would neither be firing interictally nor be recruited in the spread of ictal activity. It is further hypothesized that cerebellar stimulation also influences neuronal transmitters such as Gaba or norepinephrine in order to explain the irreversibility of action, i.e., the delay of 4 to 5 weeks in the return to pre-baseline levels of ictal and, therefore, interictal rates after stimulation ceased in our study. This explanation is compatible with the available data in the literature and appears to resolve conflicting findings of animal models of epilepsy.

Cerebellar stimulation in our monkey model did not disrupt either the sleep cycle or result in sleep deprivation. These findings are consonant with that of spastic patients ($N = 6$, Contreras et al., 1975) in which all-night sleep recordings were gathered while they were undergoing chronic cerebellar stimulation therapy. Although our data indicate that cerebellar stimulation is not generally efficacious with respect to epilepsy, it may be a very fruitful technique for the study of mechanisms of actions. Documentation (or refutation) in part or whole of our explanatory hypothesis would be of considerable importance to the understanding of pertinent neuronal pathways involved in motor seizures. If cerebellar stimulation is regarded as a research tool its continued use in the study of epilepsy may be warranted.

SUMMARY

The efficacy of cerebellar stimulation was addressed in a chronic monkey model ($N = 12$) of spontaneous focal motor and secondarily generalized seizures using 24-hr seizure frequency monitoring and all-night EEG recording. The anterior cerebellar vermis was stimulated employing the same paremeters used in man, 10 Hz, 1 msec pulses, 10 min on, 10 off, at an average current of 2.0 mA. Six weeks pre- and post-baseline periods were compared with a stimulation period of the same length. The results contribute to a clarification of conflicting findings of previous researchers by revealing an inverse relationship between seizure frequency and interictal EEG bursts during the weeks of stimulation. Seizure frequency increased significantly and interictal bursts decreased. Both of these effects (especially the former) were evident in the poststimulation period, but for different reasons than hypothesized for the period of stimulation. Whereas the therapeutic value of cerebellar stimulation on seizures may be in question, its utilization in the study of mechanisms of epilepsy may be valuable.

ACKNOWLEDGMENT

This project was supported by NIH research contract N01-NS-1-2282 and research grant NS 04053 awarded by the National Institutes of Neurological and Communicative Disorders and Stroke, PHS/DHEW. The authors are indebted to Dr. A. Basil Harris for his histological analysis of cerebellar tissue. Appreciation is also extended to Mr. William C. Congdon (research supervisor), Mr. Larry L. DuCharme (electroencephalographer), Mr. Douglas Kalk (programmer), and laboratory technicians, Mr. David Walker and Mr. Paul Franklin, for their efficient execution of the many schedules and evaluative tests in the conduction of this research.

REFERENCES

Babb, T. L., Brown, J., Soper, H. V., Strain, G. M., and Crandall, P. H. (1977): Tissue reactions to very long-term implantation of cerebellar stimulating electrodes in monkey. *Abstr. Soc. Neurosci.*, 3:393.

Bantli, H., Bloedel, J. F., and Tolbert, O. (1976): Activation of neurons in the cerebellar nuclei and ascending reticular formation by stimulation of the cerebellar surface. *J. Neurosurg.*, 45:539–554.

Bantli, H., Bloedel, J. R., Anderson, G., McRoberts, R., and Sandberg, E. (1978): Effects of stimulating the cerebellar surface on the activity in penicillin foci. *J. Neurosurg.*, 48:69–84.

Black, P., Fischell, R. E., Markowitz, S., and Powell, W. R. (1976): Cerebella stimulation: Comparison of effect on electrically induced and "spontaneous" alumina seizures. *American Epilepsy Society Annual Meeting*, Oct. 1, Dearborn, Michigan.

Boone, S. C., Nashold, B. S., and Wilson, W. P. (1974): The effects of cerebellar stimulation on the averaged sensory evoked responses in the cat. In: *The Cerebellum, Epilepsy, and Behavior*, edited by I. S. Cooper, M. Riklan, and R. S. Snider. Plenum Press, New York.

Brown, J., Babb, T. L., Soper, H. V., Lieb, J. P., Ottino, C., and Crandall, P. H. (1977): Alterations of primate cerebellar cortex induced by long-term electrical stimulation. *American Association of Neurological Surgeons Meeting*, Toronto.

Contreras, C. M., Cooper, I. S., and Fernandez-Guardiola, A. (1975): Polygraphic analysis of all-night sleep in patients submitted to chronic stimulation of the cerebellum. *Bol. Estud. Med. Biol.*, 28:327–334.

Cooper, I. S. (editor) (1978): *Cerebellar Stimulation in Man.* Raven Press, New York.

Cooper, I. S., Amin, I., and Gilman, S. (1973): The effect of chronic cerebellar stimulation upon epilepsy in man. *Trans. Am. Neurol. Assoc.*, 98:192–196.

Cooper, I. S., Amin, I., Riklan, M., Waltz, J. M., and Poon, T. P. (1976): Chronic cerebellar stimulation in epilepsy. *Arch. Neurol.*, 33:559–570.

Cooper, I. S., Riklan, M., and Snider, R. S. (editors) (1974): *The Cerebellum, Epilepsy and Behavior.* Plenum Press, New York.

Correll, J. (1977): Cerebellar stimulation. In: *American Association of Neurological Surgeons Meeting*, Toronto.

Dow, R. S. (1974): Experimental cobalt epilepsy and the cerebellum. In: *The Cerebellum, Epilepsy and Behavior*, edited by I. S. Cooper, M. Riklan, and R. S. Snider. Plenum Press, New York.

Julien, R. M. (1974): Experimental epilepsy: Cerebro-cerebellar interactions and antiepileptic drugs. In: The *Cerebellum, Epilepsy and Behavior*, edited by I. S. Cooper, M. Riklan, and R. S. Snider. Plenum Press, New York.

Lockard, J. S., Congdon, W. C., DuCharme, L. L., and Huntsman, B. J. (1976a): Prophylaxis with diphenylhydantoin and phenobarbital in alumina-gel monkey model. I. Twelve months of treatment: Seizure, EEG, blood and behavioral data. *Epilepsia*, 17:37–47.

Lockard, J. S., Levy, R. H., Patel, I. H., DuCharme, L. L., and Congdon, W. D. (1976b): Dipropylacetic acid and ethosuximide in monkey model: Quantitative methods of evaluation. In: *Quantitative Analytic Studies in Epilepsy*, edited by P. Kellaway and I. Petersen. Raven Press, New York.

Lockard, J. S., and Levy, R. H. (1977a): Efficacy of clonazepam in alumina-gel monkey model. *American Epilepsy Society Meeting*, New York.

Lockard, J. S., Uhlir, V., DuCharme, L. L., Farquhar, J. A., and Huntsman, B. J. (1975): Efficacy of standard anticonvulsants in monkey model with spontaneous motor seizures. *Epilepsia*, 16:301–317.

Lockard, J. S., Wyler, A. R., Finch, C. A., and Hurlburt, K. E. (1977b): EEG operant conditioning in a monkey model: I. Seizure data. *Epilepsia*, 18:471–479.

Meyers, R. R., and Bickford, R. G. (1974): Modulation of spontaneous and evoked chloralose myoclonus bicerebellar stimulation in the cat. In: *The Cerebellum, Epilepsy and Behavior*, edited by I. S. Cooper, M. Riklan, and R. S. Snider. Plenum Press, New York.

Ojemann, G. A., and Oakley, J. C. (1977): Effect of chronic cerebellar stimulation on seizure frequency in the alumina monkey model of epilepsy. In: *American Association of Neurological Surgeons Meeting*, Toronto.

Riklan, M., Cullinam, T., Shulman, M., and Cooper, I. S. (1976): A psychometric study of chronic cerebellar stimulation in man. *Biol. Psychiatry*, 11:543–574.

Soper, H. V., Lieb, J. P., Babb, T. L., Strain, G. M., and Crandall, P. H. (1977): *Abstr. Soc. Neurosci.*, 3:146.

Strain, G. M., Van Meter, W. G., and Brockman, W. H. (1977): Effects of cerebellar stimulation on seizure thresholds. *Abstr. Soc. Neurosci.*, 3:147.

Van Buren, J. M., Wood, J. H., Oakley, J., and Hambrecht, F. (1977): Preliminary evaluation of cerebellar stimulation in the treatment of epilepsy by double blind stimulation and biological criteria. *American Association of Neurological Surgeons Meeting*, Toronto.

Wyler, A. R., Burchiel, K. J., and Ward, A. A., Jr. (1978): Chronic epileptic foci in monkeys: Correlation between seizure frequency and proportion of pacemaker epileptic neurons. *Epilepsia*, 19:475–484.

Wyler, A. R., Fetz, E. E., and Ward, A. A., Jr. (1975): Review article: Firing patterns of epileptic and normal neurons in neocortex of undrugged monkeys during different behavioral states. Brain Res., 98:1–20.

Wyler, A. R., Lockard, J. S., DuCharme, L. L., and Perkins, M. G. (1977): EEG operant conditioning in a monkey model: II. EEG spectral analysis. *Epilepsia*, 18:481–488.

Advances in Epileptology:
The Xth Epilepsy International Symposium,
edited by J. A. Wada and J. K. Penry.
Raven Press, New York © 1980.

Central Brain Lesions for the Control of Intractable Epilepsy

F. John Gillingham, W. S. Watson, S. Chung, and C. Yates

Department of Surgical Neurology, University of Edinburgh and the M.R.C. Brain Metabolism Unit, Edinburgh, Scotland

The surgeon's approach to intractable epilepsy has evolved from observation, empiricism, and from the accumulating though scant knowledge of the dynamic pathological mechanisms underlying the origin and propagation of the epileptic discharge. In 1958 we had observed the marked reduction of frequency of attacks of "forced thinking," as Penfield might have described it, in a patient with postencephalitic Parkinsonism following a stereotactic lesion for the control of tremor (Gillingham et al., 1960). From 15 attacks a day lasting 1 or 2 min, after which the patient was somewhat withdrawn, they were reduced to two or three a week. During the operation, tremor was more difficult to control than usual but was finally abolished by a lesion that, when plotted on a stereotactic atlas, was seen to lie within the posterior limb of the internal capsule just posterior to the globus pallidus. Apart from a mild and temporary contralateral facial weakness postoperatively no motor or sensory disturbance was observed and the patient was completely rehabilitated. Before operation he had become increasingly withdrawn from his friends and relatives because of his disabilities of which the attacks of "forced thinking" were the more serious. This observation was noted but laid aside until Jinnai and Nishimoto (1963) endeavored to define conduction pathways of the focal epileptic convulsion in animal experiments and came to the conclusion that these might be interrupted with benefit at the most strategic point, namely the field of Forel. A number of patients with intractable epilepsy were treated by stereotactic lesions at this site and the reported results were favorable. The lesion in our patient included Jinnai's pathway but at a higher level than his point of interruption.

Our first deliberate attempt at stereotactic interruption of the conduction pathways for intractable epilepsy began in the field of Forel in 1968. However, two patients showed some disability after lesions at this site, mild but long-standing ataxia and dysarthria in one and some contralateral temporary weakness of the upper limb in another. This occurred in spite of such sophisticated methods as the use of depth microelectrode recording for the precise placement of lesions and careful interoperative monitoring of the patients neurological functions under local anesthesia (Gaze et al., 1964). Nevertheless, after bilateral lesions their epilepsy was reduced in frequency and severity. The field of Forel lies in a crowded area and deficits occur more readily in our experience with errors of placement of lesions than by interruption of the fasiculus lenticularis in the neighborhood of the ventral lateral nucleus of the thalamus or pallidum. We, therefore, turned to these sites in subsequent patients. We noted greater benefit from these lesions with reduction in frequency and severity of fits and with minimal side effects. These results were further improved by turning to the pallido-capsular zone at the genu of the internal capsule on the basis of our original observation in 1958. This would now seem to be the site of choice (Gillingham, 1974). Bilateral lesions are notoriously hazardous mainly because of the danger of dysarthria. It is, therefore, important not only to use sophisticated methods of target siting as already described but to enlist the help of the speech therapist in the operating theatre. With careful preoperative speech and language assessment, the therapist is particularly well-placed to detect the earliest speech disturbance as the lesion is enlarged and so prevent disability by re-siting the electrode.

For the past 5 years, 25 mg biopsies have been taken at the site of the proposed lesion before it is made and histochemical estimates made of glutamic acid decarboxylase. Thus comparative studies can be made between these and other sites with tissue from similar sites from fresh human autopsies in nonepileptic patients. This work will be the subject of a further communication when a larger series has been achieved.

Fourteen patients have now been treated with stereotactic surgery and a follow-up of 9 years had been reached in the first. Pre- and postoperative assessments were carried out by the team concerned, namely clinical, psychometric, speech, and language functions. Daily performance was charted by occupational and physiotherapists and the medical social worker. Detailed electroencephalography (EEG), skull X-ray, pneumoencephalography, and angiography (when indicated) and, more recently, CAT scan were performed. Only those patients were accepted for operation who had very frequent minor disabling attacks or severe grand mal or psychomotor seizures of not less than once a week, and who failed to respond to a prolonged, regular, and strenuous trial of antiepileptic drugs and in whom there was no demonstrable focus of discharge. The earlier results of operative treatment, neurological and psychometric studies in the light of 10 patients, have been reported elsewhere (Gillingham et al., 1976).

The practical value of stereotactic surgery in 14 patients has now been assessed on a long-term basis and the conclusions are as follows (Fig. 1):

1. Twelve of the fourteen patients have been improved. In none have seizures been abolished.

2. Younger patients have better results than older patients.

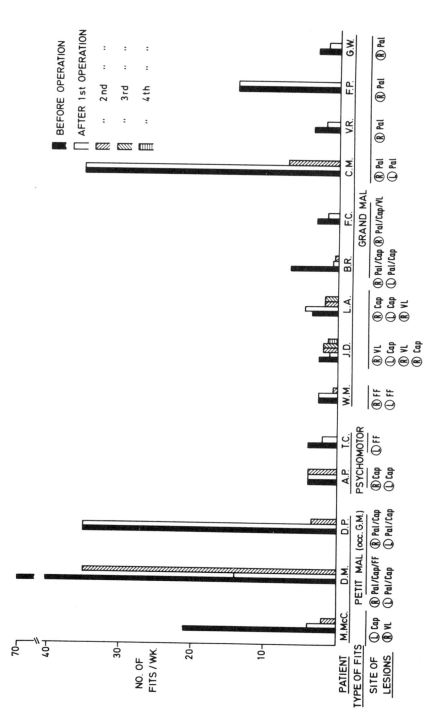

FIG. 1. Reduction in fit frequency as a result of stereotactic surgery.

3. Patients with a shorter duration of their epileptic illness have better results than those with a longer duration.

4. In this relatively small group of patients the pallido-capsular lesion would appear to be the more effective. Figure 1 illustrates the effect of operations, not only on fit frequency but also on severity. Many of the fits that occurred after operation were of a minor type of short duration. The possible greater success of the pallido-capsular lesion is supported by the fact that in three patients unilateral lesions at this site were sufficient with postoperative medication to control intractable epilepsy. At other sites bilateral operations were necessary.

5. The dosage of anticonvulsants could be reduced postoperatively in three patients, but an increase was required in four. In the three with reduced dosage two had lesions at the pallido-capsular junction, one bilateral and one unilateral. One had a unilateral lesion of the field of Forel. All had intractable grand mal seizures. In the four requiring increased medication postoperatively, all had grand mal seizures. In two of these there was considerable improvement with unilateral pallido-capsular lesions but increased medication was also necessary. In two patients bilateral lesions at the pallido-capsular junction were required with increased medication to control seizures. In one of these two there was marked improvement.

6. In six patients (four with grand mal and two with petit mal seizures) the frequency of fits was reduced but there was no improvement in the EEG after operation. In three patients (one with grand mal and two with psychomotor seizures) there was no EEG abnormality before or after operation. In two patients who had no improvement in fit frequency after operation one (psychomotor epilepsy) had no EEG abnormality before or after operation and one (grand mal epilepsy) had an abnormal EEG before and after operation.

7. There were complications from operation in eight patients but mostly with bilateral lesions. However, these were short-lived in five and recovery was complete. There was minor contralateral motor weakness of a few days duration in four and ataxia in one. Three patients were left with minor degrees of dysarthria and ataxia. Interoperative monitoring of speech and neurological function and exact location of targets by depth microelectrode recording and audiomonitoring is essential to success in stereotactic surgery.

8. Three patients had behavioral problems before operation and are now improved. Four patients had intellectual deterioration before operation and after operation one improved. One deteriorated intellectually after operation.

9. Only one patient had worked full-time before operation and he did so afterwards. After operation seven patients were working with greater or less protection. Two were working full-time in their usual occupations. In five, work potential had not improved. In one patient work capacity deteriorated some years after operation because of a cerebral vascular accident.

In summary, therefore, experience over 9 years with these patients would suggest that there is a place for stereotactic central lesions in selected epileptic patients, particularly when seizures are severe, frequent, drug resistant, and likely to be intractable. These operations might more profitably be carried out at a much earlier age and before the epileptic pattern has become so firmly established. The lesion of the pallidum close to the capsule is probably the most effective in our hands.

The thoughtful surgeon's potential in furthering the knowledge of the basic mechanisms underlying epilepsy is considerable, not only by the use of continuous survey with multiple deep microelectrodes, but perhaps in particular in the field of neurotransmitter imbalance (e.g., GABA, dopamine, etc.) and the metabolic changes occurring during a seizure. We now have most of the tools and the opportunity may occur when a seizure takes place (with the biopsy needle in position in the target area) to obtain tissue immediately.

The recent work of Caveness and the team at the National Institute of Health in Bethesda being reported in this volume indicates the significance of the metabolic activity of the globus pallidus that occurs in the more major focal seizures. This work tends to confirm our own interest in the conduction pathways of the globus-pallidus as an important surgical target for the control of intractable epilepsy.

The fascination of the hypothesis of neurotransmitter imbalance extends also to other chronic neurological disorders and the fact that epilepsy does not associate easily with them.

REFERENCES

Caveness, W. F. (1978): *Personal communication. Proceedings of the 10th Epilepsy International Symposium*, Vancouver, 1978.

Gaze, R. M., Gillingham, F. J., Kalynaraman, S., Porter, R. W., Donaldson, A. A., and Donaldson, I. M. L. (1964): Microelectrode recordings from the human thalamus. *Brain*, 87:691–706.

Gillingham, F. J., Watson, W. S., Donaldson, A. A., and Naughton, J. A. L. (1960): The surgical treatment of Parkinsonism. *Br. Med. J.*, 2:1395–1402.

Gillingham, F. J. (1974): Accidents in stereotaxy—side effects or bonus? *Acta Neurochir. (Suppl.)*, 21:5–12.

Gillingham, F. J., Watson, W. S., Donaldson, A. A., and Cairns, V. M. (1976): Stereotactic lesions for the control of intractable epilepsy. *Acta Neurochir. (Suppl.)*, 23:263–269.

Jinnai, D., and Nishimoto, A. (1963): Stereotaxic destruction of Forel-H for treatment of epilepsy. *Neurochirurgica*, 6:164–176.

Advances in Epileptology:
The Xth Epilepsy International Symposium,
edited by J. A. Wada and J. K. Penry.
Raven Press, New York © 1980.

Long-Term Follow-up Results of Posteromedial Hypothalamotomy

Keiji Sano and Yoshiaki Mayanagi

Department of Neurosurgery, University of Tokyo, Tokyo, Japan

In order to ameliorate behavior disorders, particularly those of a violent or aggressive nature, a small lesion was made stereotactically in the posteromedial hypothalamus, which is actually a continuation of the periaqueductal gray in cases of epileptic seizure and of mental retardation. Since the first operation in 1962 (Sano, 1962) for the treatment of this condition, 60 cases have been accumulated. Among them, 59 cases have been followed up for more than 2 years and 58 cases for as long as 5 to 16 years. This chapter deals with long-term follow-up results of these cases insofar as their behavioral, endocrinological, and epileptic condition is concerned.

METHODS

After radiographic demonstration of the third ventricle, a fine concentric bipolar electrode, 0.8 mm in outer diameter with an interpolar distance of 0.5 mm, is stereotactically inserted through a frontal burr hole into the target point, which is usually 2 mm below the midcommissural point and 2 mm lateral from the wall of the third ventricle. Endotracheal general anesthesia with nitrous oxide-oxygen-halothane is used. EEG, EKG, and EMG of the neck muscles, blood pressure, and respiration are monitored. High-frequency stimulation (50–100 Hz, 10–20 V with square pulses, 1 msec in pulse duration for 5–10 sec) of this point usually causes marked sympathetic responses, such as elevation of blood pressure, increase in pulse rate, mydriasis, or short respiratory arrest followed by hyperpnea or tachypnea (Sano, 1975; Sano et al., 1970). When the patient is under a light stage of general anesthesia, diffuse delta waves appear on the EEG and continue for several minutes even after cessation of stimulation. A downward and inward movement of the eyeball on the stimulated side is seen and sometimes the neck tilts toward the side of stimulation. Stimulation of this point in an awake state usually causes a very unpleasant sensation (patients reported that they felt fear or horror during strong stimulation).

The area where these responses are elicited by stimulation forms, in the lateral view, a small triangle in the posterior hypothalamus surrounded by lines connecting the midcommissural point, the mammillary body, and the posterior commissure (or the rostral end of the aqueduct). The authors named it the "ergotropic triangle." In the anteroposterior view, it occupies an area 2 to 5 mm from the wall of the third ventricle. When good sympathetic responses are obtained, especially blood pressure elevation, tachycardia, and mydriasis, electrocoagulation is performed with a high-frequency current (1 megaHz, 2–3 Watts for 3–4 min), using the same electrode.

The estimated size of the lesion is 3 to 4 mm in diameter. The operation is usually performed bilaterally at an interval of 1 to 3 weeks between procedures.

RESULTS

In the behavioral disorder study, there were 60 cases, 44 male and 16 female. Among them, 29 were under 15 years of age. Two cases required a second operation and there was one operative death. In the postoperative follow-up period, seven patients died of various causes: suicide (2), status epilepticus (2), hepatitis (1), pneumonia (1), and accidental drowning (1). In 38 cases, the effect of the operation on the behavioral disorders and the present status of the patients could be assessed and are summarized in Table 1. Nineteen cases (50%) showed excellent results, i.e., there were no rage attacks after the operation and the patient became so cooperative with other people that social and familial adaptation has been possible. We are encouraged by the fact that four patients have been employed. However, 10 pa-

TABLE 1. *Posteromedial hypothalamotomy for aggressive behavioral disorders (1962–1977) and present status of patients*

	Total	(males:females)	Under 15 years	(males:females)
Number of cases	60	(44:16)	29	(12:7)
Reoperation	2			
Operative death	1			
Death in follow-up period	7			

	Follow-up assessment (2–15 years)				
		Home		Center for the handicapped	Psychiatric institution
	Total	Employed	Unemployed		
Excellent	19 (50.0%)	4	10	5	0
Good	13 (34.2%)	0	7	4	2
Fair	4 (10.5%)	0	0	3	1
Unchanged	2 (5.3%)	0	1	0	1
Total	38 (100 %)	4	18	12	4

tients remain at home, economically dependent, and five patients have been accepted to centers for handicapped people.

Thirteen cases (34%) showed good results, i.e., no rage attacks, but still easily excited. In this group, seven patients live at home, four in centers for handicapped, and two are in psychiatric institutions due to marked mental retardation. In four cases (10.5%) the results were fair, i.e., they still showed rage attacks although less frequently and less intensively. Their social adaptation was not satisfactory. In two cases (5.3%) the operation was unsuccessful.

In summary, this procedure is considered to have been effective in 95% of these 38 cases. Satisfactory results were obtained in 84%. Intelligence was not impaired by this operation. On the contrary, an amelioration of the I.Q. was noted in about one-half of the examined cases.

The location of the surgical intervention in this procedure is close to the endocrine center of the hypothalamic-hypophyseal axis. Therefore, the plasma levels of various pituitary hormones were estimated during and after the operation. As reported in 1970 (Sano et al., 1970), stimulation of the posteromedial hypothalamus temporarily elevated the plasma level of the growth hormone.

In eight operations, levels of other pituitary hormones were estimated as well. Although stimulation and electrocoagulation of the target point resulted in a temporary elevation of the plasma value of various hormones (TSH, FSH, LH, prolactin, cortisol), no significant findings common for all cases can be attributed to these results.

In the follow-up period, no clinical manifestations of serious endocrine disturbances were found. Although several cases showed a relatively low value of urine (11-OHCS and 17-KS), no substitutional treatment was necessary. Physical development curves of 10 patients who were operated on in childhood could be made. There was no significant retardation of physical development, although a few cases tended to gain weight after the operation. The timing of development of secondary sexual characteristics was within normal limits. Menstruation in girls began between 10 to 13 years.

In four cases follow-up stimulation tests of pituitary hormones were performed. The insulin test for GH and ACTH, the LH-RH test for LH and FSH, and the TRH test for TSH and prolactin showed that the regulatory systems of these pituitary hormones were functioning well even after bilateral operations.

Most of these patients had epileptic seizures and mental retardation as well as their chief problem of behavioral disorders. Stimulation of the posteromedial hypothalamus sometimes provoked focal epileptic spikes in the EEG. Activation of seizures by stimulation of the target point was also observed. As these facts imply that electrical coagulation of this particular portion of the brain may have a favorable effect on the control of epileptic seizures, a follow-up study was made on this point.

Types of seizures encountered in these 60 cases were analyzed. About 65% of the cases had generalized convulsive seizures in which 10 cases had minor seizures as well. Minor seizures, that is, infantile spasm or Lennox-Gastaut syndrome, were seen in 13%. There were several cases of psychomotor seizures or focal motor seizures. In total, the combination of epileptic seizures and behavioral disorders in these 60 cases reached up to 90%.

Before the time of operation, the seizures in 15 cases were completely controlled with antiepileptic drugs. However, 29 cases still had had episodes of seizure frequently or occasionally.

In these 29 cases, frequency and intensity of seizures and the amount of antiepileptic drugs were compared before and after the operation. Some effect in controlling epileptic seizures was evident in 12 cases (41%). Seizure frequency was reduced in eight cases, intensity of seizures were reduced in two cases, and in two cases only smaller doses of drugs were required in order to control the seizures. With respect to the type of seizure, minor seizures that were seen mainly in childhood cases seemed to show the highest effect, then generalized convulsive seizure with or without minor seizures followed, and psychomotor seizures seemed to be least influenced. However, a definite conclusion may be difficult because of the small number of cases in each group.

DISCUSSION

The present study confirmed the results of the authors' previous follow-up studies on the effect of posteromedial hypothalamotomy for controlling behavioral disorders. Recently the results of other series have been reported by Balasubramaniam and Kanaka (1975), Rubio et al., (1977), and Schvarcz (1977). There seems to be a general agreement among these reports that satisfactory overall results can be expected in 80% or more. Although indication of such a procedure in childhood is still controversial, the authors' experiences with 29 children seem to support an early surgical intervention. The greatest advantage of an early operation is that it brings these children with behavioral disorders out of isolation and provides them with the opportunity of receiving special and intensive education in schools or in handicapped centers after their abnormal behavior has been reduced.

From an endocrinological point of view, the procedure only temporarily activates the hypothalamic-pituitary axis, without causing any serious dysfunction. This is understandable because the surgical intervention is limited to the posterior portion of the hypothalamus and does not include various hypothalamic nuclei in the anterior hypothalamus.

The mechanism of effect on the epileptic activities is not yet clear. The surgical lesion in a part of the diffuse projecting system may have an indirect influence on the activities of epileptic foci, which may situate mostly in the neocortex. This operation, however, has not been indicated as yet for epilepsies per se.

The mechanism of ameliorating behavior disorders is probably explained by the normalizing effect of this operation on the balance of the ergotropic and trophotropic functions (Sano, 1975).

REFERENCES

Balasubramaniam, V., and Kanaka, T. S. (1975): Amygdalotomy and hypothalamotomy—a comparative study. *Confin. Neurol.*, 37:195–201.

Rubio, E., Arjona, V., and Rodriguez-Burgos, F. (1977): Stereotactic cryohypothalamotomy in aggressive behavior. In: *Neurosurgical Treatment in Psychiatry, Pain and Epilepsy*, edited by W. H. Sweet, et al., pp. 439–44. University Park Press, Baltimore.

Sano, K. (1962): Sedative neurosurgery with special reference to posteromedial hypothalamotomy. *Neurol. Med. Chir.*, 4:112–142.

Sano, K. (1975): Posterior hypothalamic lesions in the treatment of violent behavior. In: *Neural Bases of Violence and Aggression*, edited by W. S. Fields and W. H. Sweet, pp. 401–420. W. H. Green, St. Louis.

Sano, K., Mayanagi, Y., Sekino, H., Ogashiwa, M., and Ishijima, B. (1970): Results of stimulation and destruction of the posterior hypothalamus in man. *J. Neurosurg.*, 33:689–707.

Schvarcz, J. R. (1977): Results of stimulation and destruction of the posterior hypothalamus: A long-term evaluation. In: *Neurosurgical Treatment in Psychiatry, Pain and Epilepsy*, edited by W. H. Sweet, et al., pp. 429–438. University Park Press, Baltimore.

Advances in Epileptology:
The Xth Epilepsy International Symposium,
edited by J. A. Wada and J. K. Penry.
Raven Press, New York © 1980.

A Small Study in Stereoencephalotomy for Experimental and Clinical Epilepsy

*Tadahiro Mihara, *Eiki Kobayashi, *Kunimitsu Yamamoto, *Tetsuhiko Asakura, and **Koichi Kitamura

*Department of Neurosurgery, Faculty of Medicine, University of Kagoshima, Kagoshima; and **Department of Neurosurgery, Neurological Institute, Tokyo Women's Medical College, Tokyo, Japan

For the purpose of helping medically refractory patients with epileptic seizures, a stereotaxic procedure has been employed for some time by many pioneering neurosurgeons in Japan with lesion-making in the basal ganglia and the diencephalon. However, since the neural mechanisms concerned with epileptic seizures seem to involve the lower brain stem structures as well, an attempt was made to evaluate the effect of electrolytic lesion placement in the various brainstem lesions of cats treated with thiosemicarbazide (TSC). It is well known that TSC can produce reversible electroclinical manifestations of the epileptic condition as reflected by recurrent spontaneous convulsive seizures as well as convulsions precipitated by auditory stimulation in experimental animals (Asakura and Wada, 1972; Wada et al., 1967; Wada and Asakura, 1969; Yamashita et al., 1971).

In this study, electrolytic lesions were placed in the various brainstem region of cats. The effects of TSC with respect to frequency and nature of induced seizures were observed in lesioned animals and compared with the same in TSC-treated but nonlesioned cats. The results of our experimental studies and those of our clinical observations seem to confirm the previous contention of posteromedial hypothalamotomy described by Sano (1970) as being effective for behavior disorder whereas Forel-H-tomy described by Jinnai (1970) as beneficial for medically refractory seizures.

PATIENTS AND METHODS

Electrolytic lesions were placed bilaterally in the posterior hypothalamus, the Forel-H field and the midbrain. Localization of the midbrain lesion was divided into rostral and caudal ends, each further subdivided into dorsal, ventral, paracentral and lateral groups. Three cats were assigned to each of these 10 groups. Ten to fourteen days after lesion placement, all the cats received an intraperitoneal injection of 8 mg/kg TSC and were subjected to hourly audiogenic stimulation lasting for 2 min with an electric doorbell having an intensity of about 100 decibels. The number of seizures (either audiogenic or spontaneous) were observed for 5 hr in all the animals. Ten control cats without brain stem lesion were similarly subjected to TSC treatment and the results were compared with those of the experimental group. All the animals had chronically implanted electrodes in a number of cortical and deep structures and EEG recording was obtained throughout the observation. Altogether, 58 cats were used in this study. Histological examination verified the localization of implanted electrode tips as well as lesions were in the intended structures.

RESULTS

Results were summarized in Fig. 1. Induced as well as spontaneous seizure frequency was significantly less in all of the lesioned animals when compared with the controlled group. The order of the extent of this seizure frequency reduction was as follows: paracentral lesion of the caudal midbrain, lateral region of the caudal midbrain, the posterior hypothalamus, and the Forel-H area. None of the animals, however, remained seizure-free with TSC. Judging from the electrographic pattern, the spontaneous convulsion appeared to have originated within the limbic system whereas the audiogenic seizure seemed to have originated from the lower brainstem.

The effect of brainstem lesions on the experimental epilepsy has often been studied by means of measuring electrical or pharmacological threshold that are required to initiate convulsive seizures. Our attempts to estimate the

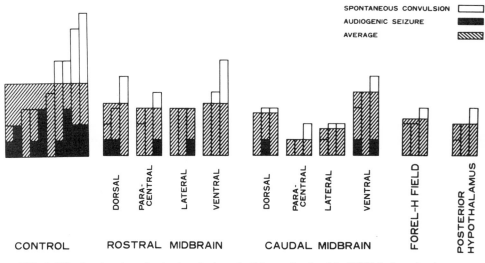

FIG. 1. Effects of various brainstem lesions to thiosemicarbazide (TSC)-induced seizures.

seizure frequencies were chosen for the purpose of obtaining a more meaningful information for the assessment of the efficacy of surgical treatment in the problem of human epilepsy. Our results are consistent with those reported by Iwata (1967). Although we have not encountered any evidence of deranged vital functions after brainstem lesioning, its application to human epilepsy requires caution. With this naturally imposed limitation, we have performed posteromedial hypothalamotomy and Forel-H-tomy in patients with medically refractory seizures with or without significant behaviour problems. Three patients each were subjected to posteromedial hypothalamotomy and Forel-H-tomy. These patients were an average of $9\frac{1}{2}$ years of age, having suffered an average of 8 years from medically resistant seizures prior to surgery. The type of seizures included generalized convulsive as well as partial seizure. Seizure frequency was documented at least for 6 months prior to surgery. Laterality of the lesion placement was determined according to the electrographic features and seizure patterns. In four cases, unilateral lesion did not produce any significant benefit and therefore, contralateral lesion was made subsequently. Only significant complication of these procedures was the transient hemiparesis in one patient after Forel-H-tomy which subsequently completely resolved.

Interpretation of results of the surgical treatment requires caution since the follow-up period is still within 2 years. However, postoperative assessment of behavior as well as seizure frequency suggests the posteromedial hypothalamotomy produced significantly beneficial results in the behavior problems, whereas Forel-H-tomy produced complete freedom from seizure in one case, and a significant reduction of seizure frequency in two cases, regardless of whether the seizure was primary or secondary generalized.

CONCLUSIONS

Results of our experimental and clinical study suggest that Forel-H-tomy in appropriately selected cases of medically refractory seizures can produce beneficial effects in terms of increasing susceptibility to medication for control of otherwise medically refractory seizures. On the other hand, posteromedial hypothalamotomy seems to exert beneficial effects primarily on behavior problems. It appears that both procedures can be expected to produce in appropriately selected cases a significant improvement in terms of increasing susceptibility to medication for better control of their medically refractory and very difficult seizure-behavior problems.

REFERENCES

Asakura, T., and Wada, J. A. (1972): Neurobiology of audiogenic seizure: A review. *Brain Nerve*, 24:513–534.
Iwata, Y. (1967): Experimental study of epileptic excitability; its intracerebral facilitation and inhibition. *Osaka Daigaku Igaku Zasshi*, 19:295–312.

Jinnai, D., and Mukawa, J. (1970): Forel-H-tomy for the treatment of epilepsy. *Confin. Neurol.*, 32:307–315.

Sano, K., Mayanagi, Y., Sekino, H., Ogashiwa, M., and Ishijima, B. (1970): Results of stimulation and destruction of the posterior hypothalamus in man. *J. Neurosurg.*, 33:689–707.

Wada, J. A., Ikeda, H., and Berry, K. (1967): Reversible behavioral and electrographic manifestations induced by methionine sulfoximine. *Neurology (Minneap.)*, 17:854–868.

Wada, J. A., and Asakura, T. (1969): Susceptibility to audiogenic seizure induced by Thiosemicarbazide. *Exp. Neurol.*, 24:19–37.

Yamashita, J., Makino, K., and Yamamoto, K. (1971): Behavioral and electroencephalographic studies on Thiosemicarbazide-induced seizure in rabbits. *Jikei. Med. J.*, 18:99–107.

Advances in Epileptology:
The Xth Epilepsy International Symposium,
edited by J. A. Wada and J. K. Penry.
Raven Press, New York © 1980.

Role of VA Lesions in the Control of Focal Motor Seizures: Experimental and Clinical Studies

Kazuo Mori, Hirohisa Ono, and Kaoru Iwayama

Department of Neurosurgery, Nagasaki University School of Medicine, Sakamotomachi, Nagasaki, Japan

Electrophysiological and anatomical studies indicate that there are two different kinds of thalamocortical relay neurons, specific and nonspecific, in the ventral anterior–ventral lateral (VA-VL) area in cats. According to the field potential analysis, these two kinds of neurons even seem to intermingle with each other in the ventral thalamic nuclear complex (Sasaki et al., 1972). Specific neurons responding antidromically to stimulation of the anterior sigmoid cortex and orthodromically to that of the cerebellar nuclei were called F neurons by Sasaki et al. Present investigations were carried out to observe the interrelationship between these two relay systems and penicillin-induced epileptogenesis on the sensory-motor cortex in cats.

Experiments were mainly performed by Dr. Iwayama, one of our co-workers.

METHODS

The animal was paralyzed with gallamine and artificially ventilated. A wide craniotomy was performed and a glass microelectrode was inserted into the VA-VL area with the aid of a stereotaxic map. Negative field potentials, elicited by stimulation of the lateral nucleus of the cerebellum, also served as a good reference to determine the location of the tip of an electrode. Extracellular unitary recording was made in the VA-VL area. The F neuron was identified by antidromic activation in which stimulating electrodes were placed on the anterior sigmoid gyrus. The epileptogenic focus was produced by application of penicillin on the pial surface near the cortical stimulating electrodes. Then the effect of cortical epileptiform discharges on activities of F neuron was observed. At the close of an experiment, the microelectrode position in VA-VL was marked by breaking off the pipette tip *in situ* so that the electrode position could be verified later histologically.

RESULTS

Behavior of F Neuron during Epileptogenesis of the Motor Cortex

Interictal Stage

The firing pattern of F neurons at this interictal stage was not identical; four types were observed (Fig. 1.) (a) In the first type, about half of the units showed simple abrupt cessation of spontaneous firing. (b) The second type of cells fired with long-latency bursts. (c) The third type fired with a short latency. (d) There were also neurons that did not seem to be involved at all.

Schwartzkroin et al. (1975) intensively studied membrane events in VL neurons in the sequence of the cortical epileptiform discharges. In view of their excellent studies, it was possible to assume that abrupt cessation of spontaneous firing observed in type A neuron was due to corticifugally induced inhibition. In some of type B units with long-latency bursts, neuronal firing might be generated antidromically by a backfiring phenomenon.

Figure 2 shows transition of the firing pattern of one and the same F neuron during seizure development. The neuron that fired indifferently at the early stage (A), transformed to an active neuron as the focus matured (C and D). This would indicate that corticifugal excitation became more and more powerful and this, in turn, produced intense positive feedback on pyramidal neurons within the motor cortex.

Ictal Stage

The majority of F neurons were involved in EEG paroxysm and fired uniformly. They responded with high-frequency burst, coinciding with a surface EEG oscillation.

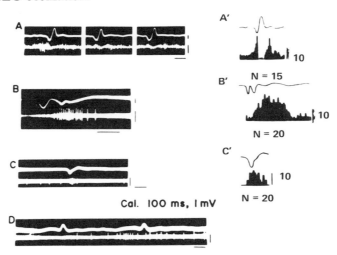

FIG. 1. Firing patterns of F neurons at interictal stage.

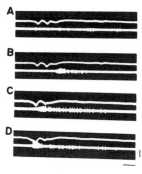

FIG. 2. Transition of the firing pattern of one F neuron during seizure development.

Cal. 100 ms, 1 mV

Effect of Additional Penicillin to the VA-VL Area on a Cortical Focus

Separate experiments were performed with a gross electrode. EEG recordings from both cortices and the VA-VL area were enhanced remarkably.

Generalization of Seizure Discharges from the Unilateral VA-VL Penicillin Focus

In another experiment, discharges were projected to both cortices diffusely. In the laminar field analysis, negative SP shift was found in entire layers of both cortices with similar amplitude; on the other hand, seizure frequency and generalization were reduced by making electrolytic lesions in the VA-VL area.

CASE REPORTS

Based on these experiments, VA lesions were placed in three patients.

Case 1. A 19-year-old man suffered from encephalitis at the age of 2. Since then, he had seizures with a frequency of five to ten times weekly. Seizures usually began with twitching of his right arm and spread quickly into a generalized convulsion and he became unconscious. He had a mild right hemiparesis and was mentally retarded. EEG was markedly slowed in the left side. At the time of surgery, seizures were occurring at a rate of four to five each day. On August 28, 1975, a radiofrequency electrocoagulation (approximately 7 × 7 mm) was made in the left ventrocaudolateral aspect of the VA extending into the VL nucleus (around the area of VPO, V.o.i and V.o.p according to Schaltenbrand's stereotaxic atlas). Since the operation, his seizure frequency has become reduced to ten to fifteen times per month (instead of per week) for about 2 years. Recently seizure frequency has increased but has remained mostly as partial seizures.

Case 2. This 28-year-old man had his first generalized convulsion at the age of 17. Since that time he has had generalized seizures and absence attacks. Seizure frequency increased until he was having one per day. Although the cause was unknown, EEG showed a right frontoparietal focus. On May 12, 1977, a lesion was placed in the medial aspect of the VA (centered to 5 mm anterior from the midpoint, 5 mm lateral and 5 mm superior from the AC-PC line). During the next 10 months, his seizure frequency was reduced from a daily seizure to seizures occurring only four to ten times per month. Then, however, seizure frequency again increased to the preoperative level but remained as petit mal attacks.

Case 3. This 16-year-old boy had a history of a difficult premature birth. He had mild right hemiparesis. Attacks were focal motor with secondary generalization. Seizure frequency was two to three times daily. EEG showed a left central spike focus. On April 18, 1978, a lesion was placed in the laterocaudal aspect of the VA extending into the VL and adjacent structures. Although this case was thought to be a favorable candidate for this type of operation, the results were not satisfactory. He has had no generalized convulsions, but focal attacks have persisted in the 3-month follow-up. His seizure frequency and EEG have not been altered in any way by this lesion.

DISCUSSION

In the experimental sphere, it has been pointed out that the VA nucleus is in a key position for nonspecific thalamic mechanisms. Effects of projected cortical epileptiform discharges on VL and VPL neurons in cats have been studied intensively by Prince and co-workers (Gutnick and Prince, 1975; Schwartzkroin, Mutani and Prince, 1975). Kusske et al., (1972) also studied the effects of stereotaxic lesions in the ventral anterior thalamus on the experimental model of focal epilepsy produced by injection of alumina cream into the monkey sensory motor cortex. From these results, together with our present findings, the VA-VL area seems to be a promising target in the treatment of intractable seizures having a focus in or around the motor cortex or being widely distributed in one hemisphere (these are cases where direct surgical excision of the cortical focus carries a risk of significant functional impairment). The destruction in this area might be efficacious in at least two ways: (a) in diminishing a positive feedback on the focus per se, and (b) in interrupting the development into generalization of seizures.

In the clinical sphere, there are not as yet generally accepted target areas in the stereotactic surgery for seizure disorders. Mullan et al. (1967) placed thalamic lesions for the control of epilepsy. In his patient group, there were three cases in which lesions predominantly involved the VA. They also had three other cases with VL lesions. VA lesions were also placed in three adult patients with medically intractable epilepsy by Ojemann and Ward (1975).

In our three cases, alleviation of seizures were all temporary. None fulfilled the criteria that are often used for evaluating resection of epileptic foci, namely the cessation or near-cessation (less than one seizure per year) of seizures for 6 months or more postoperatively. Since the operation, however, seizures were thought to have been prevented from developing into generalization. Moreover, no complications were noticed that might be attributed to the operation.

Further research and experience seem to be indicated.

REFERENCES

Gutnick, M. J., and Prince, D. A. (1975): Effects of projected cortical epileptiform discharges on neuronal activities in ventrobasal thalamus of the cat: Ictal discharge (1975): *Exp. Neurol.*, 46:418–431.

Kusske, J. A., Ojemann, G. A., and Ward, A. A. Jr. (1972): Effects of lesions in ventral anterior thalamus on experimental focal epilepsy. *Exp. Neurol.*, 34:279–290.

Mullan, S., Vailati, G., Karasick, J., and Mailis, M. (1967): Thalamic lesions for the control of epilepsy. *Arch. Neurol.*, 16:277–285.

Ojemann, G. A., and Ward, A. A. Jr. (1975): Stereotactic and other procedures for epilepsy. In: *Advances in Neurology, Vol. 8*, edited by D. P. Purpura, J. K. Penry, and R. D. Walter. Raven Press, New York.

Sasaki, K., Matsuda, Y., Kawaguchi, S., and Mizuno, N. (1972): On the cerebello-thalamo-cerebral pathway for the parietal cortex. *Exp. Brain Res.*, 16:89–103.

Schwartzkroin, P. A., Mutani, R., and Prince, D. A. (1975): Orthodromic and antidromic effects of a cortical epileptiform focus on ventrolateral nucleus of the cat. *J. Neurophysiol.*, 38:795–811.

Abstracts

FOREBRAIN COMMISSUROTOMY FOR THE RELIEF OF INTRACTABLE SEIZURES

A. G. Reeves, D. H. Wilson, M. Waddington
Hanover

In the last 7½ years we have partially or entirely sectioned the forebrain commissures in 13 patients incapacitated by seizures considered intractable to currently available medical therapy.

Surgery consisted of complete forebrain commissurotomy (division of the entire corpus callosum, hippocampal commissure and the anterior commissure) (3 patients), complete section of the corpus callosum and hippocampal commissure (5 patients), and frontal forebrain commissurotomy (division of anterior two thirds of the corpus callosum and the anterior commissure) (5 patients).

All three patients with complete forebrain commissurotomy are improved. One is seizure free 7½ years postoperatively. Two no longer have generalized seizures 5½ years after surgery.

Four patients with complete section of the corpus callosum are improved now having rare partial and generalized seizures 1-3 years after surgery. One patient had only a transient decrease in partial and generalized seizures.

One patient remains seizure free since frontal forebrain commissurotomy 5 years ago. Three patients are not improved 5 to 5½ years after surgery. One patient died 12 days post frontal forebrain commissurotomy of cortical vein thrombosis.

Ten patients continue to need anticonvulsants to prevent recurrence of seizures.

70% of our patients are improved 1 to 7½ years post-surgery. We feel that complete forebrain commissurotomy or complete section of the corpus callosum and hippocampal commissure may be reasonable alternative therapy for individuals incapacitated by intractable seizures.

RESULTS OF SURGICAL INTERVENTION IN 100 PATIENTS WITH SEVERE TEMPORAL LOBE EPILEPSIES

J. Talairach, J. Bancaud, A. Bonis, C. Munari
Paris

The following study is based on a group of a hundred acute epileptic patients who have undergone an essentially temporal cortectomy done on the basis of stereotactic exploration.

These mostly adolescent or young adult patients suffered from epilepsy beginning in nearly all cases before the age of 16 and generally, progressing for at least ten years.

Highly probable etiology was detected in more than half the cases. Approximately 75% of these patients, though correctly treated, suffered from one or more attacks a day and nearly half of them had experienced one or more status epilepticus in the course of their desease.

Surgical results, after a year's lapse, show that 62% of the patients became seizure free while another 28% have experienced several short-lived seizures.

Though there is substantial improvement in most cases, attacks persist in 16% of the patients.

The mortality rate is 2% in this series (in the last 8 years no death has been recorded).

Hence it seems to us that the new methodology in use in the last twenty years provides appreciable results even if it can only be applied to a limited number of patients.

Significantly, it thus becomes possible to bring to light the reasons for failures, and, consequently, to establish a better adapted pre-operative strategy.

STEREOELECTROENCEPHALOGRAPHY WHY SO MANY DEPTH-ELECTRODES?

J. M. Saint-Hilaire, G. Bouvier, A. Leduc
Montreal

The ease of Talairach's stereotactic method of safely implanting multiple depth-electrodes can lead to the introduction of an excessive number of electrodes in the brain of any one patient. In spite of their small diameter (less than 1.5 mm) the electrodes may cause some brain damage. One may then ask why 8 to 10 depth-electrodes when 3 or 4 could be adequate to outline the epileptic focus?

Sometimes, the epileptic zone can be easily determined from its clinical manifestations and the anomalies found in the scalp EEG recordings. But it is also well recognized that a single clinical manifestation may originate from 2 or 3 possible different foci. Therefore, with multiple primary manifestations, one has to consider so many more independent foci. Difficulties may also arise when there is no aura or other primary localizing manifestation. Furthermore, scalp EEG anomalies whether ictal or interictal are often false localizing. One important characteristic of the depth-electrode is its relative blindness in that it explores a very limited volume of the brain.

In addition to the epileptic focus, it is essential to detect the main pathways of propagation of the epileptic discharge to other brain structures. Finally, the limits of the zone for resection have to be determined precisely to spare important functional areas.

Examples will be given illustrating these problems.

THE IMPLANTATION OF MULTIPLE CHRONIC DEPTH ELECTRODES

G. Bouvier, J. M. St-Hilaire, R. Maltais,
P. Desrochers
Montreal

We, epileptologists, neurologists and neurosurgeons, must not forget how the brain is shaped but must remember that it is a 3-dimensional structure.

Early in life, the brain surface is no longer a smooth surface. It becomes very uneven with the development of sulci and gyri. Thus a great part of the cortical surface is buried in the depth of sulci: such that surface electrocorticography has a very limited application.

Talairach and Bancaud have proposed many years ago that epilepsy has a cortical origin. As they were entirely aware of the 3-dimensionality of the brain, they have developed stereotactic instruments permitting complete radiological exploration of the brain and introduction of many acute multiple leads electrodes.

Inspired by their philosophy, we from Hopital Notre-Dame de Montreal, have developed an entirely new system for safe implantation of multiple chronic electrodes, that is electrodes that stay in the brain for days or weeks. This more *physiological approach* permits a 3rd dimension anatomical definition of the epileptogenic focus: stereotactic destruction of specific structures or cortectomy is achieved with a maximum of precision and security.

So far no major complications have been encountered in over five hundred implantations.

A NEW STEREOTAXIC APPARATUS FOR PERCUTANEOUS TWIST DRILL INSERTION OF DEPTH ELECTRODES FOR SEIZURE RECORDING

A. Oliver, G. Bertrand
Montreal

In the course of our work with insertion of multiple chronic depth electrodes for the purpose of seizure recording in complex and specific problems of epilepsy, we have developed a stereotaxic device which uses an orthogonal approach combined with an X-Y system of frame coordinates.

The main advantage of such an apparatus is to give ample working space at the site of electrode insertion, through a small (3mm.) twist drill skull trephine, and the possibility of giving each pre-selected brain target an X-Y frame coordinate. In this way, the frame coordinates can be more easily handled by a computer for map display of electrodes position and of on-going abnormal electric activity at each recording site. The apparatus can also be used

for percutaneous biopsy of inoperable brain tumors.

Description: The apparatus consists essentially of a modified Leksell frame which permits INDEPENDENT bilateral vertical movement of a sliding side bar along the Y scale and on which is mounted a carrier which moves horizontally along the X scale. The depth of penetration along the mesio-lateral axis (Z) — the distance from the midline — is determined with a phantom ruler. A collet chuck on the carrier allows introduction and immobilization, within interchangeable and concentric metal cuffs, of a scalp punch, a twist drill, a screw driver for fixation of the skull hollow screws, dural coagulating electrodes and the brain canula. The carrier is also equipped with an adjustable support for immobilization of the recording electrode on target while the brain canula is withdrawn.

The frame gives an unobstructed visualization of the skull and brain during the first stage of stereotaxic localization by ventriculography, P.E.G. and angiography. The system can be used with the head supported by a sling or it can be adapted to a special base bolted to an isocentric P.E.G. chair.

The apparatus can be used with both the conventional short distance X-ray technique or with a tele-radiology system.

REGIONAL CEREBRAL BLOOD FLOW IN FOCAL EPILEPSY. A STEREOTACTIC STUDY

B. Larsen
Copenhagen
J. M. Orgogozo, A. Rougier, F. Cohadon, P. Loiseau
Bordeaux

The surgical management of drug resistant epilepsies demands a precise appraisal of the epileptogenic focus or foci. The stereotactic approach of Talairach and Bancaud has been a major advance in this respect, allowing to define the size, extent and depth of epileptic foci by intracerebral recording of spontaneous or induced seizures. But one must have strong arguments to refer patients to such a procedure which involves the implantation in the brain of several electrodes. Since the report by Hougaard el al (Arch.Neurol., 33 : 527-535, 1976) on localization of ictal and interictal epileptic foci in 10 patients, by means of rCBF studies with the Xenon 133 intracorotid injection method, we studied 15 additional patients with the same 254 channels dynamic gamma-camera. We found hyperhemic foci in all cases having a focal seizure during the study and in several "subictal" cases. To assess the potential usefulness of this technique in the selection of candidates to stereotactic investigations and surgery we adapted the rCBF system to a stereotactic frame and started to investigate that way patients with severe partial epilepsy, some of them being submitted also to electrodes implantation. The preliminary results suggest that the rCBF investigation may be helpful in the assessment of active epileptic foci, especially if they are multiple or with misleading clinical correlates.

VALUE OF A MULTIMODALITY APPROACH TO THE SELECTION FOR NEUROSURGICAL INTERVENTION OF PARTIAL SEIZURE CASES REFRACTORY TO ANTIEPILEPTIC DRUGS - A PRELIMINARY REPORT

M. Rayport, S. M. Ferguson, W. S. Corrie
Toledo

Cortical resection for the control of partial seizures refractory to antiepileptic drugs (AED) having become an established therapy, attention must be directed to the failure rate (30% to 40% of cases). Remarkable similarity in the failure rates reported by different centers around the world strongly suggests that random factors, e.g. differences of case material or operative management, play a minor role as compared with a limiting effect from a common major factor. These considerations have led to the hypothesis that the consistent failure rate of cortical resections may be associated with preoperative case selection on the basis of localization of epileptogenic gray matter by 1) extracranial recording (ecEEG) and 2) reliance on interictal EEG phenomena. Accordingly, chronic stereoelectroencephalography (SEEG), appropriate EEG and nursing personnel and facilities permitting ictal as well as interictal recording and observation were instituted *ab initio* in the epilepsy program of the Medical College of Ohio. Indications for SEEG studies were nonlocalizing ecEEG recordings in the presence of a stable partial seizure pattern. Electrocorticography was carried out during all cortical resections. All cases underwent long-term follow-up. Observations on more than 50 closely studied operated cases of whom 12 also underwent SEEG studies will be discussed in relation to the above hypothesis.

METHODOLOGY OF STEREOTAXIC INVESTIGATIONS OF SEVERE TEMPORAL LOBE EPILEPSIES

J. Talairach, J. Bancaud, A. Bonis, C. Munari
Paris

Surgical treatment of patients suffering from severe drug-resistant epilepsy relies upon an investigative procedure previously described by the authors (Talairach et al. 1974) which one can outline as follows:

1) The electroclinical work-up makes it possible to formulate hypotheses specifically as to the approximate localization of the epileptiform discharges, while the stereotaxic neuroradiological findings provide indications as to possible lesion presence and allow for a precise identification of the target areas.

2) The functional exploration of cerebral structures, particularly of the telencephalon, is done with the help of intracranial electrodes. These are implanted conciliating both the anatomical data and the technical means at one's disposal, with special attention given to the vessels so as to reduce risks.

3) The recording of the electrical activity in cortical and/or subcortical structures (S.E.E.G.) aims at identifying in the three spatial planes not only the site of origin of seizure discharges, but also their system of organization in cerebral space.

4) Recourse to a cortectomy is considered if a single epileptogenic site has been identified, one, moreover, which lies outside of cortical areas whose excision could entail severe functional disturbances.

5) The synthesis of anatomo-radiological data (made on the basis of previous stereotaxic investigations) and stereoelectroencephalographic findings provide the surgeon the means with which to program in full detail the intervention he plans to undertake.

TEMPORAL LOBE EPILEPSY AND KINDLING

R. G. Perrin and H. J. Hoffman
Toronto

A retrospective study has been undertaken involving 15 consecutive patients who have undergone temporal lobectomy for temporal lobe epilepsy (TLE) at the Hospital for Sick Children in Toronto between 1951 and 1973.

A progressive clinical deterioration was clearly documented in 6 patients prior to surgical consideration. Characteristically, staring spells were later accompanied by automatic behaviour followed (months later) by onset of motor seizures. Serial psychological testing in 2 patients showed progressive intellectual deterioration.

Five patients were seizure-free and another 7 were improved following surgery. The follow-up time was 2 months to 20 years. Calculating the average time (t̄) from the onset of seizures to surgical treatment, we found that those patients with best results (fit-free) had the shortest interval (t̄ = 9.1 years), and those who were not improved following surgery had the longest interval from first fit to surgical treatment (t̄ = 10.3 years).

Attempts made to assess the effects of chronic epileptogenic irritation on various mental phenomena had led to the conclusion that the temporal lobe epileptic suffers episodic interruptions of learning and memory process which leaves his experiential record with many unrecognized blank spaces. Such a mechanism has been held to account for the behavioural disturbances and memory impairment which often constitute a portion of the psycho-motor seizure syndrome. On this basis, it has been suggested that early definitive (i.e. surgical) treatment is indicated in children with intractable seizures. However, the kindling model analogy suggests a more nefarious underlying pathophysiology. Thus the progressive clinical deterioration is not due merely to 'interruption of experiential record' resulting in 'unrecognized blank spaces', but could be due rather to ongoing epileptogenic activity resulting in kindled seizure phenomena.

The rationale for surgery is then elimination of the kindling focus.

LIGHT AND ELECTRON MICROSCOPIC STUDIES ON SURGICALLY RESECTED SPECIMENS OF TEMPORAL LOBE EPILEPSY—WITH A SPECIAL REFERENCE TO EPILEPTOGENESIS

K. Kitamura, Tokyo
H. Awa, M. Sasahira, K. Matsuda, T. Asakura
Kagoshima

The resected epileptogenic tissues of twenty-three patients with intractable temporal lobe epilepsy were morphologically reviewed.

The results were as follows: 1) There was local devastation of the basic cell structure such as multiple necrotizing foci of neurons, numerous calcospherites and many scars. 2) As the the changes in neurons, there were frequently found degeneration and necrosis. Electron microscopy revealed devastated nucleoplasm, phagocytic lysosomes, lipofuscin granules, enlargement of RER, lamellar structure, increased numbers of presynaptic vesicles and various changes of mitochondria in synapses. 3) Reactive glial proliferation involved neuronophagia, glial rosette and gliosis. Ultrastructurally, we noticed a remarkable increase of astrocytic fibers, various phagocytic cells with abundant inclusion bodies, lysosomes and mitochondria in their cytoplasm. 4) Furthermore, various vascular malformations reached the high rate of 74% (17/23), and their adjacent tissues were accompanied by so-called sclerosis. Such findings are noteworthy concerning the circulatory disturbance of the epileptogenic tissues. Ultrastructurally, windings of the basement membrane, remarkably dense bodies of pericytes and vacuolation of endothelial cells were observed.

A discussion concerning the epileptogenesis of temporal lobe epilepsy will be made on the basis of the above observations.

INTERICTAL EEG AND RESULTS OF TEMPORAL LOBECTOMY

F. Sharbrough, E. Laws, N. Fode
Rochester, Minnesota

The preoperative and postoperative interictal EEG findings and results of surgery in 38 cases of temporal lobectomy performed during a 5-year interval and followed for 2 to 7 years are reviewed. Preoperatively, five patients showed independent spike foci; only one (20%) of this group became free of seizures causing impaired consciousness after temporal lobectomy. Of 33 patients with a single temporal focus, 23 (70%) became seizure-free after surgery. Six of the 33 patients had tumor, and only 1 (16%) became seizure-free whereas of the 27 patients with no tumor, 22 (81%) became seizure-free. Of the 27 patients with no tumor and a single preoperative focus, 12 had complete absence of spikes and sharp waves in a follow-up EEG obtained 5 months after surgery. Of these 12 patients, 11 (92%) became seizure-free, whereas only 11 of 15 (73%) with residual spike activity became seizure-free. These findings, which are important in selection of candidates for temporal lobectomy, will be compared to those in previously reported studies.

MONITORING OF PATIENTS AFTER NEURO-SURGICAL OPERATIONS WITH REFERENCE TO EPILEPTIC SEIZURES

M. Egli, H. Walser
Zurich

Prevention of epileptic fits in the early postoperative phase (up to three weeks) after neurosurgical intervention is of great importance because they may have an unfavourable influence on the patient's prognosis. We have investigated 446 neurosurgical patients undergoing operation for aneurysms (124), angiomas (47), and other space-occupying lesions (275) in an attempt to determine the incidence of epileptic fits, their risk factors, and the value of pre-operative medication.

The collected data were statistically evaluated using a log-linear technique and the risk factors for epileptic seizures in the early post-operative phase were found to be: 1) pre-existing epilepsy, 2) angiomas supratentorial site, 3) clinical complications of both cerebral and extracerebral origin in the immediate and late post-operative phase. Our study has shown that antiepileptic drugs used in the prevention of early postoperative fits as compared with "chronic epilepsy" were found to be of less value. The reason for this is presumed to be that these postoperative fits have other pathophysiological mechanisms. They may belong to "functional epileptic fits". Because of the above findings, it is our conclusion that with recurrent fits in the early postoperative phase a general anesthetic with relaxation and assisted ventilation may be incorporated in the treatment regime.

LIMBIC SEIZURES DURING THE EARLY STAGES OF NEUROSURGICAL INTENSIVE CARE

F. Miltner
Wurzburg

Cerebral bioelecrtical activity of the convexity and the base of the skull of 220 neurosurgical patients was monitored longitudinally for periods lasting up to 7 days.

With comatose patients changes in coma level were registered. Seizure patterns - often with motor events - were recorded from the basal leads (nasopharyngeal, tympanal, suboccipital). Mirror foci were detected. Those comatose patients were treated effectively by combination of hydantoin and clonazepam and drug effects on seizure patterns were investigated.

SEIZURES FOLLOWING INTRACRANIAL SURGERY: INCIDENCE IN THE FIRST WEEK

E. Matthew, A. L. Sherwin, J. Stratford
Montreal

Though it is well-established that the seizures associated with acute cranio-cerebral trauma predispose to chronic epilepsy, less attention has been paid to the seizures which occur following intracranial surgery. The present investigation addresses itself to this and establishes the incidence of "early" post-operative seizures, i.e. seizures which occur during the first week after intracranial surgery, as the first part of a prospective study which will focus on effective methods of prevention.

Consecutive craniotomies (118), drawn from two major hospitals, and performed for disorders other than epilepsy and acute trauma, were reviewed. The final diagnoses included tumour (70), subdural haematoma (13), aneurysm (10), arteriovenous malformation (7), and miscellaneous lesions (18). Eighty-seven patients (73.73%) without seizures prior to surgery constituted Group A; the remaining 31 (26.27%) had one or more seizures pre-operatively and formed Group B. Fifteen patients in Group A and all patients in Group B received anticonvulsant drugs pre-operatively.

In the first post-operative week, 11 patients in Group A (12.64%) had seizures. The final diagnoses were tumour (6), subdural haematoma (2), intracerebral haematoma (1), aneurysm (1), arteriovenous malformation (1). Six had seizures in the first 24 hours, and of these, three had further attacks. Only one of these 11 patients received anticonvulsant drugs pre-operatively. In contrast, 11 patients in Group B (35.48%%) had seizures. All patients were operated upon under general anesthesia, received steriods, and did not have metabolic derangements.

Thus, "early" post-operative seizures occur in 12.65% of patients who have not had seizures previously. Such seizures may be prevented by improving the perioperative anticonvulsant regimens currently in use. Prevention of such seizures may reduce the incidence of chronic epilepsy which may develop through mechanisms such as kindling.

SURGERY FOR TEMPORAL LOBE EPILEPSY — RESULTS IN A RECENT SERIES

N. Fode, E. Laws, F. Sharbrough
Rochester

Between 1972 and 1976, 38 patients presented with intractable temporal lobe epilepsy and, after appropriate evaluation, were considered candidates for temporal lobectomy. Etiologic factors included trauma (11), febrile seizures (9), CNS infection (4), tumor (4), cyst (2) and a number of miscellaneous conditions. All of the patients had psychomotor seizures; 6 had other types as well. Electrocorticography, with surface and depth recording, was carried out at surgery and was useful with virtually every case. Pathologic findings were "normal" in 28 cases. The remainder consisted of tumor (4), cyst (2), degenerating brain (2), inflammatory changes and chronic posttraumatic changes.

Following surgery, 70% of the patients have been free of seizures during the 2 to 7 year follow-up period. A critical analysis of this series indicates that certain prognostic features were present in most of the patients who were surgical failures. These results will be reviewed in detail in an attempt to clarify and improve the selection of candidates for temporal lobectomy.

RESULTS OF 146 CONSECUTIVE CASES OF EPILEPSY OPERATED ON FROM 1959 TO 1974. ROLE OF DEPTH EEG RECORDING

L. Ravagnati, F. Marossero, A. Franzini, G. Ettorre, and C. A. Pagni
Milano and Torino

The 146 patients of our series have been considered according to the different types of surgical treatment undergone: (a) Ablation of the epileptogenic lesion (lobectomy or topectomy), 70 cases, (b) Hemispherectomy, 19 cases, (c) Stereotactically placed lesions, 24 cases, (d) Open stereotactic exploration without surgical resection, 33 cases.

A diagnostic depth EEG study, with acute and/or chronic intracerebral stereotactically implanted electrodes, was performed in 104 cases. In 24 patients the depth EEG study was not followed by any surgical procedures, while in 80 cases cortical ablations or stereotactic lesions were performed.

The 86 followed-up patients were divided in three groups: (a) No seizures or occasional seizures (b) Worthwhile improvement (c) unimproved. The results were as follows: (i) Temporal lobectomy (30 cases): 16 in group A, 9 in group B, 5 in group C. (ii) Frontal lobectomy (12 cases): 5 in group A, 5 in group B, 2 in group C. (iii) Occipital lobectomy or topectomy (9 cases: 6 in group A, 2 in group B, 1 in group C. (iv) Other (4 cases): 3 in group A, 1 in group B. (v) Hemispherectomy (12 cases): 8 in group A, 2 in group B, 2 in group C. (vi) Stereotactic lesions (19 cases): 5 in group A, 7 in group B, 7 in group C.

A comparative analysis between cases operated on after depth EEG study and cases operated on after scalp EEG plus corticography shows that depth EEG can be of great value in partial epilepsy with extratemporal foci, and in cases of epileptogenic foci due to gross traumatic lesions. Some cases (mesial foci, lower temporo-occipital surface foci) would not have been operated on without the localizing information of depth EEG. Examples of the determinant role of depth EEG in these cases will be presented.

RELATIONSHIP OF PSYCHOLOGICAL FUNCTIONING AND SURGICAL CONTROL OF EPILEPSY IN PATIENTS WHO HAVE UNDERGONE DEPTH ELECTRODE IMPLANTATION PRIOR TO TEMPORAL LOBECTOMY

R. Rausch, P. H. Crandall
Los Angeles

In a few specialized programs, patients with medically intractable epilepsy undergo depth electrode implantation to aid localization of seizure onset. If definitive information is obtained, excisional surgery, such as temporal lobectomy, may be performed (P.H. Crandall and R.D. Walter, 1971). In a select number of these patients in our program, psychological/psychosocial profiles were performed prior to depth electrode implantation and repeated following temporal lobectomy. A comparison of psychological functioning was made for the following groups: A) patients whose seizures were controlled by definitive surgery; B) patients whose seizures were reduced 50% by surgery; C) patients whose seizures were not controlled by surgery, and D) patients who did not have definitive surgery because of failure to localize seizure onset. Preoperatively, Group A patients differed significantly from Group C patients on the Wechsler Full Scale I.Q., and psycho-social functioning (P's < 0.05), but not on interpersonal rating. One month post-operatively Group A improved in Full Scale I.Q. and interpersonal rating (P's < 0.05) but not social functioning. At one year postoperative, Group A patients improved significantly in social functioning. At one month postoperative, Group C patients showed a decrease in Full Scale I.Q. At one year postoperative, Group C patients with right-sided surgery, but not left-sided surgery, improved in intellectual functioning to preoperative level. These results suggest that preoperative psychological evaluations may be diagnostically useful. In addition, successful surgical excision for control of epilepsy can significantly improve psychological functioning.

(Supported by USPHS Grant NS 02808)

INFEROMEDIAL TEMPORAL RESECTION IN TEMPORAL LOBE EPILEPSY: LONG TERM FOLLOW-UP

H Hamada, K. Uetsuhara, T. Mihara, T. Asakura
Kagoshima
K. Kitamura
Tokyo

During the years 1970-76, 23 patients with intractable temporal lobe epilepsy underwent unilateral inferomedial temporal resection, a modification by the authors of this paper from the classic temporal lobectomy. At the time of the operation, the average age of the patients was 22 years and 10 months (4-44 years). The first seizure was noticed at 12 years and 6 months in average (10 months - 16 years).

The sex ratio of males to females was 19:4. 15 out of 23 patients had past histories; that is, 4 had had delivery troubles, 8 high fever with consciousness. The average interval from the first attack to the time of the operation was 10 years and 4 months. In the follow-up investigation between 1977 and 1978, 57% (13/23) of the patients were found to be free from seizures, and 30% (7/23) showed a remarkable reduction in the frequency of the attacks, 9% (2/23) a slight reduction and 4% (1/23) no improvement. Moreover, in the patients who showed improvement, the changes in the main type of seizures were observed; that is, automatism tended to improve more than grand mal, while minor seizures were more persistent than grand mal. Psychiatric states such as violent behavior or irritability and restlessness were found to be less prominent in 11 out of 13 patients (85%). Working ability, scholastic performance and social adaptation in general improved remarkably, although most of the patients had shown some difficulty in adapting to normal life before surgery. Postoperative neurological and psychological deficits were negligible so far as inferomedial temporal lobectomy was concerned.

In conclusion we would like to stress that surgical treatment of temporal lobe epilepsy should be applied to those patients who show resistance to medication and have a unilateral or predominantly unilateral temporal EEG focus.

HEMISPHERECTOMY FOR INTRACTABLE SEIZURES: A FOLLOW-UP STUDY

P. D. Moyes, J. Wada, H. Dunn
Vancouver

Hendrick et al reported hemispherectomies on 17 children with an average follow-up of two to three years and maximum follow-up of six years.

We have carried out hemispherectomies on seven patients ranging in age from 10 months to 20 years. The earliest was done in May 1962, the most recent in February 1977, with a mean follow-up period of nine years.

Complications included an early post-operative haemorrhage in one patient and later subdural haemorrhage in another. One patient required a shunt and another had a wound infection. One patient was investigated by pneumoencephalography and suffered increased neurologic deficit. The availability of the C.T. Scan would have avoided that problem.

Despite the complications most patients have done extremely well. All are free or nearly free of seizures and, in all, the behaviour has been remarkably improved.

It would seem from this group of patients that early improvement following hemispherectomy is well maintained over many years and later complications are rare.

NEW DRUG TESTING, MARKETING, AND AVAILABILITY

Advances in Epileptology:
The Xth Epilepsy International Symposium,
edited by J. A. Wada and J. K. Penry.
Raven Press, New York © 1980.

New Anticonvulsant Drug Testing, Regulatory Review, and Availability

Barrett Scoville

Department of Psychiatry, Johns Hopkins Hospital, Baltimore, Maryland 21205

In recent years, the processes of drug innovation and drug development have received attention from specialists in disciplines that previously were almost totally indifferent to these processes, leaving them to pharmacologists and specialized industrialized companies. Political scientists, economists, practitioners, and patients have in the last years acquired a perception that the processes are not going smoothly, and the more scholarly among them have carried out analyses and made general conclusions (Peltzman, 1974; Wardell, 1974; Grabowski, 1976; Schwartzman, 1976; Stone, 1976). It is possible that a study of a specific class of drugs, anticonvulsants, can shed light on particular problems of the whole drug development process. There are also historical reasons why this might occur.

Anticonvulsants have among the oldest histories of any modern class of drugs. Epileptologists and those working in the preclinical sciences associated with the study of epilepsy quickly became unusually sophisticated students of drug effects. Animal screening models, measures of drug concentration, and bioavailability, for example, have been of greater importance in the field of anticonvulsant drugs than in most other therapeutic classes. In the last years, epileptologists in particular have become aware, at least in the United States, that there have been very few single-entity anticonvulsant drugs brought to the market since the late 1950s. Finally, in the United States problems in the process of drug development have been highlighted by controversy surrounding the time taken to develop and approve valproate.

The process by which new anticonvulsant drugs are developed until they can be distributed as useful for a population of epileptic patients is described. Within the discussion it becomes evident that the process might be improved, and these potential improvements are considered. The process can be divided into the phases of innovation, development, review, and distribution.

FROM SYNTHESIS TO PATIENT: INNOVATION

Drug innovation is distinct from development and involves at least two parts: First, necessary but not sufficient, is the synthesis or isolation of a new chemical compound; second, the discovery that the compound has anticonvulsant activity in a living test system. Few realize that an average of 6,000 compounds may be synthesized to produce one new marketed drug (Fülgraff, 1975). Discoveries of anticonvulsant activity may be categorized into at least three groups. The most common route to discovery at present follows systematic synthesis of modifications of a molecule already known to be useful, with extensive animal screening to select the modification with the most promising anticonvulsant properties.

A second group of discoveries is the fortuitous discovery of a useful new action of a drug developed for an unrelated purpose, bromides and valproate being examples.

The third group of discoveries stems from the isolation or synthesis of an endogenous substance found to be deficient or defective in a disease. GABA may be an example in the anticonvulsant field, levodopa being the prototypical success in neuropharmacology. The first approach, that of systematic molecular modification, appears to be the most regularly productive, wasteful and clumsy as the screening process may seem.

The process of drug innovation begins by synthesis of a new molecule. One or more medicinal chemists produces a variable but large number of compounds to be screened.

The second phase of innovation, the search for anticonvulsant activity, has been rendered fairly routine for this class of drugs for over three decades. It is epitomized by the anticonvulsant screening project of the Epilepsy Branch of the National Institute of Neurological and Communicative Disorders and Stroke, implemented in Utah by Dr. Swinyard (Epilepsy Branch, 1978).

The essence of the screening test is to determine the new compound's action in antagonizing convulsions in rodents, in association with the evaluation of the drug's depressant action on behavior as an index of toxicity. If results of the first tests pass certain decision-making criteria, the drug then receives a secondary evaluation, where actions such as peak effect and median effective dose are determined, and then a tertiary evaluation, if the secondary is positive.

The use of an animal model has proven itself well, having led to the development of almost every modern anticonvulsant.

DEVELOPMENT

Once a compound is selected as promising in the innovative or screening phase, drug development proper begins. Drug development proceeds along three major lines: chemistry, animal pharmacology, and human testing. The word "development" in drug development is much more closely related to developing a photographic negative. The molecule remains the same; the prolonged testing serves to reveal characteristics of its action that were previously unknown. The length of the development process depends in large part on the extent of characterization desired.

The most important part of animal pharmacology after screening is toxicological. Long-term animal testing reveals the potential of the molecule for producing cancers or more subtle organ toxicity or effects in the offspring of pregnant animals.

Trials in humans reveal first and foremost whether the drug does, in fact, have the effect on humans that it seemed likely to have. The clinical testing then goes on to reveal more details of the indications for the drug, for example, in the case of anticonvulsants, the types of seizure disorders in which the drug will be effective. As patient reports accumulate, the most likely adverse reactions can be demonstrated. After basic efficacy is confirmed in phase 2, specialized tests are carried out in phase 3, as well as a certain number of tests aimed simply at gaining increased experience with the drug. Thus the drug might be tested in children in this phase or in specialized seizure types. Experience with chronic exposure to humans might be gained in phase 3. Specialized toxicity, for example, the toxicity involved in drug abuse potential, would be characterized in this phase. It is also in this phase that the blanks in the information necessary for prescribing can be filled in, if they have not been already. The dosage regimen should be well known.

REVIEW

After development and review, just before the drug may be distributed to the general patient population, the data are reviewed by a regulatory agency. This phase occupies an important portion of the total time between the synthesis of a drug and the time that it is generally available, 20 months or longer (FDA, 1978; Wardell et al., 1978). In this period the application for marketing the drug is prepared, submitted to a regulatory agency, reviewed there, and usually approved (about 88% of the cases in the United States). Between submission and approval there may be numerous requests for further information or even requests for further testing from the regulatory agency.

AVAILABILITY

Finally, the drug is distributed to patients. For reasons still unclear, the availability of drugs seems to vary enormously from country to country (Epilepsy International, 1976), without clear-cut correlation with size, wealth, or development of the country.

EVIDENCE OF AN IMPERFECT PROCESS

Here I wish to state specific grounds for believing that improvement is possible.

First and foremost, drug innovation seems to be decreasing. In the face of a widespread belief in progress, there have been fewer new anticonvulsants, not more.

Concern and pessimism are not restricted merely to the field of drug innovation, but currently extend to many fields of technological innovation.

The drug development process is the next major area where problems seem to exist. The evidence is only suggestive but it is of several kinds as described by Helms (1975) and elsewhere. First, the number of new chemical entities reaching the market has decreased. Second, the time from discovery to marketing has lengthened. Third, the process has become vastly more expensive. This is further complicated by a decrease in the rate of return on research investment. Fourth, the attrition rate seems very high—of drugs taken into human testing, less than 5% are successfully developed. Fifth, international comparisons suggest that the problems in drug development are not universal or inevitable, since drug development appears to meet with different success in different countries.

Some of these differences may be due to problems in the next major process in getting a new drug to patients, the government regulatory process. Evidence of problems here is of several types. First is the change in numbers of new drugs in the United States since roughly 1962, the year in which radical changes occurred in United States drug laws. The decrease has been particularly striking in the anticonvulsant field. No new primary anticonvulsant was approved in the United States from 1960 until 1974.

A second type of evidence is the increase in drug development time referred to above. Some of this increase is possibly due to "state-of-the-art" changes in pharmacology that would have occurred in any case. Another portion is probably due to the articulation by the United States regulatory agency, the Food and Drug Administration (FDA) of higher ethical and scientific standards. Still a third portion of the increase is due no doubt to the quite arbitrary imposition by government reviewers of standards that they personally established. A fairly well documented example of this is the refusal of one or two key FDA reviewers to approve any anorectic drug from 1965 until 1973 (Review Panel on New Drug Regulation, 1977).

The fourth, last, and best documented portion of the increase in drug development time is the increase in time to review applications, studied by Wardell (1978). This period itself contains many subparts. Part of the time represents time that an application is at the regulatory agency. Another part is occupied by efforts of the firm to supply information or carry out tests that the regulatory agency has requested. The period from initial submission to final approval may also be prolonged because the initial submission is not a "good faith" application but rather a trial balloon.

I have mentioned two possible types of indirect evidence that the drug regulatory process is a problem area—a decrease in new drugs and an increase in development time.

A third kind of evidence is the repeated assertions of the regulated industry that new drug development was being retarded. Recently academic scholars have joined their voices to those of industrial sponsors (Commission for the Control of Epilepsy and Its Consequences, 1977).

These assertions of a regulatory problem were seen for years by the FDA as self-serving and unrealistic without comment, then taken seriously enough to be explicitly denied, then concurred with (Crout, 1975).

A fourth kind of evidence is the kind of negative evidence that historians cherish, insofar as laws are evidence of problem areas. The FDA has increasingly been creating regulations and guidelines. These should be seen as evidence of at least two kinds of inadequacies: first, evidence of inadequacies in clinical drug development programs, but second, evidence that FDA perceives vagueness or arbitrariness in its previous decisions. Thus, guidelines should be seen not as an expansion of testing requirements, but rather as a salutary attempt to routinize testing requirements and make them predictable. This was done 10 years ago for studies of chronic animal toxicity, with generally good results. It has just been done for clinical studies (Food and Drug Administration, 1977) and results are uncertain.

Still a fifth suggestion of evidence that regulations can be a problem are international comparisons. Not only drug development times, but also drug availability varies tremendously from country to country, from as few as three anticonvulsants to as many as 25, not counting combinations (Epilepsy International, 1976). Wardell (1974) holds differences in regulatory stance responsible for many differences. Differences certainly exist (Scoville and Crout, 1978).

Finally, I wish to advance as evidence of problems in regulatory performance some stories of the internal dynamics of the FDA, as reported, for example, in the reports of the Review Panel on New Drug Regulation (1977).

AREAS FOR IMPROVEMENT

Some areas seem either more susceptible to improvement or more critical, as follows: synthesis of new chemicals; screening procedures; demonstration of chronic toxicity; quality of evidence of efficacy; data documentation and evaluation; government regulations; and incentives.

More progress in "molecular pharmacology" including better knowledge of receptor sites and drug-related subcellular changes is probably the necessary precursor to more efficient drug design. At the moment, there is not a shortage of compounds to evaluate. The United States Antiepileptic Drug Development Program has acquired some 2,400 chemical entities proposed as potential anticonvulsants and has, in fact, found that a number of them have enough potential in animal screens to merit further development.

The traditional animal screening process itself also seems rather ponderous, utilizing scores of rodents for each compound to be screened. A more effective screening model might thus be desirable.

The characterization of toxicity of compounds of anticonvulsants remains cumbersome, expensive, and at times inaccurate in predicting human toxicity.

Problems in the demonstration of efficacy in humans is perhaps the single most important factor slowing the approval of new anticonvulsants in the United States. More modern standards have been published relatively recently, first for international trials in 1973 (ILAE Commission on Antiepileptic Drugs), and more recently for United States trials in 1977 (Food and Drug Administration).

Nonetheless, the guidelines do not address questions of how to evaluate the results of tests and the assumption that controlled studies are necessary is not universally shared in practice, as the valproate controversy revealed (Commission for the Control of Epilepsy and Its Consequences, 1977). The history of anticonvulsants and the natural history of epilepsy suggests enough drugs of dubious efficacy and enough spontaneous variation in epilepsy so that clinical trials should be controlled. Yet the field could usefully elaborate further criteria on the epistemological questions involving the quality and quantity of evidence necessary before general distribution of a new anticonvulsant. This could include statements on the use of international data.

Documentation and data evaluation are an area for improvement. The manner in which drug trials are carried out and results of the trials should be recorded and coherently displayed.

New methods such as telemetry may dramatically improve documentation and thereby lead to much more efficient and elegant trials. Documentation of results should be a part of trial design, with forms designed so as to be easily interpretable and internationally negotiable.

Regulatory improvements of three kinds come to mind: (a) changes in law; (b) changes in policy; and (c) changes in organization. The last has been done repeatedly. There has been a major change in how the United States regulators settle drug controversies through the introduction of a system of outside advisory committees into a formerly closed decision-making process.

Changes in United States law are coming. They would include provisions for "drug innovation investigation" and explicit provisions for a "drug treatment investigation." But the most important aspect of the United States bill is that it challenges Congress to approve as one of the two objectives of a drug regulatory agency the avoidance of interfering with the discovery and development of new drug products.

Changes in policy or application of the law could occur without new laws and if concrete enough and well enough monitored could have major impact.

Some of these changes exist in early stages already. The simplest is the concept of sequential review, or the building block NDA. The second major concept would be to specify in advance decision-making criteria—as well as testing methodology. The last major area of potential improvements is that of incentives to discover and develop new drugs, with, as a subproblem, the development of new drugs for limited patient populations.

The cost of new drug development has increased and seems responsible in part for the decrease in new anticonvulsants. But the profit incentive remains. Dilantin still represents over 11% of Parke-Davis sales, or $15,000,000 per year (Schwartzman, 1976). If valproate sales are large, they will lure other firms into anticonvulsant research. There already appears to be more activity in the field—four commercial INDs for clinical studies and reports of three or more large firms with molecules in the preclinical development phase.

For the moment, the assumption seems accepted that anticonvulsants are of limited commercial value. The Antiepileptic Drug Development Program (ADDP) of the United States Department of Health, Education, and Welfare has thus established a program wherein the government proposes to pay one-third of development costs for new anticonvulsant drugs. The Epilepsy Branch has also provided enormous indirect support for the infrastructure of new drug development: better biochemical methods; new methods of monitoring efficacy; research centers; expert advisory groups, among many others. Other financial incentives have been proposed and include tax benefits for developing drugs of limited commercial value, or loans, to be repaid only in the case of commercial success. Still another financial incentive would be to lower costs, for example, by decreasing testing requirements.

In brief, anticonvulsant drug innovation and development are not free of problems, but there are reasons to hope for new remedies. Of interest to technologists and research scientists are screening models, better monitoring methods, improved pharmacology, and drug assay methodology. Those interested in programs will follow the ADDP and its industrial counterparts. Economists and political scientists will follow changes in administration and statute that may alter the drug regulatory climate and possible changes in economic incentives. Regulators and scholars may see changes in data evaluation, both national and international. All these should have useful effects on the availability of new anticonvulsant drugs for those suffering seizures.

REFERENCES

Commission for the Control of Epilepsy and Its Consequences (1977): *Workshop on Antiepileptic Drug Development*. DHEW Publication Nos. (NIH) 77–185 and 77–186.
Crout, J. R. (1975): New drug regulation and its impact on innovation. *Read before the Third*

Seminar on Pharmaceutical Policy Issues, sponsored by the College of Public Affairs, American University, Washington, Dec. 16, 1975.

Epilepsy Branch, National Institute of Neurological and Communicative Disorders and Stroke (1978): *Anticonvulsant Screening Project. Antiepileptic Drug Development Program.* DHEW Publication No. (NIH) 78–1093.

Epilepsy International (1976): *An International Glossary of Anticonvulsant and Antiepileptic Drugs.* International Bureau for Epilepsy, Quincy, Mass.

Food and Drug Administration (1977): *Guidelines for the Clinical Evaluation of Anticonvulsant Drugs (Adults and Children).* U. S. Government Printing Office, HEW (FDA) 77-3040, pp. 1–11.

Food and Drug Administration (1978): *New Drug Evaluation Project Briefing Book.* Project Coordination Staff, Bureau of Drugs, DHEW Typescript.

Fülgraff, G. (1975): In: *Pharmakotherapie Klinische Pharmakologie,* edited by G. Fülgraff and D. Palm. Gustav Fischer Verlag, Stuttgart.

Grabowski, H. G. (1976): *Drug Regulation and Innovation.* American Enterprise Institute for Public Policy Research, Washington.

Helms, R. B. (editor) (1975): *Drug Development and Marketing.* American Enterprise Institute for Public Policy Research, Washington.

ILAE Commission on Antiepileptic Drugs (1973): Principles for clinical testing of antiepileptic drugs. *Epilepsia,* 14:451–458.

Krall, R. L., Penry, J. K., Kupferberg, H. J., and Swinyard, E. A. (1978): Antiepileptic drug development: I. History and a program for progress. *Epilepsia,* 19:393–408.

Krall, R. L., Penry, J. K., White, B. G., Kupferberg, H. J., and Swinyard, E. A. (1978): Antiepileptic drug development: II. Anticonvulsant drug screening. *Epilepsia,* 19:409–428.

Peltzman, S. (1974): *Regulation of Pharmaceutical Innovation,* American Enterprise Institute for Public Policy Research, Washington.

Review Panel on New Drug Regulation (1977): Investigation of Allegations Relating to the Bureau of Drugs, Food and Drug Administration, DHEW, 766 p.

Schwartzman, I. (1976): *Innovation in the Pharmaceutical Industry,* Johns Hopkins Press, Baltimore.

Scoville, B., and Crout, J. R. (1978): Regulations and drug testing. In: *Principles of Psychopharmacology,* 2nd ed. Academic Press, New York.

Simon, D., and Penry, J. K. (1975): Sodium di-*N*-propylacetate (DPA) in the treatment of epilepsy—A review. *Epilepsia,* 16:549–573.

Stone, C. F. (1976): Economic effect of new drug regulation in the United States. *Background paper prepared for U.S. DHEW Review Panel on New Drug Regulation.*

Wardell, W. (1974): In: *Regulation of New Drug R & D by the Food and Drug Administration,* Hearings before the Subcommittee on Health of the Committee on Labor and Public Welfare and the Subcommittee on Administrative Practice and Procedure of the Committee on the Judiciary, 93d U.S. Congress, U.S. Government Printing Office, Washington.

Wardell, W., Hassar, M., Anaversar, S. N., and Lasagna, L. (1978): The rate of development of new drugs in the United States, 1963 through 1975. *Clin. Pharmacol. Ther.,* 24:133–145.

Advances in Epileptology:
The Xth Epilepsy International Symposium,
edited by J. A. Wada and J. K. Penry.
Raven Press, New York © 1980.

Preclinical Development of Antiepileptic Drugs

W. P. Koella

Research Laboratories, Pharmaceuticals Division,
CIBA-GEIGY Ltd., Basle, Switzerland

Most clinicians involved in the treatment of the various forms and sub-forms of epilepsy are quite aware that the currently available therapeutic armamentarium in this field is far from ideal, if not—in many cases—inadequate. Indeed, we need drugs that have and retain a generally *better efficacy and potency*; we need drugs *specially acting* on those forms of epilepsy where no or only inadequate remedies are available as yet; we need drugs that are, in general, *less toxic*; we need drugs with fewer *undesired side effects* (i.e., sedation, ataxia, dizziness); and, in turn, we need drugs that produce, in addition to their anticonvulsive action, *desired side effects,* such as a beneficial influence on the psychiatric symptoms of the epileptic patient. It is the central task of the "screening" pharmacologist, in collaboration with the "synthesizing" chemist, to perform those first and all-important steps that may lead to the development of new drugs conforming with the above-mentioned needs.

The following outline describes some of the methods used by the pharmacologist in his endeavor to develop new and better antiepileptic drugs. It describes the "start-from-scratch" method, which is a goal-directed, and a trial-and-error procedure with about a 3,000:1 chance of success. It also deals with some additional research activities on new compounds that should—albeit not always—follow the initial developmental work.

DEVELOPMENT PHASES I AND II

Development starts with the making of new compounds: The chemist may either use "leads"—derivatives of already established antiepileptic substances, and/or certain structure-activity considerations—or he may proceed "blindly" when he synthesizes new compounds. The biologist uses several simple, fast, and not very specific "models"—electroshock-, pentetrazole-, often also picrotoxin-, and strychnine-induced seizures in mice and/or rats—to obtain first indications for anticonvulsive potency and efficacy but also for obvious side effects and acute toxic (including lethal) effects. Figure 1 illustrates in two different ways the results of such "basic

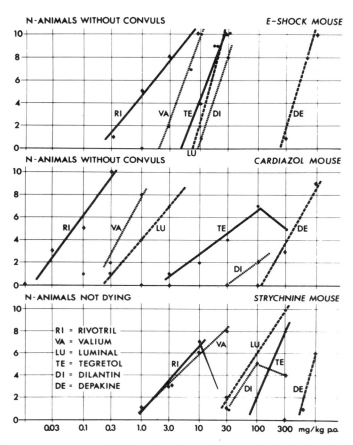

FIG. 1a: Dose-response curves in the mouse for carbamazepine (TE), phenobarbitone (LU), sodium 2-propylvalerate (DE), diazepam (VA), clonazepam (RI), and diphenylhydantoin (DI), all administered orally, in the electroshock test, the anti-pentetrazole test, and the anti-strychnine test. From Koella, et al. (1976).

screen" procedures with six well known antiepileptic drugs. Included are the findings about one particular side effect, namely sedation (Fig. 1b), and its approximate "effective" dose in relation to the "therapeutic" doses. Such relationships, i.e., the ratio between anticonvulsive doses, and the doses inducing unwanted side effects, signs of (acute) toxicity and the LD_{50}, constitute a first base for the selection of compounds to be developed further, or, more often than not, for their rejection. If the drug meets certain established standards one proceeds with the more detailed characterization (phase II).

First, one attempts a more exact definition of (unwanted) side effects including the effective dose levels and dose-effect curves for, e.g., sedative effects. One searches for "additional properties," i.e., effects in a number of

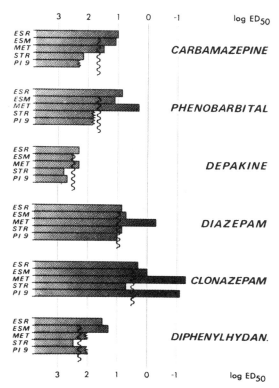

FIG. 1b: Oral "potency" profiles (ED₅₀ values) of six reference drugs in various test situations. *Abscissa:* – Log ED_{50} values (= log $1/ED_{50}$) as a measure of potency. The dose inducing sedation (in the mouse) is indicated in each instance by a *vertical wavy line*. Note the low overall potency of 2-propylvalerate and the high potency of clonazepam. ESR, Electroshock, rat; ESM, electroshock, mouse; PTM, anti-pentetrazole test, mouse; STM, anti-strychnine test, mouse; and PI 9, anti-picrotoxin test, mouse (9 mg/kg picrotoxin i.p.). [From: Koella, et al., (1976)].

commonly used neuropsychopharmacological testing procedures. Such data, among others, yield information about possible psychotropic effects such as antidepressant, antipsychotic, and antiaggressive components but also about a possible influence of the neuromuscular system (e.g., reflexes).

An additional aspect of phase II screening concerns the attempt to further characterize the new drug in a number of special test procedures representing quasi-models for special forms of epilepsy. A relative high potency against pentetrazole-induced seizures (a test used in the primary screen) has been, and still is, considered to be indicative of efficacy in petit mal epilepsy (see Woodbury, 1972). Recently a number of additional and supposedly better petit mal animal models have been developed. Penicillin, premarine (a conjugated estrogen compound), butazolidine, gamma-hydroxybutyrate and (bilateral) cobalt depots as well as electric brain stimulation are used to produce seizures characterized by a more or less typical spike-wave pattern, and, to a greater or lesser degree, behavioral signs typical for human petit mal seizures (see Prince and Farrell, 1969; Marcus and Watson, 1968; Marcus, 1972; Gloor and Testa, 1974; Schmutz et al., *this volume*). Hippocampal electrical stimulation i.e., the ensuing afterdischarge is considered to have many features in common with human temporal lobe epilepsy. Local freezing, alumina depots, and local electric stimulation can be looked at as models of focal seizures including features of secondary generalization of the seizure. Efficacy of the new compound in any one of these models to some extent suggests its effectiveness in any one of these forms of epilepsy.

Furthermore, one wants to know for how long after (usually oral) application the drug is effective. Thus, one runs time-course experiments parallel with pharmacokinetic studies. These latter investigations make it necessary at an early stage to develop methods for measuring blood and/or plasma levels of the new drug and its metabolites and, thus, to establish the basis for a first understanding of the fate of the drug in the organism, its absorption, distribution, and elimination.

To obtain an early indication of whether the new compound, during long-term use, may lead to development of tolerance, one should run a study with repeated daily applications and measurements of efficacy against, e.g., electroshock over 3 to 4 weeks. An adequate model is described elsewhere in this volume (Baltzer et al.).

A 10-day toxicology study, and a variety of additional investigations concerning circulatory, respiratory, and possibly endocrine effects, conclude phase II. If the new compound has shown good efficacy and potency in a variety of "general" and "special" epilepsy models; if it produces no or little unwanted side effects in "therapeutic" doses; if it shows no toxic (acute and subchronic) consequences; if it can be shown to have no lethal effects in doses at least 20 to 100 times higher than those producing anticonvulsive effects; if it shows no tendency to develop tolerance; if it has little or no influence on circulation, respiration, and other autonomic activities and if it even has some "desired side effects," it is considered to have a good chance to become an antiepileptic drug. It becomes a developmental compound. One of approximately 500 to 1,000 compounds reach that stage; however, additional tests are required. The so-far successful substances now have to be submitted to advanced developmental work, such as chronic toxicological studies and investigations on carcinogenicity, on mutagenicity, and on teratogenicity. At the same time, work on specific galenic forms, on stability, and a multitude of other tasks starts to prepare the new product for the most important step: clinical testing in humans.

ADDITIONAL RESEARCH ACTIVITIES

With the completion of phase II screening and the delivery of the drug for advanced developmental work, the research activities of the pharmacologist are not finished. First, and most important, he is interested in learning through animal experimentation more about the mode, locus, and mechanism of action of his new compound and about how his remedy may—or may not—differ from established antiepileptic drugs in the manner in which it combats focal and/or generalized epileptic discharge. For such studies, the pharmacologist is well advised to make use of the many recent advances in the biophysical and biochemical neuropathophysiology of epilepsy.

At an early stage, the pharmacologist should investigate whether his drug—in comparison with established compounds—acts preferentially on focal, or on spread of, epileptic discharge. Using such biophysical methods as macrorecordings, extracellular microelectrode techniques, and especially intracellular monitoring of the characteristic paroxysmal depolarization shift (PDS) (Prince, 1968, 1969; Prince and Futamachi, 1968; Ayala et al., 1970) in experimentally induced foci he will obtain important information about the effect of his drug on local epileptic phenomena. Voltage-clamp and related methods used in and around an artificial focus should advance insight into the (local) mechanisms of action of the antiepileptic compound with respect to ionic phenomena such as potassium, sodium, chloride, and calcium permeability and transport through the (focal) neuronal and glial membranes. Studies using chemical neurophysiological methodology and aiming at the detection of changes in the local levels and turnover rates of such biogenic substances as GABA, glycine, taurine, and also glutamate, aspartic acid, norepinephrine, dopamine, serotonin, and various polypeptides in response to antiepileptic drugs can well signal involvement of these "wet" transmission components in the local anticonvulsive action. Concerning investigation on a possible action of new (and established) antiepileptic agents on spread of convulsive discharge, one may make use of the "classic" method of strychnine neuronography and/or study the influence of anticonvulsants on such "new" phenomena as secondary (and mirror) focus (Morrell, 1969). Delayed or completely inhibited development of epileptic discharge in loci remote from the primary epileptogenic focus under the influence of systemically or locally (i.e., at the secondary site) applied drugs could be indicative of a preponderant activity of such drugs on spread. A similar conclusion may be drawn when drugs curtail the secondary generalization of an initially focal or partial epilepsy.

The phenomenon of posttetanic potentiation, either in its classic form (Lloyd, 1949) or demonstrated on single units, e.g., in the hippocampus (Andersen, 1978) can also be viewed as a model of a developing epileptic center. Similarly, the (slow) making of an epileptic focus around an intracerebral aluminia cream deposit and the slowly enhancing epileptic activity in response to local subthreshold electrical stimulation—the kindling phenomenon (Goddard, 1967; Morrel, 1972)—comprise many of the pathogenic aspects the spontaneously developing epileptic activity. It seems that all these "models" can and should be used in connection with drug studies. Data from such investigations could not only be indicative of the effect of (new and established) drugs on the development of experimentally induced "spontaneous" epileptic activity, but they also may well give an impetus to advance a new class of antiepileptic drugs—the epilepto-prophylactics—to be used to combat the development of epileptic activity in cases of, e.g., head traumatism, cerebral malformation, or heavy genetic loading where the eventual appearance of convulsive activity would otherwise be highly probable. Finally, it is not impossible that one of the new anti-epileptic drugs may turn out to be a true antiepileptogenic agent to be used to eliminate the epileptogenic pathology and, thus, to remove the need for a continuous symptomatic or, at best, substitutional, antiepileptic therapy. "Chronic" experimental epilepsies such as alumina- or cobalt-induced convulsions, fully kindled foci, mirror foci, or the photomyoclonic baboon, in connection with electrophysiological recordings and/or anatomical indicators (glia proliferation; structural changes in the dendrites) should constitute welcome models for the study of such possible and highly desirable true healing effects of some new drugs to be developed in the future.

REFERENCES

Andersen, P. (1978): Long-lasting facilitation of synaptic transmission. In: *Functions of the Septo-Hippocampal System*, edited by K. Elliot and J. Whelan. CIBA-Foundation, London.

Ayala, G. F., Matsumoto, H., and Gumnit, R. J. (1970): Excitability changes and inhibitory mechanisms in neocortical neurons during seizures. *J. Neurophysiol.*, 33:73–85.

Gloor, P., and Testa G. (1974): Generalized penicillin epilepsy in the cat: Effects of intracarotid and intravertebral pentylentetrazol and amobarbital injections. *Electroencephalogr. Clin. Neurophysiol.*, 36:499–515.

Goddard, G. V. (1967): The development of epileptic seizures through brain stimulation at low intensity. *Nature*, 214:1020.

Koella, W. P., Levin, P., and Baltzer, V. (1976): The pharmacology of carbamazepine and some other antiepileptic drugs. In: *Epileptic Seizures—Behavior—Pain,* edited by W. Birkmayer. Huber, Berne/Stuttgart/Vienna.

Lloyd, D. P. C. (1949): Post-tetanic potentiation of response in monosynaptic reflex pathways of the spinal cord. *J. Gen. Physiol.*, 33:147–190.

Marcus, E. M. (1972): Experimental models of petit-mal epilepsy. In: *Experimental Models of Epilepsy*, edited by D. P. Purpura, J. K. Penry, D. B. Tower, D. M. Woodbury, and R. D. Walter. Raven Press, New York.

Marcus, E. M., and Watson, C. W. (1968): Bilateral symmetrical epileptogenic foci in monkey cerebral cortex: Mechanisms of interaction and regional variations and regional variation in capacity for synchronous spike slow wave discharges. *Arch. Neurol.*, 19:99–116.

Morrell, F. (1969): Physiology and histochemistry of the mirror focus. In: *Basic Mechanisms of the Epilepsies*, edited by H. H. Jasper, A. A. Ward, and A. Pope. Little, Brown, and Co. Boston.

Morrell, F. (1972): Goddard's Kindling Phenomenon: a new model of the mirror focus. In: *Experimental Models of Epilepsy*, edited by D. P. Purpura, J. K. Penry, D. B. Tower, D. M. Woodbury, and R. D. Walter. Raven Press, New York.

Prince, D. A. (1968): The depolarization shift in epileptic neurons. *Exp. Neurol.*, 21:467–485.

Prince, D. A. (1969): Electrophysiology of "epileptic" neurons: Spike generation. *Electroencephalogr. Clin. Neurophysiol.*, 26:476–487.

Prince, D. A., and Farrel, D. (1969): "Centrencephalic" spike-wave discharges following parenteral penicillin injections in the cat. *Neurology*, 19:309–310.

Prince, D. A., and Futamachi, K. J. (1968): Intracellular recordings in chronic focal epilepsy. *Brain Res.*, 11:681.

Woodbury, D. M. (1972): Applications to drug evaluations. In: *Experimental Models of Epilepsy*, edited by D. M. Purpura, J. K. Penry, D. B. Tower, D. M. Woodbury, and R. D. Walter. Raven Press, New York.

Advances in Epileptology:
The Xth Epilepsy International Symposium,
edited by J. A. Wada and J. K. Penry.
Raven Press, New York © 1980.

Development of New Antiepileptic Drugs: Can We Do Better in the "Early Phase" Clinical Trials?

P. L. Morselli

Department of Clinical Research, Synthelabo-L.E.R.S. 75013 Paris, France

In the last 10 to 15 years, there has been a growing concern regarding drug toxicity and drug usage and at present, the problem of the correct utilization of pharmacological agents is one of the major problems that the medical profession, the pharmaceutical industry, and the governmental regulatory agencies are forced to confront. Drugs one time considered as a mean of secondary prevention have become a "factor of risk."

Such a situation, due to (a) continuous development of agents more active and more specific, and (b) an increased awareness of drug toxicity, has forced on one side the development of more precise methodologies for the correct quantification of the effects and on the other the need for recommendations and regulations for the development of new drug always more strict and severe (Kelsey, 1978; Freeman, 1977; Schriffin, 1977; McMahon, 1978).

It is useful to point out that in no case can strict regulations on clinical trials make bad clinical judgment good, and that there are no designs or magic formulas to replace numbers of patients treated over a prolonged period of time.

If we consider the situation in the field of antiepileptic agents we observe that although the need for new and better drugs is a confirmed and agreed fact, no new drug has been developed in the last 10 years (Janz, 1978). Reasons for such a "stagnation" are numerous, but they can be summarized in four aspects critical for the development of any new drug: efficacy, safety, cost, and time.

Although in fact the demands for demonstration of safety and efficacy are becoming more urgent and strict, the cost and the time necessary to develop new antiepileptic drugs are increasing due to the actual regulations.

In the present situation, the development of a new antiepileptic drug involves numerous and unnecessary repetition with disadvantages for the patients and heavy cost for the industry, which is more and more regarding the antiepileptic market as "financially unattractive" (Wardell, 1977).

In this chapter, I wish to briefly analyze the procedures usually followed for the development of a new antiepileptic drug and then put forward two propositions that appear to be useful alternatives to the present course of action.

SIGNIFICANCE OF ANIMAL DATA AND THEIR UTILIZATION AT THE HUMAN LEVEL

According to the usual procedure applied, there is a definite gap between animal and human data.

In practice in most cases, the drug is tested on animal models that have nothing in common with the human situation.

Pharmacokinetic and metabolic data are often considered as a must because they are requested by regulatory agencies, but there is very little effort to utilize them for human studies. Furthermore, in most cases, the kinetic and metabolic data are totally dissociated from the toxicity or activity data. In such a context, they become a very costly intellectual game.

SIGNIFICANCE OF PHASE I DATA AND PROCEDURES

After a drug passes animal tests it is usually studied in healthy volunteers for single dose and repeated dose tolerance, for initial dose finding, and occasionally for pharmacokinetics and metabolism.

Again because of the type of disease involved the data on single tolerance and on dose ranging may have little relevance for clinical use. For example, a compound may be administered to a healthy volunteer, free of drugs, ethanol, etc., (for at least 15 days!), or the drug may be given to a patient who is probably receiving at least two or three other compounds and, more important, whose physiological responses may be modified. Furthermore, regarding repeated doses, the doses utilized in volunteers, even if producing side effects, may not be comparable to those needed in patients.

In most cases, this is performed on a "blind basis," very empirically, without utilizing the information we may have from animal data.

EARLY PHASE II PROCEDURES

The third step consists of testing the drug in patients, according to pilot open studies, followed by short-term controlled trials, for evaluation of tolerance and dose finding.

The patients usually selected for this phase are not representative of the "user" population (Morselli, 1976). Early testing is in fact performed on very severely ill institutionalized epileptic patients, usually not responding to other antiepileptic drugs. Because of this drawback, such a testing, in most instances, is not considered valid for efficacy but only for safety. But is it meaningful for safety aspects?

If lack of efficacy in this type of population does not mean lack of efficacy in another "more normal" population, misleading data may also be obtained concerning tolerance, since in most cases subtle effects cannot be appreciated in this type of patient, in whom a large number of side effects are already present in addition.

Finally the number of patients tested is usually very limited and rarely is it possible to reach statistical significance.

TIME SPENT AND TYPE OF INFORMATION ACQUIRED

The time necessary to accomplish these steps is theoretically 2 to 3 months for phase I in volunteers and 3 to 6 months for the pilot study, but in reality often more than 1 year is required. Thus, by the actual procedure, we find ourselves, after 10 to 12 months of studies, with 20 to 30 peculiar patients treated for 2 to 3 months or more and with a very poor idea on how the drug will perform or behave in less severe forms of epilepsy.

In other words, we find ourselves at the end of these "early phases" with no real information on both range of active doses and toxicity for starting more extensive controlled clinical trials in less severe patients. And because of this, dose finding must be initiated again in this new population.

ACCEPTANCE OF FOREIGN CLINICAL DATA AND CONSEQUENCES

The aforementioned would not necessarily be a problem if the data acquired in a given country would be accepted without problems by the regulatory agencies of other nations where the product has to be developed also (Table 1).

In the present situation (Haines, 1978), it is unrealistic in terms of market size to consider developing a new antiepileptic drug for use by a single country. Unfortunately, according to the current regulations as illustrated in

TABLE 1. *Acceptance of foreign studies*

Country	Preclinical data	Clinical data
Belgium	Accepted	Accepted but local trials required
France	Partially accepted	Local trials only
Germany	Accepted	Accepted but local trials required
Italy	Partially accepted	Local trials required—published data acceptance
Spain	Accepted	Local trials required
Sweden	Accepted	Accepted
United Kingdom	Accepted	Accepted but local trials required
Brazil	Accepted	Accepted if published
Canada	Accepted	Accepted but local trials required
Mexico	Accepted	Accepted if published
United States	Accepted with reserve	Local trials required
Japan	Not accepted	Local trials only

Modified from Haynes (1978).

Table 1, clinical trials performed in another country are accepted only in Sweden, whereas in all other nations, local trials are either formally requested or strongly "suggested." This means that the same procedure must be repeated in each country concerned.

This leads in practical terms to a higher number of patients unnecessarily exposed to an investigational drug, to redundant and unnecessary studies that without leading to any gain in information entail (a) duplication of efforts by the various clinical investigators, (b) increased cost, and (c) consequent waste of human and economic resources.

The final result is a delay either in development or in withdrawal which in the first case produces a delay in possible therapeutic benefits and in the second not only an economical waste but also a loss in therapeutic benefits, since a higher number of patients were unnecessarily exposed to compounds with no therapeutic advantages.

The pooling of the data that could be a way to escape from such a waste of resources in the production of meaningless results cannot be done in most instances because of differences in attitudes of regulatory agencies, in adherence to the protocols, in nosological classification and a low degree of cooperation among various investigators, and also in several instances to a lack of adherence to internationally standardized criteria when designing protocols.

POSSIBLE ALTERNATIVES

Can we do better? Can we try to engage our activity in a less empirical way in order to arrive at the phase II double-blind studies with more meaningful information on dose ranges? Can we avoid the present wasteful repetition of data of poor significance?

I strongly believe that improvement can be obtained by: (a) a better and more complete use of animal data on activity, toxicity, and kinetics; and (b) a more efficient international cooperation coordinated by the International League.

Improved Use of Animal Data

It has been proven that primate models can be usefully utilized not only for the study and evaluation of possible anticonvulsant effects of new antiepileptic drugs but also for identifying, with a good approximation threshold, levels both for therapeutic effect and central nervous system side effects (Lockard et al., 1975; Wada et al., 1976; Weinberger and Killam, 1978; Levy et al., 1977; Lockard et al., 1977). On the other hand, from intermediate toxicity studies in two animal species, we have the possibility of knowing not only the dosages but also the plasma antiepileptic drug levels associated with biochemical disturbances, hematological alterations, endo-

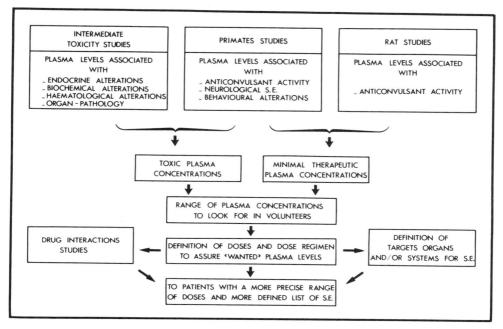

FIG. 1. Proposition for a better utilization of information derived from animal data, leading to more "rational" studies in healthy volunteers and patients.

crine effects, and/or organ functions modification. This type of study could also provide useful information on possible time- or dose-dependent kinetics.

Therefore, with an integrated approach where in the same animal the evaluation of toxicity or activity is coupled with plasma level measurement, we could arrive at our first observation in man with a more precise idea of the range of levels we should aim for (Fig. 1).

It is in fact well demonstrated that for many drugs, active plasma levels or toxic plasma levels are the same in different species, the only difference being the clearance rate, the dose, and the dosing intervals (Brodie and Reid, 1969; Morselli et al., 1971; Lockard et al., 1975; Rizzo et al., 1972; Bianchetti et al., 1977).

Improved Studies in Healthy Volunteers

With this information, studies in volunteers should be centered not on finding the maximum tolerated doses or on defining a kinetic profile on a randomly chosen dose, but on finding the dosages and the dosing intervals capable of producing plasma levels close to the one associated with acitivity on animals, and below the toxic thresholds. We should aim at attaining plasma levels that would fit the hypothetical range, at verifying similarities in metabolic degradation, and at showing the possible similarities in the plasma levels associated with production of side effects.

When such information is acquired, we could start clinical trials in patients and be in a position far better than the present one: first, aiming to obtain the "wanted" plasma levels and then, only at that stage, entering the patient in a double blind cross-over against placebo.

Necessity of International Cooperation

The approach suggested may allow a gain of a few months but does not solve the problem of unnecessary repetitions on patients not representative of the "users" population. The possibility and the necessity of an international cooperation for the development of new antiepileptic drugs was first mentioned in the reports of the First Commission on Development of Antiepileptic Drugs in 1974 (Penry, 1974) and mentioned again by Dreyfuss (1978) and by Janz (1978). It seems to be the only way to circumvent the problem. However, this international cooperation should not be left to the initiatives of single individuals, but should be viewed as an alternative in which the International League and the various national leagues play a major role.

Excellency centers or qualified investigators should be proposed and contacted by the I.L.A.E. and by the national leagues in order to establish a valid network of highly qualified clinical centers interested in the development of new antiepileptic drugs and utilizing comparable methodologies. Operative protocols should be according to the I.L.A.E. standardized criteria in order to harmonize the various phases. The I.L.A.E. and the national leagues should also encourage local administrative regulatory bodies to facilitate the studies, offering as warranty the standardized criteria and high scientific levels of the investigators.

By taking such an approach it is possible that in 6 to 8 months we easily could have a number of subjects (evaluated according to the same protocol) sufficient to express a meaningful judgment on both efficacy and safety of the new compound. Another advantage could be that the results would be evaluated by an international body of experts who would judge not only by adherence to regulations but also by the clinical relevance of the data and their possible impact on the treatment of epilepsy.

Should this early testing present a positive outcome then specific studies could be easily conducted locally to meet the various national requirements in terms of patient numbers and observation periods. Should the answer be negative, there would be a considerable saving both for the sponsoring industry and for the investigators and would avoid unnecessary exposure of other patients to an inactive drug.

Regarding the type of patient selected for the early or pilot studies, it is possible to discuss at great length the ethics involved in testing a new drug on a severely ill and brain damaged hospitalized patient as opposed to a less severely ill epileptic patient whose motivations and comprehension are surely at an higher level. Beyond the fiction of the informed consent, I think it is clear that by shifting the decision of the risk evaluation to a person who knows very little about his disease and who knows nothing about drugs, we are exploiting his ignorance and dependence as well as escaping our responsibilities.

I feel that in pilot studies we must try to include patients representative of the real epileptic population, considering not only various type of seizures but also the duration and stage of the disease. Such an approach, if impossible in a single center, should not be difficult to achieve if several units cooperate.

We must also try to include newly treated patients, since again, in a highly specialized environment, (as that of the excellency centers) the risk factor could be very limited and better controlled. In cooperative studies, each center would contribute a limited number of patients, which could have positively influenced both facility of selection and follow-up.

CONCLUSIONS

Are these propositions realistic? I think they are. As the International League Against Epilepsy should make an effort to initiate an international cooperation on "early phase" clinical testing of new antiepileptic drugs.

According to the present regulations, the requirements in terms of animal data, chemistry data, toxicity, etc., are very similar in various countries. The local requirements for early phase clinical studies also do not differ much from one nation to another. What is really missing is the acceptance of the clinical data outside each national border. On this point, I strongly feel that the International League Against Epilepsy (supported by the national chapters) should make an effort to improve the present situation in order to offer a better outlook for the future to patients suffering from epilepsy.

REFERENCES

Bianchetti, G., Bonaccorsi, A., Chiodaroli, A., Franco, A., Garattini, S., Gomeni, R., and Morselli, P. L. (1977): Plasma concentrations and cardiotoxic effects of desipramine and protriptyline in the rat. *Br. J. Pharmacol.*, 60:11–19.

Brodie, B. B., and Reid, W. D. (1969): Is man a unique animal in response to drugs? *Am. J. Pharmacol.*, 141:21–27.

Celesia, G. G., Boker, H. E., and Sato, S. (1974): Brain and serum concentration of diazepam in experimental epilepsy. *Epilepsia*, 15:417–425.

Dreyfus, F. E. (1978): The pharmacology of the newer antiepileptic drugs and perspective for the future. In: *Advances in Epileptology*—1977, edited by H. Meinardi and A. J. Rowan, pp. 232–237. Swets & Zeitlinger B. V., Amsterdam and Lisse.

Ehrlich, G. E. (1972): Guidelines for antiinflammatory drug research. *J. Clin. Pharmacol.*, 17:697–703.

Farghali-Hassan, Assael, B. M., Bossi, L., Garattini, S., Gerna, M., Gomeni, R., and Morselli, P. L. (1976): Carbamazepine pharmacokinetics in young adult and pregnant rats. Relation to pharmacological effects. *Arch. Int. Pharmacodyn.,* 220:125–139.

Freeman, M. M. (1977): The role of clinical guidelines in research: FDA's view point. *J. Clin. Pharmacol.,* 17:682–685.

Haines, B. A. (1978): Worldwide regulations and legislations; their effects on pharmaceutical product development. *Drug Dev. Ind. Pharmac.,* 4:1–30.

Janz, D. (1978): In: *Advances in Epileptology 1977,* edited by H. Meinardi and A. J. Rowan, pp. 184–186 and 243–244. Swets & Zeitlinger B. V., Amsterdam and Lisse.

Kelsey, F. O. (1978): Biomedical monitoring. *J. Clin. Pharmacol.,* 18:3–9.

Levy, R. H., Lockard, J. S., Patel, I. H., and Lai, A. A. (1977): Efficacy testing of valproic acid compared to ethosuximide in monkey model I: Dosage regimen design in the presence of diurnal oscillations. *Epilepsia,* 18:191–203.

Lockard, J. S., Uhlir, V., Ducharme, L. L., Farquhar, J. A., and Huntsman, B. J. (1975): Efficacy of standard anticonvulsants in monkey model with spontaneous motor seizures. *Epilepsia,* 16:301–317.

Lockard, J. S., Levy, R. H., Congdon, W. C., DuCharme, L. L., and Patel, I. H. (1977): Efficacy testing of valproic acid compared to ethosuximide in monkey model II: Seizure, EEG and diurnal variations. *Epilepsia,* 18:205–224.

McMahon, F. G. (1978): The effects on new federal regulations on clinical investigations. *Clin. Pharmacol. Ther.,* 23:495–496.

Morselli, P. L., Gerna, M., and Garattini, S. (1971): Carbamazepine plasma and tissue levels in the rat. *Biochem. Pharmacol.,* 20:2043–2047.

Morselli, P. L., (1976): Pediatric clinical pharmacology routine monitoring or clinical trials? In: *Clinical Pharmacy and Clinical Pharmacology,* edited by Gouveia et al., p. 277. Elsevier, New York/Amsterdam.

Penry, J. K. (1974): Report of Commission on Antiepileptic Drugs of the International League Against Epilepsy. *Epilepsia,* 15:143–146.

Rizzo, M., Morselli, P. L., and Garattini, S. (1972): Further observations on the interactions between phenobarbital and diphenylhydantoin during chronic treatment in the rat. *Biochem. Pharmacol.,* 21:449–454.

Schiffrin, M. J. (1977): The regulation of clinical research. *J. Clin. Pharmacol.,* 17:686–690.

Wada, J. A., Osawa, T., Sato, M., Wake, A., Corcoran, M. E., and Troupin, A. S. (1976): Acute anticonvulsant effect of diphenylhydantoin, phenobarbital and carbamazepine: A combined electroclinical and serum level study in amygdaloid kindled cats and baboons. *Epilepsia,* 17:77–88.

Wardell, W. W. (1977): Innovation in antiepileptic drug therapy. In: *Workshop on Antiepileptic Drug Development.* United States Department of Health, Education, and Welfare N° (National Institutes of Health) 77–185.

Weinberger, S. B., and Killam, E. K. (1978): Alterations in learning performance in the seizure-prone baboon: effects of elicited seizures and chronic treatment with diazepam and phenobarbital. *Epilepsia,* 19:301–316.

Advances in Epileptology:
The Xth Epilepsy International Symposium,
edited by J. A. Wada and J. K. Penry.
Raven Press, New York © 1980.

Principles of Screening Antiepileptic Drugs in Rodents

Ewart A. Swinyard

Departments of Biochemical Pharmacology and Toxicology,
University of Utah, Salt Lake City, Utah 84112

The potential hazards of testing new therapeutic agents in humans dictates that experimental animals be used for preliminary screening and evaluation. Ideally, such models should replicate the human disease. Unfortunately, knowledge of the underlying cause of various convulsive disorders is still incomplete and classification based on etiology is not yet possible. Consequently, most experimental models of epilepsy are designed to simulate in laboratory animals the overt manifestations of the disorder (Purpura et al., 1972).

Anticonvulsant drug activity can be studied at various biological levels, such as axons, intact single cells, groups of cells including pre- and post-synaptic events, sub-organ cellular connections including spinal cord pathways, organ systems including the whole brain, and modified intact animals in which the brain has been surgically or chemically altered (Purpura et al., 1972). Many of these models are extremely valuable, especially as penultimate tests prior to clinical drug trials and as models for the study of seizure mechanisms. Unfortunately, most of them are also tedious, time-consuming, and costly. Consequently, they do not lend themselves to the routine screening of the large numbers of chemicals one must examine in order to sort out agents with antiepileptic potential. For these and other reasons, intact normal rodents are preferred for this purpose (Krall et al., 1978).

The Anticonvulsant Drug Development (ADD) Screening Program will be used as an example of a rodent procedure. The principal objective of this presentation is to emphasize what results obtained with the ADD procedure *will* tell you and what it *will not* tell you. In addition, some discussion will be directed to what can be gleaned from the basic data obtained.

METHODS AND PROCEDURES

Methods

Male albino mice (CF No. 1 strain; 18–25 g) obtained from Charles Rivers, Wilmington, Massachusetts, and male albino rats (Sprague-Dawley strain;

100–150 g) obtained from Simonsen Laboratories, Gilroy, California, are used as experimental animals. Animals are maintained on S/L Custom Lab Diet G4.5 and allowed free access to food and water, except during the short time they are removed from their cages for testing.

Anticonvulsant activity is determined by the maximal electroshock seizure pattern (MES) test and the subcutaneous pentylenetetrazol (Metrazol) seizure threshold (s.c. Met) test. Minimal neurotoxicity is identified by the rotorod test. For information on the historical background, details, and reliability of these tests see Krall et al. (1978). Activity by the MES test correlates with ability to prevent the spread of seizure discharge through neural tissue; selective action in nontoxic doses indicates efficacy in the treatment of generalized tonic-clonic seizures. Activity by the s.c. Met test correlates with ability to raise the threshold for excitation of neural tissue; selective action in nontoxic doses indicates potential clinical efficacy against absence seizures. The rotorod test has a clear endpoint, is quantifiable, and corresponds well with the clinical assessment of minimal neurotoxicity. In addition, selected promising chemical substances are subjected to three more definitive anticonvulsant threshold tests (s.c. bicuculline, s.c. picrotoxin, and s.c. strychnine) in order to differentiate possible antiepileptic activity. Briefly, the parameters and endpoints of these tests are shown in Table 1.

Finally, a toxicity profile (general overt behavior induced by 1, 2, and 4 TD_{50}s of the test drug) is established in mice by a modification of the method reported by Irwin (1968), after which the median hypnotic dose (HD_{50}) and 24-hr median lethal dose (LD_{50}) are determined.

TABLE 1. *Anticonvulsant threshold tests*

Tests	Parameters	Endpoints
Routine		
Maximal electroshock seizure pattern (MES) test	60 Hz, 50 mA mice, 150 mA rats, 0.2 sec, corneal electrodes	Abolition hindleg tonic-extensor component
s.c. Pentylenetetrazol (metrazol) seizure threshold (s.c. Met) test	85 mg/kg, s.c., mice; 70 mg/kg, s.c., rats	Absence of threshold seizure
Rotorod toxicity test	1-inch plastic, knurled, rod rotating 6 rpm, mice; overt signs, rats	Inability to remain on rod 1 min, mice; overt signs, rats
Special		
s.c. Bicuculline seizure *threshold* test	2.70 mg/kg, s.c.	Absence of threshold seizure
s.c. Picrotoxin seizure *threshold* test	3.15 mg/kg, s.c.	Absence of threshold seizure
s.c. Strychnine seizure pattern test	1.20 mg/kg, s.c.	Abolition of hindleg tonic-extensor component

TABLE 2. *Procedures to determine anticonvulsant activity, toxicity, and potential antiepileptic efficacy*

Phase	Procedure
I	Anticonvulsant identification in mice i.p. Dose range: 30, 100, 300, and 600 mg/kg Tests: MES, s.c. Met, Rotorod, and observation of general behavior Time of test: ½ and 4 hr
II	Anticonvulsant quantification in mice i.p. TPE: MES, s.c. Met, Rotorod ED_{50}: MES, s.c. Met, Rotorod
III	Toxicity profile in mice i.p. Observation of general behavior induced by 1, 2, and $4TD_{50}s$ Determination of LD_{50} and HD_{50}
IV	Anticonvulsant quantification in mice p.o. TPE: MES, s.c. Met, Rotorod ED_{50}: MES, s.c. Met, Rotorod
V	Antiepileptic drug differentiation in mice i.p. ED_{50}: s.c. Met, direct stimulant of neuronal membrane (see phase II), s.c. bicuculline, blocks GABA receptors; s.c. picrotoxin, antagonizes GABA-mediated synaptic inhibition; and s.c. strychnine, blocks post-synaptic inhibition mediated by glycine.
VI	Anticonvulsant quantification in rats p.o. TPE: MES, s.c. Met, Rotorod and overt signs ED_{50}: MES, s.c. Met, Rotorod and overt signs

Procedures

The above tests are integrated into a six-phase procedure designed to reveal in a logical sequence maximum information on anticonvulsant activity, toxicity, and potential antiepileptic efficacy at minimum cost. These procedures are summarized in Table 2.

For convenience in the discussion of what these procedures *will* tell you and what they *will not* tell you they are grouped under four headings: anticonvulsant identification (phase I), anticonvulsant quantification (phase's II, IV, and VI), toxicity profile (phase III), and antiepileptic drug differentiation (phase V).

WHAT WILL THESE PROCEDURES TELL YOU?

Anticonvulsant identification (phase I, mice, i.p.) will identify active and relatively nontoxic substances as well as disclose inactive and/or toxic substances; it will reveal the approximate effective dose level, expose the toxic dose range, and provide a clue as to the time of peak drug action; it permits an estimate of the approximate protective index and enables one to decide if further work is justified. It is worthy of note that all this can be done with only 12 to 16 animals at a cost of approximately $40 per compound (Krall et al., 1978).

The anticonvulsant quantification procedure reveals the time of peak drug action, the median effective doses (ED_{50}s MES and s.c. Met) and median neurotoxic dose (TD_{50}) after i.p. administration in mice (phase II), oral administration in mice (phase IV), and oral administration in rats (phase VI). From these results the 95% confidence intervals, slopes of the regression lines, and protective indices may be calculated. This permits a critical comparison of times of peak drug action, potency, toxicity, selectivity of anticonvulsant and neurotoxic effects, margin of safety, routes of administration, and species differences. Data of this kind not only provide a basis for structure-activity studies, but also disclose the possible clinical application of the test substance.

The toxicity profile (phase III) is a systematic observational assessment of some 40 motor, respiratory, skin, and miscellaneous signs and symptoms. This enables one to go beyond the limitations of the mechanical rotorod procedure and establish not only a profile of the onset and duration of various toxic effects, but also to determine whether death is due to respiratory failure or cardiac arrest. These observations are essential to the subsequent determination of the HD_{50} and/or LD_{50}. Moreover, the toxicity profile is prerequisite to preclinical drug evaluation where multiple information is necessary for human prediction.

Antiepileptic drug differentiation (phase V) is designed to provide some insight into drug mechanisms and to characterize drugs within the same therapeutic group. A comparison (based on protective index) of phenobarbital, valproate, ethosuximide, and trimethadione illustrates this point (Table 3).

These data clearly establish three important facts: (a) Except for potency, all four drugs are similar if compared only by the s.c. Met test. (b) The four drugs exhibit distinct profiles of anticonvulsant action. (c) Valproate is effective in nontoxic doses by all four tests. The latter observation supports the concept that valproate probably acts by increasing the GABA level in cerebral cortical tissue (Godin et al., 1969; Schechter et al., 1978). Thus, this test is used to disclose the effects of the candidate substance on selected neurotransmitters and to gain insight into its mechanism of action and potential clinical application.

TABLE 3. *Antiepileptic drug differentiation*

Drug	Metrazol	Bicuculline	Picrotoxin	Strychnine
Phenobarbital	+++	+	++	−
Valproate	++	+	+	+
Ethosuximide	++	−	+	−
Trimethadione	++	+	++	−

Protective index: $+++ > 4$; $++ > 2 < 4$; $+ > 1 < 2$; $− < 1$.

TABLE 4. *Selectivity of antiepileptic effects in mice*

Drug	MES			s.c. Met		
	ED_{50}[a]	Slope	Protective index	ED_{50}[a]	Slope	Protective index
Phenytoin	9.5	13.7	6.89	Potentiates	—	—
Clonazepam	92.7	1.9	0.002	0.009	13.9	20.44
Primidone	11.4	3.4	59.83	58.6	3.3	11.61
Valproate	271.7	12.8	1.57	148.6	11.8	2.87
Phenobarbital	21.8	15.0	3.17	13.2	5.9	5.24
Pentobarbital	32.8	9.2	0.79	12.97	8.4	1.99

[a] mg/kg, i.p. route of administration.

The data in Table 4 will be used to illustrate how both the slope of the regression line and protective index can be used to evaluate anticonvulsant activity. A comparison of phenytoin and clonazepam provides an interesting contrast. Phenytoin is ineffective against metrazol, but has a reasonably steep slope (13.7) and a good protective index (P.I.) (6.89) by the MES test. These data suggest that phenytoin exhibits a highly selective anticonvulsant effect with a good margin of safety. In marked contrast, clonazepam has virtually no anti-MES activity (P.I. 0.002; slope 1.9) but exhibits remarkable anti-metrazol activity (P.I. 20.44; slope 13.9). Hence, clonazepam is a highly selective anti-metrazol agent. Moreover, it is extremely potent; a dose of only 180 ng is sufficient to protect 50% of mice (20 g); this latter observation suggests that clonazepam must be acting at a very discrete, molecular level. Primidone and valproate, in contrast with the two former agents, are effective in nontoxic doses by both tests. However, the relatively flat slopes for primidone (3.4 and 3.3) and its long time to peak effect (3 hr) after intraperitoneal administration reflects the fact that this substance is being converted to other active substances (Butler and Waddell, 1956; Baumel et al., 1973). In contrast, the steep slopes for valproate (12.8 and 11.8) and its very short time to peak effect (15 min), suggest that this substance, at least at this short time period, is not dependent on metabolic alteration for its action. The last two agents, phenobarbital and pentobarbital, illustrate the well known fact that anticonvulsant barbiturates are characterized largely by the margin between the effective anticonvulsant dose and toxic dose (Swinyard and Goodman, 1947; Raines et al., 1979). Thus, phenobarbital has a P.I. of 3.17 and 5.24 by the MES and s.c. Met tests, respectively, whereas pentobarbital has a P.I. of 0.79 and 1.99 by these same tests.

Finally, it is important to note the correlation between anticonvulsant activity and possible clinical usefulness. Drugs clinically useful in generalized tonic-clonic and complex partial (temporal lobe) seizures are characterized in the laboratory by marked anticonvulsant activity by the MES test and either good, little, or no activity by the s.c. Met test. On the other hand, drugs useful in generalized absence seizures are characterized in the laboratory by little or no activity in the MES test but reasonably good to marked activity by the s.c. Met test. This suggests that results obtained by these procedures correlate reasonably well with clinical usefulness in the three major seizure types. Further work with the antiepileptic drug differentiation tests (phase V) may reveal other reliable clinical correlations.

WHAT WILL THESE PROCEDURES NOT TELL YOU?

These procedures will not separate sedative-hypnotics, tranquilizers, and anticonvulsants on the basis of anticonvulsant tests alone. Attention to selectivity, as indicated by the protective index and the slope of the regression line, are helpful in making this distinction; it is the protective index that separates clearly the antiepileptic barbiturates from the nonantiepileptic barbiturates (Swinyard and Goodman, 1947; Raines et al., 1979). The two major tests, MES and s.c. Met, will tell you nothing with respect to the mechanism of action of potential antiepileptics, except for the relative effect on seizure spread and seizure threshold. However, the antiepileptic drug differentiation tests (bicuculline, picrotoxin, strychnine) will provide some information relative to the mechanism responsible for the alteration in either seizure pattern or seizure threshold. These ADD procedures will not sort out candidate antiepileptic drugs that are not anticonvulsants. This suggests that unless new screening techniques are introduced into this procedure it is quite unlikely that exciting unique antiepileptic agents with novel mechanisms of action will be discovered. The correlation between the laboratory data generated by this procedure and the use of drugs for the management of epilepsy is reasonably good in the case of generalized tonic-clonic seizures, complex partial (temporal lobe) seizures, and absence seizures. Nevertheless, precise delineation of clinical usefulness is not yet possible. Moreover, it is quite unlikely that this correlation will improve unless new techniques based on established neurochemical mechanisms are introduced into this procedure.

SUMMARY

It should be mentioned that the principles of screening antiepileptic drugs in rodents have been described and carefully evaluated. The Antiepileptic Drug Development Screening Program was used as an example of such a procedure. Thoughtful consideration has been directed to what it *will* tell you and what it *will not* tell you. Its major limitations appear to revolve about two points: (a) The tests employed are not based on known biochemical endpoints. (b) The procedure will not identify antiepileptic drugs that are *not* anticonvulsants.

The Anticonvulsant Drug Development Program is committed to develop procedures that will either remove or minimize these limitations. Until such time as these have been developed and their usefulness confirmed, the program will continue to search for new antiepileptic agents with the described tests. Ultimately, this work will not only enhance the armamentarium of the epileptologists, but it will also enable many patients to enjoy a better life through more adequate seizure control.

ACKNOWLEDGMENTS

This study was supported by a contract (NO1-NS-5-2302) from the National Institute of Neurological and Communicative Disorders and Stroke.

REFERENCES

Baumel, I. P., Gallagher, B. B., DiMicco, J., and Goico, H. (1973): Metabolism and anticonvulsant properties of primidone in the rat. *J. Pharmacol. Exp. Ther.*, 186:305–314.
Butler, T. C., and Waddell, W. J. (1957): Metabolic conversion of primidone (Mysoline) to phenobarbital. *Proc. Soc. Exp. Biol. Med.*, 96:544–546.
Godin, Y., Heiner, L., Mark, J., and Mandel, P. (1969): Effects of di-*n*-propylacetate, an anticonvulsive compound, on GABA metabolism. *J. Neurochem.*, 16:869–873.
Irwin, S. (1968): Comprehensive observational assessment: A systematic, quantitative procedure for assessing the behavioral and physiologic state of the mouse. *Psychopharmacologia (Berl.)*, 13:222–257.
Krall, R. L., Penry, J. K., White, B. C., Kupferberg, H. J., and Swinyard, E. A. (1978): Antiepileptic drug development: II. Anticonvulsant drug screening. *Epilepsia*, 19:409–428.
Purpura, D. P., Penry, J. K., Tower, D. B., Woodbury, D. M., and Walter, R. D., editors (1972): *Experimental Models of Epilepsy—A Manual for the Laboratory Worker.* Raven Press, New York.
Raines, A., Blake, G. J., Richardson, B., and Gilbert, M. A. (1979): Differential selectivity of several barbiturates on experimental seizures and neurotoxicity in the mouse. *Epilepsia*, 20:105–113.
Schechter, P. J., Tranier, Y., and Grove, J. (1978): Effect of *n*-dipropylacetate on amino acid concentrations in mouse brain: Correlations with anticonvulsant activity. *J. Neurochem.*, 31:1325–1327.
Swinyard, E. A., and Goodman, L. S. (1947): Validity of laboratory anticonvulsant tests for predicting antiepileptic potency and specificity. *Fed. Proc.*, 6:376.

Advances in Epileptology:
The Xth Epilepsy International Symposium,
edited by J. A. Wada and J. K. Penry.
Raven Press, New York © 1980.

A Chronic Petit Mal Model

M. Schmutz, K. Klebs, and W. P. Koella

Research Laboratories, Pharmaceuticals Division, CIBA-GEIGY Ltd.,
Basle, Switzerland

The development and establishment of animal models of human disease entities, particularly of neurological and psychiatric illness, is of paramount importance for a variety of reasons. First, such models, unlike the real, "spontaneously" occurring pathological state in humans, allow the intensive and detailed study of many aspects of the symptomatology, including e.g., the recording of gross neuronal activity and of single nerve cell discharges in brain areas inaccessible in humans. At the same time such studies may yield important information as to the pathogenesis of the disease (i.e., the basic causes of its overt symptomatology).

Second, and most important for the biologist interested in the development of new drugs to be used in the treatment of particular disease entities, such models constitute the necessary substrate for the testing of new compounds as to their possible efficacy in such particular diseases, in this case petit mal epilepsy.

Third, such animal models, particularly in connection with delicate biophysical and/or biochemical neurophysiological techniques, offer a welcome opportunity to study—in addition to efficacy—also mechanisms of action of newly developed and established drugs.

Basically, an animal model should include as many as possible of the symptoms and signs of the real human disease. Thus, more specifically, a model of petit mal epilepsy should reveal spaced, yet not infrequent, attacks of generalized 2 to 3/sec spike wave EEG patterns; it should show, coinciding with the "EEG seizure," myoclonic signs, e.g., in the facial area, and it should be characterized by symptoms signalling "absence," i.e., loss of consciousness or awareness. In addition, such models should "react" with a reduction or elimination of the seizure attacks in response to established petit mal remedies.

The attack elicited in mice by pentetrazole has been and still is considered by many researchers in the field to constitute a simple, albeit "incomplete," model for petit mal epilepsy. Consequently one has come to consider a good response of the pentetrazole seizure as an indication for good anti-petit mal properties of a (potential) antiepileptic drug (see Woodbury, 1972).

Recently, some promising new approaches with other chemicals such as penicillin (Gloor, 1969; Gloor et al., 1977), Premarin (Julien et al., 1975), γ-hydroxy-butyrate (Godschalk et al., 1977) and bilateral cobalt foci (Marcus et al., 1972) to elicit, on an acute, subchronic, or chronic base "petit mal" in a variety of animals, have been proposed.

In our laboratories we now use electrical brain stimulation to produce, in form of an afterdischarge, seizures that fulfill the above-mentioned criteria of a petit mal animal model.

PROCEDURE

Adult cats of either sex are chronically supplied with (bipolar) stimulating electrodes (stainless steel, 0.25 mm diameter, 0.5 mm free tip) aimed bilaterally at the white matter under the sensory motor area (coordinates: frontal, +10.0 and 12.0; lateral, 5.5; vertical, +21). Recording electrodes are placed through burr holes to rest on the sensory motor area and the suprasylvian gyrus on both sides. The electrode leads are connected to a plastic socket fastened to the skull. Connection between the socket and a swivel contact is made through a light, multilead cable.

For electrical stimulation and precipitation of the seizure the two pairs of subcortical electrodes are temporarily connected to the stimulator (100 pps, 3 msec pulses for 3 sec, 1–3 V). After cessation of the stimulus the electrodes are reconnected, together with the cortical leads, to the polygraph.

RESULTS

An usually quite proper petit mal seizure develops as an "afterdischarge," revealing a 1.5 to 3/sec spike wave pattern, attended often by myoclonic twitches of the face (rarely of the legs) and as often by a "staring" look. The attacks last, depending on stimulus strength and pattern of repetition, for 5 to 20 sec (see Fig. 1). With stronger stimuli, high repetition rates, and placement of the stimulating electrodes below the level corresponding to the plane coinciding with the dorsal boundary of the thalamus, the "absence phase" often leads into generalized seizures of the grand mal type.

To test for effects with (so far established) drugs, 2 to 4 control seizures are induced to establish adequate stimulus parameters. After the drug under investigation is administered the animal is stimulated again using the same stimulus parameters, 1, 3, 5, 7, and 24 hr after drug application and seizure parameters—duration, spike and wave amplitude, intensity of myoclonic signs—measured or gauged in a semiquantitative manner.

Ethosuximide, today's drug of first choice in human petit mal epilepsy, reduces in our model the duration of the after discharge as well as the amplitude of the spike waves in doses as small as 30 mg/kg p.o. (the ED_{40} in

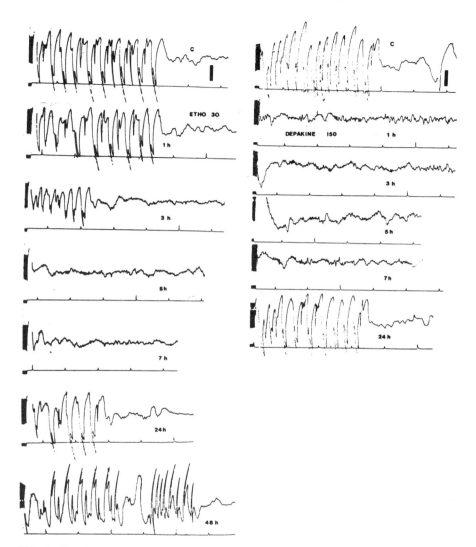

FIG. 1. Electrically induced "petit mal" attack in the cat and effect of ethosuximide (30 mg/kg p.o., **left**) and valproate sodium (150 mg/kg p.o., **right**) thereupon. *Top lines* indicate control (last of two or more at 1-hr intervals). *All other lines* indicate effect of drugs at times indicated after application. Note slow onset of ethosuximide effect and virtual temporary elimination of seizure by both drugs. Time calibration: 1 sec; voltage: 100μV.

the electroshock seizure in the mouse, ESM, one of the ordinary screening tests, is 1,000 mg/kg p.o.).

Valproate sodium shortens the electrically induced afterdischarge in our model by about 50% and reduces amplitude, in doses of 30 mg/kg p.o. (ED_{50} ESM 210–530 mg/kg p.o.). The respective figures for clonazepam, methsuximide, trimethadione, phenobarbital, carbamazepine, and phenytoin are 0.3 mg/kg p.o. (1 mg/kg p.o.), 30 mg/kg p.o. (40 mg/kg p.o.), 300 mg/kg p.o. (430 mg/kg p.o.), 10 mg/kg p.o. (13 mg/kg p.o.), 3 mg/kg p.o. (10 mg/kg p.o.), and 3 mg/kg p.o. (7–20 mg/kg p.o.).

These data clearly indicate that the two drugs most widely and most successfully used in petit mal, ethosuximide and valproate sodium, are highly effective in our model; the doses used to combat the "petit mal" epilepsy in the cat are considerably lower than those necessary to counteract the "grand mal" seizure elicited by electroshock in the mouse. This suggests a quasi-specific effect of these two drugs in this petit mal model. In turn, this indicates that our model could be a useful one to test new compounds for their potential anti-petit mal efficacy. With these attributes our model may also be quite adaptable for investigations as to mechanisms of action of anti-petit mal drugs, and finally for studies concerning the pathogenesis and the biophysical and biochemical "neuronal symptomatology" of petit mal.

REFERENCES

Gloor, P. (1969): Epileptogenic action of penicillin. *Ann. NY Acad. Sci.*, 166:350–360.

Gloor, P., Quesney, L. F., and Zumstein, H. (1977): Pathophysiology of generalized penicillin epilepsy in the cat: The role of cortical and subcortical structures. II. Topical application of penicillin to the cerebral cortex and to subcortical structures. *Electroencephalogr. Clin. Neurophysiol.*, 43:79–94.

Godschalk, M., Dzoljic, M. R., and Bonta, I. L. (1977): Gamma-hydroxybutyrate, sleep, hypersynchrony and anti-petit mal drugs. In: *Sleep 1976, Third European Congress on Sleep Research, Montpellier*, edited by W. P. Koella and P. Levin. S. Karger, Basel.

Julien, R. M., Fowler, G. W., and Danielson, M. G. (1975): The effects of antiepileptic drugs on estrogen-induced electrographic spike-wave discharge. *J. Pharmacol. Exp. Ther.*, 193:647–656.

Marcus, E. M., Fullerton, A., Losh, E., and Bowker, R. (1972): Epileptogenic effects of cobalt in *Macaca mulatta:* Unilateral and bilateral cortical foci. *Epilepsia*, 13:343–344.

Woodbury, D. M. (1972): Applications to drug evaluations. In: *Experimental Models of Epilepsy—A Manual for the Laboratory Worker*, edited by D. P. Purpura, J. K. Penry, D. Tower, D. M. Woodbury, and R. Walter. Raven Press, New York.

Advances in Epileptology:
The Xth Epilepsy International Symposium,
edited by J. A. Wada and J. K. Penry.
Raven Press, New York © 1980.

A Procedure to Detect Development of Tolerance ("Escape") to Antiepileptic Drugs: First Results

V. Baltzer, J. Baud, P. Degen, and W. P. Koella

Research Laboratories, Pharmaceuticals Division, CIBA-GEIGY Ltd.,
Basle, Switzerland

It is well known that some patients may develop tolerance to some antiepileptic drugs. Signs of tolerance may evolve or, as is often the case, may appear rather suddenly in the sense that almost from one day to the next, the antiepileptic remedy loses its efficacy. In the latter case one tends to refer to "escape" rather than tolerance. An extended comparative study in regard to what types of antiepileptic drugs, under what type of therapeutic regimen, in what types of patients are most apt to produce tolerance or escape is not available at the present time. Still, it seems justifiable to state that, particularly with acetazoleamid (Diamox®) and also with some antiepileptics of the benzodiazepine type, loss of efficacy is more likely to occur than with other drugs.

In the course of the development of new antiepileptic compounds, it seems to be of paramount importance to be able to predict, with some degree of assurance, the occurrence of such (clinical) tolerance phenomena and possibly even to stop further development of a drug if pronounced tolerance should prove to be too much of a drawback for a new compound and make it virtually useless for routine application.

In the available literature there are some indications that tolerance and/or "escape" can be detected also in animals chronically treated with antiepileptic compounds. Among others Killam et al. (1973) have shown that diazepam loses efficacy in the photomyoclonic baboon and that efficacy can be restored by increasing dosage. Frey and Kampmann (1965), using electroshock-induced convulsions (mice), noted development of tolerance to the anticonvulsive effect of both phenobarbital and diphenylhydantoin. Still, systematic studies using methods adaptable for screening procedures in the development of new compounds are not available. Thus, we thought it worthwhile to work out a relatively simple, although time-consuming, procedure that allows detection in antiepileptic compounds of tolerance development and related phenomena in animals. Based on the still limited experience thus far with a number of established antiepileptics, we think the probability of prediction of tolerance developing in humans is adequately high.

PROCEDURE

Three to five groups of 15 to 20 male rats (150–200 g) are treated daily for a period of from 28 to 31 days with the drug under investigation. Each group receives by oral route a different dose including ED_0 (vehicle) and ED_{90-100} (the minimal dose that protects on the first day all or most of the animals from convulsions). One to three intermediate doses (e.g., the ED_{25}, ED_{50}, and ED_{75}) are given to the remaining one to three groups. These various dosages must be determined before the actual long-term experiment is started. Application time of the drug must be kept constant to avoid an influence of circadian variations in susceptibility to the epileptogenic agent and to the antiepileptic drug. Every day, 1 hr (or more in special cases where preliminary experiments suggest long delays in absorption to reach maximally effective blood levels) after gavage the animals are subjected to an electroconvulsive shock (corneal electrodes, 100 V AC, 50 Hz, for 0.63 sec) and the number of animals per group are determined that are protected, i.e., that do not react with tonic extensor seizures of the hindlegs. After recovery from the seizure the animals are replaced into their home cage (one animal per cage). The experiment may be expanded to yield additional data if one routinely observes the animals shortly before application of the electroshock as to quality and quantity of side effects, i.e., sedation, motor disturbances, such as ataxia, muscular hypotonia, and/or hyperactivity. Such data can be plotted, as are the results concerning anticonvulsive effects, along a time-base as shown in Fig. 1. Statistical methods, taking into account the non-independence of the daily values, may be applied to obtain indications for significance—or nonsignificance—of possible random and/or systematic variations.

RESULTS WITH SOME ESTABLISHED ANTIEPILEPTIC DRUGS

As seen from Fig. 1, stimulation parameters were such that in all untreated groups (one separate control group for each set of experiments with any one of the six compounds) efficacy of the convulsive shock remained high; i.e., there were always between 90 and 100% responders.

With neither of the two doses of diphenylhydantoin were there signs of tolerance. In fact, in the course of the first 2 weeks of treatment efficacy increased so that even the (initial) ED_{30} attained 100% efficacy, and remained 100% efficient over the whole experimental period (Fig. 1, top left).

Carbamazepine in the two lower (submaximal) doses (ED_{40} and ED_{70}) slowly but steadily grew in efficacy. With none of the three doses tested were there any signs of tolerance (Fig. 1, top right).

However, all three doses of phenobarbital, after an initial steady period of about 10 days, started to lose efficacy. Some systematic variations with peaks on days 16/17 and 23 revealed a certain periodicity in the waxing and waning of efficacy, which in this period seems to be dose-independent (Fig. 1, middle left).

Acetazolamide, after an initial phase of growth, disclosed pronounced signs of a gradual loss of efficacy (Fig. 1, middle right).

Clonazepam yielded rather irregular results in that under this drug there occurred rather unsystematic variations from day to day. However, it appears that with this drug there is no pronounced and sustained systematic loss in efficacy over the 4-week experimental period (Fig. 1, bottom left).

Diazepam with all three doses tested showed an initial and substantial loss in efficacy, bringing down, by the 5th day, the effect of the (initial) ED_{50} by about 40% only to increase again and reach initial (50%) values by the 10th day. A systematic periodic variation in efficacy emerges leading to peaks on days 9/10, 18/20, and 27/30. This rhythmic pattern thus reveals a period of 9 to 10 days (Fig. 1, bottom right). Thus diazepam seems to be characterized—as are phenobarbital and clonazepam believed to be to a lesser extent—by a temporary and repeated but not by a sustained loss of efficacy. Two additional experimental series with this drug yielded essentially the same results, i.e., a rhythmical variation in efficacy with a period of approximately 10 days.

DISCUSSION

The one drug that probably shows clinically the most pronounced tendency toward tolerance—acetazolamide—has also been shown in the present study to lose much of its efficacy after an initial gain. In turn, carbamazepine and diphenylhydantoin, which when used in epileptic patients usually show little or no tendency toward tolerance or "escape" also reveal no signs of loss of efficacy in our animal test situation. In fact, with diphenylhydantoin there is rather an initial increase in effectiveness, which may be the manifestation of a slow build-up toward steady-state plasma levels; this, if gauged by the efficacy values, would be reached by about the 12th to 15th day of treatment.

Phenobarbital, after an initial steady period reveals a certain rhythmically waxing and waning loss in efficacy. Although signs of tolerance to phenobarbital in the course of antiepileptic treatment have been reported on many occasions, making it often necessary to increase the dose of this drug, rhythmical variations in (clinical) effectiveness have not been observed. It would be of interest, however, to record seizure incidence in patients under phenobarbital monotherapy and to look for periodically occurring "escape," i.e., temporary increases in seizure rate at intervals of several days or a few weeks.

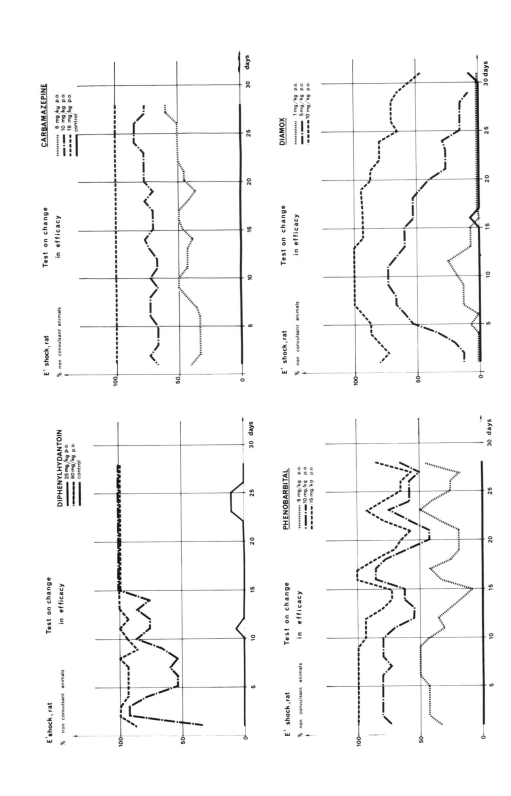

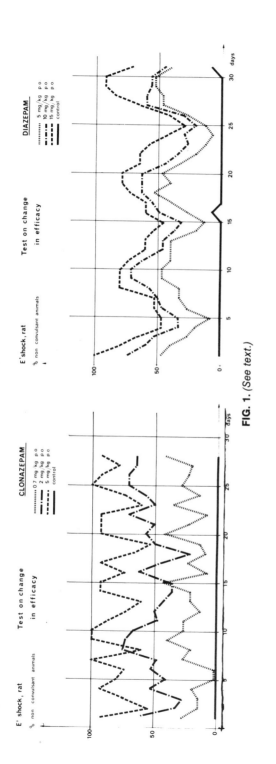

FIG. 1. (See text.)

For clonazepam our experimental results would not predict a systematic loss in clinical efficacy although submaximal doses vary considerably in effectiveness. Pinder and collaborators (1976), however, reported on occasional signs of tolerance when they used this drug in patients.

The phenomenologically most interesting data were obtained with diazepam, which produces a rapid and pronounced loss in anticonvulsive efficacy in the course of the first 4 to 5 days of treatment but also equally rapidly reestablishes efficacy during the following 5 days. As this pattern is repeated in the second and third 10-day period an almost regular rhythmical pattern of decreases and increases in efficacy emerges which, as can be judged from the present data, is dose-independent in (absolute) amplitude and in frequency. Thus, "escape," as seen under clinical conditions, may have been predicted by our experimental findings (i.e., of the first few days only). However, there is no indication as yet that patients under (continuous) treatment with diazepam reveal a waning and waxing in efficacy, i.e., a periodical increase and decrease in seizure rate that would suggest a rhythmical pattern as observed under experimental conditions.[1]

The periodicity seen with diazepam and, to a lesser extent and only after a 2-week delay, with phenobarbital may be the manifestation of similar periodical variations in drug absorption. However, determinations of plasma levels of diazepam $\frac{1}{2}$ hr after (daily) application of the drug did not reveal any systematic variations over an 11-day period. Periodic changes in efficacy thus cannot be due to changes in uptake of the drug but rather must be the consequence of either a periodically changing rate of penetration from the blood to the (central nervous) receptor sites and/or a periodically changing responsiveness of the central nervous mechanisms (including receptor site sensitivity and reactivity of secondary (tertiary, etc. messenger mechanisms) involved in the anticonvulsive activity of the drug.

REFERENCES

Frey, H. H., and Kampmann, E. (1965): Entwicklung einer Toleranz gegen Antikonvulsiva. *Arch. Exp. Pathol. Pharmakol.*, 250:250–251.

Killam, E. K., Matsuzaki, M., and Killam, K. F. (1973): Studies of anticonvulsant compounds in the *Papio papio* model of epilepsy. In: *Chemical Modulation of Brain Function*, edited by H. Sabelli. Raven Press, New York.

Pinder, R. M., Brogdon, R. N., Speight, T. M., and Avery, G. S. (1973): Clonazepam: a review of its pharmacological properties and therapeutic efficacy in epilepsy. *Drugs (Basel)*, 12:321–361.

---

[1]It is important to be aware that in a sense our data are "binary" in nature; i.e., that we measure changes in the number of reacting animals and not (day to day) changes in reactivity of individual subjects. In fact, we plan now to investigate possible changes in (individual) thresholds over extended periods.

Advances in Epileptology:
The Xth Epilepsy International Symposium,
edited by J. A. Wada and J. K. Penry.
Raven Press, New York © 1980.

Preliminary Efficacy of Experimental Anticonvulsant Cinromide in Monkey Model

Joan S. Lockard, René H. Levy, and Leonard D. Salonen

Departments of Neurological Surgery and Pharmaceutics,
University of Washington, Seattle, Washington 98195

Cinromide (3-bromo-N-ethylcinnamamide), an experimental anticonvulsant, is given a preliminary evaluation in our alumina-gel monkey model of focal and secondarily generalized tonic-clonic epilepsy. The drug had exhibited considerable protection against maximal electroshock seizures (MES) in rodents and dogs (Burroughs-Wellcome, 1976) prior to this investigation. The parent drug has a biological half-life in monkey of 1 to 2 hr and its active metabolite (3-bromocinnamide), of 4 to 6 hr (Lane and Levy, *this volume*). Since the metabolite reaches plasma concentrations approximately three times the parent drug and is some 80% as effective (Burroughs-Wellcome, 1976), it was the main point of interest in the present research. This focus seems reasonable in view of the fact that the apparent biological half-life of cinromide and its metabolite in humans (normal volunteers, Burroughs-Wellcome, 1977) are similar to monkey. Therefore, oral dosing in people on a drug regimen of four times per day (q.i.d.) would emphasize the metabolite rather than the parent drug.

METHODS

Animals

Eight subadult (4–6 kg), male monkeys (*Macaca mulatta*) were made chronically epileptic by cortical injections of aluminum hydroxide (0.25 cc) in the sensorimotor, hand and face area (verified by physiological stimulation) of the left hemisphere as described by Lockard et al., 1976. Similar to the procedures reported in that study, the animals were equipped with chronic EEG plugs and two indwelling catheters for drug administration and blood sampling, respectively. The monkeys were manifesting stable seizure frequencies and EEG paroxysms at the time of this research.

Dosing Regimen

Cinromide's insolubility and short half-life dictated its administration in a vehicle of 65% polyethylene glycol 400 (PEG) by constant-rate intravenous infusion. In phase 1 of the study, six monkeys were given the drug for a period of 5 days. The drug days were immediately preceded and followed by control days of 65% PEG 400 only (1 ml/hr, 3 days each). The PEG periods were bordered by 5 days of baseline (saline, 1 ml/hr). Three different concentrations of cinromide (12, 24, and 36 mcg/ml) were administered, respectively, at a rate of 1 ml/hr, to three groups of two monkeys each. The intent was to achieve mean steady-state plasma levels of approximately 5, 10, and 20 mcg/ml of the metabolite (i.e., about 5.0 mcg/ml of the parent drug at the highest dosage).

In phase II of the study, cinromide in a solution of 65% PEG in water was administered (1 ml/hr) for 7 days to six monkeys at the same concentration for all animals. Based on the results of phase I, the objective here was to achieve a steady-state plasma range of between 7 and 14 mcg/ml of the metabolite (i.e., less than 3.0 mcg/ml of the parent drug). Similar to phase I, baseline periods (saline, 1 ml/hr, for 7 days each) and PEG days (65%, 1 ml/hr, for 3 days each) were used as controls.

Seizure and EEG Monitoring

Seizure frequency was recorded 24 hr per day and EEG samples were gathered (as detailed in Lockard et al., 1976) of three 1-hr periods per day per animal and five night records (1900 hr to 0400 hr) per animal. The day EEGs were scheduled at a time of day to maximize the amount of recording during the initial infusion of cinromide as well as the first few hours of its subsequent withdrawal. Throughout the study, for any given animal, the time of day of its EEG sample was held constant. Several daily behavioral measures on operant tasks for food were also obtained.

RESULTS

Since each animal served as its own control, the frequency of EEG paroxysms and clinical seizures during cinromide administration were compared with periods of baseline and PEG alone using the z variant of the normal distribution (reported as a two-tail test unless specified otherwise). Parametric statistics require a considerable number of data points for comparison; therefore, EEG interictal bursts (number of spikes per minute) were relied on more heavily than the less frequently occurring clinical seizures. However, for most animals there was a consistent change in seizure duration during cinromide administration (reported in a separate section). Side effects (in terms of mean differences) were statistically analyzed by Student's t-test (two-tail).

Phase I

Cinromide appears to be efficacious at plasma levels of its metabolite of 7 to 14 mcg/ml. The mean number of EEG interictal spikes per minute of monkey 2 (Fig. 1, left side) decreased significantly during cinromide administration ($z = 2.24$, $p < 0.02$). The seizure frequency of this animal was attenuated during PEG administration and remained so throughout periods of PEG or cinromide in PEG solvent ($z = 1.95$, $p < 0.05$, one-tail test). Monkey 5 (Fig. 1, right side) also manifested a decrease in EEG interictal bursting and seizure frequency during administration of PEG alone, but seizure attenuation was significantly greater during the administration of cinromide ($z = 1.75$, $p < 0.05$, one-tail test). [In previous studies, e.g., Lockard and Levy, (1977), PEG 400 alone had been found to be efficacious and therefore was used as a control in this study].

Plasma concentrations of the metabolite less than 7 mcg/ml or greater than 15 mcg/ml were not found to be efficacious. There were no consistent changes ($p > 0.05$) in seizure frequency or mean number of EEG interictal spikes per minute in the two monkeys with plasma concentrations of the metabolite of 5 mcg/ml or less. For those two animals whose plasma concentration of the metabolite was above 15 mcg/ml, there was an *increase* in mean number of spikes per minute during cinromide administration which reached statistical significance ($z = 2.76$, $p < 0.005$) in one monkey.

Phase II

In this phase of the study, plasma concentration of the metabolite between 7 to 14 mcg/ml was achieved in four of six monkeys. For three of these animals there was a decrease in number of EEG interictal spikes per minute during days of cinromide administration as compared to baseline and PEG periods (e.g., $z = 1.74$, $p < 0.05$, one-tail test; and $z = 4.80$, $p < 0.001$, respectively). For these animals, changes in seizure frequency were not statistically significant ($p > 0.05$). For the fourth monkey, its mean seizure frequency decreased ($z = 2.46$, $p < 0.005$) during PEG administration and remained at a low value for the rest of the study; the attenuation in its mean number of EEG spikes per minute did not reach statistical significance ($p > 0.05$). For the two animals whose plasma concentrations of the metabolite were inadvertently below 7 mcg/ml, changes in either EEG paroxysms or number of seizures were also not significant ($p > 0.05$).

Seizure Duration

In both phase I and phase II, seizure duration decreased during cinromide administration for most monkeys. Only one of eight animals ($z = 1.86$, $p < 0.05$, one-tail test) manifested secondarily generalized tonic-clonic seizures while receiving cinromide; the other animals had focal seizures exclusively. The one monkey who was the exception had two small generalized seizures. On withdrawal of cinromide, generalized seizures reappeared and in greater frequency than before for some animals.

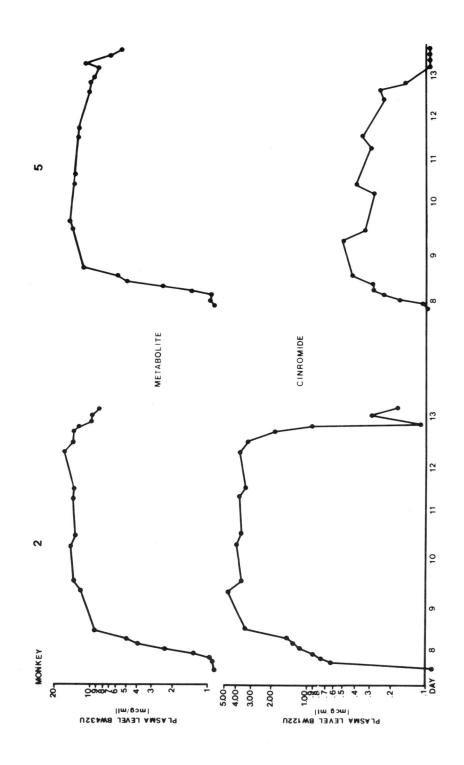

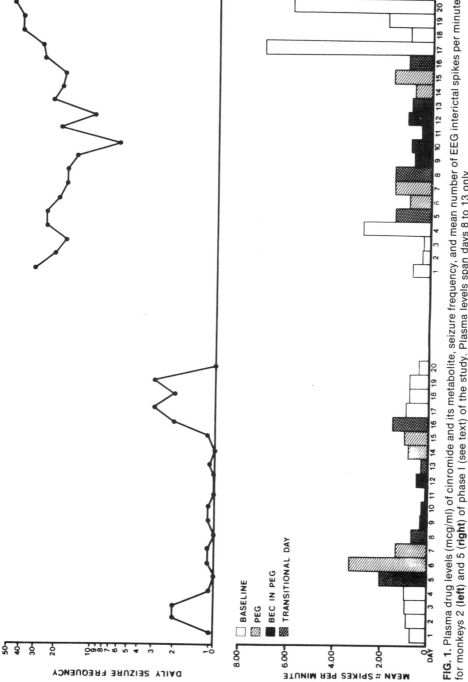

FIG. 1. Plasma drug levels (mcg/ml) of cinromide and its metabolite, seizure frequency, and mean number of EEG interictal spikes per minute for monkeys 2 (**left**) and 5 (**right**) of phase I (see text) of the study. Plasma levels span days 8 to 13 only.

Side Effects

In both phase I and phase II of the study, a significant elevation in white blood count with PEG administration was manifested (PEG versus baseline: $t = 3.26$, $p < 0.05$, and $t = 5.73$, $p < 0.005$, respectively), which was reversed on PEG discontinuance (PEG versus baseline: $t = 3.54$, $p < 0.05$, and $t = 3.58$, $p < 0.05$, respectively). Anorexia was also evident during PEG days but reached statistical significance (phase I: $t = 4.97$, $p < 0.005$; phase II: $t = 8.45$, $p < 0.001$) when cinromide was added to the regimen.

DISCUSSION

Preliminary evaluation of cinromide at plasma levels of its metabolite between 7 to 14 mcg/ml suggest that this drug may be efficacious. Both EEG interictal bursting and seizure duration were attenuated for most animals at that concentration range. Plasma levels of the metabolite at less than 7 mcg/ml or greater than 15 mcg/ml did not result in effective changes. These findings must be regarded as tentative, since cinromide's insolubility necessitated a vehicle of 65% PEG 400, which has been found to be both efficacious and toxic at this concentration in previous studies (e.g., Lockard and Levy, 1977). Appropriate control periods of the administration of PEG 400 alone did allow the influence of cinromide's metabolite on epileptic activity to be assessed. However, given the pharmacological activity of PEG 400, subtle efficacious effects of the parent drug itself were obviously obscured. This was true of side effects as well, since symptoms of PEG 400 toxicity (Lockard et al., 1978) would mask any problems of a similar nature that cinromide might exhibit. The only side effect that was attributable, in part, to cinromide's administration was anorexia, which has been reported for this drug in rodents as well (Burroughs-Wellcome, 1976). Further evaluation of cinromide as an anticonvulsant will be undertaken in our monkey model via drug administration by gastric canulation without the complication of a PEG 400 vehicle.

SUMMARY

Cinromide (3-bromo-N-ethylcinnamamide), an experimental anticonvulsant (Burroughs-Wellcome Pharmaceutical Co.) was given a preliminary evaluation in our alumina-gel monkey model. The parent drug has a biological half-life in monkey of 1 to 2 hr and its active metabolite (3-bromocinnamide) of 4 to 6 hr.

In phase I, six chronically epileptic monkeys, with focal motor and secondarily generalized tonic-clonic seizures, were administered the drug in a vehicle of 65% polyethylene glycol 400 (PEG) by constant-rate intravenous infusion. Three different concentrations of cinromide (12, 24, and 36 mg/

ml/hr) were administered, respectively, to achieve mean steady-state plasma levels of approximately 5, 10, and 20 mcg/ml of the metabolite (0.5–5.0 mcg/ml of the parent drug). In phase II, cinromide was administered for 7 days at the middle concentration for all monkeys.

The data tentatively suggest that cinromide is efficacious in the monkey model at a plasma concentration range of 7 to 14 mcg/ml of the metabolite. With the exception of one animal, *no* secondarily generalized seizures were exhibited during drug administration (but were evident in the baseline periods), and EEG bursting decreased significantly in several monkeys. Minimal side effects were manifested at these plasma levels but withdrawal seizures were evinced with cessation of the drug. Further evaluation of cinromide by gastric administration in our animal model is currently in progress.

ACKNOWLEDGMENT

This research was funded by the National Institute of Neurological and Communicative Diseases and Stroke, National Institute of Health research contract NO1-NS-1-2282 and NIH research grant NS 04053, PHS/DHEW. The authors wish to thank Mr. William C. Congdon, Mr. Larry L. DuCharme, Mr. Douglas Kalk, Mr. David W. Walker, and Ms. Julie A. Wisner for their extensive efforts in the conduct of this research.

REFERENCES

Burroughs-Wellcome Pharmaceutical Co. (1976,1977): Report on the pharmacology and toxicology of B.W. 122 μ. (*Confidential communication*).

Lockard, J. S., and Levy, R. H. (1977): Efficacy of clonazepam in alumina-gel monkey model. *American Epilepsy Society Meeting*, New York.

Lockard, J. S., Levy, R. H., Congdon, W. C., and DuCharme, L. L. (1979): Efficacy and toxicity of the solvent polyethylene glycol 400 in monkey model. *Epilepsia* 20:77–84.

Lockard, J. S., Levy, R. H., Patel, I. H., DuCharme, L. L., and Congdon, W. C. (1976): Dipropylacetic acid and ethosuximide in monkey model: quantitative methods of evaluation. In: *Quantitative Analytic Studies in Epilepsy*, edited by P. Kellaway and I. Petersen. Raven Press, New York.

Advances in Epileptology:
The Xth Epilepsy International Symposium,
edited by J. A. Wada and J. K. Penry.
Raven Press, New York © 1980.

Difficulties in Evaluating the Efficacy of an Anticonvulsant in the Presence of Other Anticonvulsants

*,**,†,†††Alan Joseph Wilensky, *,†††Linda Moretti Ojemann,
*,†††Carl B. Dodrill, and *,††,†††Nancy R. Temkin

*Departments of *Neurological Surgery, **Medicine, †Neurology,
and ††Biostatistics, University of Washington Medical School;
and †††University of Washington Epilepsy Center, Harborview
Medical Center, Seattle, Washington 98104*

The evaluation of new anticonvulsants in the United States requires add-on studies that may be open studies as part of phase II testing or double-blind as part of phase III testing (Cereghino and Penry, 1972; Food and Drug Administration, 1977). When a new anticonvulsant is added to an existing drug regimen there are major problems in measuring the efficacy and safety of the new drug because the interactions between the drugs are complex and difficult to evaluate. Because of these interactions, it is frequently difficult to distinguish effects, therapeutic and/or toxic, of the drug being studied from those of the drugs not being studied. At the University of Washington Epilepsy Center, we are currently engaged in a large double-blind study comparing the efficacy and toxicity of clorazepate with that of phenobarbital in patients already taking phenytoin who have persistent focal seizures. This chapter describes the problems we have identified in the course of this study and strategies we have developed to overcome these problems.

PROBLEMS

In order to evaluate the usefulness of a new anticonvulsant, the only factor that should change in the patient's environment is the new medication. Because of drug interactions, however, the addition of a second drug or a change in its dose will frequently affect the first drug. Thus in add-on studies a stable background for evaluating the new anticonvulsant is rarely if ever achieved.

Serum Level Changes

The most common change that investigators must deal with is an alteration in the serum level of the background anticonvulsant. Investigators are then faced with a dilemma. First, in any study of finite length only a limited number of changes can be made in the dose of medications. In general, the dose of only one drug should be changed at any one time so that the effect of that change can be observed independently of any other changes in medication. If investigators attempt to maintain a constant serum level of the non-study drug they may expend so much time and effort changing its dose that they do not adequately test the study drug at different dose levels. Effectiveness or toxicity of the new drug at high doses may be missed because there is no opportunity to raise the dose sufficiently.

On the other hand, if changes are made only in the dose of the study drug, the levels of the non-study drug will change because of drug interactions. Serum levels of the baseline drug may increase just as phenobarbital levels increase in the presence of valproic acid (Pinder et al., 1977). Serum levels may decrease as phenytoin levels do in the presence of carbamazepine (Hansen et al., 1971). Even when the probable interaction is known before the study the effect of the interaction in an individual patient may be different. Thus, although phenytoin levels are generally lower in the presence of phenobarbital than in its absence, in any individual they may increase, decrease, or remain the same when phenobarbital is added (Kutt et al., 1969; Morselli et al., 1971). Investigators are then faced with a problem of analysis. Whenever such drug interactions occur, changes in seizure frequency may be due either to the study drug or to changes in the serum level of the other drug. Similarly, toxicity may be secondary to either medication.

Free Fraction Changes

Even if the total serum level of the baseline medication does remain constant the investigators must be aware of other less obvious changes in distribution of the drug in the body. Anticonvulsant activity of a drug is thought to be related to its brain concentration. Although brain concentrations cannot be directly measured they are thought to be proportional to free serum levels and these in turn are supposed to be a constant fraction of total serum levels. The chain of assumptions that efficacy is related to brain levels and these in turn are related to free serum levels cannot, for practical purposes, be tested in a clinical study and thus has to be accepted. However, the assumption that the free level is always a constant fraction of the total serum level may not be valid. The free fraction of a drug can change because of a disease state or because of changes in other medications (Lunde et al., 1970; Hooper et al., 1974). A change in the free fraction can produce a small absolute change in the free level, which may be large in a relative sense. This change may not be reflected by significant changes in total drug level. Thus, phenytoin is usually 10% free and 90% bound with a free level of approximately 2.0 μg/ml when the total level is 20 μg/ml. A small absolute change of only 1 μg/ml in free level to 3.0 μg/ml because of a shift in binding so that 15% is free will leave the total phenytoin serum level unchanged. However, the amount of drug proportional to the brain concentration is increased by 50%. An alteration such as this in the non-study drug may produce major changes in clinical state that could be assigned to the study drug if the investigators are not alert.

Synergism

A final problem involving interactions can occur at the brain level. Two drugs may have a synergistic or antagonistic interaction on the brain. Thus, in the presence of one drug a new medication may work well, whereas it may be ineffective in the presence of some other anticonvulsant. This type of interaction is impossible to predict or detect without serially testing a new drug in combination with several other drugs. Therefore, even if a new medication produces good results in one combination, and even if these results can be shown not to be due to changes in the non-study drug, the results cannot automatically be extrapolated so as to assume the efficacy of the new medication when it is alone or when it is combined with some other drug.

STRATEGIES

When it is necessary to do an add-on study, the problems can be simplified by adding the new medication to only a single non-study drug. Even in a two-drug system, there are numerous interactions that make analysis difficult. This difficulty is much greater in a three-drug system. Only if the new drug produces spectacular results in a large percentage of cases, such as valproic acid, will the results be unequivocal in the presence of many different anticonvulsants; and even in the case of valproic acid the data have been questioned (Van Belle, 1978). The single non-study drug should be the same for all patients. If it is not, in reality, you are carrying out as many studies as you have different non-study drugs because the study drug will interact in a different way with each of the non-study drugs. Thus, in an add-on study, the experimental medication should be added to a single standard anticonvulsant and, where possible, its effect should be measured against the subject's status while he or she is on only the standard anticonvulsant, using a placebo in a double-blind manner.

Serum Level Changes

Once the proper basic study design is established, the investigators must avoid the temptation of trying to keep the non-study drug serum level constant. Even if they try, they will rarely succeed. Except when absolutely necessary, as when toxicity occurs because of increasing non-study drug levels, changes should be made in study drug dose rather than in the dose of the baseline drug. Some fluctuation in the level of the baseline drug must be accepted in order to allow for assessment of the study drug effects at various doses. At the end of the study, these fluctuations must be acknowledged in the analysis.

To make analysis practical under these circumstances, careful attention must be paid to clinical detail. Detailed, preplanned, clinical assessments are made at regular intervals. These should include seizure counts, objective measurements of toxicity, and subjective assessments by the patient of toxicity and seizure control. Changes in seizure type or quality should be noted. If a large blinded study is being contemplated, a small open pilot study should be done first to acquaint the investigators with at least some of the problems, primarily those of toxicity, which may arise during the blind study. The investigators will then be able to make management decisions that are more likely to solve the clinical problems.

Anticonvulsant serum levels must also be obtained. Because levels of medications vary with the time after each dose, they should be measured at a set time in relationship to dosing. In general, the best time is just prior to a dose, usually the first dose of the day when levels are at their lowest. Other times may be chosen depending on the information desired, i.e., peak levels versus lowest levels, convenience of the subjects, and the pharmacokinetics of the drugs being studied. Where possible, serum levels should be known before the end of the clinic visit so that drug dosage can be adjusted, if necessary, in the light of the levels. In blinded situations, the level of the drug not under study should be available at the clinic visit. Provided there is no known obvious drug interaction such that a change in standard drug level indicates the presence or absence of a blinded drug, this will not interfere with the blind nature of the study. Whenever drug changes must be made between regular visits because of toxicity or increased seizures, serum levels should be obtained if possible, so that information as to the cause of the problem is available when the data are analyzed.

Free Fraction Changes

Although accurate measurement of unbound anticonvulsant requires time-consuming procedures such as ultracentrifugation or equilibrium dialysis, for some anticonvulsants an estimate of free levels can be obtained relatively simply. Salivary anticonvulsant levels are good estimates of unbound serum drug levels for anticonvulsants such as phenytoin (Troupin and Friel, 1975). When free levels can be estimated easily in this manner, they should be measured. If there is a change in free levels that is not reflected by a change in total serum anticonvulsant level, it can then be detected. Changes in clinical status secondary to free drug level changes can then be accounted for in the final analysis.

Other Strategies

Because anticonvulsants affect neuropsychological functions, comprehensive neuropsychological evaluation of the subjects should be undertaken on and off the study drug. Each anticonvulsant tends to alter a particular set of tests (Dodrill and Troupin, 1977). Clinical changes that coincide with non-study drug level changes may be accompanied by changes in neuropsychological test results which are attributed to either the study drug or the non-study drug. Thus, the neuropsychological tests may assist the investigators in assigning clinical changes to either the study or non-study drug. The investigators then do not have to be as concerned about keeping the standard drug level constant but can concentrate on changes in the study drug.

Once the study has been completed there is no single method of analysis that can separate out the effects of the study drug from the effects of the non-study drug. This does not mean, however, that nothing can be done. A biostatistician familiar with the study should assist in the careful evaluation of the data. If, for example, the effects of blood level changes of the non-study drug are understood, the biostatistician may be able to adjust for these changes in the analysis. Thus, although extra caution in the interpretation is warranted, add-on studies can provide valuable information about the efficacy of new anticonvulsants.

ACKNOWLEDGMENTS

This project was supported by National Institutes of Health contracts NO1-NS-0-2281 and NO1-NS-6-2341, National Institute of Neurological and Communicative Disorders and Stroke, PHS/DHEW.

REFERENCES

Cereghino, J. J., and Penry, J. K. (1972): Testing of anticonvulsants in man. In: *Antiepileptic Drugs*, pp. 63–73, edited by D. M. Woodbury, J. K. Penry, and R. P. Schmidt. Raven Press, New York.
Dodrill, C. B., and Troupin, A. S. (1977): Psychotropic effects of carbamazepine in epilepsy: A double-blind comparison with phenytoin. *Neurology (Minneap.)*, 27:1023–1028.
Food and Drug Administration (1977): Guidelines for the clinical evaluation of anticonvulsant drugs (adults and children). HEW Publication (FDA) 77–3045.
Hansen, J. M., Siersback-Nilson, K., and Shoosted, L. (1971): Carbamazepine-induced accel-

eration of diphenylhydantoin and warfarin metabolism in man. *Clin. Pharmacol. Ther.*, 12:539–543.

Hooper, W. D., Bochner, F., Eadie, M. J., and Tyrer, J. H. (1974): Plasma protein binding of diphenylhydantoin. Effects of sex hormones, renal and hepatic disease. *Clin. Pharmacol. Ther.*, 15:276–282.

Kutt, H., Haynes, J., Verebely, K., and McDowell, F. (1969): The effect of phenobarbital on plasma diphenylhydantoin level and metabolism in man and in rat liver microsomes. *Neurology (Minneap.)*, 19:611–616.

Lunde, P. K. M., Rane, A., Yaffe, S. J., Lund, L., and Sjoqvist (1970): Plasma protein binding of diphenylhydantoin in man. Interaction with other drugs and the effect of temperature and plasma dilution. *Clin. Pharmacol. Ther.*, 11:846–855.

Morselli, P. L., Rizzo, M., and Garattini, S. (1971): Interaction between phenobarbital and diphenylhydantoin in animals and in epileptic patients. *Ann. NY Acad Sci.*, 179:88–107.

Pindar, R. M., Brogden, R. N., Speight, T. M., and Avery, G. S. (1977): Sodium Valproate: A review of its pharmacological properties and therapeutic efficacy in epilepsy. *Drugs*, 13:81–123.

Troupin, A. S., and Friel, P. (1975): Anticonvulsant level in saliva, serum and cerebrospinal fluid. *Epilepsia*, 16:223–227.

Van Belle, G. (1978): A statistical review of the literature dealing with the effectiveness of valproic acid in the treatment of petit mal epilepsy. Unpublished Lecture to the University of Washington Epilepsy Center.

Advances in Epileptology:
The Xth Epilepsy International Symposium,
edited by J. A. Wada and J. K. Penry.
Raven Press, New York © 1980.

A Controlled Study of Prednisone Therapy in Infantile Spasms

*,†Richard A. Hrachovy, *,†James D. Frost, Jr.,
Peter Kellaway, and **,††Thomas Zion

*Departments of *Neurology and **Pediatrics, Baylor*
College of Medicine; and †Neurophysiology Service and
††Blue Bird Clinic, Houston, Texas 77030

Since the initial report by Sorel and Dusaucy-Bauloye (1958) on the beneficial effects of corticotropin (ACTH) on infantile spasms, there have been numerous studies citing the efficacy of ACTH and corticosteroids in the treatment of the disorder. As noted by Lacy and Penry (1976), these studies have shown much variability in dosages, trial durations, and methods of evaluation. More important, since most of these studies were uncontrolled, the interpretation of the results is difficult.

Because ACTH and corticosteroid therapy are reported to be the only effective forms of treatment of infantile spasms, it has not been ethically acceptable to carry out a double-blind study. Therefore, we designed a study in which patients served as their own controls in order to determine the effectiveness of prednisone in the treatment of infantile spasms.

METHODS

During this study, patients were monitored repeatedly, using a time-synchronized polygraphic and video system (Frost et al., 1978), each session lasting 24 hr. A rigid protocol of treatment and monitoring sequencing was used as follows: Each patient was monitored prior to the institution of prednisone, to establish a baseline seizure frequency (i.e., number of ictal events per 24 hr). After the baseline recording was obtained, prednisone (2 mg/kg/day) was administered for 4 weeks; the patient was remonitored at the end of each 2-week interval. If the patient showed no objective improvement after this initial 4 weeks of treatment, i.e., had less than 50% reduction in seizure frequency compared with the baseline study, he was excluded from further monitoring studies, and the prednisone dose was tapered to zero over 4 weeks. Those patients showing improvement, i.e., a greater than 50% reduction in seizure frequency were continued in the study. Prednisone was maintained at 2 mg/kg/day for 2 more weeks (6 weeks total), reduced to 1 mg/kg/day for an additional 12-week period, and finally tapered to zero over a final 4-week interval. Monitoring sessions were scheduled approximately every 4 weeks during this treatment period and at 1 month after termination of therapy.

RESULTS

Ten patients, not previously treated with ACTH or prednisone, have been studied to date (Table 1). The ages of the patients at the time of their entrance into the study varied from 4 to 12 months, with a mean of 7.1 months. Treatment lag (the length of time from onset of infantile spasms to initiation of prednisone) varied from 1 to 24 weeks, with a mean of 8 weeks. Initially, all patients demonstrated a modified hypsarhythmic EEG pattern. Two of the patients showed "normalization" of the EEG and cessation of their seizures after institution of therapy: Patient II-5 (cryptogenic) within 2 weeks after onset of treatment, and patient II-1 (symptomatic) after 4 weeks. Both patients have been followed for more than 1 year and have shown no relapse. The remaining patients showed no change in the EEG nor improvement in seizure frequency while being treated with prednisone.

OBSERVATIONS AND DISCUSSION

The number of patients with infantile spasms who improve on prednisone is small. Steroid treatment has been reported to control infantile spasms in 60 to 70% of cases (Crowther, 1964; Harris, 1964; Jeavons and Bower, 1964). These studies were, for the most part, uncontrolled, and there were variations in dosage and duration of treatment between studies. In contrast, in our controlled study, only 20% of the patients improved while receiving prednisone. We believe these differences may be explained by the different methods of seizure detection used in our study compared with earlier ones. Studies in the past have relied heavily on parental observation to determine seizure frequency.

By comparing parental estimation of seizure frequency to the number of seizures documented by our comprehensive monitoring system, it is evident that parents grossly underestimate the number of seizures a patient is experiencing. For example, it was not uncommon in our study to have parents state that their child was having one to two seizures per day, only to discover after monitoring the patient for 24 hr that he was having 100 to 200 seizures per day. Thus, without an objective means of evaluation, it is not possible to determine whether or not a patient has improved in regard to seizure frequency.

In addition, since the natural history of this disorder is poorly understood,

TABLE 1. *Results from infantile spasm patients treated with prednisone*

Patient	Chronological age (months)[a]	Developmental age (months)[a]	Treatment lag (weeks)[b]	Etiology	Seizure Frequency/24 hr Weeks		
					Baseline	2 Weeks after prednisone	4 Weeks after prednisone
II-1	7	5	24	Tuberous sclerosis	187	94	0
II-2	5	2	1	Unknown	7	191	41
II-3	8	2	8	Downs syndrome	109	226	155
II-4	8	1	4	Premature, meningitis, intracerebral hemorrhage	126	159	265
II-5	6	5	4	Unknown	84	0	0
II-6	7	5	12	Unknown	3	38	29
II-7	8	3	8	Unknown	129	144	149
II-8	4	4	2	Unknown	38	56	69
II-9	6	6	4	Tuberous sclerosis	50	27	104
II-11	12	1	4	Viral meningo-encephalitis	77	77	43

[a]Chronological and developmental ages refer to the ages of the patients at the time prednisone therapy was instituted. Developmental age was determined by utilizing the Denver Developmental Screening Test.
[b]Treatment lag refers to the elapsed time between the onset of infantile spasms and the institution of prednisone therapy.

the possibility that the remissions seen in two of our patients were spontaneous rather than drug-induced cannot be excluded.

Treatment lag appears to be of little significance in determining which patients will improve on prednisone therapy. Some authors (Sorel, 1959; Hellström and Oberger, 1965) stated that patients with a treatment lag of less than 1 month were more likely to respond to steroid therapy. Our results seriously question the validity of this statement. Of the six patients in our study with a treatment lag of 1 month or less; only one (patient II-5) improved while receiving prednisone. The only other patient to improve had a treatment lag of 6 months.

Etiology is of doubtful significance in determining response to steroid therapy. Jeavons and Bower (1964) reported that cryptogenic patients were more likely to respond to steroid treatment than symptomatic patients. Other authors, however, have found no correlation between the two (Millichap and Bickford, 1962). Our study supports the latter premise, in that of the two patients in our study who improved, 1 (II-5) was cryptogenic and 1 (II-1) was symptomatic (tuberous sclerosis).

Developmental status prior to the institution of prednisone therapy may be an important factor in determining which patients will improve. Those patients with normal development or only minimal developmental retardation prior to the onset of infantile spasms reportedly respond more favorably to steroid treatment (Sorel, 1959; Willoughby et al., 1966). The two patients in our study who improved support this premise: Patient II-5 and Patient II-1 had only mild developmental retardation prior to the institution of therapy. None of the patients who demonstrated severe degrees of retardation showed improvement on therapy. As mentioned previously, the natural history of this disorder is not well known; therefore, it is possible that patients with little or no developmental retardation may experience spontaneous remissions more frequently and rapidly than those more severely retarded. Without untreated age-matched controls, it is difficult to determine if the cessation of seizures seen in our two patients was a spontaneous phenomenon or indeed secondary to prednisone.

Clinical relapse, reported to occur commonly in patients with infantile spasms (Pauli et al., 1960; Jeavons and Bower, 1964), has not occurred in our study. The two patients who improved have been followed for well over a year without evidence of relapse.

ACKNOWLEDGMENTS

This study was supported in part by contract NO1-NS-6-2342 and grant NS 11535 from the National Institute of Neurological and Communicative Disorders and Stroke, National Institutes of Health, United States Public Health Service.

REFERENCES

Crowther, D. L. (1964): Infantile spasm: Response of "salaam seizures" to hydrocortisone. *Calif. Med.*, 100:97–102.

Frost, J. D., Jr., Hrachovy, R. A., Kellaway, P., and Zion, T. (1978): Quantitative analysis and characterization of infantile spasms. *Epilepsia*, 19:273–282.

Harris, R. (1964): Some EEG observations in children with infantile spasms treated with ACTH. *Arch. Dis. Child.*, 39:564–570.

Hellström, B., and Oberger, E. (1965): ACTH and corticosteroid treatment of infantile spasms with hypsarhythmia. *Acta Paediatr. Scand.*, 54:180–187.

Jeavons, P. M., and Bower, B. D. (1964): *Infantile Spasms: A Review of the Literature and a Study of 112 Cases. Clinics in Developmental Medicine No. 15.* Spastics Society and Heinemann, London.

Lacy, J. R., and Penry, J. K. (1976): *Infantile Spasms.* Raven Press, New York.

Millichap, J. G., and Bickford, R. G. (1962): Infantile spasms, hypsarhythmia, and mental retardation: Response to corticotropin and its relation to age and etiology in 21 patients. *JAMA*, 182:523–527.

Pauli, L., O'Neil, R., Ybanez, M., and Livingston, S. (1960): Minor motor epilepsy: Treatment with corticotropin (ACTH) and steroid therapy. *JAMA*, 172:1408–1412.

Sorel, L. (1959): Treatment of hypsarhythmia with ACTH. In: *Molecules and Mental Health*, edited by F. A. Gibbs. Lippincott, Philadelphia, pp. 114–120.

Sorel, L., and Dusaucy-Bauloye, A. (1958): A propos de 21 cas d'hypsarhythmie de Gibbs: Son traitement spectaculaire par l'ACTH. *Acta Neurol. Psychiatr. Belg.*, 58:130–141.

Willoughby, J. A., Thurston, D. L., and Holowach, J. (1966): Infantile myoclonic seizures: An evaluation of ACTH and corticosteroid therapy. *J. Pediatr.*, 69:1136–1138.

Advances in Epileptology:
The Xth Epilepsy International Symposium,
edited by J. A. Wada and J. K. Penry.
Raven Press, New York © 1980.

The New Drug Law: How It Will Affect Development and Marketing of Anticonvulsants in the United States

Ronald Kartzinel

Division of Neuropharmacological Drug Products,
Food and Drug Administration,
Rockville, Maryland 20857

On March 16, 1978 the Drug Regulation Reform Act of 1978 was introduced in the United States Senate. This bill revises and reforms the law applicable to drugs for human use, i.e., the Federal Food, Drug and Cosmetic Act of 1936 as amended by the Kefauver-Harris amendments of 1962. It also establishes the National Center for Clinical Pharmacology. This "consensus" bill as it was originally identified, is the culmination of several years of work by the Department of Health Education and Welfare and the health subcommittees of Congress. FDA staff had considerable input into the bill, which was widely circulated in a preliminary form to regulated industry and the American medical community.

The eight major purposes of the Reform Bill are as follows:

1. To strengthen consumer protection
2. To improve consumer information and understanding
3. To encourage drug innovation
4. To make important new drugs available as rapidly as possible
5. To promote greater completion among prescription drug suppliers
6. To increase FDA openness and accountability
7. To improve FDA enforcement capability
8. To focus attention on drug sciences and to encourage research and training

In the last 6 months, extensive testimony has been given before the Health Subcommittees in both the United States Senate and the House of Representatives, which are now considering the bill. Dr. James Ferrindeli, who is currently chairman of the FDA Advisory Committee that deals with anticonvulsant drugs testified on behalf of the Epilepsy Foundation of America. It is not known whether the bill will be enacted into law this session of Congress, and if it is, what changes will be made. In this chapter I will compare and contrast the current FDA Act with the Reform Bill and discuss a few sections that I believe are critical to the development and marketing of anticonvulsants in the United States.

The current law provides the "claimed investigational exemption for a new drug" or IND as the sole means to study all drugs not approved for marketing in the United States. The Reform Bill recognizes three distinct ,types or categories of clinical investigations involving unapproved drugs. First is the "drug innovation investigation" which is intended to examine the clinical pharmacology of an unlicensed drug product in a small number of subjects, or to assess preliminarily its risks and effectiveness. This is truly the experimental phase of drug research development, the first time that a drug is introduced into humans. The objective is generally to determine how the drug functions in the human body and to assess whether there is any value in proceeding into large-scale clinical trials. It is estimated that about 90% of all drugs tested at this point do not proceed to the later development phase, because of a lack of pharmacological activity in humans, undesirable side effects, or other factors that make it undesirable or unnecessary to invest further resources into research with the drug. Under current law, too much of the scientific resources of both industry and FDA are devoted to detailed work on drugs that will be discarded shortly after their first human test. By distinguishing between the stage at which researchers make discoveries about drugs and the stage at which they seek to prove what they have discovered, the bill eliminates unnecessary and wasteful regulations of and delays in the early phase of research.

The second category of clinical investigation is the "drug development investigation." This is the phase of the drug research and development process that provides the evidence of effectiveness perceived for a drug in the innovation investigation (or during clinical trials conducted on a drug outside the United States). It is during this period also that the short-term and relatively common adverse effects of drugs are identified and evidence for assessing the risks of the drug can be gathered. Virtually every drug that enters a drug development investigation will be offered for commercial marketing in the United States, unless its risks turn out to be greater than originally anticipated, its effectiveness less than originally perceived, or commercial interest in the drug declines (because a competitor makes a better product or the cost of development and production will not be justified by forseeable revenues).

The third category of clinical investigation of unapproved drugs involves "a drug treatment investigation" which provides a drug to small numbers of patients with a serious disease, injury, or condition who are not satisfactorily treated by alternative forms of therapy. Use of the unapproved drug is primarily intended to provide treatment of the participants rather than to assess its risks or effectiveness, although information relevant to such an assessment may be derived during the investigation. These investigations are frequently characterized as "compassionate" or "therapeutic" investigations because they involve the use of an investigational drug under circumstances in which benefit to the patient is far more important than obtaining scientific knowledge.

The drug treatment investigation would have been able to handle the situation which developed last year with sodium valproate. Frequently, physicians and patients become aware of a drug under development that cannot as yet be marketed because the adequate and well-controlled studies have not been completed to justify a decision that the drug can be approved for marketing. The drug treatment investigation allows these patients to receive the investigational drug prior to official approval. Alternatively, a drug entity may have been denied approval for commercial marketing, or may be withdrawn from the United States marketplace because of a conclusion that its risk outweighs its benefits. Nevertheless, there may remain a very small group of patients to whom these risks may be acceptable because of unique benefits provided to them by the drug. This situation could be handled under the drug treatment investigation. A drug marketed in another country but not under investigation in the United States could also be made available in the same manner.

The second major area of the Reform Bill to be discussed here is what is known as the "breakthrough" provisions which provide for an accelerated approval of a new drug if certain special requirements are met as follows: (a) the drug is intended for use in a life-threatening or severely disabling disease or injury; the drug offers a major therapeutic advantage to patients with that disease or injury; and the patient population will not be adequately served by distribution of the drug under a drug treatment investigation mentioned earlier. (b) Delaying approval of the drug would present a significantly greater risk to the patients than would approving the drug for marketing. (c) The drug has been assessed for risks. (d) There is significant evidence of the effectiveness of the drug and well-controlled studies of its effectiveness are underway, if they are ethically and methodologically possible. (e) The benefits of provisional approval of the drug truly outweigh the risks for such approval.

The requirement that well-controlled clinical studies of effectiveness be completed and evaluated prior to approval for marketing of all drugs has been the mainstay of public health protection since it was enacted in 1962. That standard is maintained in the Reform Bill for the approval of all drugs except that the requirement is modified by authorizing temporary, "provisional" approval of certain drugs without completion of well-controlled studies in very limited and narrowly defined circumstances. In place of well-controlled studies of effectiveness, the breakthrough drugs would require "significant evidence" of effectiveness which consists of valid and meaningful scientific investigations, including investigations in animals and well-documented clinical experience and clinical investigations (unless such investigations are not feasible due to an absence of methodology or due to ethical proscriptions on such an investigation), on the basis of which it could be fairly and responsibly concluded by experts that the drug would have the effect represented in the informational labeling for the drug. Under this test drugs for which there is little or no scientific evidence of effectiveness could not be approved.

The third new provision of the Reform Bill is the special distribution and dispensing requirements which can be imposed if the risks of the drug are so significant that the product could not otherwise be found to be safe and no other administrative or educational action could make the drug safe for marketing. It is expected that only in rare cases will these conditions be met. These special requirements would not distinguish between physicians on the basis of training and experience or board certification, or between health care delivery facilities unless the secretary specifically determined that this distinction was needed to make the drug safe; the requirement could not be imposed without consultation with an independent advisory committee, and the requirements could only be imposed for three years.

The last provision of the Reform Bill establishes the National Center for Clinical Pharmacology. The Center will be authorized to conduct and support clinical research in pharmacology and clinical pharmacy, including investigations (a) of the safety and effectiveness of existing and new uses of drugs, (b) for the development of drugs for diseases and other conditions of low incidence, (c) of drugs of special significance or with respect to which there is substantial controversy as to the safety and effectiveness for which there have been either no or minimal animal investigations, and (d) that would otherwise facilitate breakthrough in research on drugs. The Center will report to the Secretary of HEW on promising areas of and new techniques in research on drugs and diseases or other conditions for which current research is insufficient. In other words, the National Center for Clinical Pharmacology will be authorized to investigate so-called drugs of limited commercial interest.

In conclusion, the Reform Bill allows much greater flexibility to the Agency, especially in relation to anticonvulsants. Drugs not yet marketed can be made available under a treatment investigation. Significant new drugs can be marketed at an earlier time under the breakthrough provisions. Very toxic drugs can be marketed under the restricted distribution provisions. Drugs of limited commercial interest can be investigated by the National Center for Clinical Pharmacology. Although there is probably no perfect law, the Food and Drug Administration truly hopes that the proposed Drug Regulations Reform Act of 1978 will improve on the current Food, Drug and Cosmetic Act and expedite the development and marketing of anticonvulsant and other drugs in the United States.

Advances in Epileptology:
The Xth Epilepsy International Symposium,
edited by J. A. Wada and J. K. Penry.
Raven Press, New York © 1980.

Canadian Experiences in the Introduction of New Anticonvulsants

H. G. Dunn

Department of Pediatrics,
University of British Columbia,
Vancouver, British Columbia, Canada

Since the thalidomide disaster governments throughout the world have introduced agencies controlling the manufacture, import, and marketing of drugs. In addition to performing the detailed tests required by such agencies the major manufacturers have adopted a more cautious approach to the introduction of new drugs in order to avoid the adverse publicity and possible litigation that might result from inadequate testing. Animal studies and clinical trials have become expensive, and the legal responsibility for possible toxic effects of the drug represents a possible added expense. The cost of developing a new drug appears to have risen from about $3.1 million (Clymer, 1971) to nearly $10 million in the last 7 years.

This increased cost has led to two consequences: (a) Only big pharmaceutical firms (now mostly international corporations) can afford the necessary research funds to develop new drugs. (b) Research is necessarily concentrated on drugs for which there is likely to be a large market. It may be hard to find a firm that will manufacture and distribute a drug for a limited number of patients with a rare disease, the so-called therapeutic orphans.

Canada represents a market for drugs which is said to be about one-tenth of that in the United States and about 5% of the world market, so it is relatively unimportant but not negligible for international pharmaceutical firms. The Health Protection Branch (HPB) of the National Department of Health and Welfare is responsible for the licensing and safety of new drugs and cooperates closely with pharmaceutical firms and with physicians requiring unmarketed drugs for their patients. However, it is not the function of HPB to encourage the import or manufacture of promising new drugs actively. One feature peculiar to Canada is Federal Bill C-102, passed by the House of Commons in March 1969, which lays down that in the case of a patented medicine any person may apply to the Commissioner of Patents for a license to import or make such a medicine,

and, in settling the terms of the licence and fixing the amount of royalty or other consideration payable, the Commissioner shall have regard to the desirability of making the medicine available at the lowest possible price consistent with giving to the patentee due reward for the research leading to the invention and for such other factors as may be prescribed.

After the implementation of this bill reducing patent protection, some 196 compulsory licenses covering about 59 pharmaceutical products were issued to some 24 Canadian companies during the 8 years ending December 31, 1977 (O'Connell, 1978). It seems that the Commissioner for Patents has not received guidelines to determine "due reward" for the research or to consider "other factors" that may be relevant. Evidently all royalties granted with respect to the 196 licenses have invariably been set at 4%. This would seem unfairly low. Compulsory licensing was also in effect in Great Britain, where royalties were frequently set above 15% and ranged as high as 30%, but in 1977 Great Britain reversed her patent policy and eliminated compulsory licensing. Canada is now the only developed country with this policy of compulsory licensing. In a retrospective analysis of the economic impact of Bill C-102 the Pharmaceutical Manufacturers' Association of Canada (1976) maintains that the unfavorable climate created by such legislation has had a considerable negative influence on the growth rate of research and on investment in plant and equipment by the Canadian pharmaceutical manufacturing industry and has led to a dramatic reversal in previously favorable import-export trends of the drug trade.

The introduction of new anticonvulsants into Canada has often been very slow. Sulthiame is not available; carbamazepine and clonazepam were marketed even later than in the United States; nitrazepam is not yet licensed for sale; valproic acid is on the verge of being distributed. In most of these cases the manufacturer did not choose to market the drug, presumably for commercial reasons (Law, 1977).

In general, drugs that have been unavailable in Canada may be classified into two types: (a) those of limited commercial value, e.g., 1-5-hydroxytryptophan for the treatment of postanoxic myoclonus (Such compounds are sometimes obtainable from firms producing chemicals, but it is not strictly permissible to use them as drugs unless approved by HPB.); and (b) those licensed and found useful in other countries but not yet marketed here, e.g., nitrazepam and sodium valproate. In the latter case, there may be several possible commercial reasons:

(a) The drug company may be concerned about the cost of further toxicity tests. (b) The company may plan to market a related compound, e.g., clonazepam instead of nitrazepam. (c) A foreign drug company may spend some time negotiating for a suitable distributor in Canada, where the profit margin may be limited. (d) The firm may have inadequate understanding of federal requirements for the clearance of drugs.

Before the new anticonvulsant is licensed in Canada, it is often made available to investigators. However, there has been a recent trend for pharmaceutical firms to make Canadian investigators pay for such drugs, and this causes administrative problems for physicians trying to retrieve the cost from patients. Sometimes the difficulty has been compounded by customs officers imposing a federal import duty, although this can be reclaimed.

Members of the Committee on Drugs in the Canadian Neurological Society have given considerable thought to the question of how the new anticonvulsants that have been developed in other countries could be introduced into Canada more quickly to the benefit of our epileptic patients. For instance, nitrazepam is still not licensed in the United States or in Canada, although we (Jan et al., 1971) like others have demonstrated its great usefulness in infantile spasms. Since most of the big Canadian pharmaceutical firms are subsidiaries of foreign companies (MacDonald, 1977), the federal government should be involved in negotiations to look after the needs of Canadian consumers. I could envisage useful triangular discussions between government representatives, the Pharmaceutical Manufacturers' Association of Canada (PMAC), and spokesmen of the medical profession in this respect. The following possible courses of action might be considered.

1. The cost of drug testing might perhaps be reduced by improving the predictability and relevance of *in vitro* and animal studies (FDA Committee on Drugs of Limited Commercial Value, 1975).

2. The federal government might share the cost of testing promising new drugs and recover the outlay subsequently from the company's profits. It is true that grants for quality control in the production of new drugs have already been made available by the Department of Industry, Trade, and Commerce. But we could go further and encourage small companies to have new products tested by university laboratories if their own are inadequate. Research grants might be awarded to academic investigators by government agencies in conjunction with pharmaceutical firms to encourage testing of drugs in this country.

3. Government agencies might even participate in organizing trials of new drugs, as is beginning to happen in the United States. At a Workshop on Small Clinical Trials under the auspices of the Medical Research Council (Dinsdale, 1977) the need for special funding of ancillary staff in organized drug studies was mentioned, as well as the shortage of subsidized clinical investigation units and of suitable personnel. The Medical Research Council or other agencies might more actively solicit or even organize trials of anticonvulsants. The legal liability of investigators also has to be considered. The government might share the costs of liability insurance, e.g., the deductible part of the pharmaceutical firm's insurance for injury to patients in the case of drugs of limited commercial value.

4. The government or one of the government-sponsored firms such as ConLabs might keep drugs of limited commercial value in investigational status, support their trials, and even hold a license and maintain a central store for supply to Canadian physicians. If a drug firm is unwilling to market

a useful drug in this country, the government could buy such a medication in bulk from abroad and distribute it through government-supported firms.

5. The fee for introduction of promising new anticonvulsants might be reduced, and/or tax incentives might be provided for firms developing them.

6. Government agencies might improve the information service for pharmaceutical firms and physicians with respect to correct procedures and regulations for the introduction of new anticonvulsants.

7. Ultimately one might wish that the World Health Organization could organize testing of new drugs at such a high standard of competence that all member countries would accept the findings and might cooperate in covering the expenses. This would require negotiations at a high political level. However, it would be advantageous to have international cooperation not only in the early testing of new drugs in animals and in humans but also in the subsequent surveillance of their safety.

It is questionable whether the federal government should create a special unit for the promotion of new drugs (FDA Committee on Drugs of Limited Commercial Value, 1975), but the term health protection may soon have to be interpreted more widely to include *active* participation by the Department of National Health and Welfare in the introduction of new drugs to protect the health of Canadian patients.

SUMMARY

1. The cost of developing new anticonvulsants has risen so markedly that only big pharmaceutical firms (now mostly international corporations) can afford the necessary research funds to develop new drugs without support by governments.

2. In view of this high cost, research is necessarily concentrated on drugs for which there is likely to be a large market, and although some drug firms will produce and distribute a few products without profit in the public interest, it is evident that drugs of limited commercial value are becoming hard to procure, particularly for patients with rare diseases, the so-called therapeutic orphans.

3. In Canada, Bill C-102, passed by the House of Commons in March 1969, revised the Patent Act so as to allow applications for compulsory licences by firms other than the patent holder to manufacture or import a patented drug in order to reduce prices. This appears to have caused a somewhat unfair reduction of profits for research-based companies, and the provisions of the bill should be modified (O'Connell, 1978).

4. Anticonvulsants which have been unavailable in Canada may be classified broadly into two kinds, i.e., those of limited commercial value and those licensed in other countries but not yet marketed here by pharmaceutical firms for commercial reasons.

5. It is suggested that the federal government should not confine its activities to the control of drugs for quality and safety but should take a more active part in encouraging the testing and provision of new useful anticonvulsants. A number of possible methods are suggested to achieve this purpose.

6. Communications between national medical organizations, the Pharmaceutical Manufacturers' Association of Canada, and the Department of National Health and Welfare should be improved with this aim in mind, and triangular discussions might be helpful.

7. Ultimately the World Health Organization might usefully organize the testing and surveillance of new drugs internationally.

REFERENCES

Clymer, H. A. (1971): The economics of drug innovation. In: *Proceedings of Symposium, The Development and Control of New Drug Products*, edited by M. Pernakowski and M. Darrach. Evergreen Press, Vancouver.

Dinsdale, H. B. (1977): *Report to Council on the Workshop on Small Clinical Trials, Ottawa.* Sponsored by the Medical Research Council.

Food and Drug Administration (1975): *Interim Report of the Committee on Drugs of Limited Commercial Value.* Washington, D.C.

House of Commons of Canada (1969): Bill C-102. *An Act to Amend the Patent Act, the Trade Marks Act and the Food and Drugs Act, Ottawa.*

Jan, J. E., Riegel, J. A., Crichton, J. U., and Dunn, H. G. (1971): Nitrazepam in the treatment of epilepsy in childhood. *Can. Med. Assoc. J.*, 104:571–575.

Law, C. (1977): Canada's top drug watchdog. *Med. Post.*, 13:74.

MacDonald, W. K. (1977): The role and responsibility of the pharmaceutical industry. *Can. Med. Assoc. J.*, 116:794–798.

O'Connell, M. (1978): *Improved Policy for the Pharmaceutical Industry in Canada.* Open letter to the Minister of Consumer and Corporate Affairs.

Pharmaceutical Manufacturers' Association of Canada (1976): *A Preliminary Study of the Economic Impact of Present Canadian Patent Law on the Pharmaceutical Industry.*

Abstracts

CINROMIDE: PHASE I TESTING OF A POTENTIAL ANTIEPILEPTIC

G. Cloutier, M. Gabriel, E. Geiger, L. Cook, J. Rogers, W. Cummings, A. Cato
North Carolina

Cinromide, a cinnamamide derivative designated chemically a 3-bromo-N-ethylcinnamamide, is an investigational, broad-spectrum anticonvulsant developed at Burroughs Wellcome Co.

Three Phase I clinical trials have been conducted. The first, an acute dose-tolerance, safety and pharmacokinetics study with placebo control (n=29), revealed that cinromide was safe in the subects (n=31) who received single oral doses of the drug (150mg. to 1500mg.). Mild to moderate drowsiness was reported by the subjects receiving 1200mg — 1500mg of cinromide. In a second study, 600mg. of cinromide given to subjects (n=8) every 6 hours for three doses had no clinically significant effects.

A 28-day oral dose-tolerance and pharmacokinetics study in 16 subjects (with 8 placebo controls) given up to 900 mg q.i.d. indicated that cinromide was generally well tolerated by the majority of subjects. Neurological side effects were seen in 16/16 of the treated subjects at doses of 1800mg/day to 3600 mg/day versus 3/8 of the placebo group. These included drowsiness, dizziness, lightheadedness, nystagmus and ataxia and were consistent with side effects of standard antiepileptics. Two subjects received a lower dose of cinromide (600 mg q.i.d.) because of CNS effects, while three subjects were dropped due to gastric intolerance.

Further evidence of cinromide's safety was a lack of clinically significant physical, vital signs, ECG, ophthalmologic, or laboratory abnormalities. Special tests for pituitary function (FSH/LH) and blood coagulability (PT, PTT, and fibrinogen) revealed no abnormalities.

In each of the studies, basic pharmacokinetic parameters (e.g., Cmax, Cmin, Tmax, T 1/2, and Kel) were determined for cinromide and its major de-ethylated metabolite (BW 432U72).

Statistical and clinical relevance of the dose-tolerance, safety, and pharmacokinetic data has been analyzed.

Results of Phase I clinical testing of cinromide have led to the initiation of efficacy trials in epileptic patients with partial seizures, which are now in progress. Studies in other seizure types are being planned.

ANALYZING SEIZURE DATA — CAN WE DO BETTER?

N. R. Temkin
Seattle

Clinical trials of antiepileptic drugs often use change in seizure frequency as a measure of therapeutic effect. The data are generally summarized by counting the number of patients with specified ranges of change (e.g., fewer seizures on treatment A or at least 30% fewer seizures during treatment than during the baseline period). The analysis consists of comparing the number on each treatment observed in each range to the number expected if the treatment has the same effect as the control. Analyses of this type tend to be inefficient in the sense of requiring extra patients to detect an existing difference with a specified probability at a given significance level.

We develop statistical models of seizure counts based on the experience of patients seen at the Epilepsy Center. More efficient, robust methods for analyzing the seizure data arise from the models.

A CONTROLLED PROSPECTIVE STUDY OF THE USE OF VALPROATE AS AN ANTIEPILEPTIC DRUG

J. J. Cereghino, J. K. Penry, J. T. Brock
Bethesda and New Castle

This single-blind prospective study provides data on efficacy, bioavailability, and safety of valproate (VPA) as a replacement for phenobarbital (PB) when administered with phenytoin (PHT) in up to 30 institutionalized uncontrolled seizure patients.

After pilot studies, two groups of patients participated in 6-week treatment periods with crossover. The treatment periods consisted of either PHT/VPA/placebo for phenobarbital (PLAC PB) or PHT/PB/PLAC VPA. The treatment periods were separated by 7 weeks during which the patients received their usual prestudy dosages of PHT and PB. A 5-week period was allowed to gradually increase VPA or decrease PB and to allow for the long decline in serum concentration of PB.

Nineteen of the 30 patients completed both rotations. For these patients, VPA appeared to be at least as efficacious in the control of seizures as PB and were less sedated.

Complex interactions between VPA and PB or

PHT were observed. In 3 of the 19 patients, it was necessary to increase the PHT dosage to maintain serum concentration above 10μg/ml.

VPA + PHT thus appears to be an effective antiepileptic combination in this population of institutionalized, difficult to control seizure patients.

EXPERIENCE WITH VALPROIC ACID IN PATIENTS WITH INTRACTABLE SEIZURES PREVIOUSLY TREATED WITH STANDARD ANTICONVULSANTS

L. M. Ojemann, A. J. Wilensky
Seattle

Patients with long-standing seizure disorders (of many kinds), refractory to standard anticonvulsants were treated with valproic acid. Valproic acid was added to their already established anticonvulsant program. Follow-up time was from four to eight months. In patients with Generalized Seizures (absence, myoclonic or generalized convulsive) and Generalized Epileptiform Discharges on EEG, two-thirds showed marked improvement (80 to 100% reduction of seizures). One-third were not changed. In patients with Partial Seizures and Generalized Epileptiform Discharges, one-quarter showed marked improvement. One-fourth showed no improvement at all. No patients with Partial Seizures and Focal EEG abnormalities or no Epileptiform Discharges showed definite improvement. Of all patients, 44% showed marked improvement; 31% were not helped and valproic acid was discontinued, and 25% showed no marked improvement, but were continued on the drug.

For those patients who improved, there was an initial response at the end of the first week (at 15mg/kg/day) and another increase in improvement at the end of the first month (after reaching a dose of 30mg/kg/day). Random blood samples were taken for anticonvulsant levels, including valproic acid, and these will be reported. Of note is that all of those who showed marked improvement in seizure control on valproic acid had not responded to Zarontin (ethosuximide). Side effects included transient nausea associated with taking the capsules. Liver enzymes increased slightly in a few patients but not enough to lower the dose. One patient who was also on Mesantoin (mephenytoin) experienced transient light-headedness.

Valproic acid is a safe and effective anticonvulsant in some patients with previously severe, frequent, intractable seizures. Patients with Generalized Seizures and Generalized EEG abnormalities do best but all patients with intractable seizures should be given a trial of valproic acid.

MULTI CENTRIC TRIAL WITH SODIUM VALPROATE ON INDIAN SUBJECTS

V. Virmani, E. Bharucha, J. Abrahm, S. Janaki, M.C. Maheshwari
New Delhi

This is a composite report on Sodium Valproate; a trial by five independent investigators. The selection criteria was (a) patients not responding to adequate doses of two or more anti-convulsant drugs (b) 'Absence' attacks (c) myoclonus (d) 'Absence with myoclonus (e) other generalized epilepsies (f) focal somatomotor or somatosensory, with or without generalized fits (g) psychomotor with generalized fits. The dosage varied from 15 to 60 mg/kg. Best results were obtained in cases of simple 'Absences' and myoclonus. These patients gave excellent response to Sodium Valproate given alone. The merit of this therapy over the conventional anticonvulsants in this group of cases will be discussed. Good to excellent response was seen in 45% of other primary generalised epilepsies. But in this group other anti-convulsant had to be continued. In 30% of cases the other drugs could be reduced but not discontinued. The cases with poor response were psychomotor and focal cortical. Response was particularly poor in patients with brain damage and multifocal epilepsy. The drug was found to have no effects on EEG configuration, nor was there any EEG correlation with the response to Sodium Valproate. The added benefit reported by a minority of patients was cheerfulness and improved mental efficiency. Side effects in the form of gastric irritation mild headache, itching were noted in a few cases. Role of Sodium Valproate in intractable epilepsies and minor epilepsies will be discussed.

EFFECT OF SODIUM VALPROATE ON THE CONTINGENT NEGATIVE VARIATION, REACTION TIME AND THE PHOTOCONVULSIVE LEVEL OF EPILEPTICS

G. F. A. Harding, J. J. Pullan
Birmingham, U.K.

Sodium Valproate has a known beneficial effect on the photoconvulsive range, (Jeavons and Harding, 1975). In this study over 20 patients were investigated prior to commencement of Sodium Valproate therapy or on withdrawal of therapy. In addition, a further group of patients was investigated during therapeutic change of anticonvulsant from or to Valproate.

The amplitude of the contingent negative variation (CNV) and reaction time (RT) were measured simultaneously on 4 sets of trials on each occasion. Patients who were photosensitive also had their photoconvulsive range (PCR) measured. All measures were repeated when the patients were stabilised on their new drug regime or at least 1 month following withdrawal of medication.

The majority of patients show a reduction in the amplitude of the CNV whilst receiving Valproate. Surprisingly, most patients also show a shortening of reaction time whilst receiving the drug. Improvements in Reaction time were not correlated with normalisation of the EEG. The patients initially receiving other anticonvulsants nearly all show a shorter RT when changed to Sodium Valproate.

Changes in CNV are more variable and the value of this measure in relation to behavioural scores will be discussed.

References:

JEAVONS, P.M. and HARDING, G.F.A. 1975,

Photosensitive Epilepsy. Clinics in Developmental Medicine. No. 56 S.I.M.P. London: Heinemann. Philadelphia: Lippincott.

DIPROPYLACETATE TREATMENT OF CHILDREN RELATED TO SERUM LEVELS AND EEG

O. Henriksen, S. I. Johannessen
Sandvika

100 children aged 3 - 16 years were treated with dipropylacetate (DPA). Most of the children had an intractable epilepsy and had been treated with three or more anti-convulsants.

5 patients received DPA as first drug. 31 patients ended up with DPA as the only drug.

46 patients got 75 - 100% reduction of seizure frequency (mean serum level 401 µmol/l).

22 patients got 50 - 75% reduction of seizure frequency (mean serum level 365 µmol/l), while 32 got no change, or less than 50% reduction (mean serum level 346 µmol/l).

21 of the patients on DPA alone became seizure free (mean serum level 423 µmol/l). The patients were monitored with EEG and serum levels of anticonvulsants.

Therapeutic effect was not obtained until the serum level of DPA had been adequate (300-600 µmol/l) for 2 - 4 weeks. Drug interaction often made it impossible to reach therapeutic levels of DPA before other anticonvulsants were withdrawn. Monotherapy with DPA is therefore recommended.

EEG-findings were poorly related to the effect of treatment, but patients with well organized generalized spike and wave complexes most often responded well. DPA should be the drug of choice in patients with absences and regular spike and wave complexes. DPA should also always be tried in patients with myoclonic-astatic seizures, as well as in patients with other intractable seizures. The poorest results are seen in patients with temporal lobe seizures.

SERUM CONCENTRATIONS AND THE CLINICAL USE OF SODIUM VALPROATE

M. Miyakoshi, N. Kakegawa, M. Sagisaka, M. Seino
Shizuoka

Sodium valproate (SV) serum concentrations were determined by means of gaschromatography on 150 adults and 220 children patients with epilepsy under chronic medication to assess 286 and 331 assays, respectively.

Because of rapid absorption and shorter half-life of the compound, the sampling time was set at exactly 2.5 hrs. for in-patients and 3 ± 1 hr for out-patients after the first morning dose.

Although the levels in relation to oral dosage varied to a considerable extent, they increased linearly as a function of dose increment within the range of therapeutic dosage provided the following conditions were followed:

Firstly, when SV was given alone, the concentrations attained a significantly higher level in adults compared to those of young patients under 6 years who were taking a similar dose per body weight, namely, 10-15 mg/kg/day was necessitated in adults to reach 100 µg/ml while 20-25 mg/kg/day for the young patients. Children between 7-15 years fell in between.

Secondly, while SV was maintained but concomitant use of DPH and/or PB was withdrawn, the SV concentration appeared to increase not infrequently. This fact may imply that monopharmacy by SV would be more desirable than polypharmacy when SV was chosen as a primary anti-epileptic drug.

PHARMACOKINETIC OBSERVATIONS OF DIPROPYLACETATE IN CHILDREN

S. I. Johannessen, O. Henriksen
Sandvika

Knowledge of the pharmacokinetic profile of antiepileptic drugs is of importance for a rational drug therapy.

Results of pharmacokinetic studies of dipropylacetate (DPA) in children are reported. A fixed blood sampling time, before ingestion of the morning dose, is of great importance for DPA due to extended fluctuations of the serum levels during dose intervals. The correlation between daily dose (mg/kg) of DPA and steady state serum levels is poor and is also influenced by co-medication of other antiepileptic drugs. An increase of the DPA dose gives an unpredictable increase of the serum level, especially when combined with other drugs.

Interactions of clinical importance were observed between DPA and other anticonvulsants. DPA may increase the serum levels of phenytoin, phenobarbitone and carbamazepine. DPA serum levels are even more influenced by phenytoin, phenobarbitone and carbamazepine. A twofold increase is often seen. Thus, it is often impossible to reach therapeutic serum levels of DPA (300 - 600 µmol/l) until these other drugs are withdrawn.

After withdrawal of DPA in 3 children a half-life of about 12 hours was observed.

Serum level monitoring of antiepileptic drugs is essential when using DPA.

FURTHER PHARMACOKINETIC OBSERVATIONS ON THE INTERACTION BETWEEN PHENOBARBITAL AND VALPROIC ACID IN EPILEPTIC PATIENTS

P. Loiseau, J. M. Orgogozo, B. Cenraud,
A. Brachet-Liermain
Bordeaux

P. L. Morselli
Paris

It is today generally accepted that, in patients undergoing chronic treatment with Phenobarbital (PB), the association of Valproic Acid (di-n-propylacetate=DPA) to the therapeutic regimen may lead to a significant rise in PB plasma levels. The kinetic mechanism underlying such an interaction is still poorly understood. A rise in plasma PB concentrations could in fact derive from: an increased bioavailability of PB; a reduced volume of distribution or a redistribution phenomenon; a reduced metabolic degradation of PB; a reduced urinary excretion of PB. On the basis of the actual knowledge on PB kinetics, the first two hypotheses appear very unlikely. For this reason we decided to evaluate the kinetics of PB plasma disappearance rate as well as the rate of urinary excretion of both PB and p-hydroxy PB (OHPB) in epileptic patients receiving (according to a cross-over design) either PB alone or PB + DPA. In a first series of observations, run on 10 patients, we could demonstrate that the apparent plasma half-life of PB is significantly prolonged by DPA. Mean values were 83 ± 10 hours for PB alone and 105 ± 10 hours for PB + DPA (P 0.005). In a second series of observations, still in progress, we evaluated the urinary excretion of PB and OHPB as well as the OHPB/PB ratios in patients receiving the two treatments PB and PB + DPA. A preliminary evaluation of the first five cases indicates that the amount of PB excreted in urine may either increase or decrease during DPA association. On the contrary, for OHPB, a trend toward a reduction was present. More important, the OHPB/PB appears to be constantly reduced in the case of DPA association (0.51 ± 0.15 for PB alone against 0.35 ± 0.08 for PB + DPA, $p < 0.05$). The data suggest that an inhibition of the hepatic metabolic breakdown of PB may be partially responsible for the rise in PB plasma levels during DPA association. However, due to the particular PKa of PB (7.4) modification of urinary pH, due to DPA, may further complicate the picture both by potentiating or counteracting the metabolic effect.

EFFECT OF SINGLE DOSES OF SODIUM VALPROATE ON SERUM PHENYTOIN CONCENTRATION AND PROTEIN BINDING *IN VIVO*

A Richens and A. Monks
Buckinghamshire

The effect of single oral doses of sodium valproate on steady state serum phenytoin concentrations and plasma protein binding has been studied in six epileptic patients receiving regular phenytoin maintenance therapy. Each patient was studied on two occasions, once during sodium valproate administration and once in the absence of sodium valproate in order to obtain control data. Sodium valporate (as 200 mg Epilim tablets) was administered as a single 800 mg dose at 9.00 h and blood samples were collected at intervals up to 24 h. Mean serum valproic acid concentration reached a peak of 369 ± 32 (SEM) umol/1 two hours after administration. In the presence of valproic acid the mean serum Phenytoin concentration fell from 29.2 to 24.1 umol/1 seven hours after valproate administration whereas on the control day it rose from 31.0 to 34.8 umol/1 at a similar time. The proportion of phenytoin bound to plasma proteins fell from 89.9 ± 0.4 (SEM)% to a minimum of 87.1 ± 0.7 (SEM)% one hour after valproate administration, whereas it remained constant throughout the control day at 89.7 ± 0.1 (SEM)%. Plots of serum valproic acid concentration against

percentage free phenytoin in ten patients were extrapolated linearly to a valproate concentration of 700 umol/1 in order to estimate the change in phenytoin binding at the limits of the therapeutic range of 300-700 umol/1 valproic acid. At the lower limit the percentage of phenytoin unbound rose from 10.1 ± 0.4 (SEM)% to 12.6 ± 0.3 (SEM), & at the upper limit it rose to $15.8 \pm 0.5\%$.

INTERACTION OF VALPROIC ACID WITH OTHER ANTIEPILEPTIC DRUGS

B. J. Wilder, J. Bruni, H. J. Villarreal,
R. M. Thomas, L. J. Willmore, E. J. Hammond
Gainesville

Twenty-five patients with absence seizures and other seizure types were treated with valproic acid for 6 to 10 months to a maximal dose of 17.9 to 62.5 (average 42.7) mg per kg per day. Eleven of 13 patients required a reduction of phenobarbital dose when concurrently treated with valproic acid. This reduction was necessary to prevent sedation and increasing phenobarbital plasma levels. An average dose reduction of 46% resulted in an average plasma phenobarbital decrease of 15%. Ten of 15 patients had decreased phenytoin concentrations during concurrent valproic acid therapy. Three patients required an increase in daily phenytoin dose because of tonic clonic seizure exacerbation. At the end of three months of therapy, average plasma concentration decreased from 16.4 μg/ml to 12.0 μg/ml. Average daily dose was increased from 318 mg to 328 mg. No significant interaction occurred with other antiepileptic drugs.

Lower phenytoin levels have been attributed to valproic acid competition for plasma protein binding sites leading to an increase in free phenytoin which is more readily available for metabolism by liver hydroxylating enzymes. To assess the mechanism responsible for the elevation of phenobarbital, interaction of valproic acid with phenobarbital was studied in adult cats. Plasma levels, renal excretion, and urinary pH were studied to test the hypothesis of interaction at a renal site which might result in decreased phenobarbital excretion.

EFFECT OF VALPROIC ACID ON FREE PHENYTOIN LEVELS IN EPILEPTIC PATIENTS

R. Berchou, R. Lodhi, D. Haidukewych
Detroit

The importance of monitoring the amount of free unbound phenytoin in selected groups of patients particularly those with abnormal kidney or liver function has been emphasized previously, but there has otherwise been little concern in utilizing free phenytoin levels in the clinical management of patients. One hundred consecutive samples obtained from hospitalized patients receiving a variety of chemotherapeutic agents indicated an excellent correlation ($r = .92$) between salivary and serum phenytoin. These results are in agreement with several published studies indicating salivary levels of phenytoin to be one-tenth of those of serum levels. One hundred additional samples were obtained from patients being started on valproic acid. In this group of patients, the salivary to serum phenytoin ratio varied considerably from .1 to .56. In one patient who appeared clinically intoxicated, the serum level was 12.6 μg/ml, but the salivary level 7.0 μg/ml indicating that more than 50% of the patient's phenytoin level was unbound. These data indicate that further studies are needed to determine the effect of valproic acid on free phenytoin during initiation and maintenance of therapy with valproic acid.

THE PHARMACOKINETICS OF CINROMIDE AND AN ACTIVE METABOLITE, N-DEETHYCINRO-MIDE IN THE RHESUS MONKEY

E. A. Lane, R. H. Levy
Seattle

Cinromide or bromo-ethylcinnamamide (BEC) is a new anticonvulsant drug, which has entered Phase I studies and needs to be evaluated in the epileptic monkey model. Becuase its N-deethylated metabolite, bromocinnamamide (BC), also has anticonvulsant activity, the design involved pharmacokinetic studies of both BEC and BC at several dose levels. The drugs were administered intravenously (BEC by constant infusion and BC by single bolus) to a group of five chronically catheterized monkeys. Plasma levels of both drugs were measured by HPLC. A one compartment model adequately described the precursor-successor relationship between BEC and BC. The clearance (TBC) of BEC 6.0 (6.0±2.1 L/hr) was nine times larger than the clearance of BC (0.69±0.11 L/hr). The biological half-life of BC (4.6±0.6 hr) was five times larger than that of BEC (1.0 ±0.1 hr). Twenty to fifty per cent of BEC was metabolized to BC. This study showed that: 1) BEC should not be evaluated pharmacologically without evaluating BC; 2) the low water solubility of BEC, coupled with its large TBC, limits the range of steady state levels of BEC; 3) the pharmacokinetic characteristics of BC make it potentially more useful than BEC.

Supported by NIH Res. Cont. N01-NS-1-2282 and NINCDS Res. Grant No. NS-04053.

EFFECTS OF CHRONIC ROPIZINE ADMINISTRATION ON ELECTRICALLY INDUCED SEIZURES IN THE DOG AND CAT

H. L. Edmonds, Louisville
D. M. Stark, L. G. Stark, Davis

We previously reported the ability of single doses of ropizine (RPZ) to antagonize electrically induced seizures in cats and dogs (Proc. West. Pharmacol. Soc. 17:77, 1974; Epilepsia, in press, 1978). However, to demonstrate potential clinical value as an antiepileptic, a drug must retain its anticonvul-

sant properties after continued administration. Therefore, the threshold voltage for production of electroencephalographic hippocampal afterdischarge was determined in cats and dogs bearing chronically implanted stimulating and recording electrodes. Threshold values for 7 successive days of oral RPZ administration and for 7 days following the last dose (postdrug phase) were compared to the mean value of 7 predrug stimulations by a multivariate analysis of variance. Electrical stimulation of the hippocampus in the cat generally resulted in only mild focal twitching. RPZ (15 mg/kg) raised the seizure threshold (n=7, p <.02) in the cat during the entire drug phase. Postdrug values were significantly less than drug (p <.009) and predrug (p <.03) thresholds. There were no significant day-to-day fluctuations within either the drug or postdrug phases. It is unclear whether the increased seizure susceptibility in the postdrug phase was drug-related or indicative of kindling following many repeated daily electrical stimulations. Electrically induced hippocampal seizures in the Beagle dogs were often violent generalized myoclonic episodes. Several dogs died in the predrug phase, apparently of seizure-related complications. A continuous elevation in EEG seizure threshold was seen during the drug phase in only 1 of 3 dogs receiving a fixed daily dose of RPZ (10mg/kg). By the end of the 7 day drug phase, threshold values had returned to normal in the other 2 dogs. However, RPZ virtually abolished clinical signs of seizure activity throughout the drug phase. Thus, RPZ seemed to cause a dissociation of the EEG and clinical manifestations of epileptiform activity. Since blood levels of RPZ were not determined, it is unclear whether the apparent diminished efficacy (as determined by EEG seizure threshold) in the dog was due to the development of metabolic tolerance or to the seizure kindling phenomenon. (This study was supported, in part, by fellowships to HLW from the Epilepsy Foundation of America and G.D. Searle & Co. The authors wish to thank Dr. K.F. Killam, Jr. for use of his laboratory facilities.)

PLACEBO EFFECTS IN ANTICONVULSANT DRUG TRIALS

D. Adams, R. Masland
New York

To determine the magnitude of the placebo effect in trials of anti-convulsant drugs, we compared seizure frequencies during a control period with those following administration of a placebo in three controlled studies of Sodium Valproate. We also compared response to a placebo with response to Sodium Valproate reported elsewhere in the literature. In a separate study, we have determined that in Absence Epilepsy, reported seizure frequency correlates closely with EEG seizure discharge. The placebo effect is negligible in these studies involving long-standing previously intractable epilepsy.

Comparison of Response to Placebo with Response to Sodium Valproate of Various Seizure Types.

% reduction in frequency	Placebo	% of cases					
	Placebo	Sodium Valproate					
		This Review		Simon & Penry Review			
		Absence	Mixed	Absence	GM	Compl.P	Elementary P
100 - 75	7	77	23	64	53	35	46
74 - 33	20	17	36	23	21	29	35
<33 or worse	73	6	41	12	26	36	19

DOUBLE BLIND STUDY OF THE EFFECTIVENESS OF FLUNARIZINE IN THERAPY-RESISTANT EPILEPSY IN MENTALLY RETARDED CHILDREN

A. C. Declerck
Heeze
A. Wauquier
Beerse

Flunarizine at a dose of 2 x 5 mg daily, was evaluated in 10 mentally retarded girls aged 9 -16 years, some of whom had severe behavioral disturbances; all had a therapy-resistant form of secondary generalized epilepsy, characterized by bilateral spike or polyspike wave complexes. The following parameters were evaluated before and during treatment, and after placebo: behavior, number of clinical fits, abnormal EEG phenomena observed in the routine EEG and its relation to sleep patterns (taken after one night sleep deprivation), visual evoked potentials and serum concentrations of currently taken anti-epilpetics. In order to cancel out observer bias, another group of 10 epileptic children of the same age was treated with placebo. Clinical improvement was found in three patients, epileptic fits disappeared in three others and EEG epileptic phenomena disappeared in four patients. The amplitude of the visual evoked response decreased in three patients. Sleep patterns improved in all patients whether drug- or placebo- treated. There was neither a reliable change nor a correlation between serum concentrations of current antiepileptics and clinical or electro-encephalographic improvement in the flunarizine-treated group. These results suggest that flunarizine would be a useful drug for a number of patients who have both behavioural disturbances and suffer from therapy-resistant secondary generalized epilepsy.

PROBLEMS IN THE INTRODUCTION OF A NEW ANTICONVULSANT, DIPROPYLACETATE, FOR FEBRILE CONVULSIONS

S. J. Wallace, J. A. Smith
Cardiff

121 children with their first febrile convulsion are being studied. Initially 46 were prescribed phenobarbitone 4 - 5 mg/kg/day; 48, dipropylacetate (DPA) 20 - 30 mg/kg/day and 27 no therapy, on a random basis. Information on continuance of therapy is available for 119 children for up to 1 year. The parents of

21 children placed on DPA and 8 children on prescribed phenobarbitone discontinued therapy on their own initiative. (p<0.02). Of those taken off DPA, 4 children were immediately withdrawn from the trial by their parents and in a further 5 cases newness of the drug had been remarked upon by a doctor or dispenser. Of 42 children who had estimations of plasma DPA none was found in 8. In contract, no phenobarbitone was detected in only 1 of 44 children tested. (p < 0.05, Yates correction). For an intermittent illness such as febrile convulsions, parents are more ready to accept a familiar, than an unfamiliar anticonvulsant.

THE EFFICACY OF INTERMITTENT CLONAZEPAM IN THE PREVENTION OF SIMPLE FEBRILE CONVULSIONS

J. Menkes, T. McCann, M. Spencer
Los Angeles

Recurrent febrile convulsions are a common occurrence. Their incidence is not significantly lessened by giving phenobarbital at the onset of fever. Daily phenobarbital, although a good prophylactic, induces major behaviour disorders in a significant proportion of children. Clonazepam, when given orally, enters the human central nervous system within 20 minutes, as shown by EEG changes. The drug should be capable, therefore, of preventing most febrile seizures when given at the onset of fever.

A double blind study has been designed to compare the efficacy of phenobarbital and Clonopin in preventing recurrent febrile convulsions. Children enrolled in the study were aged 6 months to 3 years and had one or more prior febrile convulsions. All patients underwent a neurological and electroencephalographic examination. Clonopin (0.01 mg/kg/ day) or phenobarbital (5 mg/kg/day) were given orally in a single daily dose during subsequent febrile episodes (rectal temperatures 100.5° or above). The current status of the ongoing study will be presented.

PRELIMINARY OBSERVATIONS ON THE EFFECTS OF SL 76002, A NEW GABA AGONIST, IN THE EPILEPTIC PATIENT

A. Baruzzi, P. Pazzaglia
Bologna
P. Loiseau, B. Cenraud
Bordeaux
E. Zarifian, M. Mitchard, P. L. Morselli
Paris

SL 76002, a new GABA agonist, has shown at animal level an interesting anticonvulsant spectrum (in test such as MES, bicuculline, picrotoxin, strichnine and metrazol) together with a very low toxicity (LD ip. 1000 mg/kg; p.o. 3000 mg/kg) and minimal sedative and miorelaxant effects.

In man the compound is well tolerated up to oral doses of 2500 mg and following oral doses of 900-1200 mg peak plasma levels of 800-2000 ng/ml are attained within 2-4 hrs. The apparent plasma T1/2 is of 8-12 hrs. The possible clinical efficacy of SL 76002 has been evaluated in an open study still in progress. Preliminary data refer to 17 epileptic patients suffering from severe seizures not responding to the pharmacological treatment despite "therapeutic AED plasma levels". In all cases SL 76002 was added to the previous treatment at doses ranging from 12 to 25 mg/kg/day. A modification of EEG activity was noticed in all cases. Clinically the drug was without effect at doses of 12-15 mg/kg/day (3 cases) while at doses of 20-25 mg/kg/day a positive reponse (reduction in intensity and frequency of seizures and/or behavioral improvement) was observed in 7 patients suffering from complex partial seizures. In other cases suffering from Lennox Gastaut syndrome (1 case) and generalized seizures (5 cases) the clinical effects were not so evident. On the basis of the severity of the cases included in the study the results appear interesting and their clinical significance will be discussed.

CLINICAL EVALUATION OF ANTIEPILEPTIC ACTIVITY OF 1-GABOB

J. Mukawa, Y. Iwata
Osaka
K. Kobayashi, A. Mori
Okayama

Since 1959 when Hayashi found that 4-amino-3-hydroxybutanoic acid (γ-amino-β-hydrobutyric acid, GABOB) was seizure inhibitory substance in his dog experiment, GABOB has been clinically tested and broadly applied on epileptic patients to control the seizures.

Following our recent basic study indicating the evidence of stronger seizure inhibitory action of 1-GABOB, an optical isomer of GABOB: (3R)-(-)-4-amino-3-hydroxybutanoic acid in comparison with d-GABOB: (3S)-(+)-4-amino-3-hydroxybutanoic acid, this substance was planned to be clinically applied on epileptic patients to evaluate its antiepileptic activity and side-effects. In this paper, recent results of the pilot study will be reported.

1. Twenty patients (4 to 42 years of age) consisting of 11 male and 9 female were given over 400 mg of 1-GABOB (maximum 1200 mg) for a period of over one and half month (maximum 15 months).
2. Seizure inhibitory activity was found in 11 out of 18 patients (61%) with the dosage of over 600 mg. Grand mal and temporal seizures were evidently inhibited.
3. No side-effects in the tests of blood count and liver function, nor aggravating effects to seizures were found.

CLINICAL TRIAL FOR THE ESTIMATION OF ANTICONVULSIVE PROPERTIES AND SIDE REACTIONS OF A NEW DRUG KETOCARBAMAZEPINE

P. V. Rai
Zurich

GP 47 680 a keto-analogue of carbamazepine from the firm Ciba-Geigy has been tried clinically in a collective of about 80 epileptic patients for a period of over 2½ years. This collective consisted of patients mostly with mixed seizures of different etiology, such ones with simple absences and 3/sec. spike-wave activity in EEG were excluded from the trial. Majority of these patients were considered therapy refractory to various anticonvulsive drugs. During the clinical trial regular clinical, electroencephalographical and laboratory controls were done to assess the antiepileptic properties of the drug as well as its side-effects.

At least 50% reduction of seizures could be recorded in over 55% of the patients. The EEG findings showed in general an improvement corresponding to the reduction of seizures. Except in one case of a severely retarded child no considerable side-reactions were noted which necessitated the withdrawal of the drug. In patients previously treated on carbamazepine, its keto-analogue showed considerably better tolerance in a dosage 30 to 50% higher.

PRELIMINARY RESULTS ON THE USE OF INJECTABLE LORAZEPAM IN STATUS EPILEPTICUS

G. Amand and P. Evrard
Brussels

Lorazepam, one of the newer Benzodiazepine derivatives, was given to 31 patients with status epilepticus. Patients ranged in age from 8 days to 78 years; they presented a total of 45 status epilepticus. When given in a rapid IV dose Lorazepam controlled 27 out of 32 status epilepticus in children and six out of eight status epilepticus in adults. The use of slow IV Lorazepam was ineffective and controlled only two out of five status epilepticus. High doses of Lorazepam, in the range of 0.5 mg/Kg can be given without compromising cardiopulmonary function.

TWO NEW ANTICONVULSANT DRUGS WITH PROLONGED ACTION

S. Rump, K. Walczyna, I. Ilczuk
Warsaw

It was stated previously that substitution of ring nitrogen atom in succinimides with amino group increased the duration of anticonvulsant activity (1,2). This observation led to the synthesis of N-amino-bromophenylsuccinimide (IL-16) and N-amino-diphenylhydantoin (IL-40). It was shown that both drugs are of similar acute toxicity as their paternal compounds, e.g. bromophenylsuccinimide (BPhS) or diphenylhydantoin (DPH) respectively. It was also stated that ED_{50} against pentetrazole-induced convulsions and against maximal electroshock seizures (MES) for IL-16, and ED_{50} against MES for IL-40 were very close to those of BPhS or DPH respectively but the durations of activity were longer than those of BPhS and DPH. It was suggested that substitution of ring nitrogen atom in anticonvulsant drugs with amino group decreased their metabolism in the body. This hypothesis was confirmed by analytical studies of the concentration of drugs in plasma.

This work was supported by a grant from the Polish Academy of Sciences in the research project No MR-I-12.2.3.18.

References:

(1) Lange, J., Rump, S., Ilczuk, I., Lapsezewicz, J., Rabsztyn, J., Walczyna, K.: Die Pharmazie 32:579, 1977

(2) Rump, S., Ilczuk, I., Walczyna, K.: Arzneim.-Forsch. (in press)

EXPERIENCE WITH CLOBAZAM AS ANOTHER ANTIEPILEPTIC DRUG

F. Escobedo, E. Otero, H. Chaparro, T. Flores, R. F. Rubio-Donnadieu
Mexico City

Following the personal communication of Dr. Gastaut during the 5th Consultation on Neuroscience organized by the WHO in Florence, April 8-10, 1978, concerning the "exceptional" results he obtained with the Clobazam — from the group of benzodiazepines — as antiepileptic drug in 21 patients with epilepsy, we decided to try a similar survey in a group of patients with different types of epileptic seizures reluctant to conventional medical treatment.

The clinical results are discussed, observing that the therapeutic action begins in a very short period and the best results are obtained when the Clobazam is used at a dose of 0.5 to 1 mgr. per Kg. per day in combination with other anticonvulsant drugs.

The favorable changes in the EEG are presented.

The secondary effects mainly in the aspect of somnolence, sedation and myorelaxation exist but in most of the cases are not very important.

The possible explanation for the pharmacological results are considered probably related to the particular chemical structure which differs partially from that of benzodiazepines and presents certain analogie in part with the diones.

EFFECT OF ROPIZINE ON THE GABAERGIC SYSTEM

D. M. Sylvester
Pullman

H. L. Edmonds
Louisville

M. A. Medina
San Antonio

Our laboratories have previously noted the ability of the experimental anticonvulsant ropizine (RPZ) to antagonize penicillin-induced convulsions (Neuropharm. 13:269, 1974). This antagonism, coupled with a slight, but significant increase in rat whole-brain GABA (Pharmacoloist 17(2):256, 1975) suggested a possible RPZ involvement in the GABAergic system. In the present study adult male albino mice and rats were treated with graded doses of RPZ. Two hours later they were decapitated. Brains were removed within 30 sec and immersed in liquid nitrogen. The activities of whole-brain glutamic acid decarboxylase (GAD) and GABA aminotransferase (GABA-T) and steady-state levels of GABA were determined. RPZ produced dose-related non-significant decreases in GABA levels, while no changes in enzymatic activity were apparent. The study was repeated in mice terminated with focused, high-intensity microwave irradiation (J. Neurochem. 24:223, 1975). Although the magnitude of RPZ-induced GABA decrease was similar in irradiated and frozen brains, the changes were significant only in irradiated animals. Apparently the microwave fixation minimized the variability in whole-brain levels associated with rapid post-mortem change. It is therefore concluded that RPZ decreases whole-brain GABA levels by a mechanism other than inhibition of GAD activity or augmentation of GABA-T activity. Our previously reported RPZ-induced increase in brain GABA appears to be an artifact resulting from a delayed freezing of brain tissue. (This study was supported, in part, by Washington State Initiative 171 Funds.)

| RPZ dose | mouse | | | | rat | |
| | microwave | frozen | | | frozen | |
(mg/kg)	GABA(1)	GAD(2)	GABA	GABA-T(3)	GAD	GABA
saline	2.3±.16	24.4±1.5	1.63±.19	54.1±2.9	18.2±2.2	1.59±.72
5	1.7±.04§	23.7±2.6	1.33±.13	55.7±5.3	17.9±1.9	1.62±.71
15	1.9±.16	24.2±1.1	1.35±.14	57.1±7.1	16.8±1.9	1.74±.51
22.5	----	----	----	----	16.9±2.0	1.46±.28
45	1.8±.08§	25.1±1.5	1.22±.15§	55.7±5.6	17.1±2.4	1.04±.25

(1) μmole $^{14}CO_2$/g wet brain/hr   (2) μmole/g   (3) μmole NADH/g/hr   § $p < .01$

THE LIVER ENZYME INDUCING PROPERTIES OF SODIUM VALPROATE

J. Oxley and A. Richens
London and Chalfont St. Peter

Most of the commonly prescribed antiepileptic drugs are potent inducers of hepatic microsomal enzymes. This property affects the metabolism of other antiepileptic drugs, drugs used for other purposes, hormones and vitamins, and may be responsible for some of the chronic adverse effects of antiepileptic therapy. Sodium valproate has been shown not to induce liver enzymes in rats. The present study was designed to assess this property in man.

Three indirect indices of enzyme induction, plasma antipyrine half-life, serum gamma-glutamyltranspeptidase and urinary D-glucaric acid excretion were measured in eight previously untreated epileptic patients on two occasions (i) before, and (ii) after at least three months' treatment with 600 - 800 mg of sodium valproate daily.

There was no significant change in D-glucaric acid excretion, or antipyrine half-life, but there was a significant rise in serum gamma-glutamyltranspeptidase.

We conclude that sodium valproate causes little, if any, hepatic microsomal enzyme induction in man, but the possibility of an hepatotoxic effect, as indicated by the rise in serum gamma-glutamyltranspeptidase, needs to be examined further.

THE COMPARATIVE EFFECTS OF SINGLE OR MULTIPLE DOSES OF SODIUM VALPROATE ON MOUSE ANTICONVULSANT ACTIVITY, PLASMA AND BRAIN VALPROATE CONCENTRATIONS AND BRAIN GABA

D. S. Walter, S. P. Boardman, E. J. R. Harry, G. M. Howe, S. Lead, M. H. Smith
Hull

Sodium valproate (EPILIM) has been shown to be an effective prophylactic drug for the treatment of epilepsy (1). Its acute anticonvulsant effects in mice, however, are not impressive. Twice daily dosing (5 doses) of sodium valproate (i.p.), however, resulted in a marked improvement in the effectiveness of the drug i.e. against pentylenetetrazol acute (A) $ED_{50}=80$, chronic (C) $ED_{50}=40$; against picrotoxin $A=416$, $C=100$, against bicuculline $A=1100$ (s.c.), $C=270$ (s.c.), against maximal electroshock $A=169$, $C=97$. Mouse plasma levels however were no different at 30 minutes following either a single or twice daily dosing of the drug at 25-400 mg kg $^{-1}$ (i.p.) giving levels of 33-601 μg valproate ml $^{-1}$ plasma (A) or 32-524 μg ml^{-1} (C). Although in mice sodium valproate causes an increase in the brain GABA concentration, no greater increase in whole brain GABA or its duration was observed after the 5th dose compared to that following a single dose. 30 minutes after dosing mice with Na [3-^{14}C] -valproate (i.p.), > 95% of the radioactivity present in mouse brain is as [^{14}C] -valproate, but the brain [^{14}C] concentration does not bear a linear relation to the dose until > 200 mg kg $^{-1}$, (i.p.). Multidosing of Na [3-^{14}C] -valproate results in no greater accumulation of radioactivity compared to a single dose. Thus, no obvious explanation was found for the increase in anticonvulsant activity observed with multidosing of sodium valproate.

Ref. (1) Pinder *et al.*, (1977) Drugs 13, 81-123.

THE INHIBITORY EFFECT OF SODIUM-N-PROPYL ACETATE (VALPROATE) ON THE GLUTAMATE EVOKED FIRINGS IN COBALT-INDUCED EPILEPTIC FOCI OF CAT

I. Koyama
Tokyo
T. Reader
Montreal

Valproate (Depakine) in a relatively new drug useful in the treatment of petit mal seizures. Protection against seizures in experimental animals has been shown to be associated with a significant elevation in the concentration of gamma-aminobutyric acid (GABA), most marked in the cerebellum, as well as a striking decrease in the concentration of cyclic G.M.P. and these changes correlate with protection in experimental seizure test. The elevation of GABA is thought to be secondary to the inhibition of the enzyme involved in its degradation; succinic semi-aldehyde dehydrogenase. We studied the DPA action on the single neurones in cortical focus of cobalt induced semi-acute epileptic brain. DPA application of 0.1-0.2 M. sol. has not an inhibitory effect on the spontaneous discharges, however, the marked inhibitory effect with a competitive fashion on the glutamate-induced firing.

ANTI-CONVULSIVE ACTION OF (3R)-(-)-4-AMINO-3-HYDROXYBUTANOIC ACID (1-GABOB)

A. Mori, Y. Katayama, M. Fujiwara, I. Yokoi
Okayama
M. Kurono
Osaka

Since Hayashi (1959) reported GABOB was able to inhibit various types of focally induced convulsion of the dog, the inhibitory effect of this substance has been studied in various kinds of experimental epilepsy, though the GABOB used in these experiments was racemate.

In the present study, 3 (R)-(-)-4-amino-3-hydroxybutanoic acid (1-GABOB) was prepared from racemic 4-amino-3-hydroxybutanoic acid amide by cystallizing with d-camphor-10-sulfonic acid. mp. 224-225°C (decomp.). [α]^{2}D3-20..71° (C=0.92·H$_2$O. 3(S)-(+)-4-Amino-3-hydroxybutanoic acid (d-GABOB) was prepared by the same way with 1-camphor-10-sulfonic acid. mp. 224-225°C (decomp.). [α] ^{2}D3+20.13 (C=1.165·H$_2$O).

We observed a stronger inhibitory action of 1-GABOB than of d-GABOB on penicillin-induced spike activity of cat cerebral cortex and on N-aminobenzamide-induced seizure activity in cat and mouse. Then, these substances were applied on the giant neurone, identified in the subesophageal ganglia of the african giant snail, and was confirmed 1-GABOB inhibited more strongly the electrical discharge of the neurone than d-GABOB did it.

On the other hand, we determined c-AMP and c-GMP in the mouse brain after i.p. injection with GABOB, and found significantly decreased level of c-GMP in the cerebellum 15 and 30 min. after the injection.

COMPREHENSIVE CARE

Advances in Epileptology:
The Xth Epilepsy International Symposium,
edited by J. A. Wada and J. K. Penry.
Raven Press, New York © 1980.

Comprehensive Care

Yngve Løyning

Statens Center for Epilepsy, 1301 Sandvika, Norway

In formulating plans for dealing with the comprehensive problems connected with epilepsy in the various communities, it is useful to make a distinction between the avoidable and the unavoidable problems.

PRESENT UNAVOIDABLE PROBLEMS

As long as we are unable to prevent the development and unpredictable bursts of epileptic brain activity, the very nature of epileptic seizures is bound to create psychosocial problems and some prejudice and superstition in any society in the world, regardless of its general level of knowledge and understanding. Furthermore, the degree to which a society can utilize its present knowledge of epilepsy in a health care program is limited by its resources and its political possibilities.

Optimism is warranted, however, for a future reduction of the present unavoidable problems. In the foreseeable future, it is probable that the rapidly increasing knowledge of epileptogenesis and pharmacodynamics from *in vivo* and *in vitro* studies of epileptic brain activity will result in more rational medication regimens, leading to a reduction in the number and the severity of seizures and thus in the alleviation of the consequences of having epilepsy.

There is hope also for a continued improvement in attitude, and in health care policy and resource allocation for handicapped persons, although the optimism is sometimes ambiguous.

In many societies, the wave of worldwide awareness and concern about discrimination toward handicapped groups has grown to the extent that health politicians are led to believe that an unrealistically high proportion of the handicapped, including persons with epilepsy, can be completely integrated into society if only our present knowledge of the subject were utilized and if prejudice were eliminated. This enthusiastic notion may in fact reduce the understanding of and the resources allocated to the handicapped in need of frequent or permanent sheltered or custodial care. Furthermore, as it becomes increasingly possible to help all handicapped, sick, and injured persons, a number of unrealistic health care plans have evolved along with a competition for resources that may result in harder times for our comprehensive epilepsy care programs. This requires an analysis of service needs and programs, maximal utilization of resources, services being provided at the lowest effective level of the health care system, and cost-benefit analysis if our clients are not to be a low-status group among the handicapped.

PRESENT AVOIDABLE PROBLEMS

In all societies a great number of the present medical and psychosocial problems connected with epilepsy are clearly avoidable if our present knowledge is fully utilized within the limitations set by local health policy and available resources. We know that globally great achievement is possible in most of the problem fields.

For instance, the very incidence of epilepsy can be substantially reduced worldwide, as evident in the chapter by E. R. Grass (*this volume*). Its prevalence can be reduced on an individual scale by operating as early as possible on all patients who fit generally accepted selection criteria. We are painfully aware of how the number and the severity of seizures and the consequences of having epilepsy can be reduced by earlier and correct diagnosis, information, and management, and by proper follow-up controls with reliable drug serum level determinations. Furthermore, the positive results of intensive observation and treatment in specialized institutions of patients with previously intractable seizures, psychological handicaps, and functional impairment are well documented, as is the fact that these positive results are easily jeopardized by improper follow-up of the discharged patient when he returns to his former environment. We have long been aware of the deleterious effects of subclinical epileptogenic activity, and, as we now are able to quantify them, it is possible to study how the total epileptogenic brain activity should be treated if, indeed, treatment is necessary. However, we are overdue in clarifying the long-term, or permanent, negative side effects of our effective therapeutic measures, including medication, surgery, and institutionalization. Even highly developed societies contain a certain degree of prejudice and superstition, resulting in serious problems for persons with epilepsy. However, much of it is due to ignorance and is thus possible to overcome.

In solving these problems all societies depend on the joint efforts of professionals, of lay organizations, and of the patients themselves. Probably the most expedient way to obtain the optimal epilepsy service each community can afford is to realistically inform both patients and the public alike of what is possible to achieve.

UNIVERSAL STRATEGIES AND ELEMENTS OF CARE

Although a universally applicable comprehensive care program is an utopianism, it should be a goal to establish generally accepted strategies for and basic elements in a comprehensive care system to back the struggle for understanding and resources in our respective communities.

A widely accepted strategy is that of having a program of comprehensive care adopted within the general system of health care. Such a program should coordinate and stimulate the efforts to establish multidisciplinary diagnostic assessment and management, training and education of medical and allied personnel for the necessary team work, a program of public education, and the initiation of research into diagnosis, treatment, prognosis, and prevention of epilepsy.

The possibilities of obtaining a comprehensive epilepsy care system vary immensely, as the chapter by Jilek-Aall et al. (*this volume*) indicates. Of the many systems described from countries with a relatively well developed general health care policy, one model that emerges as a compromise for widespread application contains the following elements: (a) Central service for both inpatients and outpatients in regional comprehensive centers connected to university hospitals. The center should have beds for short- and long-term observation and treatment localized in the regional hospital and in a close-by residential unit, respectively. (b) District service, preferably as part of the neurological, pediatric, and social-medical inpatient and outpatient service in the district hospital. A close cooperation should exist with the regional center to obtain the required special services, supervision, guidelines, and visits. (c) Local service should be available from general practitioners, neurologists, and pediatricians in private practice. (d) Visiting service to patients with epilepsy in institutions of different kinds should be available from single professionals or teams from the regional center.

EPILEPSY CARE IN NORWAY

Assuming that some of the Norwegian experiences would be of interest to others, I shall present our system of comprehensive care within the general system of health care, and an analysis of service needs we are conducting at present for further development of the epilepsy care.

The structure of our epilepsy care contains the four elements in the model just described. We have one National Epilepsy Center located in Sandvika, just outside Oslo. It has 164 beds in pavilions for long-term observation and treatment, laboratories for intensive monitoring and routine examination, sections for vocational observation and training and for occupational therapy and physiotherapy, a dental clinic, a school for children, rooming-in facilities for dependants, and a multi-professional staff of about 200. In connection with the center, there is an 18-bed unit in the department of neurology at Oslo University Hospital, for short-term observation and treatment of epilepsy and similar cerebral dysfunctions. The center supervises two affiliated homes for 68 chronic cases, and extends some, but far too little, service to institutions of various kinds.

The activity at the center also includes selection of patients for surgical treatment, studies of drug kinetics and effects on quantified clinical and subclinical epileptogenic activity and cerebral performance, and education of health professionals, patients, parents, and lay people.

At the European Symposium on Epilepsy in Amsterdam in 1971, the former director of the Center, Dr. Georg F. Henriksen, described its role in epilepsy care in Norway and presented the plans adopted by the Storting (Parliament) in 1970 for the further development of epilepsy care (Henriksen, 1972). According to the plans, regional comprehensive care centers should be established also at the other three university hospitals in Bergen, Trondheim, and Tromsø. The existing center should expand to 308 beds with a staff of 343.

Since then, the situation has changed. The general health system has been reorganized, and the primary services for persons with epilepsy have improved throughout the country with somewhat less demand on beds at the Epilepsy Center. On the other hand, improvements within diagnostics and management of epilepsy have increased the demand for specialized services within these fields for inpatients and outpatients. The enormous increase in possibilities and the resulting demand for improved health services in general has led to the absurd situation that a realization of all the regional health plans during the 1980s would burst the national budget and absorb the majority of available manpower. As a result, the government has practically stopped the allocation of more health personnel and of other resources, and is demanding better analysis of the needs and new realistic plans. In this climate the three other university hospitals are trying to establish their regional epilepsy centers.

Considering this background, we have found it necessary to analyze the different service needs to make a comprehensive care program that fits into the new general health system. I shall describe briefly the system and the analysis.

THE GENERAL HEALTH CARE SYSTEM

Our elongated country with an area equal to that of the British Isles and a population of merely 4 million, has a relatively high standard of living and of health services. The health services are mainly public, but some service is also given by health professionals in private practice.

Professional services and medicine for chronic disorders, including epilepsy, are covered by The National Insurance Scheme which, with a few exceptions, takes care of all persons domiciled in the country.

In 1975, it was decided that the public services were to be organized according to a regionalization principle, and on the principle that the services should be given to each patient at the lowest effective care level. The country was divided into five health regions, in which the health services were to be structured into three main levels:

1. *District health services*, which shall take care of the great majority of the population's health problems and include small institutions and homes for various needs.

2. *County health services*, which include specialized medical services to hospitalized or nonhospitalized patients. The county hospitals shall be of two types: type 1, which will provide all medical specialities and include psychiatric hospitals and clinics, central institutions for the mentally handicapped, and most types of small, somatic specialty hospitals; and type 2, which will provide the basic specialities in sparsely populated areas.

3. *Regional health services*, which are neither rational nor justifiable to establish in each county. Included are special institutions for patients with epilepsy and for other types of neurological disorders. Five regional hospitals are connected to the universities, and in Tromsø, Trondheim, and Bergen, and two in Oslo. They will be owned by their counties and will function also as a county hospital type 1, and they will divide between them the "national functions," which require so many resources and expertise that they should be concentrated in one or two departments serving the whole country.

A principle in this new health plan is the distribution and decentralization of responsibility by providing greater local freedom. Epilepsy care professionals fear that in the struggle for resources and understanding at the local level, epilepsy care might get a lower priority than in the past. However, to ensure even distribution of hospital services, all health plans, including building plans and staffing, must be approved by the Director-General of the Health Services.

ANALYSIS OF NEED FOR COMPREHENSIVE EPILEPSY SERVICES

The aim of our analysis of service needs is to provide data for a proper dimensioning of the different services when they are to be given at the lowest effective level within this regionalized general health system. A report of the analysis that is being conducted by myself in collaboration with Drs. Georg F. Hendriksen, Wollert Krohn, Knut Wester, and psychologist Arne Sletmo, will be published in the future. In this context it is the type of design and obtainable results that are pertinent.

The data were sampled as follows: (a) in a region with a highly developed health care system, (b) in all institutions for the mentally retarded in the country, and (c) in the psychiatric institution in the region.

The regional analysis was done in the southeast triangular tip of Norway which borders on Sweden and the sea. The region is part of a county and consists of 12 municipalities with a population in 1975 of 140,658 inhabitants, 69,000 of whom lived in three towns and the remainder in suburban and rural areas.

This region has a fairly stable population, is relatively self-contained in employment, and has a comprehensive health service apparatus (available to persons with epilepsy), which has developed to a standard considered to be a goal for all counties in the country.

A questionnaire with 84 pretested questions was sent to persons with epilepsy over 15 years of age who were refunded expenses for their anti-epileptics in 1975, assuming that patients on medication would constitute the majority of those in need of comprehensive care. The questions were designed to give us the relevant information about the patients' epilepsy, its psychosocial consequences, the extent and effect to which the regional health apparatus and our National Epilepsy Center had been utilized, and the types and degrees of possible unsatisfied care needs. The data were treated by a computer and confidentiality secured.

The response was satisfactory, as 84% of the 535 persons suspected of having epilepsy returned the questionnaire, 27 persons had no wish to participate, and 66 persons did not have epilepsy. After screening, the patients consisted of 366 adolescents and adults on medication, i.e., 2.6/1,000 of the population. The data are being checked, validated, and confirmed by information from hospital records and laboratory data.

The results appear to be satisfactorily useful for the purpose. The need for existing local and central apparatus for diagnosis and management of the epilepsy is well documented, and the different elements of it seem reasonably well dimensioned for the medical problems. It is, however, clearly underdimensioned for some of the psychosocial problems that appear to be unreasonably great compared with the severity of the epilepsies: 50% receive social benefits, and only 50% of the men and 25% of the women are employed, compared with 77% and 49% respectively in the total population. Among the unemployed there is a great desire for training, rehabilitation, and sheltered employment. The data support the belief that individual and national socioeconomic consequences would greatly diminish if society to a greater extent were to accept the less resourceful individuals for rehabilitation and for sheltered and ordinary employment.

Generally it is evident that the different elements of the service apparatus are not fully utilized according to need and capacity, neither by the patients nor by the health personnel. There is an obvious need for closer cooperation between local and central epilepsy service organizations.

The analysis in institutions for mentally retarded is based on a questionnaire filled out for each client with epilepsy. Responses from institutions covering 5,455 of a total of 5,615 beds show that about 21% of the clients have recognized epilepsy. About 12% of those had been free of seizures for the last 5 years, but a great number of the rest had severe epilepsies with frequent grand mal seizures, 6% in series, and as status epilepticus in the last year. Nearly 50% had not been seen by a specialist during the last year nor had their blood level of drugs been tested; when tested, 18 to 50% had levels outside the therapeutic levels. The personnel feels that 40% need service from an epileptologist. The service needed should be given partly at a specific unit in the Epilepsy Center, and partly by regular visits from the center to the institutions. We all know that great improvements in seizure control may be obtained by such simple measures as improved seizure observation and recording, and drug adjustments according to routine level testing.

The analysis in the psychiatric institutions in the region revealed somewhat similar conditions as in institutions for the mentally retarded. The service needed should be given within these institutions by visiting neurologists and/or epileptologists.

The analysis in general strongly supports the importance of having a program adopted for coordination and stimulation of the multitudes of services and efforts by professionals, lay organizations, and the patients themselves.

I am certain that the following section, which explores the multiple facets of needed care, will provide us with practical and inspiring information in our struggle to ensure a realization of the potential and promotion of a healthy lifestyle for individuals with epilepsy.

REFERENCES

Henriksen, G. F. (1972): The role of special centres in the care of epileptics in Norway. *Epilepsia (Amst.)*, 13:199–204.

Advances in Epileptology:
The Xth Epilepsy International Symposium,
edited by J. A. Wada and J. K. Penry.
Raven Press, New York © 1980.

Prevention of Epilepsy Worldwide

Ellen R. Grass

Grass Instrument Company, Quincy, Massachusetts 02169

Why is prevention of epilepsy important? It is doubtful that in the 20th century a universal, useful "cure" for epilepsy will be discovered, as in the case of the Salk vaccine for poliomyelitis, or the antibiotic that has essentially wiped out tuberculosis. Each has been essentially eliminated medically in our lifetime by a single medicine, simple and affordable enough to be universally used. In both cases the responsible etiological agent was a singular one, capable of inactivation by a single antagonist.

But epilepsy is not like poliomyelitis or tuberculosis. It is *multiple* in etiology. And, because each of the contributory factors it requires a different strategy for control, it is therefore illogical to expect any single universal cure for epilepsy.

Similarly, multiple etiologies require multiple strategies for the prevention of epilepsy and its consequences. Meanwhile, the intolerable cost, as was alluded to in the chapter by Løyning (*this volume*), in both human suffering and the enormous economic burden for therapy and rehabilitation continue.

In medieval times, epilepsy was believed to be due to possession by an evil spirit. We have progressed since, but to what extent? What is the magnitude of our responsibility now and in the future as compassionate medical and lay persons?

In 1950, the world population was 2.5 billion persons. By the turn of the century, the World Health Organization estimates that the world population will reach 6 billion. If, simply for convenience, one assumes a 1% prevalence rate, that means there are about 42 million persons with epilepsy now, and that there will be some 60 million by the turn of the century—more than double the number there were in 1950.

The medical manpower, the physical facilities, or the financial means to give even rudimentary care to a fraction of that number worldwide are not available. Furthermore, there are far more life-threatening problems competing for the same health manpower and dollars.

The inescapable conclusion is that we must devote more of our energies to the prevention of epilepsy.

This brings us to the question of what is meant by prevention.

Primary prevention is avoidance of a disorder altogether by a specific course of action, essentially reducing incidence. Primary prevention is possible only when the etiology is known.

Secondary prevention is reduction by therapeutic means of the severity of a disorder. The action takes place after the disorder commences. Secondary prevention, however, is possible even when the etiology is not known.

In contrast, *prophylaxis* is the administration of medicine when there is credible evidence that medicine may prevent the reasonably certain development of a disorder.

In the case of epilepsy, an example of primary prevention is action to reduce the number of persons suffering serious head injuries—a predictable number of whom will develop posttraumatic epilepsy.

An example of secondary prevention is the use of sodium valproate or other anticonvulsants to reduce the number and/or the severity of seizures.

An example of prophylaxis in epilepsy is the use of phenobarbital or other agents after a serious head injury with the objective of preventing subsequent seizures. This is currently a controversial practice.

Although a number of chapters in this volume present new ways of secondary prevention, and potential guidelines directed to prophylaxis, only few discuss means of primary prevention.

In the case of epilepsy, there is a unique primary and secondary preventive strategy for each of the multiple etiological factors and for some, prophylaxis is possible. A positive etiology for epilepsy can be established in less than one-half the cases, despite fully documented case histories and exhaustive diagnostic procedures.

It is not my intent either to present or evaluate the statistical data on posttraumatic epilepsy, perinatal influences, or infections. The Epilepsy Commission (1977) has devoted considerable time, money, and expertise in preparing a four-volume report, including such material. The report is available free for study.

Bergamini's (1977) very careful study reports that the cause of epilepsy can be identified in only 44% of patients. Therefore, primary prevention can be specifically targeted to only that group.

Can we hope then to achieve anything by primary prevention? The answer is a resounding yes. We will deal with three examples: epilepsy acquired as a consequence of head injury, perinatal care, and immunization.

Everyone is susceptible to posttraumatic epilepsy.

What is the magnitude of the association between head injury and epilepsy? One can start with a group of persons with epilepsy and look for the number whose seizures may be attributable to head injury. About one-third of patients for whom the etiology is established have seizures acquired as a result of head injury.

One can study retrospectively how many persons with well described head injuries subsequently developed seizures. Preliminary results (Annegers, 1978) show that the incidence of head injury is 286 per 100,000 for males and less than one-half that number, or 115, for females. Of the nearly 3,000 head-injured persons who qualified for the study, about 5% developed seizures, about equally divided between early and late onset.

The brain is injured in many different ways. The geography, the economy, nutrition, living conditions, customs, and modes of transportation differ widely throughout the world. But all of the following factors are universal:

Accidents involving moving vehicles. The person hurt can be the driver, a passenger, people in the other car, or pedestrians. This category includes anything that moves dangerously such as motorcycles, bicycles, skateboards, even horses and elephants!

Falls from high places, that is, accidents while working. These involve machinery that strikes the head, or that causes the person to fall and injure himself, and injuries due to farm machinery.

Injuries from sports, professional and amateur. The most frequent offenders are boxing, football, and ice hockey.

Violence. In this category fall mass violence such as both declared and undeclared war, smaller skirmishes on our streets, person-to-person violence, and suicide. All are inexcusable and preventable.

An example of preventable head injuries relates to those incurred by persons who drive motorcycles. The data are from the United States (U.S. News and World Report, 1978), but the problem is a relatively common one because motorcycles are a rather universal mode of transportation throughout the world. They involve death, serious injury, and consequently posttraumatic epilepsy.

From 1963 to 1966, when protective helmets were not required by law, there were 11.5 deaths for each 10,000 registered motorcycles. In the following 9 years during which the majority of the 50 states required protective helmets to be worn, the rate dropped steadily to one-half this number. However, in early 1976, when states began repealing helmet legislation, the death rate rose sharply again to eight deaths for each 10,000 registered motorcyclists. In 1977 over 4,000 persons died, the majority young males. The most common argument for repealing the helmet law has been that of individual rights. It is argued that the individual has the right to decide for himself whether he wants to wear a helmet. The premise is that if a person is killed because he does not wear a helmet, it is his choice.

A Massachusetts judge stated,

From the moment of injury society picks up the person from the highway; delivers him to a local hospital and doctors for which we pay; provides him with unemployment compensation if he is unable to work; and if the injury causes permanent disability, assumes responsibility for him and his family's continued subsistence. We do not understand the state of mind that permits plaintiff to think that only himself is concerned.

Prevention of posttraumatic epilepsy can be accomplished by preventing accidents that injure the brain. Complicated government programs, complex organizations, large sums of money, computers, microprocessors, or CT scans are not as important here as prevention of injury by irresponsible behavior and unsafe practices. It is also important that governments act in the best interests of preventing epilepsy, especially in areas related to highway and industrial safety.

Avoiding injury to the brain is one of the very important altruistic, compassionate, low-cost courtesies we can extend to each other.

Secondary prevention in posttraumatic epilepsy is achieved by the use of anticonvulsant drugs and surgery. However, there is little secure knowledge of why head trauma sometimes results in epilepsy. Recent basic research with animal models is providing some provocative clues (Ramsay et al., 1977: Hammond et al., 1978). When venous blood of a cat is introduced onto its own cortical surface at the upper end of the marginal gyrus near the Sylvian fissure, EEG changes, minimal during the first few months, develop into full spike foci about 9 months later, accompanied by observable clinical seizures.

What factor in the blood is responsible? It is reported that both ferrous and ferric chlorides cause similar EEG and clinical seizures when injected supially. The author states,

> A chronic epileptic focus can now be induced by quantitative chemical means that reflect the events considered possible after head injury and cerebral infarct. . . Recurrent epileptiform discharges caused by cortical injection of iron salts suggest that the development of human post-traumatic epilepsy may depend in part on the neurochemical alterations induced by metallic ions found in whole blood.

This series of experiments still leaves uncertain the precise responsible agents in blood that produce the electrical and behavioral seizure-like activity. Future reports may contribute to an understandable rationale for more effective secondary prevention of posttraumatic epilepsy.

Recent work by Dennis Feeney and Earl Walker (1977) permits computerized prediction of human posttraumatic epilepsy. They studied carefully the published data from eight series of studies, about 1,100 cases, and they entered into the computer, both for those who developed epilepsy and those who did not, data with respect to the causative agents. The computer then determined the factors that bore higher risk than others: injury in the central parietal area, penetration of the dura by either a bone fragment or a missile, the presence of hemiplegia, hemiparesis or aphasia, and the occurrence of hemorrhage. Feeny and Walker state:

> Simple mathematical equations which can be used to estimate the probability of post-traumatic seizures are described. The equations give results that predict with approximately 95% confidence the chances of post-traumatic epilepsy for group data as well as single cases.

Such work leads to more certain prophylactic strategies.

A second preventive strategy in the area of primary prevention is the reduction of insults to the immature central nervous system by improved perinatal care, including programs of immunization and vaccination.

The chapter by Masland (*this volume*) emphasized the enormous importance of high standards of perinatal care. Improvements in perinatal care not only reduce the incidence of epilepsy, but a host of other associated disorders of the central nervous system (CNS). In these efforts, we have common cause with many others in the medical and public health community. Estimates of epilepsy resulting from perinatal injuries range from 15 to 30%. Bergamini (1977) has said: "Such data enhance the possibility that many cases of epilepsy can be prevented."

The Epilepsy Commission staff (1977) states:

> The same factors responsible for the brain injury that may subsequently lead to epilepsy are also causative factors in other neurological conditions, such as cerebral palsy and the organic forms of mental retardation. The preventive measures applicable to one of these conditions are also applicable to the others. They are all dependent on the level of maternal and child health care provided. There are few national objectives which should have higher priority.

Use of the means now available for prevention of perinatal problems could bring about a significant reduction in CNS crippling. These improvements will not materialize without determination on the part of individuals in their home communities.

International attention should be given to better control of infections of the CNS, including those that invade the brain itself (encephalitis), and those that primarily attack the brain coverings (meningitis). The offending organisms are both bacterial and viral. Childhood infections rank third among the known causes of symptomatic epilepsy. In spite of available vaccines, epidemics of these preventable diseases are still occurring. Thirty-five percent of children in the United States were inadequately vaccinated in 1974, and only 5% of the poor urban and rural children were protected. This is unpardonable for, generally speaking, such vaccination programs are available at no charge.

Again it is an individual responsibility. Parents must care enough to bring their children to the physician or clinic. Physicians must insist that they do. Health officials should not permit children to start school until there is evidence of satisfactory vaccination. Lists of the recommended vaccines and other agents are available.

Amil Gotschlich reports 20,000 cases of bacterial meningitis (Epilepsy Commission, 1977). One in 200 newborn infants in the United States will experience neonatal meningitis, and one in 430 will not be normal afterward. The mortality rate is 40% and one-half of the survivors have some type of neurological deficit. Twenty-eight percent of the survivors need treatment for seizures. In developing countries, the rates are even more alarming.

Antibiotics reduce the mortality but not the morbidity. The bacteria involved are all of the encapsulated types. Special research has been yielding very useful information about their control.

Certainly primary prevention should include strenuous efforts to make sure that children are properly immunized. Additionally, the research toward developing better vaccines should be strongly supported.

It is true that we do not know all the potential ways to prevent people from getting epilepsy in the first place, or of limiting its devastation, but we do know many quite useful and effective ways to bring this about. With time, more information will be discovered. However, as Løyning (*this volume*) stated, we are not taking full advantage of what is known.

It is everyone's responsibility to help reduce the epileptic population to well under the predicted 60 million at the turn of the century.

REFERENCES

Annegers, J. F. (1978): The epidemiology of head trauma and post-traumatic epilepsy and EEG findings in head trauma—A preliminary study. In: *Central EEG Society Meeting*, Omaha, Nebraska, May 19.

Bergamini, L., Bergamasco, B., Benna, P., and Gilli, M. (1977): Acquired etiological factors in 1,785 epileptic subjects: Clinical anamnestic research. *Epilepsia*, 18:4.

Epilepsy Commission (1977): *Plan for Nationwide Action on Epilepsy, A Report of the Commission for the Control of Epilepsy and its Consequences.* DHEW Publication 78-276 (Four volumes. Obtainable from the Office of Scientific and Health Reports, Room 8A08, Building 31, NINCDS-NIH, Bethesda, Maryland 20014 at no charge. Head Trauma, Post Traumatic Epilepsy and their Prevention are discussed in Vol. 1, Sect. IV, 23–38; Vol. II, Sect. 111A, 122–123; Vol. II, Part 1, Sect 111A and B, 245–253, followed by reference, 254–255).

Feeney, D. M., and Walker, A. Earl (1977): The prediction of post-traumatic epilepsy: A mathematical approach. (*in press*.).

Hammond, E., Ramsay, R. E., Villareal, H., and Wilder, B. J. (1978): Blood Induced epileptogenesis: Effects of various blood components. In: *American EEG Society Meeting*, San Francisco. Abstr.

Ramsay, R. E., Hammond, E., Wilder, B. J., and Willmore, L. J. (1977): Blood induced epileptogenesis: A physiologic model of epilepsy. *Personal communication.*

U.S. News and World Report (1978): Sept. 4, pp. 35–36.

Advances in Epileptology:
The Xth Epilepsy International Symposium,
edited by J. A. Wada and J. K. Penry.
Raven Press, New York © 1980.

Definitive Evaluation of Multihandicapped Children with Seizures

Penelope K. Garrison and James R. Schimshock

Good Samaritan Hospital and Medical Center, Portland, Oregon 97210

Literature to date describes the plight of families with multiply handi-capped children (Ounsted, 1955; Hartlage and Green, 1972; Livingston, 1972). The Children's Neuropsychiatric Unit (CNPU) has been developed to study and treat these children, combining the services of a general hospital and the model of a psychiatric unit. During a carefully planned intensive hospitalization, the child is assessed from the perspectives of child neurol-ogy, child psychiatry, neuropsychology, education, speech pathology, and social service. Treatment trial is implemented during the hospital stay. The family is strongly encouraged to participate and/or room in. The family and community agencies are enlisted as advocates for the child.

This unit excludes acute pediatric medical emergencies and is separate from the general pediatric unit. The setting permits careful and accurate clinical observation requiring a stability of environment, ample time, and receptiveness to subtle unexpected behaviors (Ounsted, 1974). Although brief hospitalization on a general pediatric ward may prove helpful for some children in a crisis, a stable sensitive milieu is required for definitive evalua-tion of complex seizures and related behavior problems, and for thorough psychiatric assessment of the complicated family reactions thereto.

The philosophy and design of staffing provides both a multidisciplinary team approach and primary nursing care. The primary worker, a nurse or a child development therapist, has responsibility to provide direct, consistent patient care on a one-to-one basis. Prior to admission, this individual gathers all information from previous medical records, the educational system, and other agencies, and makes pre-admission contacts with the families. He or she acts as an advocate for the patient and the family, coordinates involve-ment with outside professionals during the hospital stay, and also arranges follow-up plans and contacts. This protects the patient and family from the experience of dealing with the entire team at once without satisfactorily having questions answered. The primary person functions to insure that the work-up is continually relevant to the patient's needs and that the patient and family are aware of results as the work-up is in progress. The complex needs of this patient population demand versatility, as each work-up must be tailored individually. The purpose of this chapter is to describe the methodology employed to study these patients and their families, and report our experience in the care of the first 112 patients.

PATIENTS AND METHODS

Description of the Children's Neuropsychiatric Unit

Our referral patterns indicate a utilization of unit services by a cross-section of professionals, including referring physicians, school, and state welfare agencies. Before admission, a pre-staffing conference is held to acquaint all staff with the child and permit orderly planning of the work-up. Early in the hospitalization there is a rapid initial evaluation and development of data base, including medical, neurological, neuropsychological, psychiatric, social, and family assessments. Additional neurological study, including computerized axial tomography (CAT), EEG, anticonvulsant level determinations, and EEG videotelemetry, as well as appropriate metabolic studies, are done as indicated. Detailed data for evaluation of behavioral strategies, medication, and EEG progression are collected. Families of the children are extensively involved in the diagnosis and treatment throughout the hospital stay. Parents' participation, including rooming in at no charge, is vigorously encouraged, as this may be especially valuable in diagnosis. Because the child's problem affects the entire family, the evaluation of the family unit is regarded as pivotal in planning treatment.

After the initial assessment, a planning and approach staffing is held and a trial treatment program devised. During the treatment trial, the patient's medical progress and response to the program is evaluated daily to permit necessary changes in treatment. This period allows the family and staff to assess the adequacy of recommendations before the child is discharged and to make appropriate modifications. There is a strong emphasis on close communication with both the family and the referring physicians and agencies because it is assumed that the usefulness of the CNPU evaluation to the patient rests on its usefulness to these people. The child returns to the care of the primary physician in his community. Follow-up surveillance by telephone, questionnaire, and outreach visits are also offered by the CNPU staff after discharge.

Characteristics of the Patient Population

Patient diagnoses are presented in Table 1. The primary diagnostic categories are displayed vertically. Secondary diagnostic categories are displayed horizontally. As evident, the majority of patients had more than one problem. This reflects the complexity and severity of the handicaps of all our patients and indicates why they required intensive inpatient evaluation. For

TABLE 1. *Children's neuropsychiatric unit: patient diagnoses*

Diagnostic category	Mean age (years)	Mean duration of illness	Number of patients	Secondary seizure type	Other neurological problem	Psychiatric diagnosis	Other medical illness
Neurological diagnoses with seizures							
Generalized							
Tonic-clonic	9.1	7.3	25	13	7	10	3
Myoclonic	9.6	4.1	10	5	0	1	1
Absence	9.4	7.4	5	2	0	4	0
Partial							
Partial complex	8.5	3.9	16	5	4	10	2
Partial elementary	7.0	1	1		0	1	0
Neurological diagnosis without seizures			5	0	1	5	0
Mixed neuropsychiatric problems	8.6	5.1	16	0	16	9	2
Psychiatric[c]	9.9	4.4	17	(9)[a]	11[b]	10	1
Psychosomatic	11.4	4.8	17	0	0	17	5
Total	8.0	4.4	112	34	39	67	14

[a] Seizures quiescent.
[b] Developmental delay or learning disability.
[c] No identifiable medical neurological illness and codable psychiatric diagnosis.

57 children, seizures were the first diagnosis and predominant problem. Thirty-three children had other neurological diagnoses (e.g., Sturge-Weber or cerebral palsy) without seizures, or had mixed, less definable "neuropsychiatric" problems. Of these, some had seizures in the past or had currently controlled seizures. The distribution of seizure types does not reflect typical office practice. Our children often had a secondary seizure type, and admission to the hospital was necessary only if (a) their seizures were intractable and had evaded clear definition and medical management in the outpatient setting, or (b) psychiatric problems had eluded diagnosis and/or obstructed smooth medical management.

Sixty children had discharge diagnoses of psychiatric illnesses, i.e., even in the absence of medical problems they would have merited a codable psychiatric diagnosis. The 17 children with only psychiatric diagnoses had no identifiable medical or neurological illness. Each child and family had psychiatric assessment, including evaluation by questionnaire, interview, and direct observation of the impact of seizures on the patients and families.

Criteria were developed to rate mild, moderate, or severe impact of seizures on finances and family. Financial impact was rated moderate if there were very heavy medical expenses and consequent alteration of family decisions. Financial impact was rated severe if the family had declared bankruptcy, placed the child out of the home for financial reasons, or gone on welfare. Family impact was rated moderate if there was obvious marital strain, reactive stress in other family members, or if the child had been subjected to repeated work-ups or other help-seeking maneuvers. Family strain was considered severe if the child's illness had contributed substantially to divorce, to psychiatric decompensation of either parent, or to the child's leaving the home. A majority of families with children in all seizure categories had moderate or severe financial and family impact.

Neuropsychiatric evaluation disclosed that a substantial portion (61%) of our youngsters with seizures had developmental delays: I.Q. scores of 15% fell in the borderline (70–80), 20% in the mild (55–70), and 26% in the moderate (30–55) range. For some youngsters, educational placement had previously been unsuccessful because developmental delays and/or specific learning disabilities were not recognized and the child's learning problems had been ascribed to seizures or to medications with which they were treated. Educational consultation with the school, as part of the hospitalization, resulted in placement in an educational setting where the child's learning needs were met and where he could begin to experience success.

Multidisciplinary Analysis of Seizures

The diagnostic and treatment approaches to seizures took full advantage of the multidisciplinary staff. All children had careful clinical observation by nursing staff who collaborated closely with the families to develop a neuropsychological data base and to identify target behaviors for closer study. This was the single most useful function of the hospitalization.

In addition to clinical and free-ranging telemetry approaches to understanding seizures, the psychological assessment of the child and family specifically analyzed the question of interaction of seizures with the vicissitudes of ordinary childhood development and parenting a handicapped child. This yielded useful recommendations in the majority of cases.

EEG Telemetry

Fifty to seventy percent of all children in all seizure groups were referred for free-ranging EEG video telemetry study, which differs from traditional approaches (Penry and Porter, 1977; Porter, et al., 1976) as described elsewhere in this volume. The telemetry consultant then devised an individually tailored protocol with a specific approach to the clinical question specifying montage, duration, and timing of the recording, and the inclusion of specific activating procedures or continuous performance tasks.

In designing each individual EEG telemetry investigation, specific goals of the study were determined and grouped into five categories: (a) definition of seizure type; (b) determination of seizure frequency; (c) correlation of seizures with environmental and metabolic precipitants; (d) correlation of seizures with target behaviors; and (e) parent education. The percent of youngsters for whom telemetry attained goals were attained through telemetry varied within each seizure category from 25 to 100%. Children were commonly referred for telemetry to attempt to correlate unusual, automatistic, stereotyped, or noncompliant behaviors with a known mixed seizure disorder. This goal was successfully met in 100% of children with absence seizures, but only in 50% of children with partial complex seizures. The goal of establishing the existence of precipitants of seizures met with success in 86% of children with myoclonic seizures and only in 25% of children with partial complex seizures. Parent education was the most frequently attained goal.

RESULTS

Seizure Control

Traditional approaches to seizure control were employed. Change of drug, i.e., subtraction or addition of medications, was used in 74% of tonic clonic, 80% of myoclonic, 40% absence, and 63% of partial complex. Carbamazepine and sodium valproate were the most frequent drugs added. Change of drug delivery includes such factors as teaching administration of liquid medications to an embattled toddler, changing times of doses using information gained from serial serum anticonvulsant levels, and altering to better absorbed preparations. This occurred in 48% of tonic-clonic, 40% of myoclonic, 20% of absence, and 56% of partial complex seizures.

Change in child management includes diagnosing and dealing with child noncompliance, and diagnosing pseudoseizures that might interfere with accurate parental recording, determining existence of stresses precipitating seizures. This contributed to seizure control in 74% of tonic-clonic, 40% of myoclonic, 20% of absence, and 56% of partial complex.

The majority of children shifted from poor or very poor control to good control during hospitalization, and maintained this improvement for the period after discharge with gradual improvement thereafter in three seizure groups. Success was ascribed to two factors: (a) Close clinical observation enabled more sensitive anticonvulsant applications and adjustment. (b) In families where poor comprehension, noncompliance, or psychiatric factors (such as grief, conflict, and denial) were contributory, these were rapidly worked through during the hospitalization.

Follow-up

Children were followed by their referring physician and seizure frequency post-discharge was evaluated from their office records. Objective follow-up was derived from telephone reports by parents and from questionnaires returned after discharge. Short- and long-term effects of the admission on the children's seizures, education, psychiatric adjustment, family adjustment, and development were questioned. There was improvement in seizures in all groups, with greater variability in children with partial complex seizures and less success in that difficult group in attaining social and educational goals.

DISCUSSION

This unit was designed and staffed to be flexible so that children with a wide variety of problems and with multiple problems can be simultaneously assessed and undergo treatment trial. This permits children with poorly defined problems, e.g., (a) latent behavioral problems; (b) uncontrollable seizures; (c) subtle interactions between family and child that cannot be teased out and understood in the traditional office or clinical practice setting, to receive both intensive evaluation and a variety of secondary and tertiary preventive services. Because such children may not have been accurately described by previous diagnostic categories, they may not have been adequately directed toward available services. The hospitalization is financed as a medical surgical hospitalization with third party payment. The unit is designed to function effectively in a society where intensive diagnostic facilities for handicapped children are insufficient and where about one-half of children live in rural areas. Follow-up liaison is vigorously developed during hospitalization to encourage effective implementation of recommendations. Discharge conferences are attended by personnel from the child's school and routine prompt contacts are made with referring physicians during hospitalization and at the time of discharge.

Despite rising hospital costs, this population is seriously compromised. Failure to understand and adequately treat both the patient in terms of his seizure disorder and his family in terms of their perception or accommodation to his problem may have long-term consequences that are more costly. The controlled, nonthreatening environment that permits the staff to see both the child's behaviors and seizures and the families' strengths and liabilities functions as an "incubator" where psychiatric growth may occur even more rapidly than neurophysiological adjustment.

Utilizing EEG telemetry and sophisticated staff observations to more accurately diagnose and treat the child's seizures, as well as intensive psychiatric observation, analysis, and treatment, we have produced an impact on the lives of a group of seriously impaired children. Complete seizure control has been achieved in 60 to 100% of children depending on the seizure type. Overall, the seizures of 95% of children were significantly improved, although partial complex seizures have proven relatively refractory. Initial follow-up indicates that the psychiatric, social, and educational impact of the hospitalization is also beneficial and has lasting effect.

REFERENCES

Hartlage, L. C., and Green, J. B. (1972): The relation of parental attitudes to academic and social achievement in epileptic children. *Epilepsia*, 13:21.

Livingston, S. (1972): *Comprehensive Management of Epilepsy in Infancy, Childhood and Adolescence*, pp. 6–7 and 584. Charles C Thomas, Springfield, Illinois.

Ounsted, C. (1955): The hyperkinetic syndrome in epileptic children. *Lancet*, 269:303–311.

Ounsted, C. (1974): A special center for children with seizures. *Health Trends*, 6:69–71.

Penry, J. K., and Porter, R. (1977): Intensive monitoring of patients with intractable seizures. In: *Epilepsy: The Eighth International Symposium*, edited by J. K. Penry. Raven Press, New York.

Porter, R. J., Penry, J. K., and Wolf, A. A. (1976): Simultaneous documentation of clinical and electroencephalographic manifestations of epileptic seizures. In: *Epilepsy: Quantitative Analytic Studies in Epilepsy*, edited by P. Kellaway and I. Peterson, pp. 253–268. Raven Press, New York.

Advances in Epileptology:
The Xth Epilepsy International Symposium,
edited by J. A. Wada and J. K. Penry.
Raven Press, New York © 1980.

Comprehensive Treatment of Intractable Seizures

R. J. Gumnit, D. Jacome, V. Ramani, J. Johnston, S. Reuben, and S. Whalen

Minnesota Comprehensive Epilepsy Program and the Department of Neurology, University of Minnesota, Minneapolis, Minnesota 55455

Most patients with seizures respond to conventional therapy. That is, their seizures are brought under control by their family physician with the help of a general neurologist. A significant number of patients, however, still have difficulty. Twenty-five years ago, it was acceptable medical practice to conclude that these unfortunate people would have to resign themselves to their condition and adjust as best they could. Today, however, with the increase in effectiveness of medical treatment, and particularly with the increased social expectations of our population, this attitude is no longer acceptable. Even an occasional seizure is socially disabling. Seizures prevent patients from having a driver's license and obtaining insurance. They interfere with employment opportunities and create social isolation. Therefore, we must aim for complete seizure control with a drug regimen that produces the least possible side effects.

A COMPREHENSIVE TREATMENT MODEL

In order to help persons with persistent seizures, the Minnesota Comprehensive Epilepsy Program has organized a multidisciplinary Diagnostic Treatment and Rehabilitation Program (DTRP). Neurologists who specialize in epilepsy, electroencephalographers, nurses, pharmacists, psychologists, social workers, and various counselors each play an important role. The DTRP functions in a variety of inpatient and outpatient settings. It cooperates closely with family physicians, neurologists, and social agencies. It also operates model outpatient comprehensive seizure clinics and has close working relationships with a variety of residential facilities.

The heart of the DTRP is the Diagnostic Treatment and Rehabilitation Unit at University of Minnesota Hospitals, where intensive medical and social/psychological diagnostic and treatment activities are carried out. Definitive long-term therapy is performed on an outpatient or a residential basis.

Each potential patient is screened prior to admission to the DTRP. The team evaluates the adequacy of previous care and may refer a patient to a general neurologist if this level of care seems to be appropriate. The team also carefully evaluates the motivation of each patient. Patients who are too passive, or who have so great a vested interest in being permanently disabled that they are not suitable candidates for help, are not accepted. The essential criterion for admission to the DTRP is whether the team believes the program can be effective in significantly improving the quality of life of the patient.

Once a patient is accepted for treatment, the following specific objectives are pursued:

(a) The team seeks a precise diagnosis. Combined video/EEG monitoring, telemetered EEG, and walk-about EEG tape recorders are used as necessary.

(b) Observation of the number and type of seizures in a quantitative manner;

(c) Precise monitoring of anticonvulsant levels;

(d) Psychological evaluation and especially identification of motivating factors;

(e) Evaluation of vocational potential and interest, and preparation of vocational rehabilitation prescription;

(f) Evaluation of social problems and preparation of a plan for social intervention.

It is mandatory that a physician have a precise diagnosis if patients with intractable seizures are to be adequately treated. These patients frequently have several different types of seizures or a mixture of genuine and hysterical seizures. Prolonged, combined, video EEG monitoring has proven to be very helpful in making the proper diagnosis. Telemetered EEG and walk-about EEG tape recorders have more limited but definite indications. Although the severity of epilepsy cannot be completely described by counting the number of seizures, it is only with precise quantitative determination that one can judge the efficacy of anticonvulsant prescriptions. A variety of techniques including observation by nurses, automatic analysis of EEG data, and patient reporting are used to count seizures. The effectiveness of anticonvulsants is measured by counting seizures as a function of anticonvulsant blood levels. Patients with intractable seizures are frequently on multiple anticonvulsants, and drug interactions are such that very frequent monitoring is needed if we are not to be misled. A small but significant number of patients have been found to be intractable because of unusual pharmacokinetics. Here, precise and frequent measurement of serum anticonvulsants is absolutely essential if one is to find the proper prescription.

To achieve these objectives, patients are hospitalized for approximately 4 to 6 weeks on the unit. An intensive program of patient education and individual and group counselling is carried out. Each patient is encouraged to set realistic goals and to actively participate in treatment efforts directed to increasing independence in all aspects of life. Conventional contracting and behavior modification techniques are used. Members of the patient's family are involved in planning, and are taught how they can best support the patient in his or her efforts to achieve independence.

Discharge planning begins as soon as a definitive diagnosis has been made, and community agencies are involved in planning while the patient is still in the hospital. Patients may be discharged to a variety of outpatient settings while the program continues to supervise treatment. Some return home or to their own apartments. Those who are mentally retarded, mentally ill, or physically handicapped are discharged to an appropriate community residential facility whose personnel receive inservice training and continuing supervision from DTRP staff. A residential program for patients with sei-

TABLE 1. *Data on the first 74 patients to complete the Diagnostic Treatment and Rehabilitation Program*[a]

A. Minor seizures

Number of seizures per week	Admission	Time at which measurement was taken after discharge		
		3 Months	6 Months	12 Months
More than 100	8	4	0	0
31–100	11	4	0	5
15–30	7	4	4	5
8–14	6	4	7	0
1–7	8	14	18	5
Less than 1	3	0	14	23
None	57	70	57	62
Total	100	100	100	100

B. Major seizures

Number of seizures per week	Admission	Time at which measurement was taken after discharge		
		3 Months	6 Months	12 Months
More than 100	0	0	0	0
31–100	4	0	4	0
15–30	16	0	0	10
8–14	10	4	4	0
1–7	40	30	25	10
Less than 1	4	9	14	10
None	26	57	53	70
Total	100	100	100	100

[a]All results are expressed as percentages.

zures who do not have other handicaps is being developed in which the transition to fully independent living can be assisted.

OUTCOMES AND CONCLUSIONS

The DTRP is being evaluated independently by David Brings of the Minnesota Center for Social Research. Thus far, data on the first 74 patients to complete the program have been gathered and analyzed via a series of regression tables (Table 1). For evaluation purposes only, seizures were divided into minor and major categories. Pre-tests indicated that this corresponded to the patient's perception of his or her experience. Minor seizures were those that did not create severe interruption in the patient's ongoing activities and included brief absence, partial, or complex partial attacks. Major seizures included drop attacks, prolonged partial or complex partial seizures, and generalized tonic-clonic seizures.

Seventy-four percent of the patients had major seizures on entering the program, but only 30% had them 1 year later. Only 20% had one or more per week. Forty-three percent had minor seizures on entering the program. Forty percent had one or more per week. A year after discharge, 38% still had minor seizures but only 15% had one or more per week. There has been a substantial and a sustained improvement in seizure control. Similar results were obtained in an analysis of the severity of seizures. Measures of patients' independence in activities of daily living, frequency of social activities, and level of employment showed sustained improvement at the 50 to 75% level.

These results show that a substantial number of patients whose seizures were intractable to conventional therapy can benefit from an intensive program of medical and social/psychological intervention. The Minnesota Diagnostic Treatment and Rehabilitation Program has proven to be effective and can serve as a model for a small network of tertiary referral centers to treat this particularly difficult group of patients.

ACKNOWLEDGMENT

This study was supported in part by the National Institute of Neurological and Communicative Disorders and Stroke, contract N01-NS-5-2327.

Advances in Epileptology:
The Xth Epilepsy International Symposium,
edited by J. A. Wada and J. K. Penry.
Raven Press, New York © 1980.

Training of Community Epilepsy Teams by the Georgia Comprehensive Epilepsy Program

R. A. Mercille, J. B. Green, G. Katter, and H. Deaver

Department of Neurology, Medical College of Georgia, and The Division of Vocational Rehabilitation, Georgia Department of Human Resources, Augusta, Georgia 30912

The Georgia Comprehensive Epilepsy Program is charged with demonstrating to physicians and other professionals the newest advances in epilepsy research and treatment and with establishing a broad program for public education. In order to carry out this responsibility, the strategy developed was tailored to fit the characteristics of the state of Georgia. Georgia, the largest state east of the Mississippi River, is rural, sparsely populated in many areas, and poor. Per capita income in Georgia is among the lowest of the 50 states. Georgia is undersupplied in physicians, nurses, and other health professionals. Great distances and lack of public transportation compound the problems of delivering health care. Neurological services are mainly available in the metropolitan areas of Atlanta and Augusta where medical schools exist. There are no neurologists in the southern part of the state and only one in the central area.

In approaching the problem of providing comprehensive care, it was decided to enhance the capacities of local communities to deal with the problems of persons with epilepsy. The guiding principle was to help local people help local people, rather than increase dependence on the services at the Medical College of Georgia, which are expensive, distant, and subject to the vagaries of funding. A training program was designed to increase the level of knowledge of health and social service professionals about epilepsy and to improve the quality of service to persons with epilepsy throughout Georgia. Training a network of professionals would provide the means by which all persons with seizures might receive comprehensive services. This network would be accessible in local communities, would enable a person to assess his or her own needs, and would provide a package of available local services and referral to agencies outside the local communities.

The training program was developed by an interdisciplinary team within the department of neurology and consisted of eleven faculty members representing psychology, nursing, counseling, vocational rehabilitation, social work, special education, community development, speech pathology, occupational therapy, and neurology. This team had been well prepared by 3 years' experience in providing consultation and training to agencies serving the developmentally disabled in Georgia. The training process was planned by answering the questions of who was to be trained, and where and how the program was to be implemented.

Even in a small community, a public health department, a department of family and children's services, a public school system, and a division of vocational rehabilitation usually exist. The nurses, social workers, teachers, and counselors of these agencies who are likely to contact persons with epilepsy needed to be included in the training. Thirteen population centers were selected as training sites because the adjacent rural populations had traditionally traveled to these cities for health care (Fig. 1). During the first year of the Georgia Comprehensive Epilepsy Program, training was held in Augusta, Savannah, and Statesboro encompassing 13 counties. By the end of the second year (June 1978), the population centers of Macon, Albany, and Rome had been included, reaching 32 more counties.

An important decision was made to conduct the training both at the Medical College of Georgia and in the local communities (population centers). This had the effect of forging a network of communication among the local

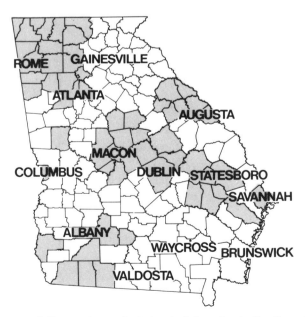

FIG. 1. Thirteen population centers selected as training sites in the Georgia Comprehensive Epilepsy Program. Fifty-eight counties were served, 181 people were trained, 15 serving multiple counties.

professionals and between local professionals and faculty at the Medical College of Georgia. Local professionals and Medical College of Georgia faculty become aware of each others' facilities and resources. The training sessions are conducted for a total of 4 days with the first day at the medical college in Augusta and the last 3 days in the local community.

A month before each planned 4-day session a faculty member makes extensive advance preparations at the designated population center. During his visit he talks with agency supervisors about the goals and objectives of the proposed training in epilepsy. He suggests that staff of the agency volunteer to participate and that supervisors recognize that participating in the training commits the agency to increased activity on behalf of persons with epilepsy. The advance visitor makes arrangements for professionals to be enrolled from the metropolitan area and also from the surrounding rural counties. In recruiting such trainees, there is a deliberate mixing of agency personnel and in more populous areas two training sessions are given, one for the urban and another for the surrounding rural counties. At the time of the advance visit, contact is made with newspapers, television, and radio stations to arrange for publicity about epilepsy. The support of local civic groups is enlisted. The final task of the advance visitor is to choose a site for the training in the local community. Often a nonmedical facility such as a bank or hotel meeting room is used. This has the advantage of influencing the community beyond the group of health professionals and aids in the dissemination of educational information to the public.

Each training session is initiated at the medical college with a pre-test in epilepsy. The trainees receive a source book of selected references. A social event aids in introducing the trainees to each other and to the interdisciplinary team of preceptors. The first day of training is used to familiarize the trainees with the clinics and the diagnostic and treatment unit for epilepsy. The steps in the diagnosis of epilepsy are presented with demonstrations of the electroencephalogram and the neurological examination. The treatment of seizure disorders is discussed with emphasis on anticonvulsant blood levels. The trainees discuss the epilepsies with neurologists who have a special interest and expertise.

Also on the first day, the trainees are assigned to activity groups, each of which is given the task of completing an outline on one of the more frequent seizure types. The trainees must identify the type of epilepsy by the International Classification, describe the typical clinical manifestations, and list the possible etiologies, hereditary factors, possible triggering mechanisms, and so forth. They review the positive physical and neurological findings and laboratory tests. They hypothesize the anatomic pathology. They outline medical treatment with possible side effects, indications for surgery, and a comprehensive program of management with follow-up procedures. This practical exercise is carried on throughout the entire training session and copies of the completed outlines are given to each trainee. The first day of training ends with the knowledge that the program will continue in the trainee's home community 1 week later.

The second day of training has as its objectives the development of skills in observing, recording, and reporting seizures; learning correct first-aid procedures for the major types of seizures; acquiring a basic understanding of the anatomy and physiology of the brain in respect to seizure disorders; and recognizing the effects of epilepsy on personality. Still another objective is to develop interpersonal relationships among the trainees and to continue the group activities in developing outlines on the assigned seizure types.

The third day includes a further elaboration on the diagnostic process and aims at achieving greater familiarity with components of comprehensive treatment including anticonvulsant drugs. The trainees are introduced to a panel of "consumers," persons with epilepsy and their families. Specialists cognizant of the life problems of persons with epilepsy such as insurance underwriters, lawyers, and personnel managers are included on this panel.

On the fourth day of training, the groups present their completed outlines to all participants. There is a general discussion about how the training received might be applied to the local area and follow-up is planned. A post-test of knowledge about epilepsy is administered and the trainees answer an evaluation questionnaire about the training experience. Certificates indicating that they have completed the training in epilepsy successfully are awarded in a formal ceremony.

The interdisciplinary team of preceptors continues to maintain contact with all of the participants by providing educational materials on epilepsy and assisting in developing services for epileptics in local communities. Local physicians are notified of the names and agencies of the professionals in their area who have completed the training and are available to assist them in the management of patients with epilepsy.

In 2 years 187 professionals have been trained from 58 counties in Georgia. Included were 38 social workers from the Department of Family and Children's Services, 48 counselors from the Division of Vocational Rehabilitation, 32 mental health workers, 29 public health workers, 28 educators, 13 hospital workers, two from voluntary epilepsy organizations, eight from youth development centers, one from the Mayor's Committee on the Handicapped, one from Crippled Children's Clinic, and three graduate students. Comparison of pre- and post-test results indicate learning of factual information and analysis of the evaluation questionnaires shows a rating of "excellent" for the educational experience.

Beginning in the summer of 1978, a complete evaluation by individual interview of every professional trained was scheduled. A standard set of questions was developed so that the data collected would aid in the evaluation process. Each professional trained is asked the number of persons with epilepsy who are served, the number of interagency contacts on behalf of persons with epilepsy, physicians contacted, public education news programs in epilepsy, patients referred outside the community and location of that referral, contacts with fellow trainees, feelings of adequacy in dealing with epilepsy (persons and subject), and areas in which help was needed for further professional and personal development. This evaluation has as a goal encouragement of further community development and fostering of cooperative services in the local areas. Meanwhile the training program is proceeding and it is planned that by the end of the third year 345 professionals will have been trained.

ACKNOWLEDGMENTS

This project was supported by the National Institute of Neurological and Communicative Disorders and Stroke contract N01-NS-6-2340 (Department of Health, Education, and Welfare) and by grants from the Office of Developmental Disabilities (Department of Health, Education, and Welfare) and The Georgia State Council on Developmental Disabilities.

Advances in Epileptology:
The Xth Epilepsy International Symposium,
edited by J. A. Wada and J. K. Penry.
Raven Press, New York © 1980.

Comprehensive Care of the Adult Epileptic Patient: An Objective Method for the Evaluation of Social and Psychological Problems

Carl B. Dodrill, Lawrence W. Batzel, Henne R. Queisser, and Nancy R. Temkin

Epilepsy Center, Department of Neurological Surgery, University of Washington School of Medicine, Seattle, Washington, 98195

Despite abundant evidence for social and psychological difficulties among epileptic patients, the evaluation of such problems is most frequently done in a subjective manner. Furthermore, even when objective measures are utilized, such measures routinely have been developed and standardized with populations other than epileptic persons. Only rarely has any attempt been made to develop as much as a single scale to evaluate psychological and social problems among epileptic persons. Apparently no one has developed a multi-scale test or inventory specifically for epileptic patients. Such an instrument is required for a comprehensive assessment of their special psychosocial problems.

In this chapter, the development of such an inventory is presented. This inventory is designed solely for adults having seizure disorders. It permits an evaluation of the psychological and social concerns frequently found among epileptic persons and provides standardized findings that approximate those that would be obtained from a detailed professional evaluation of psychological and social problems.

METHODS

Prior to the execution of the formal study reported here, extensive preliminary work was undertaken that resulted in the identification of (a) the psychosocial areas to be evaluated, (b) an item pool that covered each of these areas with items tested for clarity and for minimal overlap, and (c) the development of rating sheets on which judgments of psychosocial functioning might be recorded. Space will not be taken to detail these efforts, but it should be noted that they included two complete pilot studies and involved approximately 100 patients. After all of the materials had been prepared, the administrative procedures worked out, and human subjects' approval obtained, the formal validational study reported here was undertaken.

Subjects

Subjects selected for this study were all adults (age 18 and over) who were patients at the Epilepsy Center, Department of Neurological Surgery, University of Washington School of Medicine. All subjects for this study were drawn from outpatient clinic schedules and an effort was made to obtain a representative sample of individuals utilizing such services. To do so, clinic days were chosen in advance with no knowledge of the patients who would actually be scheduled on those days and whenever possible, all adults seeing all neurologists that day were approached for possible participation in the study.

By employing the above procedures, a total of 154 adult epileptics were approached over a five month period. Of these, 127 (82%) actually completed the study. Sixty-seven were males and 60 were females. They ranged in age from 18 to 56 years, with a mean age of 29.16 years (SD = 9.02). They averaged 12.58 years of education (SD = 2.24). Primary seizure diagnoses were as follows: elementary partial, 16; complex partial, 73; generalized non-convulsive, 4; minor motor (akinetic, atonic, tonic or clonic), 6; more than one of these types, 10; and generalized convulsive, 18.

Procedure

Each participating patient was approached at the time of the clinic visit and paid $5.00 for participation. This consisted of two separate activities: (a) a psychosocial interview by a social worker or psychologist; and (b) completion of the Washington Psychosocial Seizure Inventory. The order of these two activities was approximately counterbalanced.

Professional ratings of adequacy of psychosocial functioning were used as the basis for developing scales for the inventory. After establishing interrater reliability, the professionals rated adjustment in each of the following areas: (family) background; emotional; interpersonal; vocational; financial; adjustment to seizures; medicine and medical management; and overall psychosocial functioning. In order to determine which inventory items best evaluated these areas, an item-by-rating correlational approach was used. An item was considered for an inventory scale if it had a significant point-biserial correlation with professional ratings of that psychosocial area. A significance level of 0.01 was used for the individual clinical scales and 0.001 for Overall Psychosocial Functioning. When an item correlated to this extent with more than one psychosocial area, it was included only in the area with which it correlated highest. In this fashion, each scale was composed on a purely statistical basis regardless of the content of the items.

From the earliest work on this inventory, it was concluded that a series of

Validity scales was needed to determine the probable accuracy with which the responses to the inventory represented the person completing it. Three scales were developed. The first (Scale A—No. Blank) merely consisted of the number of items that was left blank (in standard administration, no more than 10% or 13 items are allowed to remain blank). The second scale (Scale B—Lie) was designed to detect obvious tendencies to make one's self look better than is warranted. It consisted of items such as, "Is your life free from problems?" and "Have you ever felt tense or anxious?" An answer of "yes" for the former question or "no" for the latter question would be scored on the Lie scale. The third scale (Scale C—rare items) consisted of all items in the inventory endorsed by less than 15% of the patients. Such a scale has previously been shown to be helpful with respect to the Minnesota Multiphasic Personality Inventory (Dahlstrom et al., 1972) because of its sensitivity to random responding, whether by intent on the part of the patient or due to poor understanding, visual difficulties, confusion, etc. Taken together, all three scales were designed to be of assistance in determining the acceptability of any inventory completed.

Profile Development

Early in the work on the inventory, it was determined that a visual display of the patient's scores was of assistance in grasping the significance of the patient's responses. Because many questions in the inventory specifically asked about seizures, it was not possible to use a normal or control sample as a reference group. An initial attempt was made to report patients' scores as percentiles. However, this was clinically misleading because the prevalence of problems varied widely over the different areas. Consequently, the final profile was based directly on the professional ratings for each area. The actual placement of scores on the profile corresponded to the best prediction of the professional rating that could be made for each area based on the simple linear regression of the rating on the inventory scale. These then were more comparable from one scale to the next and one could determine the areas in which the patient was having the greatest difficulties by noting the highest elevations on the profile. Furthermore, to assist in making judgments as to the absolute level of problems in any area, clinical work provided for the establishment of four regions of profile elevation: (a) no significant problems; (b) possible problems, but of limited significance; (c) distinct and definite difficulties with adjustmental significance; and (d) severe problems having a striking impact on adjustment.

RESULTS

Application of the above procedures resulted in the development of eight Clinical scales (Background, Emotional, Interpersonal, Vocational, Financial, Adjustment to Seizures, Medicine and Medical Management, Overall Psychosocial Functioning) with from 7 to 57 items each as well as three Validity scales. Stability of measurement was evaluated by having 21 persons retake the inventory 1 month after initial administration. Correlation of the same Clinical scales from the two administrations resulted in coefficients ranging from a low of 0.70 to a high of 0.87 with a median of 0.82. Internal consistency of the scales as evaluated by the split-half technique with all 127 participants resulted in coefficients ranging from a low of 0.69 to a high of 0.95 with a median of 0.88. Similar coefficients for interrater reliability determination based on 10 joint interviews were 0.80, 0.95, and 0.90.

Turning from statistical indications of reliability to those of validity, it was observed that the correlations between the clinical scales and the respective professional ratings ranged from a low of 0.58 to a high of 0.75 with a median of 0.70. Furthermore, it was demonstrated that these correlations were consistent over various subgroups of the sample.

Figure 1 presents the profile that was developed for plotting the results of individual patients. The line plotted on the figure represents the average scores of the 127 patients used in the development of the inventory.

DISCUSSION

The reliability and validity correlation coefficients appear to be within acceptable ranges with especially satisfactory coefficients pertaining to agreement among professional raters. The scales of the inventory itself appear to be both stable and consistent in measurement. The validity correlation coefficients are somewhat lower than is desirable on certain of the scales. It was observed that such correlation coefficients were most often found on scales having only a few items and also on scales such as Medicine and Medical Management, where a restriction in range of scores was found with scores tending to cluster toward one end. These factors may at least in part account for the lowered coefficients.

The average profile presented in Fig. 1 is consistent with our clinical work with this patient population. Definite emotional problems have most often been noted by us in this patient group but interpersonal, vocational, and financial problems have also been frequently seen as well as those pertaining to acceptance of the seizure disorder. Less frequent are problems pertaining to family background, at least from the point that they are substantially detrimental to present adjustment. Finally, almost all our patients are very positive about their physicians and this of course is likely to be at least in part a matter of selection.

At present, we have completed only one study in addition to the investigation reported here on the inventory (Batzel et al., *this volume*). This study demonstrated that the inventory effectively differentiated between groups of fully employed, partially employed, and unemployed epileptic persons. Furthermore, it did so more clearly than did the much longer Minnesota

Date_____ No_____ Name_____

WASHINGTON PSYCHOSOCIAL SEIZURE INVENTORY

Profile Form

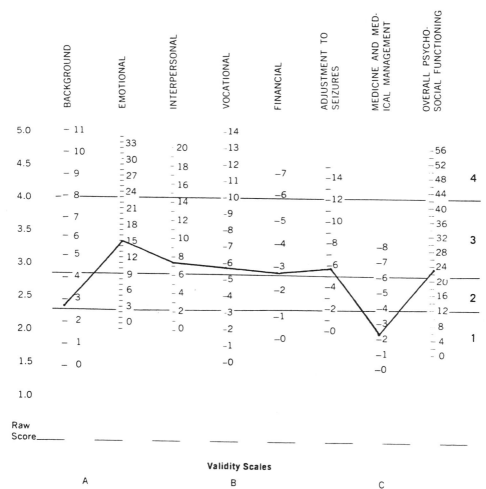

FIG. 1. Profile sheet for the Washington Psychosocial Seizure Inventory with the average scores of 127 epileptic persons plotted.

Multiphasic Personality Inventory. At the present time, we are applying the inventory to the evaluation of various treatment procedures for epileptics, including the effects of anticonvulsants, surgery for epilepsy, and operant conditioning. These and many other research applications are apparent as one attempts to evaluate treatment effectiveness and change in this patient population.

Our clinical work has also led to several other findings. First, the majority of these patients can complete the inventory in 15 to 20 min and can use the standard written version if they are able to read. If they are not able to read, they can listen to the inventory read over a standard tape cassette, which requires 21 min. Individuals with I.Q.'s less than 60 or 65 are not able to be tested by this means and are therefore beyond the scope of this instrument. Furthermore, it has been found useful to develop a list of critical items that represent particularly important areas pertaining to each of the first seven Clinical scales. These are noted on the back of the profile sheet. Thus, attention is immediately drawn to matters deserving special consideration as when individuals positively respond to questions such as, "Do you often wish you were dead?" and "Have seizures ruined your life?"

The Washington Psychosocial Seizure Inventory is easy to administer and score and is received well by patients as relevant to their problems. Our clinical work suggests that it is of assistance in rapidly obtaining an overview of difficulties in psychosocial adjustment. Research with it to date has been very limited, but it would appear to be useful in the evaluation of treatment programs, in identifying epileptics with special needs, and, in general, wherever an objective assessment of psychological and social difficulties is needed. Work toward the identification of the potentials of this Inventory is underway at our Epilepsy Center.

ACKNOWLEDGMENTS

This investigation was supported by a grant from the Epilepsy Foundation of America and by NIH contracts N01-NS-0-2281 and N01-NS-6-2341, awarded by the National Institute of Neurological and Communicative Disorders and Stroke, PHS/DHEW. Sincere appreciation is expressed to Alan J. Wilensky, M.D., Ph.D., for his assistance in providing the neurological information on the patients used in this investigation. Appreciation is also gratefully acknowledged to David Frazer, computer programmer, for his untiring assistance with the numerous analyses required for all parts of this study.

REFERENCES

Dahlstrom, W. G., Welsh, G. S., and Dahlstrom, L. E. (1972: *An MMPI Handbook, Vol. 1,* revised ed. University of Minnesota Press, Minneapolis.

Advances in Epileptology:
The Xth Epilepsy International Symposium,
edited by J. A. Wada and J. K. Penry.
Raven Press, New York © 1980.

Public Relations and Epilepsy

Johannes N. Loeber

Instituut voor Epilepsiebestrijding, Heemstede, Holland

Great progress has been made recently in the fight against epilepsy. Compared with only a few years ago, many improvements in medical aid have taken place, most notably the development of computerized axial tomography (CAT). The therapeutic armamentarium has been enlarged by several new drugs. The social and psychological approach has become more comprehensive and more effective. Occupational opportunities have been created for people with epilepsy in various countries. Nevertheless, the prejudice against epilepsy, and against those who suffer from it, persists. How can assistance in the medical, social, and occupational field for the patient with epilepsy be fully effective as long as the patients feel themselves surrounded by opinions that are so hostile that they feel the only way to live with their condition is to conceal it from others? Thus, the person in question lives with a constant fear of detection and of rejection. This prejudice is well-known, but takes different forms in different countries. However, the principal attitude is the same: Someone with epilepsy is different. He is not quite to be trusted, because he may lose control. Not only do fears exist of the seizures that may occur, but also beliefs that, for instance, a person with epilepsy may suddenly set fire to the house, run away with all the money, or suddenly commit a sexual misdemeanour. Moreover, there is the expectation that the patient eventually will become mentally deranged.

A striking proof of existing prejudices was recently published by Hanssen and Duffield (1976) and demonstrated the stereotype that holds that people with epilepsy have unattractive personalities and that their condition can be read from their faces. Students were shown a series of photographs of people chosen at random (none of them had epilepsy as far as was known). These photographs were given a score for attractiveness by means of a proven scale. The pictures ranged from very attractive to very unattractive. Each student was shown two sets of 10 photographs and he was told that in each set was a person who had been diagnosed as having grand mal epilepsy. The students were told that the purpose of this experiment was to assist medical personnel in emergencies such as motor accidents to identify unconscious patients suffering from epilepsy. Sixty-nine percent selected an unattractive female as epileptic and 83% an unattractive male.

It is certain that the positive achievements in the medical field, which currently ensure that seizures taking place in public are rare, have a negative effect as well. It means that most people suppose that they do not know anyone with epilepsy. Usually the only people with epilepsy known to their associates are those who have a mental handicap as well, or those with certain striking behavioral deviations. Thus the small group of people with epilepsy easily recognizable on account of mental abnormalities tends to account for the image of the group as a whole. This effect is reinforced because it appeals to the deep-rooted negative feelings that surround the inexplicable and unpredictable.

PUBLIC RELATIONS

All that is done and achieved in the sociomedical field must be accompanied by efforts to change society. The need for public education is stressed in the recent Plan for Nationwide Action on Epilepsy of the (American) Commission for the Control of Epilepsy and Its Consequences (1977). It states, "Public misunderstandings about epilepsy are so deep and the age-old 'stigma' that shrouds the condition so thoroughly ingrained, that efforts to provide the public with a realistic and up-to-date awareness of epilepsy will present a formidable challenge." The role of public relations (PR) is thus significant, in that it can provide much useful information. Public relations are a result of the changes in society, which at the same time has become more complicated and interdependent. It originated in the world of business and industrial organizations, where it was discovered that making good products was not sufficient, certainly not after technical developments led to innovations. About 100 years ago a firm could operate independently. In present society this is impossible. For its functioning such a firm is dependent on its surroundings to such an extent as would have been unimaginable before. Consider trade unions, pressure groups for the environment, legal regulations, governmental actions, and so on. All these must be taken into account if one wishes to sell one's products. Thus PR is far more than advertising alone, although there are points of similarity. The definition of PR accepted by the PR society in Holland is as follows: PR is the systematical promotion of mutual understanding between organizations and their "publics" in society. PR is an applied part of sociology and social psychology. The words "public opinion," "image," "attitude," "stereotype," and "message" are key words in this context. Here we find connections between PR in the usual sense, i.e., applied in the world of organizations, and PR for a special group of people, as in our case: the people who are handicapped by epilepsy. We can say that PR for epilepsy is the systematical promotion of mutual understanding between the group of people with epilepsy and the social groups that are relevant to them. PR provides methods and makes us aware of obstacles.

METHODS

1. There is no such thing as "the public," although in some cases we can speak of "public opinion." It is necessary to divide the general public into different groups, each of which needs its own approach, because it is considering the object, i.e., epilepsy, from a different angle. Thus we can distinguish the medical profession, social workers, employers, teachers, ballot committees of, e.g., sport associations, people with epilepsy, and other groups. They are all distinguishable subgroups.

2. What do our target groups require? Thorough investigation of their opinions, their misunderstandings and their relationship to people with epilepsy is important.

3. It is then necessary to formulate a message intended for the specific subgroups (related to what we wish to impress on them).

4. We should set up a planned action program and leave nothing to chance.

5. Finally, it is necessary to have an evaluation of the results of the actions and, if necessary, adapt the message and the approach as a result of this feedback.

COMMUNICATION

The theory of communication is central to the process. It can be helpful to keep the SMCRE-model in mind, which means that there is a source (S) which formulates a message (M), sends it through a channel (C) to a receiver (R) to obtain a certain effect (E). Each of these stadia has its specific requirements.

The *source*, the sender of the message, is responsible for starting the action. What does he want to achieve? How does he prepare for what follows? It is also very important for the effect to know who is sending the message.

The *message* should contain what the sender wants to transmit in a code which can be decoded by the receiver. If there is a gap between the meaning a sender gives to a word (or another symbol he uses for the transmission) and the interpretation by the receiver, no effective communication is possible. Here a continuous feedback is necessary to make certain that no misunderstandings will arise between the meaning of the sender and what the receiver makes of it.

The *channel* (the medium used) can vary between a direct personal talk, a lecture, a letter, a book or leaflet, a radio or television transmission, and other forms. The choice of the right channel for a specific situation is important.

The *receiver* is different from the sender; otherwise the exercise would be unnecessary. It is useful to appreciate how great the difference may be. It is necessary to form an opinion about the receiver, to try to visualize his preconceived ideas, to know something about the interest he has in the matter in question, and to know his possible defenses.

The *effect* the communication has had must be found out and used as a feedback to the sender. The effect is the aim of the communication. Therefore, it is remarkable that evaluation of the result is sometimes neglected and that the effect is taken for granted.

OBSTACLES

The effects of (mass) communication must not be overstressed. In 1960 Joseph T. Klapper showed that the effects are more often a reinforcement of existing opinions than a conversion to new ones. Which influences play a role?

The receiver tends to close his ears (and mind) to anything that does not fit into his world. Three processes of selection can be distinguished: (a) *selective exposure*: the receiver selects the medium or the communication with which to be acquainted (e.g., the kind of newspaper he reads); (b) *selective perception*: The receiver refuses (sometimes unconsciously) to let a message penetrate. He closes his mind, eyes, and ears to the things he does not want to know, see, or hear and at the same time opens them for the things that confirm him in his existing opinion. (c) *selective retention*: the receiver only remembers the things he "wants" to remember. In summary, the main effect of communication is to confirm the ideas the receiver already had.

Much communication works indirectly. It finds its way from sender to receiver by way of intermediaries. All types of mediating factors play a role in this process. The acceptance of a message does not depend so much on the independent opinion the receiver forms for himself as on the opinion of those who are opinion leaders for him (politicians, clergymen, teachers, doctors, TV personalities). This is called the two-step flow of communication. Also, the things said in a café, in an office, or in the barbershop have more impact than an official document. The message lands in a specific social climate, where group norms can have a great influence.

PLANNED ACTION

Plans to change opinions about epilepsy involve all of the aforementioned factors. At present in Holland there is a research project in progress that aims first at the clarification of the social obstacles confronting people with epilepsy. A representative group of 100 people with epilepsy are interviewed. Part of the interview is free—patients can bring out the problems they feel most acutely. A long questionnaire is completed in collaboration with the person interviewed. This is to be a basis for further planned action. We hope to have concluded this phase during 1979. Then we hope we will know more about our target public. The next phase is to develop the instruments by which change in attitudes and behavior can be effected. Put in our framework, they are the channels we must use. We have not only to formulate the message but also to find out what are the most effective media for our purpose. This next phase will start soon. Much remains to be done, but we think it important to do it thoroughly. For people with epilepsy this action is just as important as the developments in the medical field or in the social approach. It certainly is just as difficult when we bear in mind the barriers to changes in attitude and of prejudice. Cooperation between workers in different countries is vital. I make an appeal to them to communicate their results and to work together in these new ways in the fight against epilepsy and its consequences.

The most effective way to achieve changes in opinion, however, should come from people with epilepsy themselves. They have to play an increasingly active role in this battle against prejudice and misunderstanding. It is up to them to show that they are normal effective people, with nothing really wrong with them as long as they are under the right medical treatment. They must have the courage to drop their protective shield of secrecy, because—notwithstanding all that is said by professionals—only their message will gain credibility.

REFERENCES

Hansson, R. O., and Duffield, B. J. (1976): Physical attractiveness and the attributions of epilepsy. *J. Soc. Psychol.*, 99:233–240.

Klapper, J. R. (1960): *The Effects of Mass Communication.* The Free Press of Glencoe, Illinois.

Plan for Nationwide Action on Epilepsy (1977). The Commission for the Control of Epilepsy and its Consequences. *DHEW Publication (NIH) 78–276.*

Advances in Epileptology:
The Xth Epilepsy International Symposium,
edited by J. A. Wada and J. K. Penry.
Raven Press, New York © 1980.

Epilepsy-Specific Educational Needs of Medical and Allied Health Professionals: An Intervention and Utilization-Focused Assessment

David M. Brings

Minnesota Center for Social Research, University of Minnesota,
Minneapolis, Minnesota 55454

An important and difficult task for health educators concerned with epilepsy is the development of educational programs and materials that provide accurate information about epilepsy and improve the lives of persons with epilepsy. Even when adequate resources are available for such programs and materials, educators can fall short of their objectives. One reason for this is that these programs and materials do not reach people who need them, or when they do, they are not useful (Larson and Nichols, 1972; Gutek el al., 1974). Educators do not always address the needs of the potential consumer of educational information, or translate that information into practical action alternatives (Havelock, 1976; Zaltman and Duncan, 1977).

The Minnesota Comprehensive Epilepsy Program (CEP) has been engaged in a number of formal and informal educational efforts designed to be responsive to these concerns. Noteworthy have been the educational programs and materials directed to medical and allied health professionals. The research described here was undertaken to assess the epilepsy-specific educational needs of medical and allied health professionals so that effective educational interventions could be planned, implemented, and evaluated. It is an example of a utilization-focused evaluation (Patton, 1978), designed to answer the following questions:

1. Is there a set of sensible criteria that can serve as the basis for assessing the epilepsy-specific educational needs of medical and allied health professionals, and also be used to evaluate educational interventions directed to them?

2. Are there identifiable groups of medical and allied health professionals that represent workable target populations for educational interventions?

3. If there are identifiable target populations and sensible assessment criteria, are there systematic relationships between them, such that indi-

vidualized educational programs and materials can be developed to satisfy unique epilepsy-specific needs?

MATERIALS AND METHODS

A questionnaire was constructed to survey medical and allied health professionals' knowledge about epilepsy and Minnesota state laws pertaining to epilepsy, attitudes toward epilepsy and persons with epilepsy, procedures for serving persons with epilepsy, contacts with epilepsy or persons with epilepsy, and personal and organizational demographic characteristics.

Questionnaires were mailed to 527 medical and allied health professionals in Minnesota. These health professionals worked for organizations that CEP had previously identified, via a feasibility study, as potential intermediaries, through which persons with epilepsy could be identified for medical and social services. Two weeks after the initial mailing, a follow-up letter was sent to nonrespondents reminding them of the importance of their responses and giving them the opportunity to request another questionnaire, in the event that they had misplaced or never received their original copies. A total of 343 persons returned completed questionnaires, giving a response rate of 65%.

The 343 health professionals who responded represented eight types of services as follows: day activity (23%), public health nursing (20%), welfare (18%), mental health (11%), advocacy (8%), vocational counseling (8%), employment (7%), and rehabilitation (5%).

With regard to work roles, 34% of the respondents were administrators, 32% were direct service providers, and 34% performed some combination of both. Of the total group of respondents, 42% were directors of their respective organizations.

Respondents held the following academic degrees: Bachelor of Arts or Science (51%), Master of Arts or Science (25%), Registered Nurse (8%), High School diploma (7%), Doctor of Philosophy (3%), Associate of Arts (3%), Doctor of Laws (2%), and Doctor of Medicine (1%).

Females composed 50% of the total group of respondents.

Data analysis began with the construction of composite dependent variables from the knowledge, attitude, and procedure items. Knowledge items were those that had correct and incorrect response choices. If a correct response was selected, one point was awarded. If an incorrect or "don't know" response was selected, no points were awarded. A composite knowledge score was then computed for each respondent by summing their scores across all knowledge items.

Attitude items were those that asked respondents to make positive or negative value judgements about epilepsy, persons with epilepsy, or services for patients with epilepsy. Procedure items were those that asked respondents to describe procedures employed by themselves, their own organizations, or other organizations to serve persons with epilepsy. Construction of composite dependent variables for these items was carried out via two separate factor analyses—one on the attitude items and one on the procedure items. The alpha method of factor analysis was used for each of these procedures. The objective here was to generate one set of attitude factors and one set of procedure factors that would be maximally generalizable to the actual, but previously unknown, dimensions underlying the attitudes and procedures of medical and allied health professionals. For each of these factor analyses, an orthogonal Varimax rotation was used to approximate a simple factor structure. Factor scores were then calculated for each of the factors generated.

Next, a set of independent variables was selected from among the demographic and contact items. The fundamental criterion for selection was relevance for assessing the epilepsy-specific educational needs of medical and allied health professionals so that educational interventions to meet those needs could be planned and evaluated. That is, a demographic or contact item was selected as an independent variable if a confirmed relationship between it and a dependent variable would have practical social action implications for health educators.

To explicate underlying relationships in the data, each composite dependent variable was tested with each of the independent variables. All of the dependent variables were analyzed as interval variables. Independent variables were analyzed as either nominal variables or ordinal variables, depending on whether they designated categories or amounts of a certain characteristic, respectively. Correlation coefficients were calculated between each dependent variable and each ordinal independent variable and tested for statistical significance. Analyses of variance were carried out for each dependent variable with each nominal independent variable. For each analysis of variance, a multiple classification analysis was also carried out to rank values for independent variable categories around the grand mean of each dependent variable.

RESULTS

Significant results emerged to answer each of the research questions. First, 19 dependent variables were identified as criteria for assessing the epilepsy-specific educational needs of medical and allied health professionals, and evaluating the impact of educational interventions appropriate to those needs. Eight of these were found to be particularly useful. They were as follows:

Knowledge: High scorers gave correct responses to items about epilepsy and Minnesota state laws pertaining to epilepsy.

Prejudice: High scorers expressed prejudicial attitudes toward persons with epilepsy.

Social problem orientation: High scorers interpreted the problems facing persons with epilepsy as social problems.

Relevance: High scorers felt that it is important that they know something about epilepsy in order to perform their job well.

Avoidance: High scorers reported that they feel uneasy around persons with epilepsy and that they are hesitant to have social contact with them.

Identification action: High scorers reported that they make an effort to identify persons they serve who have epilepsy.

Referral action: High scorers reported that they refer persons they serve, who identify themselves as having epilepsy, to services available to them in other organizations.

Procedural action: High scorers reported that they, or their organizations, have special procedures for serving persons with epilepsy.

Second, 15 independent variables were identified for focusing educational interventions on specific target populations. Each of these described an aspect of one of the following eight general characteristics: *service type, work role, job tenure, educational background, sex, age, previous experience with epilepsy,* and *previous exposure to epilepsy-specific educational information.*

Third, individual differences in performance on the assessment criteria were found to vary in a lawful manner with respondents' target population.

DISCUSSION

On the basis of these findings, each of the research questions can be answered affirmatively. These findings also reveal a number of important implications for the development, dissemination, and utilization of epilepsy-specific educational information.

With regard to the development of educational programs and materials, this research suggests that grouping informational content according to knowledge, attitudes, and procedures is a sensible means to understanding and addressing educational needs. With regard to the dissemination of epilepsy-specific educational information, this research shows the importance of matching programs and materials to target population needs. Finally, this research demonstrates the efficacy of utilization-focused evaluation for planning educational interventions.

ACKNOWLEDGMENTS

This project has been funded, at least in part, with federal funds from the Department of Health, Education and Welfare under contract number N01-NS-5-2327.

REFERENCES

Gutek, B. A., Katz, D., Kahn, R. L., and Barton, E. (1974): Utilization and evaluation of government services by the American people. *Evaluation*, 2, 1, 41–46.

Havelock, R. G. (1969): *Planning for innovation through dissemination and utilization of knowledge*. Institute for Social Research, Ann Arbor.

Larson, J. K., and Nichols, D. G. (1972): If nobody knows you've done it, have you. . . ? *Evaluation*. 1, 1, 39–44.

Patton, M. Q. (1978): *Utilization-Focused Evaluation*. Sage Publications, Beverly Hills.

Zaltman, G., and Duncan, R. (1977): *Strategies for Planned Change*. John Wiley & Sons, New York.

Advances in Epileptology:
The Xth Epilepsy International Symposium,
edited by J. A. Wada and J. K. Penry.
Raven Press, New York © 1980.

The Development of Self-Help Groups

Shelagh McGovern and Owen M. Jones

British Epilepsy Association, London, England

Epilepsy is a word familiar to everyone reading this volume, and sometimes familiarity can breed a kind of contempt, in that it can cause us to accept the *word* and overlook the ramifications. Unless one is a physician, or more specifically, an epileptologist, the diagnosis of epilepsy tells us practically nothing except that the individual has a tendency to fits. To know that he has epilepsy is to possess information that is, in itself, practically useless. It does not specify the type of fits he has; how often, or how rarely they occur; and to what extent, if any, they affect his ability to live a full life. These are facts that we have to discover; otherwise we risk doing thousands of people a grave disservice.

This philosophy was the basis for the British Epilepsy Association's decision to set up self-help groups throughout the country.

What has bedevilled people with epilepsy, certainly in Great Britain, and surely internationally, is the problem of "not knowing"—why it has happened to them, how to cope with the diagnosis, not knowing when a fit will occur, where to go for nonmedical help, not knowing what reaction they will evoke from their friends, neighbors, and even family if they have a fit. The family's and the public's lack of understanding about what it *is*, or what to do, or what the person with epilepsy is able to do, add to the problem. The British Epilepsy Association has a vital and imaginative program of health education designed to replace the ignorance with an enlightened awareness. Nevertheless, we recognize that the surest way of getting a message home to anyone is to have it illustrated and demonstrated in his own village or town.

In 1974 we devised a formula that was both simple and fraught with dangers. We formed groups of people, in villages, towns, and cities who were prepared, for whatever reason, to work for epilepsy. This aspect was not difficult. The danger lay in the tendency of each member of the group to become involved solely with his own interest, exacerbating an already poor situation.

We solved this problem by deciding what the aims of the groups should be and then building, within each group, the expertise necessary to fulfill the needs efficiently and effectively.

Briefly, the aims are two-fold: (a) to provide support and information for those with epilepsy and their families and offer them the therapy of shared involvement; and (b) to present an enlightened focal point for the local community whose work or leisure brings them into contact with the problems of epilepsy.

Groups vary in composition both numerically and in ability, and so any structure that is to contain them all must be flexible. Any rigidity will hinder development at some point. Even so, a structure must be present, as well as guidance. It must constantly be remembered that we are probably dealing, in every group, with a small percentage of people who, because of their epilepsy, have never before "belonged." To some of these there is little difference between freedom and license. We realized we were in our early, inexperienced stage, but even then there were very few calamities and no disasters. Most of the problems that arose sprang from difficulties in personal relationships and from feelings of inadequacy that became apparent through aggression, dominance, or negative reactions. These difficulties continue in spite of our efforts because we are dealing with people, some of whom have been damaged by constant rejection, some of whom have become embittered by seeing a member of their family struggling for a foothold in a society that did not understand, and some of whom are only now, through contact with a group, learning the social skills that enable people to be accepted in society.

Such people illustrate the need for the first aim of groups. They need support, information, and therapy. The British Epilepsy Association provides groups, through films and tapes, information about various aspects of living with epilepsy and it encourages groups to undertake events that will absorb the efforts of all members to the degree of which they are capable. To provide enlightened support for existing members and for individuals or families newly diagnosed, the association trains group members in "skills in helping," and provides a constant back-up service, accepting the ultimate responsibility for any action taken.

To strengthen the authority of the group, the association trains suitable members as speakers. The standard is high and those who pass the test are accredited, by the association, to speak on its behalf to local, non-professional audiences. We provide refresher courses, and the more able speakers are asked to attend advanced sessions to update their knowledge and increase their expertise.

The British Epilepsy Association is aware of the need to unite groups throughout the country in a common campaign; we call this aspect of our work "Action for Epilepsy." The campaign is centrally administered and organized and although we aim for flexibility, there are certain statutory requirements that groups must fulfil. Any material prepared for the media must first be passed by the association unless it deals only with domestic matters. Secretaries of groups are required to send regular reports of meetings and events. Support members and speakers liaise with, and work through, the campaign staff, and group treasurers send statements of the financial situation with cash returns every quarter. The campaign staff send out a bi-monthly newsletter to all groups and there are two national conferences a year to which each group sends delegates.

The "Action for Epilepsy" campaign is the means by which the Association establishes a presence in villages, towns, and cities throughout the country. The groups are our representatives locally, and with their help we are in touch with local views and reactions about which we might otherwise be unaware. In addition they provide a channel through which the association can present its message and its policy to local communities. The value of this network of self-help groups to the parent body is undeniable, and it alone would be sufficient.

But there is a more significant consideration that is demonstrated in each of the 100 areas in which groups operate: the effect of the campaign on the lives of individuals and families living with epilepsy. The local educational program eventually promotes the type of public understanding that can differentiate between epilepsy and fits, that recognizes the intensely individual nature of the condition, and seeks to learn about each individual case. In many cases this enlightened attitude locally has caused people to come forward and join a group after living in secrecy and isolation for as long as 20 to 30 years. The enlightenment spreads to local employers, who are encouraged to review their policy with regard to people with epilepsy. General practitioners have often told us that the knowledge gained by their patients has challenged their professional expertise. This may be considered a mixed blessing, but hopefully in the final analysis greatly benefits the patient.

There is no doubt in the collective mind of the British Epilepsy Association that self-help groups work. People with personalities damaged by constant rejection gained stature and regained confidence and self-respect through group work. We have seen overprotective parents gradually relax their hold on the life of a child, and the family unit begin to operate without strain. We have seen energies channeled, abilities developed, and skills discovered as a result of group work.

Groups offer the means of rehabilitation for socially damaged people by presenting various types of challenge in a familiar atmosphere. To be fully effective they need a strong, informed and efficient committee and it is the responsibility of the parent body to train able people to take office within the group. Within the British Epilepsy Association we have learned the need to provide an efficient back-up service, a steady stream of ideas and encouragement, and a structure that is both flexible enough to contain the more avant garde thinkers, and firm enough to inspire confidence in those who habitually need support.

The Action for Epilepsy Campaign is our answer. In 4 years we have recruited into action groups, 3,000 people who are living with epilepsy. Once they have been helped to come to terms with their problems, they are ready to offer help to others, and to pass on their knowledge and understanding to a wider public.

The development of self-help groups, therefore, is the development of ever-increasing enlightenment and tolerance, which we are confident must eventually benefit all those with epilepsy in Great Britain.

NOTE ADDED IN PROOFS: Alterations to Miss McGovern's original text were made by the editors.

Advances in Epileptology:
The Xth Epilepsy International Symposium,
edited by J. A. Wada and J. K. Penry.
Raven Press, New York © 1980.

Public Awareness and Attitudes Toward Epilepsy in Finland

*M. Iivanainen, **A. Uutela, and **I. Vilkkumaa

*Department of Neurology, University of Helsinki, Helsinki, Finland; and
**Department of Social Psychology, University of Helsinki, Helsinki, Finland

There are many difficulties in the relationships between epileptic people and others. Usually this is attributable to negative attitudes toward epilepsy in the general population (Bagley, 1971; Ekermo, 1976). In recognition of needed change in these attitudes, the Finnish League for Epilepsy started its Attitude Forming Program in early 1977. Its purpose is to try to eliminate the stigma of epilepsy, and to prevent discrimination of epileptic persons in society. Just prior to the start of this program, a survey of attitudes in Finland was undertaken; the results are reviewed in this chapter. The major goals of this first part of the program were: (a) to obtain an initial estimate of public awareness and attitudes toward epilepsy, allowing later assessment of the effectiveness of the attitude forming program, and (b) to correlate, if possible, awareness and attitudes of the responders with two variables: social background and contacts with epileptic people. We report here the results of the survey and its analysis.

PATIENTS AND METHODS

In early 1977, 3,000 names were randomly selected from the population registry, with ages ranging from 15 to 64 years. Of these, 2,789 were contacted in two mailings; 2,272 (81%) responded. Twenty-eight epilepsy-related questions were asked. These concerned social background, contacts with epileptic persons, awareness of epilepsy, and general opinions and attitudes of the interviewees toward the disorder. The style of the questions was obtained in part from studies in the United States (Caveness et al., 1974); the questions were modified to reflect the characteristics of Finnish society.

---

*Dr. Iivanainen's present address is: National Institute of Communicative Disorders and Stroke, Bethesda, Maryland 20014.

This chapter appears in expanded form in *Epilepsia*, 21(4), 1980 (*in press*).

RESULTS

The social background of those who answered did not deviate significantly from that of the population as a whole in this age range. Late responders appeared to have more negative attitudes than those who answered more quickly. Only a few, however, had a distinctly negative attitude; only 0.9%, for example, would resign from their jobs if an epileptic co-worker were hired. There were 19 epileptic persons among the responders. This is 0.7% of those contacted and 0.8% of those answered. Of the responders, 95% had heard of epilepsy, 50% knew an epileptic person, 40% had seen an attack, and 12% knew how to aid a person having a generalized convulsive seizure. Fifteen percent offered a reasonable opinion regarding the cause of epilepsy, e.g., disease of the nervous system, trauma, and heredity. The attitude toward children with seizures was more charitable than toward adults.

The ability to help an epileptic person having an attack was explained by three variables: (a) knowing an epileptic person, (b) education, and (c) age of the responder. Variables such as social background and contacts with epileptic people were unimportant in explaining attitudes toward epilepsy.

Knowing an epileptic person correlated with potential for assistance; this potential varied considerably between different age and educational groups. It was highest (good in 61%) in older, well-educated individuals who know an epileptic person and lowest (good in 1%) in younger, less educated persons who did not know an epileptic person (Table 1). Furthermore, three trends were evident: Potential for assistance was highest among (a) those who knew an epileptic person, (b) persons with high education, and (c) persons of older age groups.

The material could be divided into three subgroups on the basis of the correlation between knowing an epileptic person and potential for assistance related to age and education. This correlation was very small (1–4%) in the best educated groups of young (15–29) persons and in the best educated group of middle-aged (30–49) persons. The correlation was strong (25%) in the 50- to 64-year old group with advanced education; the effect was moderate in other groups.

Generally, there was a positive correlation between age and favorable attitudes. However, the amount of favorable attitudes decreased in very old persons. Another exception to the trend was that the attitudes related to work and hobbies were more favourable in younger than older individuals. In addition to the close association between favorable attitudes and knowing an epileptic person, education and age, persons who had better jobs and who lived in an urban society also tended to have favorable attitudes. In general, females had better attitudes than males.

DISCUSSION AND CONCLUSIONS

A questionnaire on public awareness and attitudes toward epilepsy in Finland showed that 95% had heard of epilepsy, 50% knew an epileptic

TABLE 1. *Potential for assistance correlated with education, knowing an epileptic person, and age*[a]

	High education				Low education			
Knows an epileptic person:	Yes		No		Yes		No	
Age:	15–29	50–64	15–29	50–64	15–29	50–64	15–29	50–64
Potential for assistance	(N = 58)	(N = 23)	(N = 77)	(N = 12)	(N = 91)	(N = 193)	(N = 131)	(N = 135)
Good	22	61	21	8	10	14	1	4
Some	66	35	51	67	55	69	35	39
Lacking	12	4	29	25	35	17	64	56
Total	100	100	100	100	100	100	100	100

[a]Middle-aged (30–49 years) persons with average education fell mostly between the extreme values below. Values expressed in percent of N in each column.

person, and 45% had seen an attack. Thus Finns recognized the term epilepsy as well as Americans, but fewer Finns than Americans knew an epileptic person or had seen an attack (Caveness et al., 1974). The observation that only a few of the responders had a very negative attitude toward epilepsy is interesting, since impressions from medical practice contrast with this. It is known that questionnaire methods tend to produce socially acceptable answers. This bias is likely to have affected this study. Another factor that might have affected these figures is the poor economic climate at this time. The observation that only 1% of the responders would leave their jobs if they had to work together with an epileptic person may be related to economics rather than fundamental attitudes toward the epileptic person. Ignorance and negative attitudes were correlated with delayed response time. It seems likely that negative attitudes may even have prevented some from answering at all. The prevalence of epilepsy (0.7%) in the present small sample corresponds rather well to the prevalence measured in larger studies, which generally report figures of about 0.5%. Many forms of epilepsy, however, especially nonconvulsive forms, are underdiagnosed, and the actual prevalence may be considerably greater.

Epileptic persons themselves appeared to effectively disseminate information about epilepsy. Besides actually providing information, their very existence also necessitates the spread of information. Also, certain processes in Finnish society such as rising educational level and aging of the population are factors promoting the dissemination of such information. Knowing an epileptic person seems to be the most significant factor in the ability to help. Level of education and age appear to be less important in this respect.

The National Epilepsy Association and its many local chapters have even more effective opportunities for spreading information than private persons. To have a job is also important to the epileptic person, as it offers an opportunity to form a positive and active self-esteem. Furthermore, fellow epileptics, in cooperation with physicians, psychologists, social workers, and others can be of great help in solving difficult problems. The legal position of epileptic people, for example, could be improved faster if efforts were made in a cooperative manner with appropriate associations. We should also emphasize cooperation with other countries in this field.

Education should be directed especially toward the younger age groups, where awareness of epilepsy was astonishingly poor. We need laws to ensure equality between epileptic people and healthy persons in educational and vocational areas of life. Premises will thus be set forth for the development of real human relationships; the epileptic stigma and its negative content will gradually be removed.

ACKNOWLEDGMENTS

This study was supported by the Slot Machine Association (Rahaautomaattiyhdistys) and Research Foundation, Orion Group Ltd.

REFERENCES

Bagley, C. (1971): *The Social Psychology of the Child with Epilepsy*. Routledge and Kegan Paul, London.

Caveness, W. F., Merritt, H. H., and Gallup, G. H., Jr. (1974): A survey of public attitudes toward epilepsy in 1974 with an indication of trends over the past twenty-five years. *Epilepsia*, 15:523–536.

Ekermo, C. (1976): What it means to have epilepsy. Emotional experience and social reality. In: *Epileptology. Proceedings on the Seventh International Symposium of Epilepsy*, edited by D. Janz. West Berlin.

Advances in Epileptology:
The Xth Epilepsy International Symposium,
edited by J. A. Wada and J. K. Penry.
Raven Press, New York © 1980.

A Pilot Project to Forestall Chronic Unemployment Among Young People with Epilepsy

Harold A. Benson, Jr. and Susan A. Dabbert

Epilepsy Foundation of America, Washington, D.C.

The recent report of the United States Commission for the Control of Epilepsy and its Consequences (1977) identified the search for employment as one of the major problems faced by persons with epilepsy. Until now, the working community has not welcomed persons with epilepsy with open arms. On the contrary, it has been an uphill and often futile struggle for persons with this disorder to break into the working world. To complicate this, current rates of employment in the United States have provided employers with a virtual army of nonhandicapped persons from which to select employees. Finally, of the handicapped persons who are hired, persons with epilepsy are the last on the list to be chosen. These facts encourage persons with epilepsy to hide their disability, further complicating employer attitudes. It is time that steps were taken to tear down some of these barriers.

Over the past 25 years, the attitude of the United States public toward epilepsy and the person with epilepsy has improved quite significantly. However, in 1974 there still remained an estimated 10 million people who were opposed to persons with epilepsy being part of the working force. Generally, the surveys indicated that the more favorable opinions toward persons with epilepsy were expressed among the better educated, better employed, younger, and urban members of the population. Yet despite the improved attitude, the Commission reports that the unemployment rate for persons with epilepsy is somewhere between 17 and 25%. Most rehabilitation workers identify employer resistance to hiring persons with epilepsy as the significant factor barring rehabilitation. Undoubtedly, the biggest obstacle to rehabilitation of people with epilepsy can be traced to this continued employer resistance. Furthermore, the emotional roots of this prejudice have proven to be resistant to appeals to logic or intelligent reasoning.

Another aspect to be considered in employment of those with epilepsy is the effect of psychosocial difficulties on overall job performance. In many instances, these problems relate to the childhood environment. Certain parental attitudes and child rearing practices may negatively affect the child's achievement. Overprotectiveness or the emotional smothering of a child with epilepsy by his parents may impair his work performance. Thus, a rehabilitation counselor should include the parents within the individual written rehabilitation plan, if possible, to determine the influence of the home and family and to secure their full support for the program. Even if the parents have not been overly protective of the child, it is quite likely that the child has had difficult experiences in school relating to the disorder. The counselor should be prepared to deal with low expectations and lack of confidence in some students.

Underemployment was identified as another major problem for people with epilepsy. One reason given by the Commission investigating epilepsy was that, after suffering repeated rebuffs from employers, people with epilepsy tend to accept employment from which they are overqualified. The Epilepsy Foundation of America's Training and Placement Service (TAPS) project has been successful in assisting these individuals in obtaining employment more suitable to their individual skills and training.

Cooperative working agreements have been reached with other service providers such as vocational rehabilitation agencies to complement rather than compete with their services.

Referrals are carefully screened during the intake process to assure the appropriateness of providing services. On occasion, referrals are made to state rehabilitation systems for assessment and vocational testing. Referrals are also accepted from rehabilitation systems and other service providers to assist in the placement process.

A lifetime of rejection and excuses because of misunderstanding on the part of others can hinder an individual's realistic approach to employment. Constant referral to the disability as a reason for refusal to hire may cause these persons to become defensive in many ways. These are problems that rehabilitation counselors and employers alike must be aware of and be prepared to address. One difficulty is the possible unwillingness of co-workers to accept persons with epilepsy. Such attitudes may be due to a lack of understanding of what the disability *is* and what it *is not*. Feelings of fear, uncertainty, and even superiority on the part of the person with epilepsy may have to be dealt with by the rehabilitation counselor and the employer.

Studies have shown that the person with epilepsy can be a successful and contributing member of the community when these problems are dealt with effectively and realistically. These studies were a basis for the development in 1976 of TAPS of the Epilepsy Foundation of America (EFA), a program funded by the United States Department of Labor under the Comprehensive Employment and Training Act. Since that time, local prime sponsors have also been engaged to provide additional support to five local project sites (Atlanta, Cleveland, Minneapolis-St. Paul, Portland, San Antonio), as well as to interest local business, industry, and schools for endorsement of the

TAPS program within the community at large. A prime sponsor is a local agency designated by the Department of Labor to administer and distribute federal funding within the community. Since the start of the project, Boston has been added as a sixth Department of Labor funded project, and several other cities and states have been funded by other resources such as vocational rehabilitation, developmental disabilities, and state manpower monies. The program, including community development, job development, and the need for appropriate preemployment procedures will be discussed.

At the time of its inception, the TAPS project target population was limited by the United States Department of Labor to young people with epilepsy seeking employment. EFA realized early that, in addition to efforts of the local prime sponsor, each project would have to embark on its own campaign to heighten and improve public awareness and acceptance of the employment needs of persons with epilepsy. Toward this end, the responsibility of TAPS staff and volunteer advisors in each city has been to forge linkages with, and elicit the cooperation of, various community manpower and support services. Extensive contacts have been made with such organizations as the National Alliance of Businessmen, local boards of education, chambers of commerce, state employment services, committees on the employment of the handicapped, state and local legislators, personnel management associations, and vocational rehabilitation agencies. Local media are also utilized; newspaper articles, radio announcements, and television coverage help to highlight the employability of persons with epilepsy.

TAPS provides a wide spectrum of employment service from job seeking and job keeping skills classes to job development, on-the-job training, and job placement and follow-up. Services are always geared to the individual, taking into account his/her personal problems, goals, and current level of job-related skills.

Enrollment in TAPS is completely voluntary. Some local schools identify potential clients and then notify their parents regarding the TAPS program, or may refer clients directly. In certain cities, CETA offices and department of rehabilitation agencies also identify eligible applicants and refer them to TAPS. Physicians, medical clinics, and social service programs refer as well.

Once an individual expresses an interest in TAPS, personal data are obtained and a training agreement is established between the project and the trainee. After trainees are enrolled, the coordinator evaluates their employment-related problems, interests, and abilities, and devises a suitable employment plan. This plan may include subsidized on-the-job training, as well as job preparation and training in job retention skills.

Since the early months of the TAPS program, national and local staff have become aware that certain socioeconomic problems, coupled with generally low skill or training level, impede on-the-job training for some enrollees. Project staff estimate that approximately 68% of clients have little or no knowledge of how to look for a job. Moreover, some enrollees suffer from poor self-image, lack of independence and self-confidence, and inability to compete. Consequently, in some cities, employers were receptive to providing training but the clients simply were not ready to take advantage of it. To remedy this situation, all projects are now providing some form of job-seeking and job-keeping skills to their clients.

This program, which may be described as job readiness training, encourages the development of an objective approach by the client to self-evaluation, realistic career information, campaigning for a job, development of applications and/or resumés, interview techniques, and employer/employee relationships. It is up to the counselor to make an exceptionally careful and intelligent placement for each client. Job development must be approached focusing on the clients' employment objectives and goals based on their needs. Job development is much more than the solicitation of a job opening. It is a complex process that requires team effort, taking into consideration the needs of both employers and clients; that places persons in the jobs most suitable to them, jobs that provide career development; and that provides employers with productive workers to fill their manpower needs. Job development involves reducing artificial barriers as mentioned heretofore, while close cooperation among all involved would be crucial to ensure successful retention of the client on the job. Approaches to employers will differ depending on the type of placement being sought; direct placement in an unsubsidized position for a "job ready" person or partially subsidized employment as an initial step.

Recognizing that job retention is often a serious problem for persons with epilepsy, another support group entitled Retain and Increase Salaries Efficiently (RAISE) was formed. RAISE meets monthly and is designed to give employed persons with epilepsy a chance to discuss problems that arise in the job situation.

Job development can be effective only in the context of the local labour market conditions. Information must be obtained by the coordinator regarding present anticipated job openings utilizing certain criteria such as the skills required and the industry involved; plant expansions or contractions; characteristics of the local labor force, particularly of the unemployed as to age, sex, race, and geographic concentration; skill level; average hourly earnings and hours of employment, and so forth. Counselors must develop strategies to contact employers and establish good relationships with them. The counselor should be fully aware of services that are available to clients and to employers, and should know the employment market. Counselors should be required to make a minimum number of contacts per day or week, based on the distance to be travelled and on contract obligations. Goals should be established for the number of referrals expected from the contacts.

The success of any job development effort depends on an accurate diagnosis of the decision making patterns, employment practices, and interpersonal approach for job development. The counselor can save a lot of time by going directly to the person in the company who will make the ultimate hiring decision. Personnel departments primarily perform a screening function and should be considered for the purpose of job solicitation. Supervisors, department heads, or foremen are generally the people who make the decision to hire. The hiring practices of individual employers must be addressed, particularly the job mobility ladders and training opportunities within the companies.

Workers' compensation and insurance are often used in the United States and Canada as reasons for denying employment to persons with epilepsy. Many employers express concern that insurance rates will escalate if employees with epilepsy are on the job. Studies conducted by the Epilepsy Foundation of America and others have shown that these notions are untrue.

The activities of the TAPS coordinator do not end with the placement of a client, but must be continued to ensure successful retention on the job through continued supportive services; provision of onsite crisis intervention; exploring possibilities of job restructuring to create new positions; follow-up, including the provision of advisory and supportive service to management and to client, i.e., emergency transportation or mediating a dispute, social services, and so forth; and arranging "rap" sessions with employer and employees to alleviate tensions that may have developed and discuss mutual problems.

In order to alleviate tensions felt by co-workers, it would be beneficial for the training and placement coordinator to discuss personally the disorder with them and dissipate any fears or uncertainties they may have about their co-worker's disability. The "buddy system" is often employed by the TAPS project at the outset of employment or with individuals who have a hard-to-control seizure disorder. The "buddy system" involves pairing up one co-worker with the person with epilepsy who can assist with the basic first aid procedures should a seizure occur on the job. It is similar to the "buddy system" utilized by the labor unions.

Although TAPS was originally funded as a 1-year demonstration project this first year was completed so successfully that a second-year contract was approved, an additional project site was added, and services were expanded to assist *all* vocational age groups, broadening the original specifications emphasizing youth.

The project has approached the community in an innovative way in an effort to integrate school systems, community systems, and employment systems into a comprehensive support system for the client. The coordination of these resources, i.e., community agencies, social service programs, vocational rehabilitation, media, local and state government, school systems, self-help groups, and so forth, has developed a strong support network within the community in order to provide employers and clients with new and positive attitudes and assistance regarding successful placement of persons with epilepsy.

By developing public awareness, public acceptance, and public involvement within a community, we have provided the client with an adequate support system to enable him to enter and remain in the employment market in a meaningful position.

Advances in Epileptology:
The Xth Epilepsy International Symposium,
edited by J. A. Wada and J. K. Penry.
Raven Press, New York © 1980.

Placement of Multiply Handicapped Epileptic Clients into the Open Job Market

*Barbara Rader, *Howard L. Shapiro,
and *,**,†Ernst A. Radin

*Epilepsy Center of Michigan, Detroit, Michigan 48201; *Department of Neurology and Electroencephalography, Detroit, Michigan 48207; and †Department of Neurology, Wayne State University School of Medicine, Detroit, Michigan 48201*

From October, 1974 to October, 1975, the Epilepsy Center of Michigan (ECM) participated in a joint project with the Michigan Bureau of Rehabilitation (BR) and the Jewish Vocational Services (JVS) in order to ascertain how many chronically unemployed, multiply handicapped epileptic clients could be successfully placed into the competitive job market when maximum resources are made available to them. It was also an opportunity to demonstrate interagency coordination and a team approach to meeting the employment needs of individuals with epilepsy. Clients identified for the project were severely disabled as a result of their seizure disorder along with concomitant other problems and had employment difficulties.

METHODOLOGY

Each client received a comprehensive evaluation consisting of social history, neurologic, psychiatric, psychologic, and electroencephalographic investigations, in addition to other laboratory tests as indicated. After a complete evaluation, representatives of BR, JVS, and the staff of ECM met in joint conference to decide whether a given client was a suitable candidate for the special rehabilitation project. In case of doubt, a decision was made to admit the client to the project on a trial basis in order to maximize the client's chances in life. Only individuals with severe psychiatric handicaps, profound intellectual problems, or severe neurological disabilities, e.g., spastic triplegia in addition to epilepsy, were excluded. A client who was accepted into the program was then referred to JVS for a 4-week period of work evaluation that included assessment of work-related behavior and a work adjustment training phase designed to prepare the individual for competitive employment. During the workshop phase, individuals were involved in both individual and group counseling. Candidates who successfully completed the workshop were then placed by the JVS placement specialist into a work exposure program in the community lasting up to 6 weeks. The employers subsequently had the option to either hire the person or to return the client to JVS with a letter regarding the individual's job performance.

SUBJECTS

A total of 91 individuals were initially identified for the project; however, 33 either dropped out or were screened out prior to having had contact with ECM. Fifty-eight clients were evaluated and considered by ECM for the program and, at the staff conference, 44 were found to be suitable candidates for the workshop, keeping the previously mentioned criteria in mind. All clients who were accepted into the program were closely followed medically, either at ECM or at Lafayette Clinic (LC) with frequent anticonvulsant blood level determinations. The sample description is given in Table 1 and an attempt is made in the table to compare some data with the Three Cities Study conducted by Frank (1969) containing a much larger client population. Table 1 compares the socioeconomic characteristics of the sample of those clients who participated in either of the two projects. As can be seen from Table 1, although the ECM sample contained more males and more members of the white race, ECMs clients were less commonly married, had lower educational attainment in terms of college but higher educational attainment in graduations from high school, and lower occupational standings. The diagnostic characteristics of the ECM study shown on Table 1 cannot be compared with the Three Cities project; however, it is apparent that the mean I.Q. of our clients was in the dull-normal range and that the additional handicaps the clients were experiencing were predominantly of a psychiatric and/or intellectual nature.

RESULTS

On completion of the project, 10 of the 44 clients who had been recommended by ECM for the work evaluation phase of the project did not enter the program at JVS. Nine others did not complete the workshop evaluation at JVS. Of the remaining clients, 15 were hired after the work exposure program, although not necessarily after the first one. Up to four different employers (average two employers) were tried in some instances before the client could be regarded as employed at the time of termination of the project. Four additional clients found work through their own efforts after they had failed the work exposure programs. This brings the total of employed clients at the time of termination of the project to 19. If one calculates the employment rate by considering only those clients who had successfully completed the JVS workshop program (*N*25), it would be 76%. Considering the 34 clients who had in fact made initial contact with the JVS workshop program, the success rate is 56%. If one, however, considers the sample that

TABLE 1. Socioeconomic and diagnostic characteristics of participants (N58) in ECM study and comparison with Three Cities study participants (N115)

	ECM	Three Cities
Median Age	27	28
Sex (%)		
Male	71	61
Female	29	39
Marital status (%)		
Married	12	26
Single	78	57
Separated	5	9
Widowed	—	2
Divorced	5	—
Educational attainment (%)		
0–4 Years	3	6
5–8 Years	14	20
9–11 Years	28	32
High school graduate	48	25
Some college	7	14
College graduate	—	4

ECM Study Participants

I.Q.	Range	Percent
Superior	120–129	2
Bright normal	110–119	—
Average	90–109	40
Dull normal	80–89	29
Borderline	70–79	20
Defective	Under 70	9
	Range: 55–122	
	Mean: 85.7	

Epilepsy and related disabilities	Percent
Epilepsy associated with intellectual or organic mental changes, but no psychiatric problems	7
Epilepsy associated with psychiatric problems, but no intellectual or organic mental changes	15
Epilepsy associated with psychiatric problems and intellectual limitations and/or organic mental changes	78

was regarded as potentially suitable for employment and referred to JVS (N44), the rate of employed clients dropped to 43% and, finally, when the total number of clients discussed at the staff conference (N58) are used in the calculations of the success rates, the figures drop further to 35%.

Inasmuch as it was anticipated that these initial figures might not represent long-term success or failure, follow-up efforts continued for the 25 clients who had completed the workshop phase. As of June, 1977, contact had been made with 21 of the 25 clients and only 11 of them were working full-time, although not necessarily within the same company. Part-time employment was not included because these individuals were still receiving financial assistance. This means that only 52% of the 21 were still employed and, therefore, a drop of success of 24% from the time of completion of the project. In January, 1978, all 44 clients who had initially been referred to JVS were sent letters to inquire about their current status with regard to employment. Of these, two were returned "undeliverable" by the post office and only 19 clients replied. Most of the information regarding current status on the others was obtained from other knowledgeable sources.

From this 2-year follow-up, information was available on 18 of the 25 clients who had completed the workshop phase. Of these, seven who were employed at the termination of the project were still employed and one additional individual who was not employed at termination was now employed as the result of her own efforts after the project. Therefore, eight of 18 were employed which yields a success rate of 44%, a drop of 8% from the June, 1977 follow-up, and 32% from the termination of the project. There was not a structured or statistical review of factors, which resulted in failure at obtaining or maintaining employment. However, it should be noted that all individuals in this project had concomitant organic or psychiatric problems that interfere with employability. In regard to organicity, motor slowing appeared to be a major influence in the failure of clients to achieve employment. The successes, although few, were striking. For example, one man who had been receiving disability for 20 years has been employed at the same job for the last $2\frac{1}{2}$ years after participation in this project. Another man who had no prior gainful employment and who had a long history of incarceration has also been employed in the same job for the past $2\frac{1}{2}$ years.

DISCUSSION

It is of interest that the percentage of clients regarded as unsuitable for the second phase of the project was very similar between the ECM and the Three Cities study, i.e., 24% versus 29%. It is also important to mention that the initial success rate of multiply handicapped individuals who participated in the Three Cities project was 57% and ECMs was 56%, when one considers those clients who had actually made contact with JVS. This means that the findings obtained by ECM, although generated by a small number of clients, are representative for a larger epilepsy population who experience employment difficulties. Our study extends beyond these observations, however, because it demonstrates quite clearly that the results decay with time and points to the necessity of having to work with the client over several years before one can make a final judgment of failure or success.

Only a few studies are available in the literature that give success rates for employability of epileptic clients and nearly all of them suffer from the problem that final assessment is made when the project terminates. Since most of the projects cover only a 1- or 2-year span, the follow-up is correspondingly short and the figures that are being generated are not likely to hold up on a long-term basis. In the Three Cities study, the follow-up was done at 1 month, 3 months, 6 months, and 1 year after placement, but no figures are provided as to relative number of clients in the various follow-up categories. Since the entire project lasted only from August, 1966 to March, 1968, it is likely that in the majority of cases, clients had been followed less than 1 year. Schwartz (1975) who provided an extensive review of the literature and bibliography on the topic of rehabilitation of epileptic clients, noted that nationally an estimated 36% of the total handicapped population was successfully rehabilitated into jobs in 1974. Not only is this figure disturbingly low, but also it contained only 0.15% of epileptic clients who are known to be difficult employment placement problems. De Torres (1963) in Minneapolis showed an employment rate of 50% after rehabilitation efforts, but follow-up was likewise short due to termination of the project, and the same applies to the Massachusetts project (Pigott, 1969). The latter was planned for 4 years and started in 1967. The first-year report dated February, 1968 covered June, 1967 through January, 1968, but the final report was dated September, 1969, which can only mean that the total project covering 210 clients was cut short after 2 years. At the time of closure, 42% of clients were employed; the rest were either still in workshop evaluation training, other forms of rehabilitation or phased out due to poor cooperation. Similar findings were also available in Europe. Porter (1968), with length of follow-up unspecified, reported that 59% of 100 registered disabled clients who were referred for intensive rehabilitation efforts were subsequently employed within the open market. Feuerstein and Verdier (1974) reported 36% employment after rehabilitation and Juul-Jensen (1963), 31%. While these figures indicate that rehabilitation of epileptic clients does indeed represent a major challenge to rehabilitation agencies, it must be emphasized very strongly that the clients who have vocational problems usually suffer not only from epilepsy, but also from additional associated handicaps. As Dennerll et al. (1966) have stated previously, it is the intellectual/organic as well as the psychiatric components of the client that usually decide unemployability of a given client rather than the frequency of type of seizures. This finding is in agreement with other published data, especially those of Juul-Jensen (1961) and Hakkarainen (1973) who stressed likewise that the mental state of the client is the decisive factor in whether or not employment can be found and held. Since rehabilitation of epileptic clients is frequently difficult, time-consuming, and expensive, a careful assessment should be made at the onset in regard to the suitability and motivation for competitive employment for a given client. Where placement with a severely disabled epileptic population is concerned, a team approach such as has been demonstrated in this project is required. It is also necessary that employers have the disciplines involved in the composition of the team available as consultants in the initial stages of employment. In addition, there is a need for continuing supportive services for this population to assure that the person's medical and psychosocial problems do not interfere with maintaining employment. This will require a specialized resource that can provide continuity of care and will follow the client indefinitely to maximize his chances of maintaining employment. Finally, we must recognize that some individuals will never be able to compete in the labor market and that the use of alternative forms of employment such as the sheltered workshop may be the only feasible solution.

REFERENCES

Dennerll, R. D., Rodin, E. A., Gonzalez, S., et al. (1966): Neurological and psychological factors related to employability of persons with epilepsy. *Epilepsia*, 7:318–329.

De Torres, T. (1963): *Employment problems of epileptics*. Research and Demonstration Grant 382, Office of Vocational Rehabilitation, Department of Health, Education and Welfare, Washington, D.C.

Feurerstein, J., and Verdier, P. (1974): Follow-up of severe epileptics discharged from a professional rehabilitation center (French). *Readaptation (Paris)*, 208:24–28.

Frank, D. S. (1969): *The multi-troubled jobseeker: The case of the jobless worker with a convulsive disorder.* Three Cities Employment-Training Program. Epilepsy Foundation of America, Washington, D.C.

Hakkarainen, H. (1973): Rehabilitation of patients with epilepsy. *Acta Univ. Oul.*, D5, Neurology 1, Oulu, Finland.

Juul-Jensen, P. (1961): Vocational training of epileptics. *Epilepsia*, 2:291–296.

Juul-Jensen, P. (1963): Epilepsy: A clinical and social analysis of 1,020 adult patients with epileptic seizures. *Acta Neurol. Scand. (Suppl. 5)*, 40:1–148.

Pigott, R. A. (1969): *Evaluation of a service program focused on vocational rehabilitation as prototype for an urban voluntary epilepsy agency*, Boston, Massachusetts. Research Grant No. RD2592-G, Rehabilitation Services Administration, Department of Health, Education and Welfare, Washington, D.C.

Porter, R. (1968): Epilepsy and employment. *Irish J. Med. Sci.*, 7:83–90.

Schwartz, R. P. (1975): Epilepsy employment: An historical perspective. *Unpublished study*, San Diego, California.

Advances in Epileptology:
The Xth Epilepsy International Symposium,
edited by J. A. Wada and J. K. Penry.
Raven Press, New York © 1980.

Socioeconomic and Demographic Characteristics of Childhood Epilepsy in the New Haven Area

Sherry L. Shamansky

University of Washington School of Nursing, Department of Community Health Care Systems, Seattle, Washington 98195

During this past century, there has been increasing awareness of epilepsy as a major medical and socioeconomic problem, and numerous epidemiologic studies have been accomplished. However, little information is available on socioeconomic and racial status as risk factors for epilepsy. No study in the United States literature has reported incidence rates for epilepsy among Blacks. The only information concerning differences in rates for epilepsy according to race was provided in a detailed analysis of death certificate data from the United States for the years 1959 through 1961 (Kurtzke, 1972). Non-Whites consistently had a rate for epilepsy more than twice as high as that for Whites, and the male preponderance was much greater among non-Whites than Whites. In the United States, data from the 1973 National Health Survey (1977) suggest that there is an inverse relationship between family income and education of the head of the family and the prevalence of epilepsy. In addition, rates for epilepsy are higher either in the central city or rural areas than in the suburban areas of Standard Metropolitan Statistical Areas.

PATIENTS AND METHODS

Region Studied

This epidemiological investigation was designed to provide an estimate of the incidence of childhood epilepsy in the New Haven, Connecticut area. The 11 towns in the New Haven Standard Metropolitan Statistical Area were grouped into four areas according to indices of socioeconomic status—income, occupation, and education—obtained from the 1960 and 1970 census information. The towns in area I comprised the highest socioeconomic area. Area IV, the central city of New Haven, was the lowest socioeconomic area.

EEG requisitions and reports were reviewed to identify the children who were being evaluated for possible epilepsy. Information available from the requisitions and reports included name, address, date of birth, sex, race, date of EEG, history of illness, age at onset of symptoms, description of the seizures, possible etiology, physical and neurological findings, medications, tentative clinical diagnosis, and the results of the EEG. Whenever the EEG requisition forms were incomplete, every attempt was made to obtain missing information from the hospital record if the patient had been assigned a unit number.

It appeared that review of the EEG requisitions and medical records from the two major hospital EEG facilities would provide nearly complete identification of children with diagnosed seizure disorders in the New Haven Standard Metropolitan Statistical Area. A patient met the residency requirements if he or she lived in the New Haven Standard Metropolitan Statistical Area at the time of the initial EEG and had not reached the 15th birthday at that time. The date of the first EEG was considered the date of diagnosis; the date of the first known symptoms and/or seizure was considered to be the onset of the seizure disorder.

Classification of Cases

The definitions and classifications used in this study were similar to those of Hauser and Kurland (1975). Cases were classified into three categories: (a) definite epilepsy; (b) probable epilepsy; and (c) neonatal seizures.

Category 1 included children with historical or clinical evidence of at least two episodes of seizures, without an identifiable causative metabolic or acute structural abnormality.

Category 2 included children with clinical or historical evidence of a single convulsion from any cause, recurrent convulsions occurring within 3 months of an acute process that produced an identifiable structural alteration of the brain, or repeated convulsions, each related to a recurrent systemic metabolic disease, e.g., hypoglycemia, uremia, or to exposure to a toxic agent. Patients in this category might or might not have been treated with anticonvulsants.

Category 3 included recurrent severe generalized seizures that occurred in the neonatal period, designated as the first 28 days of life.

In all categories the EEG was considered an adjunct in making the diagnosis; the report of abnormal cerebral electrical rhythms in the absence of clinical findings of epilepsy did not result in a ''case'' for this study any more than a normal EEG in a patient with an appropriate history would rule out such a diagnosis. Each case was classified on the basis of the clinical history; whenever questions arose with regard to classification of a case, the requisition and record were reviewed by an epileptologist whose clinical inference prevailed.

RESULTS AND DISCUSSION

Study Population

After the requisitions for more than 45,000 EEGs had been examined, 733 individuals met the age, residency, and significant medical criteria necessary for the inclusion in the study population. The "definite" category included 557 patients; 123 children comprised the "probable" group; and 53 infants were included in the "neonatal" category.

Sex Ratio

There was a slight excess of males among diagnosed epileptic children ($p = 0.08$), with a ratio of males to females of 1.2. For White children, the male to female ratio was 1.08; for Black children, 1.36.

This finding was consistent with findings reported in other studies (Crombie et al., 1960; Krohn, 1961; Gudmundsson, 1966; Leibowitz and Alter, 1968; Ounsted and Taylor, 1972; Brett, 1974; and Brown et al., 1974). Several explanations for the male excess have been postulated. Males seem to be more susceptible to many diseases at any given chronological age than do females because of a different rate of development of the immune system (Ounsted and Taylor, 1972). Male children are reported to have more accidents, episodes of head trauma, and ingestion of toxic substances during childhood, factors that contribute to the development of secondary epilepsy.

Age at Diagnosis

Analysis of the data according to age at diagnosis and sex revealed that the mean age at diagnosis for children under 15 was older for females than for males, 6.5 years and 5.9 years, respectively ($p = 0.11$). This trend was consistent when race was held constant; the mean age at diagnosis for White females was 6.6 years; for White males, 6.2 years; for Black females, 6.4 years; and for Black males, 5.4 years.

The later age at diagnosis of epilepsy in females is apparently related to the onset of menarche. It has long been known that there is a direct relation between epileptic seizures and menstruation (Livingston, 1958). The precise physiologic change or changes that occur during the menstrual cycle and that are responsible for the precipitation of seizures are not clearly understood; they are thought by some to be related to complex hormonal changes, disturbances with pre-menstrual edema, and/or cerebral circulatory changes. The mean age at diagnosis was younger for Blacks than for Whites; it is of interest to note that age at onset of menarche is younger for Black females than it is for Whites.

Race

Evidence that Blacks were consistently at greater yearly risk than Whites, both among males and females, was abundant. There was a statistically significant increase in the case rate among Black males in both the 1960 through 1964 and 1965 through 1970 time intervals ($p < 0.01$ and $p < 0.0001$, respectively). Similarly, the excess of cases among Black females was statistically significant for both time intervals ($p < 0.05$ and $p < 0.01$, respectively). When sex and time were held constant using Cochran's method, the difference in the proportion of epileptics among Blacks and among Whites was still highly significant ($p < 0.0001$).

This is the first United States study that has estimated the incidence of epilepsy among Blacks. No incidence or prevalence study reported in the literature has given good evidence of racial differences, since the communities and study populations have had very small numbers of Blacks.

The data in this study did show an excess of Blacks regardless of the variable considered, and the consistent differences between Whites and Blacks would be difficult to explain by extraneous variables or possible errors during the coding process. From 1960 through 1970, Black males were at greatest risk, followed by Black females, White males, and White females. Overall, the rate for Blacks (1.17 per 1,000) was nearly twice that for Whites (0.62 per 1,000). There is some evidence that the census underestimates the size of the Black population in Connecticut, but it is doubtful that this could account for the nearly twofold increased rates among Blacks. The conclusion was therefore reached that Black children were more susceptible to epilepsy than were White children.

When all cases were considered for the eleven years, 1960 through 1970, the cumulative incidence rate of 11.03 per 1,000 implied that 1 in 91 children in New Haven Standard Metropolitan Statistical Area would suffer from epilepsy before the fifteenth birthday.

Socioeconomic Status

The distribution of epilepsy was next examined according to economic area. For 1960 through 1970 holding race or sex or age at diagnosis constant, there was a significant association between epilepsy and economic area, i.e., children from the lower socioeconomic areas had an increased risk for epilepsy.

There was a total of 733 cases of epilepsy diagnosed for the eleven year period. Numbers of cases per year ranged from a low of 42 in 1962 to a high of 101 in 1967, with an average yearly number of 66 and a mean annual incidence rate of 0.73 per 1,000 population under 15 years of age.

Cumulative Incidence of Diagnosed Epilepsy in the New Haven Standard Metropolitan Statistical Area

The annual age-sex-race-specific incidence rates were summed to calculate the cumulative incidence or attack rate.

In this study, the prevalence of epilepsy in children at 15 years of age was considered to be equivalent to the cumulative annual incidence up until that age. The cumulative incidence rate was seen as a useful measure of the frequency of a condition that affects a narrow age range (Molloy and MacMahon, 1966) and was used in this study under the following assumptions: (a) Epilepsy occurs predominantly during childhood (Brett, 1974). (b) The age-specific mortality rate for epilepsy is minimal (0.46 per 100,000 in children under 15 in Connecticut, 1970). (c) The incidence rate for this condition remains relatively constant over the time interval considered in this study. The prevalence rate found in this study at age 15 was 11.03 per 1,000 population, a rate consistent with those reported above, although different study methods and somewhat different populations were used.

The ethnic derivations of the populations showed considerable variation and could have accounted for part of the difference in the prevalence of epilepsy. It was also possible that the differences noted could have reflected true variations in the frequency of seizures between geographic regions. Data from the National Health Survey (1977) indicated that the prevalence of convulsive disorders was somewhat higher in the northeast regions of the United States.

Epilepsy, like some other chronic disorders, is of multiple etiology. However, there is a dearth of information about factors leading to a high risk of epilepsy. In spite of the absence of definitive information, it is believed that the incidence of convulsive disorders is high in medically indigent urban populations (Wiygul, cited in Alter and Hauser, 1972). Lack of medical care in such individuals may lead to neurological complications from common diseases. Other populations with a high risk of epilepsy may include those with high infant mortality, groups with high accident rates, and groups in which prenatal care is poor or lacking. Still other groups that would be expected to have a high rate of convulsive disorders include those with nutritional deficiencies, a high rate of premature births, birth defects, and birth injuries that might be expected to accompany poor nutrition. There is a known relationship between lead intoxication and convulsive disorders, and it has been well documented that lead poisoning is more common among inner city children.

In the New Haven Census Use Study (1971), it was noted that populations in areas of New Haven City characterized as low socioeconomic status were noticeably remiss in the adequate surveillance of health care. Pregnant women in low socioeconomic areas had fewer prenatal visits, more anemia during pregnancy, more prematurity, and more complications of pregnancy. It is noteworthy that the twofold risk for epilepsy among Black children parallels the infant mortality rate for Blacks, which is twice that for Whites. It is possible, then, that some aspects of epilepsy may have social causes.

REFERENCES

Alter, M., and Hauser, W. A. (editors) (1972): *The Epidemiology of Epilepsy: A workshop. NINDS Monograph No. 14, DHEW Publication No. (NIH) 73–390*, Washington, D.C.

Brett, E. M. (1974): Some aspects of epilepsy and convulsions in childhood. *S. Afr. Med. J.*, 48:705–707.

Brown, J. K., Purvis, R. J., Forfar, J. O., and Cockburn, F. (1974): Neurological aspects of perinatal asphyxia. *Develop. Med. Child Neurol.*, 16:567–580.

Crombie, D. L., Cross, K. W., Fry, J., Pinsent, R. J. F. H., and Watts, C. A. H. (1960): A survey of the epilepsies in general practice: A report by the Research Committee of the College of General Practitioners. *Br. Med. J.*, 2:416–422.

Gudmundsson, G. (1966): Epilepsy in Iceland: A clinical and epidemiological investigation. *Acta Neurol. Scand. (Suppl 25)*, 43:1–124.

Hauser, W. A., and Kurland, L. T. (1975): The epidemiology of epilepsy in Rochester, Minnesota, 1935 through 1967. *Epilepsia*, 16:1–66.

Krohn, W. (1961): A study of epilepsy in northern Norway: Its frequency and character. *Acta Psychiatr. Neurol. Scand. (Suppl. 150)*, 36:215–227.

Kurtzke, J. (1972): Mortality and morbidity data on epilepsy. In: *The Epidemiology of Epilepsy. A Workshop*, edited by M. Alter and W. A. Jauser, pp. 21–31. *NINDS USDHEW Monograph 14.*

Leibowitz, R., and Alter, M. (1968): Epilepsy in Jerusalem, Israel. *Epilepsia*, 9:87–105.

Livingston, S. (1958): Convulsive disorders in infants and children. *Adv. Pediatr.*, 10:113–195.

Molloy, M., and MacMahon, B. (1966): Incidence of Legg-Perthes disease (osteochondritis deformans). *N. Engl. J. Med.*, 275:988–990.

National Health Survey (1977): Prevalence of chronic conditions of the genitourinary, nervous, endocrine, metabolic, and blood and blood-forming systems and of other selected chronic conditions United States—1973. *Series 10, No. 109 DHEW Publication No. (HRA) 77-1536, National Center for Health Statistics.*

Ounsted, C., and Taylor, D. C. (1972): *Gender Differences: Their Ontogeny and Significance.* Williams & Wilkins, Baltimore, 273 pp.

NOTE ADDED IN PROOFS: Much of this data previously published in: Shamansky, S. L. and Glaser, G. H. (1979): Socioeconomic characteristics of childhood seizure disorders in the New Haven area: an epidemiologic study. *Epilepsia*, 20:457–474.

Advances in Epileptology:
The Xth Epilepsy International Symposium,
edited by J. A. Wada and J. K. Penry.
Raven Press, New York © 1980.

Lay Association Movement for People with Epilepsy in Japan

Ryo Matsutoma

Japanese Epilepsy Association, Suginami-ku, Tokyo, Japan

The problems relating to epilepsy in Japan are complicated by the conflict and imbalance between our changing economic and social structures and our Japanese traditions and conventions. Rapid changes after World War II in Japan's industrial structure and major reform of the social system have stimulated a gravitation of population to the cities, causing the conventional community and family system to collapse. Our traditional interrelationships among regional communities based on "soil" and "blood" are facing dissolution, and policies of the central and local governments are powerless to cope with the situation.

However, it is not easy to change the customs peculiar to Japan, which is a united nation consisting of one race on a small island country. Our history of communities founded on a rice crop agriculture in a temperate monsoon climate, with cultural influences in religion, philosophy, and politics from China and India, dates back more than 2,500 years. We still observe the proprieties of respecting harmony within our own group while at the same time disliking exceptions and differences, and being clannish to other groups.

In our country, prejudice and discrimination toward people suffering from epilepsy do not appear collectively or violently. We have no history of religious persecution of epilepsy. On the contrary, prejudice and discrimination are individualistic, psychological, and latent. The Japanese word "ten-kan," meaning epilepsy, is a medical term originating in ancient China. Today, however, it is also used to ridicule and insult and may be used in a teasing manner referring to acts having no relation to epilepsy itself. It is enough to say, "He has epilepsy" if you want to keep a sufferer away from school, from his job and community, and sometimes even from his relatives. This stems from the fact that the sufferer and his family consider epilepsy shameful and they will become withdrawn and self-accusing because they know they cannot be a part of any community without mental acceptance and mutual bonds.

In addition to mental pressures and rejection by other members of the group to which they belong, the limitations of the nuclear family in support of a patient often prevents him from taking advantage of the appropriate treatment and thus the possibility of social independence. Government policy in certain areas also hinders the movement to reform discriminating procedures that keep patients from acquiring various qualifications, such as a driver's license. These conditions force the sufferer and his family to face secondary problems, often leading to character change, family collapse, poverty, and suicide, which in most cases means mass suicide of a whole family.

ORIGINS OF THE MOVEMENT

Considering this background of Japanese society, the movement on behalf of epileptic patients was negligible and carried out by small bodies working for mental patients and retarded persons. In fact, it was not until 1973 that the first and true fight got underway.

In 1973 two bodies were founded separately. One was the Association of Parents of Children with Epilepsy, which consisted mainly of parents of children with West's syndrome. The other was the Volunteers Association for People with Epilepsy, which was made up of medical specialists on epilepsy and the families of adult sufferers. In the development of both organizations we found overlapping membership and problems. As a result, the need for unification of the two associations was apparent and concrete discussions to achieve this end were held.

In October 1976, after more than 6 months of consultation, the two bodies were formally unified as the Japanese Epilepsy Association, also known as Nami no Kai, meaning association of waves. Our movement now entered a new stage. More than 350 sufferers, their families, physicians, and volunteer workers gathered from all over the country for the founding meeting held in Tokyo. Dr. Haruo Akimoto, President of the Japanese Epilepsy Society, emphasized in his commemorative address the importance of the fight against epilepsy and the significance of the new organization. In December of the same year (1976), the Japanese Epilepsy Association formally joined the International Bureau for Epilepsy as an association representing Japan.

ORGANIZATION

The association has eight branches with about 2,000 members throughout the country, the most recently established branch having opened on October 1, 1978. Irrespective of belief, occupation, religion, or thought, anyone may become a member and be registered with the head office. The membership fee is approximately $15 a year, but this is sometimes excused depending on the member's circumstances. With the help and guidance of the head office, each branch carries on its own activities and maintains an independence and character of its own.

An approximate breakdown of the association's membership is: patients,

15%; their families, 65%; physicians, 5%; non-medical professionals, 5%; and volunteers, 10%. The overwhelmingly high proportion of patients and their families is indicative of the weakness of our social assurance system, poor awareness of specialists, especially social workers, and the short history of voluntary activities in Japan. It shows also that it is the persons most directly concerned who most strongly desire the existence of the organization and who spare no effort on its behalf. This is true of every association for handicapped people. All activity funds, approximately $7,500 a year, are derived from membership fees, individual contributions, and income from bazaars and publications. Physicians and officials provide their services at no cost.

ACTIVITIES OF THE ASSOCIATION

Our association's aims are to abolish ignorance, prejudice, and discrimination toward people with epilepsy, and to this end we appeal to the public, to government, and to self-governing bodies to foster a system with sufficient medical services, education, and welfare for these individuals. A further aim is to resolve the uneasiness and problems of sufferers and their families by providing them with useful information and the opportunity to make contact with each other. Our activities are of a social nature; however, participation in each concrete activity provides an opportunity for training and counselling. Therefore, our activities fill the role of on-going, comprehensive care in the field of human relations.

Our chief activities during the past 5 years were as follows:

1. More than 150 regular meetings for suffers and their families have been held in various places, with 10,000 participants. Lectures on medical treatment and case counselling take up most of the time of our meetings, although we sometimes meet for recreational activities such as hiking.

2. Four thousand copies of our association's 20-page publication are published every month. The 52nd issue has recently appeared. We have more than 200 regular subscribers and copies are sent to the central and local governments and to medical institutions. The contents of this publication are topical and contain information on medical treatment, education, welfare and job opportunities, notices and reports of our activities, and personal experiences of sufferers and their families.

3. Two annual summer camps are held every year in the country. One is a 4-day camp for parents and children. Five camps of this kind have been held. With the help of volunteers and specialists, children are trained at camp to support themselves in everyday life in such things as how to dress themselves, etc. At the same time, parents study and have discussions with each other apart from their children. The other camp is for adult sufferers, planned and carried out voluntarily by the sufferers themselves and aimed at fostering a voluntary spirit and cooperation.

4. At all times we conduct counselling by telephone and by letter covering

a few thousand cases a year. Our counselling covers many areas; e.g., introduction to medical institutions, explanation of medical treatment, and advice on therapy. This information is provided by officers of the association, voluntary workers, and physicians.

5. Every year, lectures to enlighten the public and to educate volunteers are held, along with study groups for non-medical professionals. The former are free and participation in the last three lectures totalled more than 1,000. The latter, which started last summer, gathered participants from all over the country. In spite of a $30 registration fee, applications were received from more than twice the number who could be accommodated (250).

6. Appeals are made regarding swimming for children with epilepsy. We have appealed to government offices, school teachers, and to the public for approval of swimming for children with epilepsy. In conjunction with this, we opened swimming schools in various locations. The main reason that prevents children with epilepsy from swimming is the question of who will be responsible if there is an accident. This sort of thinking comes from ignorance and prejudice toward epilepsy. Unfortunately, most people believe it is harmful for persons with epilepsy to participate in sports of any kind, to say nothing of swimming. Our swimming schools were held in five places this year, with 350 participants. One of the classes was broadcast over the radio to reach a wider audience.

7. We believe that the real situation of people with epilepsy is still unknown to the public, and we have carried out studies into the actual conditions of our members. The first study was done in 1974 and the second one is now in progress. Within the year, we are planning a publication on studies into epilepsy and have invited papers. It will be the first of its kind in Japan.

8. Public enlightenment is continually carried out by means of pamphlets, posters and mass-communication appeals. On occasion, we are compelled to take stronger action. For example, last year a newspaper in Japan with a circulation of 8 million carried an article written by a criminal psychiatrist in which he conjectured that an unarrested criminal who had committed a bizarre murder might have been an epileptic. Because the article linked epilepsy with crime, we protested and succeeded in having the newspaper subsequently publish an apology.

9. We have appealed to the central and local governments for better understanding of epilepsy and for the start of a comprehensive care policy. This kind of activity has been carried out by various means, such as presentation of demands, meetings with responsible persons, petitions, and so forth.

IMMEDIATE GOALS

The following problems still confront us:

First, in order to strengthen our organization we must increase the number of members and branches. It is especially necessary to appeal to more volunteers and non-medical professionals to join and build up our movement with a broad, long-term perspective.

Second, we must continue our persistent appeal to the national and local governments to make them recognize epilepsy in its proper light and to make appropriate policies.

Third, and most important, the establishment of a sound financial basis for maintaining and development of the above activities is indispensable.

In conclusion, we believe that the history of people with epilepsy in Japan will be changed by our efforts, which are paving the way for a new era. We thus proudly declare that our persistent fight will continue toward achievement of this worthwhile goal.

Advances in Epileptology:
The Xth Epilepsy International Symposium,
edited by J. A. Wada and J. K. Penry.
Raven Press, New York © 1980.

Mobile Delivery of a Comprehensive Program Multidisciplinary Team

Malcolm J. Cant

Director of Special Education, Vancouver Neurological Center,
Vancouver, British Columbia, Canada

The philosophy of the Vancouver Neurological Center is unique in that it endeavors to provide a comprehensive and decentralized program for its clients; that is, treatments are conducted in the home and at school/preschool wherever possible, instead of the center proper.

PATIENTS AND METHODS

Of the 197 clients with epilepsy who have been with the center since 1974, 45 clients were randomly sampled to be the recipients of a survey questionnaire. There was a 75.5% return of the questionnaires; i.e., 34 of the original 45 that were mailed out. The questionnaires were constructed so that there was no way in which the client (respondent) could be identified by the investigator.

For the years 1975 through to a pro-rated 1978 year, the professional staff time-statistics were compiled so that an investigation of actual staff member/client interaction time could be pursued. The statistics were compiled for the epilepsy caseload, the cerebral palsy caseload, Parkinson's caseload, and the total caseload in order that the total statistical picture could be presented—this being a more realistic overview of the value of a decentralized program.

RESULTS

The statistics contained in Table 1 represent the staff member/client interaction time on the basis of individual sessions, group sessions, and family conferences inclusive. They reflect the working days that are lost per year due to annual vacations, statutory holidays (11 per year), professional advancement time, and staff turnovers when there is less than the normal staff complement in a given department. The statistics do not reflect the working time that is lost per year due to: sick leave, open days, lectures for student groups, staff meeting time, and telephone contacts.

TABLE 1. *The staff member client interaction time for individual, group, and family conference sessions per working day*

Social work	Epilepsy	Cerebral palsy	Parkinson's	Total
1975	3.15	2.03	0.03	5.48
1976	3.24	1.41	0.33	4.98
1977	3.39	1.74	0.36	5.49
1978	3.72	1.11	0.56	5.39
Occupational therapy	Epilepsy	Cerebral palsy	Parkinson's	Total
1975	1.05	2.30	—	3.35
1976	1.47	3.24	—	4.71
1977	2.40	3.58	—	4.98
1978	2.56	3.72	—	6.28
Speech therapy	Epilepsy	Cerebral palsy	Parkinson's	Total
1975	2.06	2.95	0.00	5.01
1976	0.70	3.85	0.03	4.58
1977	1.37	4.04	0.30	5.71
1978	1.25	3.58	0.34	5.17
Educational consultant	Epilepsy	Cerebral palsy	Parkinson's	Total
1975	1.11	2.95	—	2.26
1976	1.89	0.96	—	2.85
1977	3.21	1.29	—	4.50
1978	4.11	1.72	—	5.83
Physiotherapy	Epilepsy	Cerebral palsy	Parkinson's	Total
1975	0.25	5.19	—	5.44
1976	0.20	4.77	—	4.97
1977	0.28	4.85	—	5.13
1978	0.26	6.09	—	6.35

It can be seen that, for a regular working day, the social worker spends 5.39 hr per day in 1978 in actual client contact, 3.72 hr being for clients with epilepsy. The occupational therapist spends 6.28 hr per day in 1978 in actual client contact, 2.56 hr being for clients with epilepsy. The speech therapist spends 5.17 hr per day in actual client contact, 1.25 hr being for clients with epilepsy. The educational consultant spends 5.83 hr per day in 1978 in actual client contact, 4.11 hr being for clients with epilepsy. The physiotherapist spends 6.35 hr per day in 1978 in actual client contact, 0.26 hr being for clients with epilepsy.

The results that were obtained from the survey questionnaire are as follows:

The five most important factors about the services given by the center that help to meet the total needs of the client

No. responders	Percent of responses
(30) Involvement with home and school	88.2
(30) Open communication with staff members	88.2
(28) Informed about client's progress	82.4
(26) Cost of treatment is based on income	76.5
(24) The variety of services	60.6
(16) Individual home treatments	47.1
(6) Personal relationship built up with staff	17.6
(2) Can select the location for treatment	5.9
(2) No other center available in the city	5.9
(0) Staff members are like one of the family	0
(0) Other	0

The five most important factors about the services given by the center that fail to meet the total needs of the client

No. responders	Percent of responses
(28) Not enough staff	82.4
(18) Lack of communication with doctors[1]	52.9
(14) Not enough treatment sessions	41.2
(6) Parents not informed of client's progress	17.6
(4) Lack of communication with parents	11.8
(4) More pressure should be put on fathers to help	11.8
(2) Not enough practical advice given	5.9
(0) Too demanding of parents	0
(0) Invasion of family privacy	0

[1]All physicians receive the written reports of staff members who are involved with their particular referred patients, so this may be a case of physicians not reading their mail!

What are the benefits of treatment at the home for your child and yourself?

No. responders	Percent of responses
(24) Program is more personal in nature	70.6
(24) Program builds a better relationship between staff member and child	70.6
(16) Child cooperates much better at home	41.1
(16) Do not have transportation or parents unable to drive	41.1
(14) More carryover by the parents of what staff member demonstrates	41.2
(2) Program adapted to facilities at home	5.8
(0) It is not different from treatment at the center	0

What are the benefits of treatments at the center for your child and yourself?

No. responders	Percent of responses
(16) The opportunity to meet other parents, see other children	47.1
(16) A group treatment better suits the needs of the child	47.1
(8) Have no babysitting or transportation problems	23.5
(4) It is more professional to go to the center	11.8
(2) The opportunity to get out of the house	5.9

It is interesting to note that 47.1% of the respondents have transportation problems whereas only 23.5% of the respondents have no babysitting or transportation problems.

What are the benefits of treatments at the school/pre-school for your child and yourself?

No. responders	Percent of responses
(26) Teacher will know what staff member is doing with the child	76.5
(26) There is better communication between the school and center staff	76.5
(26) Potential problems in class can be avoided	76.5
(20) Closer personal relationship develops between teacher, staff member, and parent	58.8
(16) Parents are better informed of child's progress in school	47.1
(14) Child misses less school work than if he/she has to go in to the center	41.2
(4) Teachers learn more about the child's special problems	22.8
(0) It is no different from treatment at the center	0

At what location do you feel that your child benefits most from his/her treatments with staff members?

No. responders	Percent of responses
(20) Home	58.8
(8) School/Pre-school	23.5
(4) Location isn't a factor	11.8
(2) Center	5.9

It can be seen that, with 58.8% of the responses, the respondents felt their child benefits most from home treatments with the staff members. This fits in with the 88.2% response rate for "involvement with home and school" as the most important factor about the services that are given by the center (Question 1).

Have you learned more about your child's epilepsy through . . . ?

No. responders	Percent of responses
(16) Home treatments	47.1
(12) Film and lecture	35.3
(3) Physician	8.8
(2) Center treatment	5.9
(1) School/Pre-school treatments	2.9

It is interesting that 47.1% of the respondents indicated that they had learned more about their child's epilepsy through home treatments, whereas 35.3% felt that they learned more from the film and lecture presentation. The neurologist in charge of the epilepsy case load of the center makes a public film and lecture presentation three times per year at the center. All parents, clients, and interested members of the public are invited to attend these presentations.

Have you learned more about your child's developmental progress (0–5 years) through . . . ?

No. responders	Percent of responses
(16) Home treatments	47.1
(6) Pre-school treatments	17.6
(0) Center treatments	0
(0) Other locations	0

It must be pointed out that referrals that come in to the center are not all of the early age at which we would prefer to commence our work. As a result of this, not all the respondees (64.7%) could check a response to this question.

Have you learned more about your child's school functioning through . . . ?

No. responders	Percent of responses
(22) School/Pre-school treatments	64.7
(4) Home treatments	11.8
(4) Center treatments	11.8
(0) Other	0

An overwhelming 64.7% of the respondents were of the opinion that they learned more about their child's school functioning through school/pre-school treatments.

Do you feel that you can contribute more to your child's treatment and thus progress, from staff treatments that are given as . . . ?

No. responders	Percent of responses
(24) Home treatments	70.6
(8) School/Pre-school treatments	23.5
(2) Center treatments	5.9
(0) Other	0

Does a closer bond develop between the staff member and child as a result of . . . ?

No. responders	Percent of responses
(26) Home treatments	76.5
(6) School/Pre-school treatments	17.6
(2) Center treatments	5.9
(0) Other	0

It was felt by 76.5% of the respondents that a closer bond developed between the staff member and child as a result of home treatments. This question was included in order to assess the validity of the responses to the question of "the benefits of treatments at the home for your child and yourself." To this question 70.6% of the respondents felt that "the program was more personal in nature," and the "program builds a better relationship between staff member and child."

What professionals should be included in a team that is to serve the total needs of the child with epilepsy and his/her family?

No. responders	Percent of responses
(30) Neurologist	88.2
(28) Family physician	82.4
(28) Educational psychologist	82.4
(26) Special education consultant	76.5
(25) Occupational therapist	73.5
(20) Social worker	58.8
(20) Speech therapist	58.8
(17) Play therapist	50.0
(12) Recreation therapist	35.3
(10) Child and adolescent psychiatrist	29.4
(9) Vocational psychologist	26.5
(8) Music therapist	23.5
(4) Pediatrician	11.8
(3) Nurse	8.8
(2) Clinical psychologist	5.9
(1) Physiotherapist	2.9
(0) Other	0

The medical professionals lead the list with 88.2% and 82.4% of the responses for neurologists and family physicians, respectively. The educational and developmental professionals follow with 82.4%, 76.5%, and 73.5% of the responses for educational psychologists, special education consultant, and occupational therapist, respectively. The next three response-ordered choices have their involvement more in the home and social situation (as well as the school to a degree!). They are the social worker, speech therapist, and play therapist with 58.8%, 58.8%, and 50.0%, respectively. The latter response was very surprising to the investigator.

DISCUSSION

One of the most frequently used arguments against the implementation of a decentralized or mobile program of any type is the lack of actual client interaction time. However, it can be seen that a well structured, decentralized program can have a very acceptable number of hours per day of client interaction for all the departments within a comprehensive center.

Admittedly, there has not been an investigation of the comparison between the cost in dollars and cents for the operation of a centralized service and a decentralized service. A comparison of this type should look at the long term results of this investment of public monies.

There has been definite evidence presented that the clients of the center are justly satisfied with the program, which meets their needs in the home, the school and the community, and with the composition of the team that is utilized to serve their needs.

I will conclude this chapter by reiterating the remarks that Dr. Feindel made during his Guest Lecture at the Opening Ceremony of this Epilepsy International Symposium . . . "there is a need for comprehensive programs for persons with epilepsy."

Advances in Epileptology:
The Xth Epilepsy International Symposium,
edited by J. A. Wada and J. K. Penry.
Raven Press, New York © 1980.

United States Commission Report on Epilepsy: Social Aspects

*Richard L. Masland and **Patsy M. Owens

*Neurological Institute, College of Physicians and Surgeons of Columbia
University, New York, New York 10032; and **National Institute of Neurological
and Communicative Disorders and Stroke, National Institutes of Health,
Bethesda, Maryland 20014*

In 1976, the United States Congress established a Commission for the Control of Epilepsy and its Consequences to study the state of the art of medical and social management of epilepsy in the United States, to make recommendations regarding the role of federal and state governments and public and private agencies, and to develop a comprehensive national plan (USDHEW, 1978). In so doing, the Congress recognized that measures for the control of epilepsy are not limited to the administration of drugs, or the application of surgical procedures, but include also a broad spectrum of social and rehabilitation services.

Whether or not seizures are controlled, the psychological and social consequences of epilepsy must be negated if the individual is to take his appropriate place in society. Unfortunately, this aspect of the control of epilepsy is frequently overlooked. Rodin et al. (1976) document that the disabilities of epileptic persons relate less to their seizures than to their psychological and emotional concomitants, and that only 23% of their clients suffer from "epilepsy only"—48% exhibited intellectual impairment and 54% significant changes of behavior.

Intervention to ameliorate the consequences of epilepsy relates to a number of areas.

SOCIAL ADJUSTMENT AND MENTAL HEALTH

Mental health care systems in the United States include various state institutions for those who need psychiatric and psychological services and community mental health centers that provide mostly outpatient care and include some short-term, local hospital, inpatient care. People with epilepsy are traditionally served by these mental health systems only if a psychiatric or psychological problem is present and is the predominant reason for requesting the service.

The person with epilepsy faces a unique constellation of psychological insults: his own and society's reaction to his illness; the effects of depressant drugs; the direct effect of the seizure on the brain; and the impact of underlying brain disease. Recent data suggest that some forms of epilepsy are associated with a special psychological impact, but all must cope with environmental stresses, which can be devastating. There is need for more counselors trained to help persons with epilepsy. Not only should such help be available in epilepsy centers, but community mental health centers should also be prepared to deal with the mental health problems of persons with epilepsy.

The adolescent and the young adult with epilepsy face emotional problems of special severity. Many cannot flourish within an overprotective home environment. There is a great need for semi-sheltered or group living environments where young persons can achieve independence yet receive the benefit of mutual support. The United States has no centers such as those of Holland, Belgium, and Norway, within which young people with epilepsy can have the benefit of a total rehabilitation effort.

At an older age, psychosis is not uncommon in epilepsy. Twelve percent of those in our state mental institutions suffer from epilepsy. Early intervention and appropriate manipulation of anticonvulsant and ataractic drugs may reduce this figure. This problem is urgently in need of greater attention.

EDUCATION AND EMPLOYMENT

Recent years have seen notable changes regarding the education of handicapped children in the United States. The "Education Amendments of 1974" mandated that no child could be denied public education without due process of law, that handicapped children should receive their education within the "least restrictive environment commensurate with their needs," and that each state must establish a goal and a plan to provide full education for all children however handicapped. A new act in 1975 (PL 94-142) goes beyond this: It authorizes education of handicapped children starting at age 3; it mandates a continuing effort to locate and identify all handicapped children, preferably at pre-school age; it requires that an individualized treatment program be developed for every handicapped child; and it requires that wherever possible education be provided within the public school environment and classroom. Children will be placed in special classes "only when the nature or severity of the handicap is such that education in regular classes, even with supplementary aids, cannot be achieved."

This legislation will greatly strengthen the hand of those seeking to assure the education of epileptic children. Data reported to the Epilepsy Commission reveal that learning problems are common among children with epilepsy. They appear to be especially prominent in children with partial epilepsy. Boys with left temporal lobe disorders are especially prone to exhibit hyperactive behavior and specific reading disability (Stores and Hart, 1976). Within the Chicago school systems 17% of children with epilepsy require special education. Children with epilepsy should be removed from their regular classroom only if the nature and extent of their associated intellectual or behavioral problems make it impossible for them to learn within that environment. Counseling should be available for those showing evidences of social or emotional maladjustment. Special vocational training programs should be developed at the high school level.

However, vocational training will have limited value unless persons with epilepsy can be assured that they will find employment. Here also, important developments are taking place in the United States. For many years, the United States has had a well organized vocational rehabilitation program to provide special training for injured or otherwise handicapped persons. Unfortunately, its value for persons with epilepsy has been limited because employers do not hire persons with epilepsy, and for this reason rehabilitation agencies have been unwilling to undertake the rehabilitation of epileptic applicants unless their seizures are under almost complete control. (A lack of focus on the medical aspects of the rehabilitation of epileptic persons has also prevented effective seizure control.) To remedy this problem new provisions of Sections 501, 502, and 503 of the 1974 Amendments of the Rehabilitation Act (PL 93-516) emphasize *employment* as opposed to *rehabilitation*. These provisions make it illegal for a government agency or contractor to deny employment to a qualified handicapped employee or applicant, and require that the employer make reasonable accommodations to render his facilities accessible and useable by handicapped employees. This "accommodation" refers not only to the physical characteristic of the workplace but also to such matters as working hours and other special provisions. The full impact of this legislation remains to be assessed. It will depend on the definition of "qualified applicant," and what is considered "reasonable accommodations." However, the existence of this legislation provides valuable ammunition for rehabilitation agencies which emphasize job development and *job placement*. This effort is also being enhanced by activities of the Department of Labor. Under the Comprehensive Education and Training Act (CETA), the Epilepsy Foundation of America has developed in a number of cities a Training and Placement Service (TAPS), which is proving very effective in placing epileptic trainees in suitable jobs. Many persons with epilepsy, because of repeated rejections, have developed hostile or defensive attitudes that interfere with employment. Special training in job finding skills and techniques is proving helpful in overcoming these attitudes.

It may be that the opportunity now exists also to encourage the development of the equivalent of "sheltered workshops" actually within the framework of industry. This might be preferable to, or at least complement, costly efforts to expand the existing sheltered workshop program in this country. Accurate data are not available in the USA on the number of persons with epilepsy employed in sheltered workshops or other noncompetitive work situations. Data from Florida and Minnesota—states with active epilepsy rehabilitation programs—suggest that these states have about half as many persons in noncompetitive employment as are reported, e.g., from Holland.

INDEPENDENCE AND EQUALITY

The United States has no system of national health insurance comparable to that in England and other countries. Persons who receive medical and/or rehabilitation therapies and counselling services through federal and state resources must "qualify" for these services by a low income and/or severe disability.

Appropriate medical and surgical therapy, including appropriate reimbursement for drug costs, should be freely available to all persons with epilepsy.

Transportation is an essential requirement for independence. In many communities, the ability to drive is almost essential to achieve access to employment and services. In the development of services for persons with epilepsy, accessibility to public transportation is an important consideration.

Many persons with epilepsy are capable of driving safely. There is a need for more precise data on the characteristics of the safe driver. From this can be developed uniform drivers' licensing laws. Such laws should also include and publicize an appeal mechanism to protect against capricious or arbitrary denial of license.

Language barriers and cultural differences often interfere with use of United States governmental systems of medical and rehabilitation services. Regulations to implement new anti-discrimination laws are to obviate this problem. Service agencies and providers must include minority personnel on staff.

LIVING ARRANGEMENTS

In spite of the best of modern medical management, many persons with epilepsy are incapable of living independently—either because of the frequency and devastating character of their seizures or because of associated mental retardation or psychosis. In the United States, there are an estimated 58,000 persons with epilepsy in institutions for developmentally disabled persons, and over 20,000 in mental hospitals. One community survey documented that an equal number of severely handicapped persons are being cared for in the community. There must be a much larger number of less severely afflicted persons living dependent lives with their families.

The great humanitarian movement of the 19th century developed the concept of the "asylum." In the case of epilepsy, this was a special colony in which persons with epilepsy could live and work in a protected environment. Unfortunately, the large size and isolated environment of the large state institutions and colonies led to social isolation and neglect. In addition, the development of improved anticonvulsants made that type of institutional care unnecessary for uncomplicated epilepsy. In recent years, the colony concept has been abandoned.

In the 1970s, severely handicapped persons with epilepsy were grouped legislatively with those with mental retardation, cerebral palsy and autism and are referred to as "developmentally disabled." Most institutionalized persons with epilepsy are now grouped with individuals with these other types of developmental disabilities. The person with epilepsy is unique among the developmentally disabled, in respect to his greater dependence upon close medical supervision. This is not likely to be provided where he is living within an environment that does not focus on his personal and individual needs.

Currently, vigorous efforts are being made to create small community-based facilities and to remove developmentally disabled persons from large residential facilities. To do so, however, requires the creation within the community not only of the place of residence for the person with epilepsy, but also of a constellation of accessible medical and other supportive services. Two parallel programs are required.

The isolation of the large scale institutions should be obviated by integration of their medical, educational, and vocational services with those of the general community. For example, special neurological supervision should be achieved by affiliation with university departments of neurology, or other available neurological clinics. Education should be provided in the community schools, as mandated under pending legislation. Vocational training and sheltered workshops should be developed and shared with noninstitutionalized residents in the community.

Paralleling this must be a vigorous effort to develop a spectrum of smaller community-based residential facilities so diversified as to provide not only for the severely afflicted, but also for those who require only the minimum protection afforded by group living accommodations. There is a particular need for activity and employment centers to provide a central focus for a constellation of small, cooperative homes or hostels for those capable of semi-independent living. Within the United States, pending legislation (Congregate Housing Services Act of 1978), if enacted, would provide special funding to assist in the creation of such facilities.

Residential facilities, whether large or small, should meet minimum standards of medical care (Table 1), and should be staffed by persons trained in the management of epilepsy.

TABLE 1. *Medical services: minimum standards of care*

Initial medical evaluation
  To determine the cause and nature of the epileptic process
    Medical history
    Accurate subjective and objective description of seizures
    Developmental history
    Family history
    Physical and neurological examination
    Diagnostic tests
      Biochemical, hematologic, and serologic studies
        Complete blood count
        Urinalysis
        Serum calcium and phosphorus
        Studies to exclude tuberculosis and syphilis
        Fasting blood sugar
      Electrophysiologic studies
        Electroencephalogram (EEG)
      Radiologic studies
        Computed tomogram of brain
        Angiogram or pneumoencephalogram (if indicated)
  The following additional studies may be required in selected cases
    Five-hour glucose tolerance test for atypical seizures
    Chromosome studies for congenital malformations
    Amino acid screen for metabolic disorders
    Spinal fluid examination for infection of nervous system
    Special EEG activation procedures
      Sleep deprived
      Telemetered
      Chemical activation
  Application of International Seizure Classification
  Data base entry of medical problems not directly related to epileptic process

To achieve control of seizures
  Reliable and accurate record of seizure frequency
  Charting of anticonvulsant drug consumption
  Periodic anticonvulsant drug levels
  Case review
    For incompletely controlled patients
      Weekly by technical specialist
      Monthly by medical specialist
    For patients having less than one seizure per month (for patients in community-based
    living arrangements, periodic review by a physician no fewer than two times per year)
      Monthly by technical specialists
      Quarterly by medical specialists

To protect against medical emergency
  Appropriate observation by trained attendant or companion
  Institution of ongoing and detailed training for families, associates, attendants, or health
  professionals responsible for the care of patients with epilepsy
  Health professional availability on an emergency 24-hr basis
  Access to emergency hospital-type care within 20 min

Referral for special study
  Persons with atypical or "focal onset" seizures, or having evidence of underlying neurological disease, or with uncontrolled seizures (more than one per month) should be
  referred for special evaluation, preferably to a center specializing in epilepsy for special
  services as follows:
    Twenty-four hour video and EEG monitoring
    Angiography
    Supervised inpatient drug control
    Special consideration for surgical intervention

EDUCATING THE INDIVIDUAL/FAMILY WITH EPILEPSY, THE PROFESSIONAL, AND THE PUBLIC

Ignorance—including that of persons with epilepsy and their families—poses a formidable hurdle to their positive integration into society and its service systems and to public acceptance.

The United States, as do other countries, must currently rely on its voluntary epilepsy organizations to improve the public's understanding of epilepsy, inasmuch as there is little governmental intervention in this problem. The voluntary role must be strengthened. A national information center on epilepsy is needed to provide public information, develop training programs, and serve as a clearinghouse.

A minimal number of hours of instruction on epilepsy is included in neuroscience, medical school, and nursing curricula. National board examinations for these professionals must, as curricula are expanded, eventually include more emphasis on seizure disorders. Allied health professionals, paraprofessionals, public servants, and others must have access to current materials and organized training on the special needs of persons with epilepsy.

Many types of services that are needed by persons with epilepsy are already available in the United States through various federal, state and private mechanisms. It is the expertise on epilepsy which is lacking among service providers that most often leads to inability to meet that person's needs. It may well be that education about epilepsy at all levels is the key to solving the problems of the social aspects of epilepsy.

REFERENCES

1. Rodin, E., Shapiro, H. L., and Lennox, K. (1976): *Epilepsy and Life Performance.* Lafayette Clinic, Detroit.
2. Stores, G., and Hart, J. (1976): Reading skills in school children with generalized or focal epilepsy. *Dev. Med. Child. Neurol.*, 18:705–716.
3. United States Department of Health, Education, and Welfare Plan for Nationwide Action on Epilepsy (1978): Publication (NIH) 76-278 NINCDS, Bethesda, Maryland 20014.

Advances in Epileptology:
The Xth Epilepsy International Symposium,
edited by J. A. Wada and J. K. Penry.
Raven Press, New York © 1980.

Comprehensive Care of Epilepsy in the Changing Medical Climate of North America

Robert J. Gumnit

Comprehensive Epilepsy Program, University of Minnesota,
Department of Neurology, St. Paul-Ramsey Medical Center,
St. Paul, Minnesota 55101

This chapter reviews what a patient with seizures can reasonably expect regarding care and introduces the practical problems of obtaining it.

Our best evidence indicates that 3% of the population will have more than one seizure during their lives and are at risk to develop the problems that accompany epilepsy. Perhaps only one-third of this group, or 1% of the population, are seriously affected. That means that two million people in the United States alone need special attention.

One does not measure the seriousness of epilepsy simply by counting the number of seizures. Very brief seizures may not seriously interrupt what a person is doing. Others are severe and may cause serious trouble and injury. Furthermore, it is not the presence or absence of the seizure alone, but also the implication of having seizures that we must be concerned about. Epilepsy is the best example of a disease in which disability is a function of the social environment of the patient. A patient may be incapacitated by seizures for only a few minutes a year and have complete disability for a modern society.

The patient should demand that a physician have definite and clearcut therapeutic goals. We must attempt to stop the seizures completely. Neither the patient nor the physician should be satisfied to reduce the occurrence of seizures to only a few each year because this leaves the patient with severe social handicaps. At an early stage, the patient should expect that someone will help him avoid disability and the secondary problems that accompany seizures. At the very least, he needs help coping with the embarrassment that attends having a seizure. Similarly, because the way in which society views a person with seizures tends to destroy the individual self image, this problem should be dealt with openly and early. But the task does not fall on the patient alone. While he should be encouraged to hold his head up, society must be equally encouraged to change its image of the patient with epilepsy.

Early consideration should be given to employment. Without a job, one does not have a place in society. Anxiety is an inevitable part of having seizures. The patient and his relatives should demand that they be given a good knowledge of the facts of epilepsy, both in general and as they refer to the specific case. The physician and society must maximize the areas in which the patient has control over the situation. Knowledge and control are part of the essential emotional support needed in the treatment of epilepsy. Without early intervention in this area, the patient with epilepsy will have fear and anxiety, tends to withdraw socially and, thereby, isolates himself from society. Thus, the patient becomes frustrated, angry, and alienated.

There are a series of related practical problems. It is almost impossible to live in all but a very few cities in North America without having a car. If one cannot drive, he is severely limited in opportunities for social life, recreation, and employment. There *are* practical problems that limit employment opportunities. Some situations are simply too risky. However, since an automobile is a potentially lethal weapon, if it is safe to give a patient a driver's license, it certainly is safe to allow him to operate most industrial and production line equipment. In addition, there are problems with life and health insurance. Many patients cannot obtain insurance at all, and others, only at very high rates. However, there is little actuarial evidence to support this discrimination.

How do we go about wrestling with these problems as the entire organizational pattern and funding of health and social services undergo rapid change? The physician is frustrated. There are proven therapeutic methods of increased effectiveness that are denied his patient because the resources have not been made available or because of cost. At the same time, patients are demanding more medical and social services than our society delivers or perhaps can afford to deliver. Under these circumstances, we must perform a careful analysis of the problems and develop an appropriately organized system. The report of the National Commission on the Epilepsies and Their Consequences is a major step in this direction.

The allocation of resources or funds to the care of people with epilepsy is really a political problem. How are these resources allocated? How does one obtain funds?

We are no longer in a marketplace where the individual patient decides whether something is worth the price and pays it. Perhaps only the Arab sheiks still fall into that category. In North America, we have fallen out of the habit of paying for medical and social services on an individual basis. We have been told that health care and social services are a right, not a privilege and that they should be provided for us, either by mandatory insurance or by governmental funds. Therefore, physicians and patients are continuously dealing with health insurance schemes or legislatures and health commissioners in the allocation of resources. That means we are dealing with organizations. The health insurance plans are as much a bureaucracy as the ministry of health or the ministry of transport.

There are lessons to be learned about dealing with bureaucracies. First, goals must be defined, implying the need for a sensible plan. Second, it is necessary to convince the bureaucrats that action can and should be taken regarding the plan.

Politics is a business that solves problems that cannot be solved scientifically and rationally. Politicians are in business to resolve conflicting demands for money for diverse necessities; e.g. money for transportation and money for patient care. They must always add apples and oranges.

Politicians have a different way of looking at the purpose of spending funds. In this regard, we are talking about more than those politicians who stand for election. Civil servants, management people, and insurance people fall into the same category. When one works in a bureaucracy, this is a most important lesson to be learned.

How do we influence the decisions and behavior of these people? We cannot do it as isolated members of society. Patients and relatives, friends and physicians alike must join forces. In North America at present, there are two basic ways of obtaining services. One is in a free market economy, and the other is by bureaucratic decision. A classic example of the use of the free market economy was the introduction of the Papanicolau smear for the detection of cancer of the cervix. When women learned about it from the Cancer Society, they found that many family doctors were not interested in providing the service. Therefore, they went to an obstetrician, or some other physician, to be tested. Subsequently, local family doctors very rapidly began to provide those services. The same will result from telling the family physician, "I want you to pay more attention to my seizures and my needs." If he does not, one should seek a more responsive physician.

Bureaucratic action can be obtained by lobbying. In order to lobby effectively, one must have clearly delineated goals. Once the plan is decided upon, it is necessary to educate the men and women who make the decisions. They must be convinced that the plan is sensible and to dispense the funds. The main problem, however, is getting their attention.

In the legislative area, we can learn a lesson from the activity of motorcyclists. The death rate for riders of motorcycles was so high that most legislatures in the United States passed a mandatory helmet law. The death rate fell 60%. The motorcyclists felt this was an infringement on their basic human freedoms. They came in groups of hundreds and circled the state houses on their motorcycles, gunned their engines, mobbed the corridors, and called for their rights. The legislators, in their wisdom, began to repeal the helmet law. The death rate rapidly climbed up again. But this does illustrate how one gets a politician's attention. If he runs for office, go down with friends who vote in his district and talk with him. It is amazing how few people who vote in a given district are needed to get a politician's attention.

If he does not run for office, i.e., he is a bureaucrat in or out of government, it becomes more difficult. There are certain rules that can be followed.

First, let him know that you are persistent, and will be coming back again and again. The first defense of a bureaucrat is to stall and delay in hopes that the petitioner will tire and disappear. Secondly, attempt to involve him in planning and decision making. If he can be made to believe that your plan is his plan, you are much more likely to get favorable action. Thirdly, lobby him in the same way that you lobby someone who runs for office, but in a slightly more subtle fashion. If you can bring along a bureaucrat of equal or higher rank, or an influential citizen, or in some other way bring about peer pressure, you are much more likely to succeed. If all else fails, let him know that you are prepared to go over his head to his superior. There is nothing that is less pleasing to a bureaucrat than to know his behavior will be brought to the attention of his boss. Choose your timing carefully. The year to work hard for maximum gain is the year that the prime minister in office discovers he has a relative with seizures.

We live in an era of increasing governmental regulation of health and social services. What services will be available will depend largely on money that is allocated by bureaucratic decision. The decision to allocate funds will be based on the needs perceived by the bureaucrat, not the needs as perceived by the physician or the patient. All of us—patients and doctors, relatives and friends, nurses and social workers—must be united in support of clearcut plans and work together to help the bureaucrat see that our need is their need.

Abstracts

THE ESTABLISHMENT AND THE ADMINISTRATION OF A PROGRESSIVE EPILEPSY ASSOCIATION

J. B. Kent
Toronto

Effective Epilepsy Associations have been established in many countries; in others, no social services exist for epileptic persons.

Epilepsy Association, Metro Toronto has experienced outstanding grówth phenomena over a four year span. Evaluation of this development suggests that careful application of certain administrative procedures results in high quality services for persons with epilepsy. Trial and error methods have also clarified the consequences of lesser known innovations in this meaningful field.

We propose to show systematically the marked advantages to the epileptic client with respect to progressive and appropriate administration systems. An example of this would be the achievement of greater membership participation through improved internal record keeping.

Statistics will be used. Relevant resource material includes analysis of: realistic goals, service programs, volunteers, membership, community education, public relations and the use of the media, funding and financial management.

We wish to illustrate that a definite, provocative, and frequently overlooked relationship exists between the administration profile and the quality of service offered by an existing social service organization.

Our theme suggests that more specific attention might be paid to this important connection.

THE ROLE OF PHYSICIANS IN NON-MEDICAL ASSOCIATION MOVEMENTS

T. Soga
Tokyo

The first impulse and the growth of the non-medical Association in Japan have been driven by a group of physicians for the past five years. Nonetheless, the majority of the members are patients or their relatives. This tends to result in a sort of strained and hierarchical state between the volunteering physicians and the lay members, because both of them are inevitably involved in epilepsy. Therefore, doctor-patient relationship spontaneously formed in a clinic should be avoided intentionally in the lay association activities.

The main part of physicians was to give appropriate knowledge and information about medical aspects of epilepsy. Meetings and the newletters are efficient mass-media. However, a logic of generalization, a fate of medical sciences, is not always happily accepted by lay members who are in position of longing to individualize their own concerns personally.

Unless patients themselves become well aware of the necessity of *active* participation in a long-term treatment program, any trial in the comprehensive care would not have succeeded. Thus, psychotherapeutic or self-supporting approach is believed to form a core part of physicians' role for lay members who are inclined to a *passive* beneficiary of the miracle of medicine.

"HANNE" (FILM)

To be presented by: J. N. Loeber
Heemstede

This film has been produced by Rebrofilms, Breda, Netherlands, under the direction of Maartje van der Heyden, and is provided with English subtitles. Its duration is about 30 minutes.

Contents:

A 19-year-old girl is followed during her daily life at home, in her job, with her friends. One sees the difficulties she experiences because of her epilepsy, in her relation with a boy-friend, with her family, and in obtaining a job. In flash-backs she figures as the little girl of 13 at the time when her epilepsy became manifest. She had a seizure in church, which is misunderstood. Her feelings of alienation, her struggle for a life of her own are shown. She goes to a hospital for epilepsy and undergoes different clinical examinations. Afterwards she has another seizure in the middle of a busy street (this event was staged but passers-by did not know that, so their reactions are authentic). An ambulance is called and she is transported to hospital, which she regrets.

The film has an optimistic end. Her relation with the boy-friend is continued and she expresses her own outlook on life in general in the words: "I am a very happy girl". The film is widely used in Holland for general audiences, and especially appeals to youth.

TAKE A LOOK AT US, MAMMIE, WE COULD SWIM! (FILM EXHIBIT)

K. Nagai
Tokyo

This is a movie by the Japanese Epilepsy Association, 1977, illustrating exciting night and day of a

467

summer camp for children with epilepsy.

Twenty-five pairs of children ranged 4 to 15 years of age with seizure as well as behavioral problems and their parents went into an outdoor training program at a rural village. Thirty volunteers including physicians lived together with them to encourage the overprotected children to run about in the forest and have a dip in the water. Day by day, parents became aware that oversolicitous care in the past was as a matter of fact meaningless and needless.

The 3 night 4 day excursion, laborious but worthwhile endeavour, has been carried out for different groups of clients for 5 years every summer. As the children have been getting through, not only the parents but volunteers grow up to learn how to cope with these difficult children.

(A 30 min. roll of 8 mm color film with magnetic recording in English narration.)

COUNTERACTING EMPLOYER BIAS AGAINST HIRING QUALIFIED EPILEPTICS

R. C. Reilly
Toronto

"Epilepsy" is frequently the main reason given by clients for their failure to obtain employment. Job placement experience over the past four years suggests that there are significant underlying reasons for this failure, the identification and analysis of which could direct placement efforts into a more manageable and relevant methodology.

One such reason for job search failure, the variable nature of epilepsy, will be investigated in the light of placement data. We will show that its effect upon employer evaluation and upon the establishment of a general hiring policy is a significant determinant of employer bias.

The role of the epileptic job seeker in counteracting this bias will be assessed.

LEGAL REMEDIES FOR EMPLOYMENT DISCRIMINATION AGAINST PEOPLE WITH EPILEPSY

G. Downs, M. Hardin
Portland

This paper is designed to give information to non-legal professionals about legal remedies for unemployment discrimination against persons with epilepsy. The paper explains what constitutes employment discrimination against persons with epilepsy and discusses the role of the non-legal professional person in spotting discrimination and assisting clients to utilize the most effective legal remedies.

The principal legal remedies existing in the United States are outlined, including when they apply and how each may be enforced. The paper describes gaps in statutory prohibitions against discrimination and suggests ways that private attorneys can sometimes bring suit where no clear statutory remedy exists.

COMPREHENSIVE CARE OF THE EPILEPTIC PATIENT: STEPS TOWARDS THE EVALUATION OF EMPLOYABILITY THROUGH OBJECTIVE PSYCHOSOCIAL ASSESSMENT

L. Batzel, C. Dodrill, R. Fraser
Seattle

Substantial numbers of epileptics are chronically unemployed at least in part due to numerous social and psychological problems. Efforts to increase client employability have been only partially successful. Tests evaluating emotional problems have been used as indicators of employability but have been of limited utility. The study reported here evaluated the employment correlates of a new psychosocial assessment inventory, the Washington Psychosocial Seizure Inventory (WPSI) and compared them with those of an older test, the Minnesota Multiphasic Personality Inventory.

Forty-six adult epileptics were administered both inventories and were classified as 1) Employed, 2) Partially Employed, or 3) Unemployed. Statistically significant differences were found across the groups with both inventories. However, the WPSI rendered larger differences and more uniformly demonstrated increasing psychosocial problems with a lessening in employment status. In addition, the WPSI Vocational Scale provided the clearest discrimination between groupings among all variables considered. Multivariate analyses indicated that this was the best predictor among all such variables. These findings and the ease with which the WPSI is administered suggest that the WPSI may be of value in assessing employability among clients with epilepsy. A consequence could be early identification of those who will need more intensive vocational services.

This project was supported by a grant from the Epilepsy Foundation of America and by NIH Contracts N01-NS-0-2281 and N01-NS-6-2341, National Institute of Neurological and Communicative Disorders and Stroke, PHS/DHEW, USA.

THE JOB PERFORMANCE OF EPILEPTICS IN THE BRITISH STEEL INDUSTRY

M. Saunders and A. Das Gupta
Cleveland, U.K.

There are little objective data concerning the job performance of epileptics in heavy industry. This study reports the findings on 45 patients with epilepsy employed by the British Steel Corporation compared with matched controls.

Each patient was interviewed and an assessment made of the severity of the epilepsy, the type of medication and associated general medical and psychiatric disorders. An independent assessment of job performance on patients and controls was carried out by Works' Managers. The hospital records of all patients with epilepsy were reviewed.

There was no significant difference in sickness absence, or accident frequency and severity between patients and controls. There was no overall difference in job performance between epileptics and controls. However, patients with epilepsy assessed as aggressive had a significantly poorer attitude to work. There was also a highly significant association between the presence of a personality disorder amongst the epileptic population and a poor attitude to five work factors analysed. A significantly smaller proportion of epileptics eligible for shift work worked shifts compared with controls.

It is concluded that the job performance of epileptics in heavy industry is not significantly impaired compared with controls, unless there is an associated psychiatric disorder.

THE ROLE OF SPECIALIZED VOCATIONAL SERVICES IN COMPREHENSIVE TREATMENT OF THE INDIVIDUAL WITH EPILEPSY

R. Fraser, K. Erikson, J. Thompson
Seattle

The job frustrations encountered by many individuals with epilepsy are well-documented in the literature. A recent national survey by the National Epilepsy League (Perlman, 1977) indicates that 51% of those with the disability feel that it has presented problems in obtaining a job. Wright (1975) indicates that the State-Federal program rehabilitated a smaller percentage of clients in 1973 than it did in 1962. Based on statistical data from the late 60's and early 70's (Epilepsy Foundation of America, 1975), the unemployment rate among people with epilepsy in the labor force varied between 20 to 25%. This paper describes the activities of a specialized vocational unit within the context of a comprehensive team approach to epilepsy rehabilitation during the initial 18 months of services.

Referral procedures, interactions with other disciplines within the Center, and characteristics of the vocational unit's client populace will be described early in the presentation. Various aspects of the vocational unit program will also be described. Client characteristics will span areas such as seizure-related information including prior impact upon work activities, previous employment, financial status, history of contacts with rehabilitation or placement agencies and outcome of these contacts, and client availability to transportation. In addition to intake data, follow-up information has also been secured on clients handled by the unit (seizure activity post-employment, etc.). These data will be reviewed and contrasted among the various outcome groups (the employed, those enrolled in school programs, those currently involved with the program, and negative program exits). Modifications which the program has undergone in order to improve services will be explained, and implications of client-related data relative to new components for the vocational program (e.g., systems of client job maintenance and career enrichment) will be outlined.

The program and research activities described above are supported under contract N01-NS-6-2341, National Institute of Neurological and Communicative Disorders and Stroke, PHS/DHEW, USA.

HEALTH EDUCATION ON EPILEPSY IN THE U.K.

A. Craig and O. M. Jones
London, U.K.

To enable the person with epilepsy to fulfil his potential in the community all professional persons who will have to deal with those who have epilepsy must be aware of the social problems faced in connection with epilepsy, and the general public, particularly such groups as employers, landlords and fellow employees, must be taught what epilepsy is and how it can affect the life of those who have it. The Association mounts its programmes of courses for doctors, nurses, social workers, Disablement Resettlement Officers, Health Visitors, Day Centre Workers and many others in the community. It works with teachers, senior pupils, ambulancemen, firemen, community workers, members of the legal profession and others, to teach about epilepsy and its problems of adjustment within the community. Recent developments include a course for the legal profession; co-operation with the Trades Union Council in providing training information for safety officers and extension of courses for General Practitioners.

Conclusion: The widest possible programme of health education and dissemination of information is essential if attitudes are to change.

TEACHING SCHOOL AGE CHILDREN ABOUT EPILEPSY

Sister A. V. Walton, M. R. Hammer
Minneapolis

The Comprehensive Epilepsy Program for the State of Minnesota, recognizing the need for education of all ages, developed a one hour program for junior/senior high school students. Behavioral objectives were set, learning activities designed, and a systematic evaluation conducted to determine the program's effectiveness. The evaluation question examined was: Did the program increase students' knowledge about and develop more postitive attitudes toward epilepsy?

Specifically two major research questions are being investigated:
1) What is the level of knowledge and attitudes of participants toward epilepsy prior to participation in the program?
2) Are there significant differences in the participants' level of knowledge and attitudes after participation in the program.

To date a program evaluation questionnaire has been developed and administered in a junior high school setting. A pre-post test design which also assesses pre-test learning effects was employed. Initial results indicate that students 1) scored significantly higher on the knowledge measure ($p \leq .001$); and 2) had significantly more favorable attitudes toward epilepsy ($p \leq .001$) after participation in the program.

A more rigorous evaluation design is being used in the senior high setting (a pre-post test, control group design) which also assesses pre-test learning effects.

An outline of the program and results of evaluation will be presented.

THE IDENTIFICATION OF CHILDREN WITH EPILEPSY AT SPECIAL RISK OF EDUCATIONAL AND OTHER BEHAVIOURAL PROBLEMS

G. Stores
Oxford

Although there is evidence that educational and other behavioural problems are over-represented in children with epilepsy attending ordinary school, there has been no clear indication of which particular children are handicapped in this way. Four studies have been carried out in a search for high risk factors in this group. Measurements of reading retardation, inattentiveness of various types, dependency and other aspects of disturbed behaviour in epileptic schoolchildren suggest that male sex and the presence of persistent left temporal lobe spike discharge are consistently associated with these problems. The possibility is also raised that certain types of antiepileptic drug treatment can adversely affect intellectual function. It is suggested that detailed neurological and behavioural assessment can help identify those children with epilepsy at special risk of behavioural problems and that prevention or remedial measures can be introduced at an early age in order to minimize the adverse psychological and social effects of recurrent seizures.

CAN SEIZURE OBSERVATION BE TAUGHT TO A HEALTH PROFESSIONAL?

J. Beniak, M. R. Hammer
Minneapolis

The Comprehensive Epilepsy Program discovered through community education programs that health professionals had difficulty documenting the occurrence of a seizure accurately. A teaching unit on seizure observation was necessary to meet this deficit. This unit was developed using a competency-based model of instruction which included the development of behavioral objectives by having the participant observe actual seizures and complete a seizure record.

This unit was one of six presented at an all day workshop on epilepsy for health care professionals. Criteria were developed which assigned points to specific behaviors that needed to be recorded for a particular seizure. A pre-post test design which also assesses pre-test learning effects was employed to evaluate the effectiveness of this unit.

Preliminary results of the study indicate that:
1) Participants were significantly more accurate in observing and documenting a seizure after completing the unit (p ≤.01) than they were before the unit began.
2) The effects of the pre-test on participants learning was not significant. Replication studies have been completed at other workshops.

The methodology for the unit and results will be presented.

TEACHING HEALTH CARE PROFESSIONALS ABOUT EPILEPSY

J. Soderberg, M. R. Hammer
Minneapolis

A one-day workshop is being conducted in four different locations for health care professionals in Minnesota by the Comprehensive Epilepsy Program to: 1) increase participants' knowledge of current concepts about epilepsy and its management; and 2) to encourage the development of more positive attitudes towards epilepsy. Systematic research is being conducted to assess the effectiveness of the workshops on participants' cognitive and affective learning. Three questions are being examined:
1. What is the level of knowledge and attitudes of participants toward epilepsy prior to participation in the epilepsy workshop?
2. Are there significant differences in the participants' level of knowledge and attitudes after participation in the epilepsy workshop?
3. Do any changes in the level of knowledge and attitudes of the participants that result from their participation in the workshop persist over time?

To date, a questionnaire has been developed and pilot tested. At one site, a pre-post-followup test design has been employed. Initial results of the pre-post test analysis indicate that the workshops significantly increased participant knowledge about epilepsy (p ≤.001) and significantly encouraged more favorable attitudes toward epilepsy (p ≤.001).

A second more rigorous pre-post-followup test design that assesses the effect of the pre-test on participants cognitive and affective learning is presently being used. Information concerning workshop objectives, program modules, and evaluation results will be presented.

NURSE TRAINING PROGRAMS IN EPILEPSY

J. Ozuna
Seattle

The evolution of nurses into expanded roles has logically meshed with the need for more and better care of people with epilepsy in the United States. To follow Ms. Hawken's paper, two epilepsy nurse training programs currently in progress in the Seattle Area will be discussed.

The first is the Epilepsy Nurse Clinician Training Program sponsored by the Epilepsy Center. Six registered Nurses (4 from Neurologist's offices and 2 who are Stroke Nurse Clincians) were recruited from various communities in Washington State. After attending a 1½ day symposium on epilepsy, they each attended a one-week preceptorship at three epilepsy clinics in Seattle, under the direction of Judy Ozuna, R.N. Each nurse was asked to explore and define her potential role as an Epilepsy Nurse Clinician in areas such as medical management, psychosocial management, patient and family teaching, community liaison and advocacy work. Follow-up with these nurses will be discussed.

The second program is offered by the Department of Physiological Nursing, School of Nursing, University of Washington. This program produces Master's prepared nurses with knowledge of nervous system disorders and, particularly, epilepsy. This program will be discussed. Job potentials for nurses from both programs will be discussed.

EXTENDED ROLES FOR NURSES IN THE MANAGEMENT OF THE EPILEPTIC PATIENT

M. Hawken
Seattle

As the needs of consumers regarding health care have increased and medical technology has become more sophisticated and complex, specialization in medical and nursing practice has become a necessity. The physician is not longer able to be the sole provider of primary care. As a result, the past fifteen years has seen a gradual change in traditional nursing practice which now includes primary care and other extended roles.

The extended role is based upon the interest, clinical expertise and educational preparation of the nurse. The nurse clinician, nurse practitioner and clinical nurse specialist are all examples of the new dimensions in nursing. Differentiation of these positions and their credentials will be further discussed.

Nurses in extended roles in epilepsy have numerous different functions and responsibilities. These include primary care of the hospitalized and ambulatory care patient, teaching patients and families about epilepsy, coordinating epilepsy wards and clinic activities. In addition, there are professional responsibilities within the community, in all levels of the educational system and in continuing education to professional counterparts. The nurses roles as related to these functions will be discussed. The role of the Clinical Nurse Specialist in Epilepsy will be discussed.

A STUDY ON THE SOCIAL ADAPTATION OF EPILEPTICS

K. Suwa
Tochigi
H. Moriya
Tokyo
Y. Mori
Kanagawa
T. Tokizawa
Ibaragi

We compared the status of social adaptation of epileptics in an out-patients clinic ten years ago (1967) with that at the present (1978). All subjects were adult patients and included wives and students. We divided these patients into a socially adaptable group and a non-adaptable group. The former consisted of patients capable of economically self-supported living, and the latter consisted of patients incapable of this aspect of daily living. As a result, the ratio of the adaptable group at the present time was larger in comparison with that ten years ago. The factors that increased the ratio of the adaptable group at the present were studied. We

studied a number of biological factors, such as onset of seizures, clinical type, length of course, effect of therapy, character disorder and intelligence disorder, and social factors, such as educational career, occupation, personal relationships at work, attitude of the neighborhood to the disease, patient's attitude to the disease, and regularity of taking medicine. It was found in this study that onset of seizures, clinical type, length of course, intelligence disorder, attitude of patients to the disease and regularity of taking medicine did not correlate, but the effect of therapy, character disorder, educational career, occupation, personal relationship and attitude of surroundings correlated with improvement of social adaptation.

ASSESSMENT OF ALTERED NEUROBEHAVIORAL FUNCTION IN EPILEPTICS

R. M. Pinnas, L. J. Willmore
Gainesville

Accurate documentation of the impact of epilepsy upon behavior has been hampered by selection of inappropriate examination instruments for evaluation of neuropsychological function, by improper classification and differentiation of seizure types, and by selection of epileptic patients for study based upon a history of behavioral problems. In the present study, we assessed neurobehavioral function in 93 unselected seizure patients. The test, designed on the quantitative approach of the Halstead-Reitan test battery and the qualitative analysis of Luria, evaluates auditory discrimination, and memory span, visual reversals/inversions, expressive language, fine motor skills, spatial judgement, and portions of the WAIS. Functional observations were quantitated by a questionnaire response.

Of 93 patients, 33 had generalized convulsive seizure, 22 had nonconvulsive seizures (absence), 20 had complex partial seizures and 7 had mixed seizure patterns. Eleven patients appearing in the nonselective sequence may not have had seizures.

Conceptualization, phonemic and retrieval language performance constituted the most common neurobehavioral dysfunction in this population. Functional scoring identified prominent feelings of inadequacy, groundless worry and helplessness as most common in this outpatient population.

THE STIGMA OF EPILEPSY AS A SELF CONCEPT

R. Ryan, A. Emlen
Portland

Much of the literature on the social consequences of epilepsy regards stigma as a major culprit in problems of social adjustment and employment. This paper describes the factor analytic construction of an attitude scale measuring stigma as a self-concept, and reports correlates of the scale. Findings are based on the responses of 445 persons residing in Oregon. Men and women are equally represented. Respondents range from the successfully employed to the chronically unemployed.

The results reveal a low sense of stigma. Most

study participants feel that others, including employers, react reasonably to their disorder.

Twenty-two variables are examined for their relevance to perceived stigma. While no relationships with age, age at onset, education, and disclosure attitudes emerge, awareness of one's seizure condition, having experienced discrimination, and type of occupation do correlate with stigma. Frequency and type of seizures are also related, but only among men over 25.

Findings indicate that while stigma does exist, perceived stigma is not as pervasive as the literature suggests. The authors argue that over-emphasis by concerned professionals may actually foster stigma by creating among persons with epilepsy, the expectation of being considered deviant.

YOU DON'T GET EPILEPSY FROM MASTURBATION, DO YOU?

J. Soderberg
Minneapolis

How do people feel when they first receive a diagnosis of epilepsy? What do people with epilepsy feel they need to know to assist in the management, over time, of their disorder?

The Comprehensive Epilepsy Program for the State of Minnesota was interested in the responses to these questions when staff set out to develop patient and family education programs and begin to encourage other human services providers to do the same.

To obtain answers to these questions, 35 people with epilepsy (21 males, 14 females, age range 16 to 60, variety of seizure types, frequencies, and age of onset) were interviewed in a group situation.

The interviewer, using a set of structured questions, asked people if they could remember the day they received their diagnosis, what questions or feelings they had at the time, what they felt people with epilepsy needed or wanted to know to live more effectively with their epilepsy, and finally, what suggestions they had to give us in developing epilepsy education programs.

The results to these interviews serve to alert the health care professional to the great need for epilepsy education in both the affective and cognitive domain.

Results, conclusions and practical suggestions to deal with need will be presented.

DETERMINATES OF PATIENT EDUCATION IN THE TREATMENT OF EPILEPSY: VETERAN POPULATION SURVEY

W. Graham and A. Mayersdorf
Minneapolis

Epilepsy is a chronic disorder requiring lifetime adherence and lifestyle change. Baseline data at the Epilepsy Treatment Center, Veterans Administration Hospital, Minneapolis, Minnesota, of responses of veteran population to questions related to problem areas in their life were collected. Many patients indicated areas of family, financial and employment problems; difficulty in expressing self, control of anger and depression; and medication and seizure problems as areas of concern in their life. In response to these concerns, four separate sessions for patient education were developed and presented in an informal setting.

In a random sample taken one year after the initiation of the program, the patient responses were essentially the same. This seems to indicate a need for continuous ongoing education in our population. The results of this survey propagated a wider base study that includes formal, continual ongoing classes with patient and health care provider contracting. The contracting is for specific, health related, attainable goals in return for specific, patient identified, rewards from the health care provider.

Results of these surveys will be presented correlating increased knowledge of treatment regimen with behavior change and their influence on seizure control.

Address correspondence to: Winnie Graham, R.N., Epilepsy Treatment Center (127C), Veterans Administration Hospital, 54th Street and 48th Avenue South, Minneapolis, Minnesota 55417

GROUP TRAINING IN PROBLEM-SOLVING FOR PATIENTS WITH EPILEPSY

W. R. Smith, H. R. Queisser
Seattle

The University of Washington Epilepsy Center has undertaken an innovative approach to alleviating the psychosocial problems experienced by many individuals who have chronic seizure disorders. The approach utilizes a psycho-educational model which emphasizes teaching a variety of social, tension management and mood management skills. The format of the intervention is a series of 8-12 hour classes which are taught by a clinical psychologist and social worker.

The emphasis of the paper submitted for presentation focuses on a class which teaches problem-solving skills. There are ample data indicating that epilepsy patients suffer deficits in basic problem-solving skills such as inhibiting immediate responses to situations demanding action, discriminating relevant from irrelevant features of a problem situation, and judging the possible consequences of alternative courses of action. Class materials used to teach these skills are outlined. Also presented are objective group data on the impact of the classes and selected case histories illustrating the effect of the class on patients' psychosocial problems and seizure disorder. The paper concludes that such classes show promise as a cost-effective adjunctive treatment in the rehabilitation of individuals with epilepsy.

INPUT AND OUTPUT OF A SPECIAL CENTRE FOR EPILEPSY

H. Meinardi
Heemstede

Certain characteristics will be analysed of patients who came under the care of the Instituut voor Epilepsie-bestrijding respectively in the years 1972 and 1976.

These characteristics are: maximal seizure frequency before admission; type of previous care; final diagnosis; level of education; anti-epileptic drugs used on admission and on discharge; type of follow-up care; prognosis at the time of discharge with respect to the medical, social and occupational spheres.

The significance of the special centres in the total care of epilepsy will be discussed.

LONG-TERM HOSPITALIZATION ON A MULTI-DISCIPLINARY EPILEPSY UNIT

V. R. Jones, M. Ragland, N. Santilli,
J. C. Sackellares, F. E. Dreifuss, and J. Q. Miller
Charlottesville

Fifty patients with poorly controlled epilepsy underwent intensive multidisciplinary hospitalization for periods of four to twenty-eight weeks. The goal was to minimize the disruptiveness of epilepsy on their lives. Attention was directed toward optimal anticonvulsant therapy, and educational, social, psychological and vocational needs. The effects of treatment were determined by comparing subjective and objective performance at admission, discharge and six months later.

This paper enumerates and quantitates the changes and their permanence. Outcome was influenced by choice of anticonvulsants, drug side effects, patient's intelligence, patient's emotional state and ability of family and social agencies to provide appropriate support services. The utility of careful observation including combined telemetered EEG-videotaping of seizures and frequent blood anticonvulsant determination is discussed.

Patients experienced significant reduction in seizure frequency and severity after discharge from hospitalization. They were better informed about epilepsy and their capacity to be productive in society increased. They left the unit, generally on different medications than they entered; they were on the same number of medications at discharge.

This project intends to examine the results of long-term hospitalization in a multidisciplinary setting. It should provide basic information helpful in determining the allocation of society's finite resources between research and service.

COMPREHENSIVE CARE OF INSTITUTIONALIZED PERSONS WITH EPILEPSY*

J. M. Freeman, K. R. Holden, E. Schoenfeld
Baltimore

Institutionalized persons are our most neglected population. Those with epilepsy are the most neglected of the institutionalized. A five state collaborative study of 6488 institutionalized individuals identified 2028 (31%) with epilepsy. Problems varied by institution but showed significant under-recognition of seizures and under or over medication of those who were recognized.

Involvement of medical school personnel interested in epilepsy with institutional staff, and the use of trained paramedical personnel made significant and cost-effective changes in the life of the institutionalized epileptic. A decrease in toxicity and seizure frequency, a decrease in episodes of status epilepticus and seizure related deaths, was documented. The use of blood levels to document toxicity and inadequate therapy played a major role in improving seizure control. In two institutions 20-25% of patients could be taken off medication. Medication could be given on a once or twice daily schedule decreasing nursing requirements. The cost of this project, less than $200/year/person with epilepsy, was more than compensated by decrease in medication, nursing and medical costs.

*Funded by DHEW, Office of Human Development, D.D. Office, Region III, Grant 51-P-15485-02.

SEIZURE CONTROL IN MENTALLY RETARDED INSTITUTIONALIZED PATIENTS: EFFECTS OF INTERVENTION

B. D'Souza, J. Murphy
Milwaukee

The authors established a weekly seizure clinic at an institution for mentally retarded persons, to improve seizure control there. A preintervention survey described drug usage, and seizure frequency in the first 62 patients evaluated there (American Epilepsy Society Meeting, Nov. 1977). This report describes the changes that have been noted in this original sample six months after their initial evaluation.

Initially 39% of the sample were taking 4 or more drugs, and 2 of the 62 were receiving 6 anticonvulsants daily. Six months later 6% of these patients were on 4 drugs, and none were receiving 5 or 6. (Drugs were discontinued in 2 of the original patients.) Initially only 21% were receiving 2 or fewer anticonvulsants daily, presently 57% of the sample receive 2 or less drugs. Concurrent with this drug reduction, 8% patients are seizure-free, 28% have at least an 80% reduction in their monthly seizure frequency, 36% have had no change in the number of seizures, and 18% are having more siezures.

Twelve patients were selected by the nursing personnel of the clinic as being markedly improved re: alertness, gait, etc., and their records were studied. In 10 of these 12, the number of anticonvulsants had been markedly reduced, 4 had fewer seizures (2 had more seizures) and 3 had toxic serum concentrations of anticonvulsants reduced to therapeutic concentrations.

This report indicates that an on-site seizure clinic may be more effective than utilization of a referral center, and that such institutionalized patients can be more handicapped by their drugs than their seizures.

AN EVALUATION OF THE STATUS OF EPILEPSY IN THE MENTAL HEALTH SYSTEMS*

H. Sands, W. Young
New York

Psychological and social problems associated with epilepsy have been reported as being more difficult to deal with than seizure problems and as being the most neglected and least understood.[1] This, coupled with the opinion that many mental health professionals — psychiatrists, psychologists, and social workers — have not had specific training to deal with the specialized psychological and behavioral problems of epilepsy (XI-21), has led the Commission to recommend specialized training for mental health professionals in the social and psychological aspects of epilepsy. The Commission's report also notes the lack of information about epilepsy in texts and training materials (XI-21).

The absence of hard data regarding the level and kind of information members of mental health teams have about epilepsy in general and the psychosocial aspects in particular is a serious gap in the literature. Further, such data are required if a meaningful curriculum for graduate and continuing education is being prepared. This investigation is designed to provide these data.

The investigation emphasizes an assessment of knowledge about epilepsy of mental health practitioners. In addition, the status of a variety of counseling, psychotherapy and psychiatric services available to people with epilepsy was investigated. Hence, the investigation consists of two components:

1) Using a 50 item questionnaire, the knowledge of mental health practitioners about epilepsy and their attitudes toward treatment of clients and/or patients with epilepsy was assessed. The data were collected at a major community mental health clinic, The Postgraduate Center for Mental Health. Further, knowledge and attitudes were analyzed for their demographic relationship to the population.

2) Information about and attitudes toward epilepsy were gathered in a nationwide survey. The data and statistical analyses from both the questionnaire and survey are discussed. Both sources of data are regarded as essential for the development of a continuing education program for mental health practitioners, and increasing the availability of mental health services to patients with epilepsy.

1. Commission for Control of Epilepsy and Its Consequences, Report: Plan for Nationwide Action on Epilepsy, volume 1, August 1977.

*The research described was funded by a grant from the Klingenstein Foundation.

THE NEED FOR A HEALTH SYSTEM WITH CONTINUOUS CARE IN DEALING WITH EPILEPSY

H. Smits, H. S. M. Bakker
Heemstede

Very often to have epilepsy means to have it all one's life. That is to say that the threat of "having a seizure" is always there.

In 1974 an advisory committee of the Minister of Health in the Netherlands stated that primary responsibility for the treatment of people with epilepsy should be with the general practitioner. However, at least once a year a so-called second echelon should give a check-up with the help of electroencephalography, estimation of serum levels of the antiepileptic drugs, and so on.

If the seizures are resistant to therapy or if there are problems with diagnosis or if there are problems in the social and occupational spheres, the patients should be referred to specialized neurologists, who are often called epileptologists, even though this is not an officially registered specialization. These epileptologists are attached to one of the three special centres for epilepsy in the Netherlands. Apart from their intramural activities these centres also maintain ten polsocs (policlinics and social advisory bureaus). In the concept of a continuous health care system they form a network together with the independent specialists (neurologists and paediatricians).

The present research is concerned with the effectiveness of an exemplary polsoc. By means of MSO rating scales the condition of the patient group under its care is followed over a period of time. Structure and functioning of the polsoc are analysed. Some of the findings and the scope of this investigation will be discussed.

EXPERIMENTAL SEIZURES AND MECHANISMS

Advances in Epileptology:
The Xth Epilepsy International Symposium,
edited by J. A. Wada and J. K. Penry.
Raven Press, New York © 1980.

Comparative Effects of Phenytoin, Phenobarbital, and Carbamazepine on Cyclic Nucleotide Regulation in Brain

James A. Ferrendelli and Dorothy A. Kinscherf

Department of Pharmacology and Department of Neurology and Neurological Surgery (Neurology), Washington University School of Medicine, St. Louis, Missouri 63110

Most of the anticonvulsant drugs presently used to treat epileptic patients can be distinguished by their effects on clinical and experimental seizures. For example, phenytoin and carbamazepine, and several others, have selective activity against maximal electroshock seizures (MES) and are particularly effective for the treatment of generalized tonic-clonic convulsions. In contrast, ethosuximide, trimethadione, and valproic acid, drugs of choice for treatment of absence seizures, have preferential activity against pentylenetetrazol (metrazol) seizures but have less potent or no anti-MES activity. Some drugs, especially barbiturates, possess both anti-MES and anti-metrazol activity and may be used to treat several types of clinical seizures.

Recently we compared some biochemical effects of several anticonvulsant drugs and found that many have distinct neuropharmacological actions that correlate well with their selective effect on clinical and experimental seizures. Initially we found that phenytoin and phenobarbital, two drugs with similar potent anti-MES activity, inhibited accumulation of calcium by isolated nerve terminals (synaptosomes), but ethosuximide, which is devoid of anti-MES activity, had no effect (Sohn and Ferrendelli, 1976). More recently we observed that drugs with anti-MES activity, i.e., phenytoin, carbamazepine, phenobarbital, primidone, aromatic substituted succinimides and high concentrations of clonazepam, inhibited depolarization-induced accumulation of both adenosine 3',5'-monophosphate (cyclic AMP) and guanosine 3',5'-monophosphate (cyclic GMP) in incubated slices of mouse cerebral cortex (Ferrendelli and Kinscherf, 1979). In contrast, ethosuximide, trimethadione, valproic acid, and low concentrations of clonazepam, drugs with predominant anti-metrazol activity, were ineffective in this system or inhibited accumulation of only cyclic GMP. Additional studies, reported here, reveal that anticonvulsants with anti-MES activity can be further characterized by their differential effect on veratridine- and K^+-induced accumulation of cyclic nucleotides, and these biochemical effects appear to distinguish drugs devoid of any anti-metrazol activity.

PATIENTS AND METHODS

As previously described (Ferrendelli et al., 1973), 6 to 8-week old female Swiss Webster mice were decapitated and their brains removed and placed in ice-cold Krebs Ringer bicarbonate buffer, pH 7.4, containing 121 mM NaCl, 4.7 mM KCl, 2.5 mM $CaCl_2$, 2.4 mM $MgSO_4$, 1.2 mM KH_2PO_4, 25 mM $NaHCO_3$, and 10 mM glucose. Pieces of cerebral cortex were dissected and cut into slices 0.30 mm wide with a Brinkman McIlwain Tissue Chopper. The slices from two mice were dispersed in 30 to 35 volumes of fresh Krebs buffer and then incubated for 1 hr at 37°C. During all incubations the slices were gently agitated by bubbling 95% O_2–5% CO_2 through the incubation medium. At the end of this hour of incubation, the slices were divided into eight samples containing 10 to 30 mg of tissue each and placed in 2 to 3 ml fresh buffer for 5 to 10 min. Small volumes (0.5–300 μl) of test substances were then added to the individual samples and the samples incubated for another 10 min. To achieve a K^+ concentration of 64 mM, buffer containing 121 mM KCl and 4.8 mM NaCl (and the other salts and glucose listed above) was mixed with an equal volume of regular Krebs buffer. Veratridine was dissolved in 0.006 N HCl prior to use. Phenobarbital and barbituric acid were readily soluble in aqueous solutions at a physiological pH. Phenytoin and hydantoin were dissolved in dilute NaOH prior to addition to the brain slice suspension; the pH of the buffered incubation media was not altered by the addition of the small amount of base, and at concentrations less than 1 mM, the drugs remained in solution. Carbamazepine was first dissolved in either 100% or 30% polyethyleneglycol prior to addition to the incubation media. The concentration of polyethyleneglycol in the incubation media never exceeded 3%, and at this and lower concentrations it did not alter basal levels or depolarization-induced elevations of either cyclic AMP or cyclic GMP. Experiments were terminated by the addition of 1.1 ml cold 10% trichloroacetic acid (TCA) to the slices after the removal of the bathing medium.

The TCA-treated samples were centrifuged at 20,000 × g for 10 min. The clear supernatant fluids were washed four times with four volumes of water-saturated ethyl ether, and the residual ether left in such extracts was removed by heating the samples to 80°C. The samples were then buffered with sodium acetate to achieve a final concentration of 50 mM NaAc and assayed for cyclic AMP and cyclic GMP by the radioimmunoassay described by Steiner et al. (1972). Pellets from the TCA-treated samples were dissolved in 1 N NaOH and assayed for protein by the method of Lowry et al. (1951).

All mice were purchased from Eldridge Laboratory Animals, Barnhart, Missouri. Phenytoin (Na-Dilantin), phenobarbital (Na-Luminal), and carbamazepine (Tegretol) were generous gifts of Parke-Davis & Co., Winthrop Laboratories and Ciba Pharmaceutical Co., respectively. Hydantoin was obtained from Aldrich Chemical Co., Inc. Veratridine was purchased from ICN·K & K Laboratories, Inc. and Aldrich Chemical Co., Inc. Barbituric acid was obtained from Eastman Kodak, and polyethyleneglycol was purchased from Sigma Chemical Co. All chemicals used in these studies were of the highest grade available.

RESULTS

Preliminary studies revealed that maximally effective concentrations of veratridine (20 μM) or K^+ (64 mM) increased cyclic GMP levels approximately tenfold from 0.7 to 0.8 to 6 to 10 pmoles/mg prot and elevated cyclic AMP levels approximately 100-fold from 7 to 18 to 400 to 700 pmoles/mg prot in incubated slices of mouse cerebral cortex.

Only phenytoin altered basal levels of cyclic nucleotides; this drug increased cyclic AMP levels twofold. However, all three drugs tested—phenytoin, phenobarbital and carbamazepine—inhibited veratridine-induced accumulation of both cyclic AMP and cyclic GMP in a dose-dependent manner, and all exhibited a statistically significant effect at concentrations of 1 mM or less (Fig. 1). Hydantoin (1 mM) and barbituric acid (1 mM), the nonanticonvulsant parent compounds of phenytoin and phenobarbital, respectively, were ineffective, however. Phenytoin and carbamazepine were equi-potent and produced 50% inhibition (ID_{50}) of cyclic AMP and cyclic GMP accumulation at concentrations of approximately 0.1 to 0.2 mM. These concentrations of phenytoin and carbamazepine are near their median effective doses for preventing maximal electroshock seizures (MES ED_{50}) and less than their median toxic dose (TD_{50}). Phenobarbital was only one-tenth as potent as phenytoin and carbamazepine; its ID_{50} concentration is more than 10 times its respective MES ED_{50} and also somewhat higher than its respective TD_{50}.

We previously reported that concentrations of phenytoin up to 0.3 mM inhibit veratridine-induced elevations of cyclic nucleotide levels, but have little or no effect on the elevations produced by high concentrations of K^+ (Ferrendelli and Kinscherf, 1978). A similar selective effect was also seen in the present experiments; 50% inhibition of K^+-induced elevations of cyclic GMP levels required 0.75 mM phenytoin, more than six times that necessary to produce an equivalent inhibition of veratidine-induced elevations of cyclic GMP. Carbamazepine also exhibited a more potent effect against veratridine-induced accumulation of cyclic GMP, and four times more drug was required to inhibit the effect of K^+. In contrast, phenobarbital had no significant differential effect. Phenytoin and carbamazepine, but not

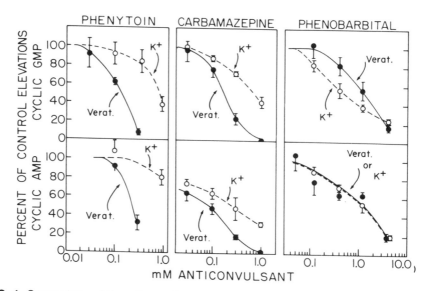

FIG. 1. Comparison of the effects of phenytoin, carbamazepine, and phenobarbital on K^+-induced and veratridine-stimulated elevations of cyclic GMP and cyclic AMP in slices of mouse cerebral cortex. Samples were incubated with either 64 mM K^+ or 20 μM veratridine together with the indicated concentrations of anticonvulsants. Results are expressed as the percent of elevation produced by each depolarizing agent after control (undepolarized) levels have been subtracted. Each symbol represents the mean of 3 to 8 samples.

phenobarbital, also exhibited a selective inhibitory effect against veratridine-induced elevations of cyclic AMP levels (Fig. 1). Interestingly, the concentrations of phenytoin and carbamazepine necessary to inhibit the K^+-induced elevations of cyclic AMP and cyclic GMP were similar to the concentrations of phenobarbital required to inhibit K^+- or veratridine-induced accumulation of cyclic nucleotides.

DISCUSSION

The present results confirm previous reports that phenytoin, carbamazepine, and phenobarbital can inhibit the effects of depolarizing agents on cyclic AMP accumulation in brain tissue *in vitro* (Lewin and Bleck, 1977) and further demonstrate that they also inhibit depolarization-induced accumulation of cyclic GMP. In addition to the three drugs studied here, primidone, aromatic substituted succinimides, and very high concentrations of clonazepam also inhibit depolarization-induced accumulation of both cyclic AMP and cyclic GMP in incubated slices of mouse cerebral cortex (Ferrendelli and Kinscherf, 1979). All of these drugs are particularly effective in the treatment of generalized tonic-clonic convulsions and are especially potent in the prevention of MES. In contrast, anticonvulsant drugs, viz., trimethadione, ethosuximide, valproic acid, and low concentrations of clonazepam, which have less or no effect against MES and tonic-clonic convulsions but readily prevent metrazol seizures and are especially useful in the treatment of absence seizures, do not inhibit depolarization-induced accumulation of both cyclic AMP and cyclic GMP. Instead, these drugs have no effect, or, in the case of ethosuximide and valproic acid, only inhibit accumulation of cyclic GMP. These observations have led to the hypothesis that inhibition of depolarization-induced accumulation of both cyclic AMP and cyclic GMP is somehow related to an anticonvulsant drug's ability to prevent MES. Conversely, the lack of this particular biochemical effect may be characteristic of drugs that are inactive against MES or those with predominant activity against metrazol and absence seizures.

Most published data indicate that elevated levels of cyclic AMP and cyclic GMP produced by depolarizing agents such as veratridine, ouabain, and high concentrations of extracellular K^+ in brain slices are consequences of cellular depolarization and are not a direct action of the depolarizing agent on cyclic nucleotide synthesis or degradation (Daly, 1977; Ferrendelli, 1976). It is well known that cellular depolarization augments influx of calcium into intracellular spaces (Katz, 1966; Rubin, 1970); it has been suggested that the increased intracellular concentration of calcium leads to accumulation of cyclic GMP (Ferrendelli et al., 1973), perhaps as a result of calcium activating guanylate cyclase. In addition, cellular depolarization increases neurotransmitter release, which is also a calcium-dependent process. The released neurotransmitters act on nearby cells to produce many effects. It is probable that released adenosine and biogenic amines activate specific membrane-bound adenylate cyclases and thereby increase cyclic AMP levels (Daly, 1977).

Obviously, elevations of cyclic nucleotide levels produced by depolarizing agents could be inhibited by several different mechanisms. Prevention of their depolarizing action would prevent the elevations of both cyclic nucleotides. Inhibition of changes in calcium conductance, either by attenuating depolarization or blockade of calcium channels, would prevent the elevations of cyclic GMP, and if calcium-coupled neurotransmitter release is blocked, cyclic AMP increases also would be prevented. Marked reduction of neurotransmitter release (especially adenosine or biogenic amines) by other means or blockade of the postsynaptic receptors of these neurotransmitters would prevent accumulation of cyclic AMP, but should have no effect on cyclic GMP. Finally, inhibition of guanylate cyclase or adenylate cyclase activity or activation of cyclic AMP or cyclic GMP phosphodiesterases would also be expected to prevent accumulation of the appropriate cyclic nucleotide.

The observation that phenytoin, carbamazepine, and phenobarbital inhibit both cyclic AMP and cyclic GMP accumulation induced by K^+ and veratridine suggests that these drugs somehow inhibit or prevent some of the actions of the depolarizing agents. One possibility is that all three may modify membrane function and reduce transmembrane ionic fluxes. In support of this contention, there is ample evidence indicating that they all alter intracellular ionic concentrations and/or modify conductance of various cations across cell membranes (Lipicky et al., 1972; Pincus, 1972; Schauf et al., 1974; Sohn and Ferrendelli, 1976; Swanson and Crane, 1972; Woodbury, 1969). The finding that phenytoin and carbamazepine are capable of inhibiting veratridine-induced accumulation of cyclic AMP and cyclic GMP at much lower concentrations than those necessary to inhibit the effect of K^+ suggests that these two drugs have a selective effect on ionic conductances. Previously we proposed that phenytoin selectively inhibits veratridine- (and ouabain-) induced accumulation of cyclic nucleotides in brain slices by blocking sodium channels in membranes of excitable cells and reducing Na^+ influx during depolarization (Ferrendelli and Kinscherf, 1977, 1978). This hypothesis is supported by the fact that tetrodotoxin, a known specific blocker of sodium channels, also selectively inhibits veratridine- and ouabain-induced accumulations of cyclic nucleotides (Ferrendelli and Kinscherf, 1978). Furthermore, phenytoin has been reported to block influx of Na^+ into several nervous tissues (Lipicky et al., 1972; Perry et al., 1978; Pincus, 1972). We now suggest that both phenytoin and carbamazepine have a similar mechanism of action and selectively block sodium channels, since they both have a similar effect on depolarization-induced accumulation of cyclic nucleotides.

Of particular interest is the fact that phenytoin and carbamazepine, although potent anti-MES drugs, are essentially devoid of anti-metrazol activity. In fact, these two drugs potentiate clonic seizures in metrazol-treated animals. In contrast, phenobarbital has both anti-MES and anti-metrazol activity and is equipotent against both of these experimental seizures. The present results demonstrate that phenytoin and carbamazepine preferentially inhibit veratridine-induced accumulation of cyclic nucleotides, whereas phenobarbital inhibits veratridine- and K^+-induced accumulation equally well. This suggests that selective inhibition of veratridine-induced, and probably ouabain-induced, accumulation of cyclic nucleotides is characteristic of drugs with anti-MES activity but lacking anti-metrazol activity. In support of this contention, preliminary studies in our laboratory reveal that mexiletine, an anticonvulsant that prevents MES but not metrazol seizures, also selectively inhibits veratridine-induced accumulation of cyclic AMP and cyclic GMP, but methsuximide, an anticonvulsant drug that prevents both MES and metrazol seizures, has an equipotent inhibitory effect on veratridine- and K^+-induced accumulation of cyclic nucleotides. Possibly, blockage of sodium channels (see above) is responsible for both selective inhibition of veratridine-induced accumulation of cyclic nucleotides and the ability of a drug to prevent MES, but not metrazol, seizures.

Hydantoin and barbituric acid are parent compounds of antiepileptic drugs but have no antiepileptic activity themselves and do not inhibit depolarization-induced accumulation of cyclic nucleotides. This suggests that inhibition of cyclic nucleotide accumulation produced by anticonvulsant drugs with anti-MES activity is related to their neuropharmacological action and is not a nonspecific effect. However, whether or not inhibition of cyclic nucleotide accumulation by these anticonvulsant drugs is specifically related to their antiepileptic activity is difficult to ascertain. Inhibition of K^+-induced elevations of cyclic nucleotides requires concentrations of phenytoin, carbamazepine, and phenobarbital that are higher than their TD_{50} doses, and inhibition of veratridine-induced elevations of cyclic nucleotides by phenobarbital also requires concentrations greater than the median toxic dose of this compound. Therefore, it is possible that these effects may not be related to the anticonvulsant actions of the above drugs but may be involved in mechanisms responsible for their toxic or sedative actions. On the other hand, both phenytoin and carbamazepine inhibit veratridine-induced accumulation of cyclic AMP and cyclic GMP at concentrations that are near their median effective doses for the prevention of MES and less than their median toxic doses. This suggests that phenytoin's and carbamazepine's inhibition of veratridine's effect may be related to their antiepileptic action. Whether their presumed blocking action at sodium channels or their inhibition of cyclic nucleotide accumulation or both contributes to their anticonvulsant effect is uncertain and will require further investigation.

REFERENCES

Daly, J. W. (1977): *Cyclic Nucleotides in the Nervous System*. Plenum Press, New York.

Ferrendelli, J. A. (1976): Cellular depolarization and cyclic nucleotide content in central nervous system. In: *Advances in Biochemical Psychopharmacology, Vol. 15, First and Second Messengers—New Vistas*, edited by A. Costa, E. Giacobini, and R. Paoletti. Raven Press, New York.

Ferrendelli, J. A., and Kinscherf, D. A. (1977): Phenytoin: Effects on calcium flux and cyclic nucleotides. *Epilepsia*, 18:331–336.

Ferrendelli, J. A., and Kinscherf, D. A. (1978): Similar effects of phenytoin and tetrodotoxin on cyclic nucleotide regulation in depolarized brain tissue. *J. Pharm. Exp. Ther.*, 207:787–793.

Ferrendelli, J. A., and Kinscherf, D. A. (1979): Inhibitory effects of anticonvulsant drugs on cyclic nucleotide accumulation in brain. *Ann. Neurol.*, 5:533–538.

Ferrendelli, J. A., Kinscherf, D. A., and Chang, M. M. (1973): Regulation of levels of guanosine cyclic 3',5'-monophosphate in the central nervous system: Effects of depolarizing agents. *Mol. Pharmacol.*, 9:445–454.

Ferrendelli, J. A., Rubin, E. H., and Kinscherf, D. A. (1976): Influence of divalent cations on regulation of cyclic GMP and cyclic AMP levels in brain tissue. *J. Neurochem.*, 26:741–748.

Katz, B. (1966): *Nerve, Muscle and Synapse*. McGraw Hill, New York.

Lewin, E., and Bleck, V. (1977): Cyclic AMP accumulation in cerebral cortical slices: Effect of carbamazepine, phenobarbital, and phenytoin. *Epilepsia*, 18:237–242.

Lipicky, R. J., Gilbert, D. L., and Stillman, I. M. (1972): Diphenylhydantoin inhibition of sodium conductance in squid giant axon. *Proc. Natl. Acad. Sci. USA*, 69:1758–1760.

Lowry, O. H., Rosebrough, N. J., Farr, A. L., and Randall, R. J. (1951): Protein measurement with the folin phenol reagent. *J. Biol. Chem.*, 193:265–275.

Perry, J. G., McKinney, L., and De Weer, P. (1978): The cellular mode of action of the anti-epileptic drug 5,5-diphenylhydantoin. *Nature*, 272:271–273.

Pincus, J. H. (1972): Diphenylhydantoin and ion flux in lobster nerve. *Arch. Neurol.*, 26:4–10.

Rubin, R. P. (1970): The role of calcium in the release of neurotransmitter substances and hormones. *Pharmacol. Rev.*, 22:389–428.

Schauf, C. L., Davis, F. A., and Marder, J. (1974): Effects of carbamazepine on the ionic conductances of *Myxicola* giant axons. *J. Pharmacol. Exp. Ther.*, 189:538–543.

Sohn, R. S., and Ferrendelli, J. A. (1976): Anticonvulsant drug mechanisms: Phenytoin, phenobarbital and ethosuximide and calcium flux in isolated presynaptic endings. *Arch. Neurol.*, 33:626–629.

Steiner, A., Parker, C., and Kipnis, D. (1972): Radioimmunoassay for cyclic nucleotides. I. Preparation of antibodies and iodinated cyclic nucleotides. *J. Biol. Chem.*, 247:1106–1113.

Swanson, P. D., and Crane, P. O. (1972): Diphenylhydantoin and movement of radioactive sodium into electrically stimulated cerebral slices. *Biochem. Pharmacol.*, 21:2899–2905.

Woodbury, D. M. (1969): Mechanisms of action of anticonvulsants. In: *Basic Mechanisms of the Epilepsies*, edited by H. H. Jasper and A. A. Ward, pp. 647–681. Little, Brown and Co., Boston.

Abstracts

HYPERTHERMIA AND THALAMOCORTICAL INSTABILITY: A COMPARISON WITH THE EFFECTS OF OTHER CONVULSANT AGENTS

R. N. Johnson, S. R. Quint, W. J. Nowack, G. R. Hanna
Charlottesville

Febrile convulsions of childhood may occur as an isolated event without sequelae. However, exacerbation of chronic seizure disorders during febrile illness throughout life is also common. Attempting to further elucidate the mechanisms involved in this relationship, the present study compares the effects of hyperthermia with other convulsant agents on the cat thalamocortical system.

In previous studies, we have demonstrated complex modulation of excitability levels in this system by administration of anticonvulsant drugs, anesthetic agents and cerebellar stimulation. Using similar methods, animals were operated under chloralose anesthesia. Stimuli were delivered in pairs to ventrolateral thalamus, varying both the amplitude of the second stimulus and the stimulus pair interval. The resultant evoked responses from the computer generated stimuli were quantified and stored on-line. A three dimensional evoked response profile (ERP) was generated to characterize the thalamocortical system in its resting state and under various experimental conditions. These included hyperthermia induced with an electric heating pad, contralateral homotopic penicillin, and systemic convulsants.

During prolonged hyperthermia, the ERP demonstrated marked threshold shifts and oscillatory behavior strikingly similar to that seen following topical application of penicillin to the contralateral cortex. In other experiments, hyperthermia produced marked regional enhancement of the ERP, suggesting increased excitability similar to that seen after subconvulsive doses of the convulsants bicuculline and methohexital. Based on these observations, it is clear that hyperthermia produces multiple effects, both temperature and time dependent. These parallel not only those seen with systemic epileptogenic agents, but also those seen from topical penicillin.

A BEHAVIOURAL EVALUATION OF 6 ANTI-CONVULSANTS IN AMYGDALOID KINDLED RATS

D. Ashton, A. Wauquier
Beerse

10 male Wistar rats implanted with a bipolar electrode in the basolateral amygdala and kindled to a stage 5 motor-seizure (Racine 1972) were selected for a behavioural study of the effects of anti-convulsants on seizures provoked by a 100 μA 4 sec train of biphasic square-wave 1 msec pulses at a rate of 100 pulses per sec. The drugs selected were clonazepam, flunarizine, depamide, methsuximide, mephenytoin, and acetazolamide. Doses were chosen from ED_{50} values obtained in the maximal metrazol test. On a test day two control convulsions were triggered with an interval of 30 minutes; the drug or saline was then administered I.P. and 30 minutes and 24 hours later a further stimulation was given. The presence of ipsilateral-turning, closing of the ipsilateral eye, rearing, falling-over, facial clonus, fore-limb clonus, hind-limb clonus, and "wet-shaking" was tabulated; and the duration of fore-limb clonus was measured. All drugs significantly reduced the duration of the fore-limb clonus 30 minutes after administration, whereas only flunarizine and mephenytoin were effective 24 hours after administration. Acetazolamide and flunarizine have no effect on clonic seizures in the metrazol test, their effectiveness against predominantly clonic kindled seizures suggests that the kindling preparation may be useful in anti-convulsant screening.

EFFECT OF ANTI-ABSENCE DRUGS ON INHIBITORY PATHWAYS IN THE CENTRAL NERVOUS SYSTEM

G. H. Fromm, A. S. Chattha, D. J. Glass, J. D. Alvin
Pittsburgh

A conditioning stimulus to the contralateral coronal gyrus or to the periventricular gray matter of cats inhibits the response of spinal trigeminal neurons to stimulation of the maxillary nerve. Sodium valproate, ethosuximide, trimethadione and imipramine decrease the cortical inhibition of the spinal trigeminal nucleus, while carbamazepine and phenytoin primarily decrease the response to maxillary nerve stimulation alone. Clinical trials showed imipramine to be effective against absence and myoclonic seizures in some patients, showing that our experimental model accurately predicts the effect of drugs against absence and myoclonic seizures. We have now found that sodium valproate, ethosuximide, and imipramine also decrease the periventricular inhibition of the spinal trigeminal neurons without significantly affecting the response of these neurons to maxillary nerve stimulation alone. On the other hand, carbamazepine and phenytoin again decreased the response to maxillary nerve stimulation alone. Our results therfore provide further support for the hypothesis that an important characteristic of drugs effective against absence seizures is their ability to selectively depress inhibitory pathways in the central nervous system, while drugs effective against tonic-clonic and partial seizures primarily depress excitatory pathways.

L-DOPA, L-5HTP AND BROMOCRIPTINE IN EPILEPSY AND KINDLED CONVULSION

S. Nakanishi, H. Kumashiro, T. Aono, E. Ohno, S. Uemura, N. Mori, T. Fukatsu, Y. Numata, K. Maruko
Fukushima

The present study deals with the effects of amine precursors and dopamine receptor stimulant on the clinical seizures of epileptic patients and on the electrical convulsions of amygdaloid kindled rabbits. The results are as follows:
1) L-DOPA
In a 17 year old boy (Lennox's syndrome), administration of L-DOPA (800 mg/day) diminished his convulsions for three months. In four kindled rabbits, pretreatment of L-DOPA (200 mg/kg) elevated their convulsion threshold.
2) L-5HTP
When the abovementioned boy was administered L-5HTP (100 mg orally), clinical convulsions and EEG spike discharges were activated. In another 17 year old boy with epilepsy (grand mal), L-5HTP (100 mg) activated only EEG spike and wave discharges. This phenomenon was not observed when he was administered L-5HTP (100 mg) and L-DOPA (200 mg) simultaneously. On the other hand, in four kindled rabbits, pretreatment of L-5HTP (50 mg/kg) did not change the convulsion threshold. However, it was suggested that the kindled convulsion was of a shorter duration.
3) Bromocriptine (dopamine recptor stimulant)
When bromocriptine was administered to the boy with Lennox's syndrome, much improvement was observed for three weeks.
In kindled rabbits, it appeared that bromocriptine suppressed the EEG after-discharges.

5-HYDROXYTRYPTAMINE METABOLISM IN E1-MOUSE

A. Mori, M. H. Hiramatsu
Okayama

E1-mice are an inbred strain with a convulsive disposition. Convulsions are produced in adult E1-mice by postural stimulation i.e. a violent tonic-clonic convulsion will occur after a mouse is gently thrown up in the air several times.
We have reported that brain dopamine and norepinephrine concentrations of "stimulated" E1-mice are lower than those of "non-stimulated" control E1-mice, and administration of L-DOPA and MK486, a peripheral decarboxylase inhibitor, to the mice had no effect on the convulsion.
In this experiment the mice were divided into two groups: the non-stimulated control and "stimulated" group, and 5-hydroxytryptamine (5-HT) and 5-hydroxyindolacetic acid (5-HIAA) levels in the brain were determined in these groups. The experimental results show the 5-HT and 5-HIAA levels at the resting stage of the "stimulated" series were significantly lower than those of the non-stimulated control.
In another series of experiments, 5-hydroxytryptophan (5-HTP) and MK 486 were administered to the "stimulated" animals, and marked elevation of the convulsive threshold (throwing times needed to induce convulsion) was observed in these mice. This finding suggests that the seizure mechanism in E1-mice could be closely related to the low brain level of 5-HT.

THE CSF- AND SALIVA-SERUM RATIO OF PHENYTOIN IN EPILEPTIC PATIENTS WITH AND WITHOUT IMPAIRMENT OF THE BLOOD-CSF-BARRIER

U. Hartmann and H. J. Lehmann
Essen

The CSF- and saliva-serum ratio of phenytoin was determined with a modification of the benzophenone procedure described by Dill, Chucot, Chang and Glazko 1971. Two groups of patients were compared:
1. Patients suffering from idiopathic epilepsy,
2. patients with symptomatic epileptic siezures for instance in brain tumors, meningitis.
Examination of the CSF- and saliva-serum ratio of phenytoin in these two groups of patients gives information on the validity of saliva phenytoin determination in patients with blood-CSF-barrier-impairment.

EPILEPTIC FOWL AS A PHARMACOLOGICAL MODEL OF EPILEPSY

D. D. Johnson, H. L. Davis, R. D. Crawford
Saskatoon

The evaluation of epileptic fowl as a pharmacological model of human epilepsy has been based on the premise that, to provide an acceptable model, the seizures must be sensitive to the common antiepileptic agents within the range of plasma drug concentrations known to be effective in human epilepsies. Groups of 8 to 10 chickens were used in a cross-over experimental design to determine the effect of the drugs on the incidence and severity of seizures in response to photic stimulation. Plasma samples were obtained for determination of drug concentrations by GLC at several time intervals following drug administration and the latter were correlated with observed changes in seizure susceptibility. Seizures were abolished or reduced in severity by phenobarbital (PB), phenytoin (PH), primidone (PR), diazepam, clonazepam and valproate, but not by ethosuximide. Complete protection was afforded by PB at mean plasma concentrations between 13 to $16 \mu g/ml$ and a significant reduction in seizure susceptibility occurred at $5 \mu g/ml$. PH significantly reduced the incidence of seizures (8-14 $\mu g/ml$) but higher concentrations appeared to activate the seizure process as evidenced by the production of the first stage of the motor seizure. Exposure of these chickens to photic stimulation did not produce a major seizure. This toxicity did not occur in heterozygotes at plasma concentrations in excess of those required to produce significant protection in epileptics. PR abolished seizures but was metabolized to PB. Pre-treatment with SKF-525A to prevent the metabolic production of PB revealed that PR itself had anticonvulsant activity. PEMA, a second metabolite of PR, had no effect. Ethosuximide had no anticonvulsant activity in acute and subacute studies although plasma concentrations in excess of 400 μg/ml were achieved. The finding that the seizure process in epileptic fowl is sensitive to PB, PH and PR at plasma concentrations equivalent to or slightly lower than those required to control generalized tonic-clonic and cortical focal seizures in humans whereas ethosuximide was ineffective suggests that this model is a relatively specific pharmacological model for those types of seizures.

Supported by the MRC of Canada.

ABNORMAL PLASTICITY IN THE MUTANT EL MOUSE OF A SENSORY PRECIPITATING EPILEPSY

J. Suzuki, Y. Nakamoto
Tokyo

Seizures of El mice are mainly induced by a paraboloid movement. Provoking stimuli are repetitively given once a week since the age of 3 weeks. At the age of 6 weeks abortive seizures occur, and fully developed seizures of tonic-clonic convulsions are formed gradually until about 20 weeks. The seizure thresholds are lowered markedly after the age of 15 weeks. In the EEGs of seizures initial spikes of discharges are recognized at a unilateral parietal area and after a while spikes generalize and fire continuously. The time between the initial spike and the first component of the bursting is an average of about 13 sec at the first seizures, and becomes shorter at successive seizures. The time between the initial spike and the generalization of the discharge also becomes shorter as seizures occur repetitively. The most suitable frequency of stimulation is once a week. An absolute refractory period of seizures is about 15 sec. In the El mice with fully developed seizures of low threshold, no seizure occurs after no stimulation period of 8 weeks. Accordingly, the occurrence of seizures needs to be given reinforcement stimulations. The occurrence of seizures of El mice is considered as plastic phenomenon by the development of the animals and the repetitive stimulations.

TIME COURSE OF CREATINE KINASE (CK) ACTIVITY IN SERUM AFTER GENERALIZED SEIZURES

F. L. Glötzner, M. Gaab, M. Planner
Wurzburg

Total CK activity in serum was increased postictally in 14 out of 17 patients (82%) being admitted to

hospital in the wake of one or more generalized seizures. No correlation was found between increased CK levels and ictal injuries. A highly significant negative correlation exists between regular antiepileptic treatment and elevated levels of the enzyme (p < 0.01).

The maximum value of CK activity was found on the third or fourth postictal day in 10 out of 14 patients. In some cases a smaller initial peak was seen within 24 hours after the seizure.

In cats two maximum values of CK activity in serum were found after experimentally induced seizures, one within 24 and the second after 48-96 hours.

In animals protected from convulsive muscle movement by relaxant drugs, only the initial postictal peak was found. The biphasic course of enzyme levels may be helpful in the diagnosis of generalized convulsions. The late peak of CK activity seems to be related to the intensity of ictal muscle contractions.

SPECIFIC RECEPTOR BINDING OF PHENYTOIN: A NEW PROPOSED MECHANISM OF ACTION

W. M. Burnham, L. Spero
Toronto

In recent years, studies utilizing the radioreceptor assay technique have demonstrated that a number of potent therapeutic drugs (*e.g.* the neuroleptics) exert their effect by binding to and activating specific receptor sites in the brain. Preliminary studies utilizing 3H-Diphenylhydantoin (3H-DPH) and a modified filter-assay technique suggest that phenytoin may work via a similar mechanism. A high-affinity, saturable binding site has been found in rat whole-brain homogenate. Spirodilantin 790 A, an active anticonvulsant enantiomer, competes for the specific 3H-DPH site, whereas Spirodilantin 790 B, the inactive stereoisomer, does not. Research now in progress will attempt to determine the regional distribution of specific 3H-DPH binding, and also to indicate which of the other anticonvulsant drugs and endogenous transmitters compete for the specific 3H-DPH site.

The possible significance of these findings relative to future developments in anticonvulsant therapy will be discussed.

ENZYME ACTIVITY IN KINDLED BRAINS

M. E. Corcoran, D. P. Reedy, E. G. McGeer, W. A. Staines
Vancouver

Intermittent application of localized electrical stimulation to the amygdala or certain other areas of brain results in the development of generalized seizures (kindling). In an attempt to identify possible neurochemical correlates of kindling, we measured the regional activity of neurotransmitter-synthetic enzymes in the brains of amygdaloid kindled rats and of yoked control rats that either received non-epileptic low-frequency stimulation of the amygdala or carried amygdaloid electrodes and were handled but not stimulated. In addition to measuring the activity of enzymes involved in the synthesis of GABA, glutamate, acetylcholine, catecholamines, and taurine, we also measured the regional high-affinity uptake of glutamate in kindled and control rats. All rats were killed 24 hours after the fifth fully generalized seizure in the kindled group.

The results were negative. There were no changes in enzyme activity or glutamate uptake that were reliably related to amygdaloid kindling. The mechanisms underlying the lasting increase in seizure susceptibility produced by kindling thus may not be expressed at the levels of enzyme activity or uptake of glutamate.

DC POTENTIALS OF TEMPORAL LOBE SEIZURES IN THE MONKEY

Y. Mayanagi
Tokyo
A. E. Walker
Albuquerque

In 8 monkeys made epileptic by alum or penicillin injection into temporal lobe structures, 40 seizures were studied by both DC potential and EEG recordings.

Eighteen seizures of lateral temporal origin had an abrupt negative DC potential shift of 0.5 to 2.0 mV in and around the focus. The frontal, parietal and occipital cortices did not develop DC potential changes, perhaps due to the limited propagation of the neocortical seizures.

Twenty-two seizures of medial temporal origin showed negative shifts of the anterior, inferior or lateral temporal cortex in 85% of seizures. The other 15% has a positive shift or none at all. In hippocampal seizures, a positive shift was sometimes seen prior to the main negative shift in the lateral temporal cortex. The remote cortex developed only a minimally positive shift in 30% of the mediotemporal seizures.

A markedly negative shift in the frontocentral cortex was the first sign of impending generalization which may result from a series of chain reactions with seizure propagation, involving more and more structures of the brain.

Registration of DC potentials in temporal lobe seizures may give insight into the nature of abnormal EEG activities and to some extent into the origin of seizures.

DEVELOPMENTAL SEIZURE PATTERNS AND SPIKE AND WAVE COMPLEX IN RAT

Y. Hirabayashi, N. Kataoka, Y. Takasaka
Sapporo
T. Yamauchi
Bethesda

Experimental seizures were produced in rats by the subdural or intracortical application of tungstic acid gel on the left sensorimotor area, and behavioral and electroencephalographic changes were monitored. Electrocorticograms (ECoG) were recorded from the cortical surface on frontal, central and occipital regions. In some other rats, the subcortical activities of the hippocampus, thalamus and caudate nucleus were also recorded. Ontogenic studies of the epileptogenic process were carried out from birth to 45 days of age.

1) In 30 to 60 minutes after gel application, the animals showed rhythmic or clonic jerks of the contralateral forelimb. These movements corresponded to high voltage slow waves accompanied later by some small spikes on the EEG.

2) In 60 to 90 minutes, the rats showed a specific posture of the body with increased muscle tone, standing up with the hindlimbs widely open. During the episode, there appeared spike and wave complexes on the ECoG, and generalized spike and wave complexes in the subcortical nucleus.

3) In the more advanced stage, the seizure developed further into a generalized major convulsion. The ECoG showed multiple spikes, multiple spike and wave complexes.

4) Ontogenetically, spike and wave complexes were observed after 20 days of age.

MODIFICATION OF SOMATO-SENSORY EVOKED POTENTIALS /SSEP/ DURING KINDLING IN CATS: ANALOGON OF LEARNING?

J. Majkowski, O. Kwast
Warsaw

In our previous studies and in literature there are suggestions that mechanisms of kindling and learning have some similarities. Also, we and others were able to correlate a particular change in shape of EP with learning. The purpose of the experiments was to study an effect of kindling on modification of cortical SSEP. The kindling was performed on right somato-motor cortex with usual procedure. The averaged SSEP were recorded before kindling and every 3rd week during every day formation of chronic epileptic focus. During one session left and right anterior paw was biopolary stimulated by electric shocks of 1 msec duration and at frequency 1 Hz. For each side stimulation, 64 averages were taken simultaneously from ipsi — and contralateral somato — sensory cortex. The averaged 3 to 7 SSEPs recorded during different stages of kindling were analyzed and compared.

The visual inspection clearly showed that during kindling there was distinctive shape modification of the SSEP in left and right kindled cortex. The main modification was within the late component about 150 msec and later. The relation of the shape modification to kindling itself and its epileptic effect is discussed.

RETICULAR MULTIPLE UNIT ACTIVITY DURING THE ONSET OF ADVERSIVE SEIZURES INDUCED BY ALUMINA CREAM IN CATS

M. Velasco, F. Velasco, C. Cepeda, and F. Estrada-Villanueva
Mexico

In this work, we quantitatively determined changes in multiple unit activity (MUA) of the mesencephalic (central tegmental field) and pontine (giganto cellular tegmental field) reticular formation concomitant to the onset of EEG and EMG tonic clonic discharges during wakefulness and sleep of cats with adversive epileptic seizures induced by alumina cream.

Mesencephalic and pontine reticular formation MUAs showed parallel changes during wakefulness (W), slow wave sleep (SWS) and paradoxical sleep (PS). During W and SWS, EEG and EMG tonic clonic discharges and a significant increase in reticular MUA were observed simultaneously. In contrast, during PS, EMG contractions occurred 7 sec. after the onset of EEG clonic discharges and reticular MUAs showed a significant initial increase 4 sec. before, a decrease 3 sec. after and a second increase 7 sec. after the onset of EEG tonic Clonic discharges.

These results suggest that during PS, the onset of EEG epileptic activity is related to an activation-deactivation reticulo cortical rather than to an activation of the reticulo spinal mechanism.

STUDIES ON NEURONS IN CHRONIC EPILEPTIC FOCI IN MONKEY
PART II ULTRASTRUCTURAL STUDY

T. Hori
Tokyo
B. Ishijima, N. Yoshimizu
Tochigi
H. Hirano
Mitaka

It was attempted to see whether or not one can detect the Morphological alterations in the fine structures in the neurons related to the epileptogenesis induced by the alumina cream injection in the motor cortex of adult java monkeys using the recently developed technique of horse radish peroxidase iontophoretic injection.

The experiments were made on three adult java monkeys. Epileptic focus was made in the left motor cortex by injecting the 0.2 ml of alum intra-cortically. After about 4 weeks the animal became epileptic. The epileptic discharge related neurons were identified by the physiological study and horse radish peroxidase (type VI, Sigma) was injected iontophoretically into this neuron (0.1 μA, 5 sec.). After several procedures the marked neuron was identified light-microscopically and studied electron-microscopically.

Up to present time, any conclusive data has not

been definitely obtained. Their cell membrane, mitochondria, lysosomes, synapses attached to them, synaptic vesicles have revealed no peculiarities. Further study will be required.

HIPPOCAMPAL SEIZURES AND BRAIN MONO-AMINE CONCENTRATIONS

T. Higuchi, Y. Kobayashi, Y. Igarashi, T. Noguchi
Saitama

For studying the correlations between convulsive processes and brain monoamines, biochemical analysis of regional brain monoamines was carried out by the acute experimental models during and after hippocampal seizures. Sprague-Dawley male rats at 6-7 weeks after birth were anaesthetized with nembutal. Electrodes were implanted stereotaxically in the bilateral hippocampus and bilateral frontal cortices. Seizure discharges were produced by local electrical stimulation of the left hippocampus. At various stages of hippocampal seizures, the enzyme system in the brain was inactivated by the microwave irradiation. After decapitation, the brains were regionally removed by the method of Glowinski (cortex; striatum, hippocampus; hypothalamus; midbrain; medulla oblongata; cerebellum). The levels of norepinephrine, dopamine and serotonine were determined by means of high performance liquid chromatography with electrochemical detection. The sensitivity of these assays is 100pg for norepinephrine and dopamine and 1ng for serotonine.

Recent investigations by the chronic models have indicated that the brain catecholamines are important functionally in the convulsive seizure mechanism. But it is difficult to determine whether the participation of the brain monoamines to the seizure mechanism is primarily or secondarily. Therefore we studied by the acute models above mentioned and analyzed the levels of norepinephrine, dopamine and serotonine.

CHRONIC EPILEPTIC FOCI IN MONKEYS: CORRELATION BETWEEN SEIZURE FREQUENCY AND PROPORTION OF PACEMAKER EPILEPTIC NEURONS

A. R. Wyler, K. Burchiel, A. A. Ward, Jr.
Seattle

This study sought to determine if a relationship exists between the number of epileptic neurons recorded within epileptogenic cortex and the frequency of ictal events. A total of 1,617 neurons from 15 alert, undrugged, Macaca mulatta monkeys was studied in detail. Thirteen monkeys had chronic epilepsy induced by subpial alumina injections in precentral cortex. Precentral neurons were judged epileptic by the magnitude and variability of the percentage of interspike intervals less than 5 mS during periods when the monkeys were awake. This method of quantifying epileptic single neuron activity appears highly reliable in distinguishing epileptic neurons from precentral neurons in either normal cortex, cortex contralateral to, or within the focus. For the 13 epileptic monkeys, the relative proportion of strongly epileptic neurons found within the foci was *logarithmically* correlated with the mean number of daily seizures. Because of the similarity between the physiology of the alumina focus in monkeys and the epileptic foci in humans, these data imply that the severity of focal human epilepsy is a function of epileptic neuronal mass.

STUDIES ON NEURONS IN CHRONIC EPILEPTIC FOCI IN MONKEY. PART I: UNITARY ANALYSIS IN THE DEVELOPING PROCESS OF EPILEPSY

B. Ishijima, N. Yoshimizu, F. Sato
Tochigi, Japan

Chronic unitary recording was done in the chronic alumina cream epileptogenic foci of awake, unanesthetized monkeys.

Epileptic discharges in the EEG were first recognized within 2 to 3 weeks, and spontaneous seizures developed around the end of the 4th week after injection.

Neurons with epileptic discharges increased in number with the development of epileptic activity. Some neurons (Type A) were related to EEG spikes in some degree in the interictal stage, while others (Type B) were not.

The structure of burst discharges was variable and the bursts of lobg first interval were rare and inconstant.

The unitary recordings during more than 20 spontaneous seizures were made. Type A neurons often participated in the seizures from the beginning, but on some occasions, they were not included at all, or involved only in the late stage.

Seizure may not always develop from some specified neurons. A given cell in the focus may be a trigger of seizure on some occasions and, on others, may be secondarily involved in it occurred from the other point.

Morphological study was made by labelling the bursting neurons with horseradish peroxydase at the end of the experiments.

IONTOPHORETIC AND TOPICAL PENICILLIN APPLICATION TO THE HIPPOCAMPAL PYRAMIDAL CELLS AND THEIR INHIBITORY SYSTEM

T. Yamauchi, S. E. Newman
Bethesda

Mechanisms for penicillin (PCN) induced epileptogenesis in the CNS have been investigated by various routes of PCN administration; systemic, topical, local infusion, and by microelectrode iontophoresis (Walsh; Ebersole; Macon and King). Extracellular recording from the feline hippocampus following topical and iontophoretic PCN application was investigated.

Stable cells (n=144) in the CA1 and CA3 regions of 45 cats were identified as pyramidal (n=36), or non-pyramidal (n=34) types by electrical stimula-

tion; the remainder were untested (n=74). PCN iontophoresis increased the unit firing rate, and decreased the duration of electrically induced post-discharge inhibition. Conversely, following topical PCN induced interictal surface discharges, unit firing was inhibited for a longer duration (2-10 sec) than following electrically induced post-discharge inhibition (50-370 msec). GABA suppressed homocysteine induced and spontaneous unit firing, but failed to completely suppress topical PCN induced unit firing occurring between surface interictal discharges. Similar findings were noted in the three cell groups.

These findings suggest that topical PCN induced surface interictal discharges are associated with diffuse hippocampal population synaptic effects, whereas PCN iontophoresis may be related to direct excitation/inhibition of the pyramidal cell/basket cell circuitry, respectively.

SLOW POTENTIAL SHIFTS AND POTASSIUM CLEARANCE IN PENICILLIN FOCUS IN CATS

K. Mori, M. Kaminogo, K. Yamashiro, K. Iwayama
Nagasaki

Slow potential (SP) shifts associated with paroxysms have been shown to correlate with changes in glial membrane potential which was, on the one hand, proportional to the amount of extracellular potassium ($[K^+]_o$).

To further clarify this thesis, simultaneous recordings of SP, $[K^+]_o$ and neuronal activity were made by a double-barreled electrode (Prince et al.) in a Penicillin focus in paralyzed cats.

Most of paroxysms, either interictal or ictal, were associated with transitory increases in $[K^+]_o$ and negative SP shifts. These took a heavy neuron density of 1000-1500 μm. These also showed limited values. Regardless of the type paroxysms, $[K^+]_o$ rose to peak levels no higher than approximately 8 mu and clearance after termination of the seizure was also rapid, indicating that the buffering capacity was well preserved in our acute experimental model.

However, a unique paroxysm was observed occasionally in which electrocorticogram showed a characteristic figure and $[K^+]_o$ increased periodically without accompanying marked SP shifts. Neuronal firing was also not remarkable.

Although the cause of the unique paroxysm is obscure, increases in $[K^+]_o$ do not elucidate, without exception, negative SP shifts associated with paroxysms.

BEHAVIOR OF CEREBELLAR CORTICAL NEURONES DURING SPIKE-WAVE PAROXYSM IN CAT

H. Yuasa, N. Kageyama
Nagoya
S. Watanabe
Gifu

The relation between generalized, synchronous spike-wave paroxysm and neuronal activity of cerebellum was studied using "spontaneous" spike-wave rhythm which was elicited by parenteral Penicillin G (200,000 - 300,000 Unit/Kg) to adult cats. Unit recordings from the cortical neurones of the cerebellar vermis and that of the pericruciate area were made. Approximately 3/sec spike-wave paroxysm appeared about 30 min. after Penicillin administration. There was no certain pattern of cerebellar cell discharge prior to the beginning of spike-wave paroxysm. Purkinje cells showed the burst of discharge in coincident with the spike phase of the corticogram and decreased firing during the wave phase. Some cerebellar neurones did not decrease firing during the wave phase. Simultaneous recording from cerebral and cerebellar cortical neurones showed similar discharge pattern to each other during paroxysm. Usually cerebral neurones started discharge 5-20 msec earlier than Purkinje cells, but occasionally Purkinje cells fired earlier than cerebral neurones. In the case of generalized tonic-clonic seizures, cerebellar neurones showed increased firing, particularly at the beginning of seizures.

Cerebellar cortical neurones were strongly influenced from the spike-wave paroxysm but there was little evidence to show that cerebellum exerts influence on the spike-wave paroxysm.

ALTERATIONS IN EXTRACELLULAR POTASSIUM CONCENTRATION DURING STIMULATION OF HIPPOCAMPAL SLICES

C. K. Benninger, J. L. Kadis, D. A. Prince
Stanford

Extracellular potassium rises ($[\Delta K^+]_0$) have been demonstrated following repetitive stimulation of the *in vivo* hippocampus and following spontaneous epileptiform discharges. These rises have a characteristic ceiling level and topographic distribution. This study was conducted to determine the suitablity of using a more accessible *in vitro* preparation to investigate these phenomena. Guinea pig hippocampal slices maintained *in vitro* were studied using potassium ion-sensitive microelectrodes prepared by standard techniques. The baseline tissue potassium level in "healthy" slices was similar to that of the bathing solution which was varied from 3 to 10 mM $[K^+]_0$. $[K^+]_0$ reached equilibrium with the bath within 20 min. of change in bath $[K^+]$. Spontaneous sustained increases in $[K^+]_0$ were an early sign of slice deterioration. Stimulation of orthodromic pathways in CA1 stratum radiatum produced $\Delta[K^+]_0$ which had a number of characteristics similar to those seen *in vivo*. The $\Delta[K^+]_0$ was greatest in stratum pyramidale with a progressive fall off in stratum oriens and stratum radiatum. Maximum rise from a baseline of 5 mM was to about 10 mM depending upon the intensity and frequency of the stimulus, with 10 Hz or higher being optimal. During long stimulation trains a plateau in $[K^+]_0$ was reached in about 5 sec., followed by a fall toward baseline levels. The largest $\Delta[K^+]_0$ was seen when baseline $[K^+]_0$ was 5-6 mM and increments were far smaller in 3 mM and 10 mM $[K^+]_0$ for

comparable stimuli. There was a strong correlation between the $[K^+]_0$ level reached during various portions of a stimulus train and the field potentials generated. The field potential amplitude increased and repetitive firing occurred as the potassium level increased to the plateau value. As the stimulus continued and $[K^+]_0$ fell, the field potentials fell toward control levels. Introduction of penicillin (2,000 U1ml) into the bathing medium produced no change in resting $[K^+]_0$ but did produce spontaneous and evoked epileptiform field potential bursts similar to those previously reported. $\Delta[K^+]_0$ in the penicillin solution was larger than that evoked in the normal medium and a maximum rise of 7 mM from a resting baseline of 5 mM could be recorded. The magnitude of the stimulated $\Delta[K^+]_0$ in penicillin was comparable to that reported *in vivo*, but the ½ rise times and ½ fall times were shorter. We conclude from these experiments that much of the phenomenology of potassium change during activity previously described *in vivo* can be duplicated in the *in vitro* situation independent of circulatory system influence. (Supported in part by NIH grant NS 12151 to DAP and by the Deutsche Forschungsgemeinschaft to CKB.)

THE ACTIVATED ASTROCYTES. AN HISTOCHEMICAL MARKER OF SOME CAUSAL FACTORS OF FOCAL EPILEPSY

J. A. Dresse,
M. A. Gerebtzoff
Liège

In previous works, we demonstrated the histochemical characteristics of a special class of reactive astrocytes, which we have named "ACTIVATED ASTROCYTES". We have postulated a link between these cells and human or experimental epileptic foci. We can now determine the epileptic potential of a given focus of gliosis, by the presence or absence of activated astrocytes.

In order to determine if the activated astrocytes are the consequence of seizures or if they represent a morphologic marker of some causal factors, we performed two types of experiments:

a) kindling phenomenon in 20 rats, some of which presented more than 150 seizures, never induced the appearance of activated astrocytes. The absence of these cells defends the thesis that activated astrocytes are not the consequence of repeated motor and electrical seizures.

b) Cobalt-induced epilepsy in 115 rats allowed us to study pre-convulsive states. We found, near the mplantation site, activated astrocytes in those animals presenting electrical anomalies, such as spikes, on the electrocorticogram, without motor seizures. Moreover we found a precession of enzymatic modifications on electrical signs. We conclude that activated astrocytes are not the consequence of seizures but that they serve as morphologic markers of some causal factors of focal epilepsy.

THE DEVELOPMENT OF SECONDARY FOCI IN THE MONKEY: THE ROLE OF THE COMMISSURES

G. Ettlinger
London

We have attempted to identify the pathways responsible for the spread of the primary focus to the contralateral (secondary) hemisphere. Unexpectedly we found that deep commissure section did not prevent the development of secondary (mirror) foci in parietal cortex of the monkey. Secondary transmitted and also independent events could be recorded from the mirror foci after commissure section. Subsequently we widely ablated either the primary or the secondary foci in such monkeys: ablation of the primary focus eliminated primary and secondary transmitted events; ablation of the secondary focus eliminated secondary independent (but not secondary transmitted) events. These findings suggest that the secondary transmitted events reach the contralateral focus by volume conduction; but that the independent events have a neural origin in the parietal cortex of the secondary hemisphere — even when they develop after deep commissure section. (However, we have not yet been able to control for the passive spread of the epileptogenic agent, aluminium hydroxide, from the primary to the secondary hemisphere.) This work was done in collaboration with M. V. Driver, M. B. Lowrie, J. J. Maccabe and V. Nie, and was financed by the M.R.C.

THE DEVELOPMENT OF SECONDARY FOCI IN THE MONKEY: THE EVIDENCE FROM MICRO-ELECTRODE RECORDINGS

G. Ettlinger
London, U.K.

Our aim was to follow the changes in the pattern of discharge of units in inferotemporal cortex during the development of secondary foci. Primary foci were induced by application of aluminium hydroxide to one inferotemporal cortex. Then, at intervals varying for different monkeys from 2 to 26 months, wells were implanted bilaterally to permit microelectrodes to be inserted simultaneously into both inferotemporal regions. Unitary activity was recorded extracellularly from both electrodes while the monkey was undrugged and only lightly restrained. Ictal or interictal events were identified in the scalp EEG and/or from the mass activity recorded with the microelectrode. Unit activity in the secondary inferotemporal cortex (contralateral to the primary epileptogenic lesion) was frequently time-locked to ictal or interictal events recorded from the primary focus. The changes time-locked to ictal events were seen as early as 2 months after the epileptogenic agent was applied to the primary cortex, and to interictal events as late as 21 months. The predominant (but not sole) change in unit activity in the secondary hemisphere was a decrease in the rate of discharge. This work was done in collaboration with O. Holmes

and V. Nie, and was financed by the M.C.R. and Wellcome Trust.

PROPAGATION OF FOCAL MOTOR SEIZURES IN THE MONKEY

W. Caveness, M. Kato, S. Hosokawa, B. Malamut, S. Wakisaka and R. O'Neill
Bethesda

Focal seizures were induced in 3.5 Kg. Macaca mulatta by injecting 25,000 units of Penicillin in 0.25 ml water into the face-hand area of the right cerebral motor cortex. The paroxysmal activity was monitored by electroencephalography and electromyography. After thirty minutes each head was removed, frozen and serially sectioned. The cortical and subcortical metabolic activity was then determined by the Sokoloff Method: 2-deoxy-D-[^{14}C]glucose, injected by vein at the beginning of the seizure, competes with glucose for transport across the blood brain barrier and for the enzyme hexokinase. While glucose completes its metabolic cycle, the deoxyglucose is trapped in brain tissue at the phosphorylated phase where its [^{14}C] label may be quantitatively measured by autoradiography. Using these measurements with those of the isotope in arterial blood, the actual rate of local glucose utilization may then be calculated in mg per 100 grams of brain per minute.

The pattern of glucose utilization in four control monkeys was bilaterally symmetrical with a range in individual brain components from 8-9 mg/100 gm/min to 2-3 mg/100 gm/min. The right-left difference, %(R-L)/L, was negligible. With contralateral *face* seizures, in four monkeys, there was a distinct though uneven increase in activity with a right-left difference of 90-100% in the lateral globus pallidus, VPM of the thalamus, and motor cortex, with somewhat less difference in VPL, VL and medial globus pallidus. With extension to contralateral *face and hand* seizures, in four monkeys, there was a dramatic change in pattern, predominantly unilateral, with values as high as 22-28 mg/100 gm/min. The right-left difference was 400% in medial, and 340% in lateral globus pallidus, twice that of any other structure; 120-160% in the motor and sensory cerebral cortex; 90-120% in VL, VPL and VPM; and a left-right difference of 50-60% in the cerebellar cortex.

These data provide fresh insight into the location and extent of increased neuronal activity in focal motor seizures, that must be accommodated when considering basic mechanisms. Further they provide the location of targets, that may be suitable for stereotactic surgery.

THE ACTION OF INHIBITORY AMINOACIDS ON ACUTE EXPERIMENTAL MODELS OF EPILEPSY

R. G. Fariello
Madison

Epileptiform activity was induced in adult cats under general or local anesthesia. Acute models of focal epilepsy were created by application of various epileptogenic agents to neocortical or limbic structures. Intramuscularly injected penicillin was used as a model of generalized epilepsy. Inhibitory aminoacids were i.v. injected and their effect on epileptiform discharges monitored for two hours after administration. Aminoacid solutions were adjusted at variable pH from 5.5 to 8. Glycine (up to 200 mg/kg) did not induce any change. Short lasting inhibitory effects (5 sec. - 5 min) were noted with Balanine (> 80mg/kg), GABA and Taurine, (> 50 mg/kg) and 3 aminopropanesulfonic acid (APS, > 10 mg/kg). Particularly powerful was the action of APS capable of abolishing cortical spiking with only moderate depression of the background EEG activity. Moreover APS transiently inhibited unitary epileptic firing of pyramidal neurons at a threshold concentration of 2 mg/kg. GABA, Taurine and APS also induced depression of respiration in animals under barbiturate anesthesia. APS in addition caused a 20% drop in systolic blood pressure. Similar and even greater pressure drop was caused by various control drugs which however did not affect the epileptic firing rate. The inhibitory action of the aminoacids was better evident on models of focal epilepsy than on the generalized one. APS seems to deserve further investigation as a possible antiepileptogenic agent.

FOREBRAIN NORADRENALINE AND METRAZOL-INDUCED SEIZURES

S. T. Mason, M. E. Corcoran
Vancouver

The results of a previous experiment (Corcoran et al., *Exp. Neurol.*, 1974, 45:118-133) suggested that central catecholamines act to suppress seizures induced by the convulsant drug Metrazol (pentylenetetrazol). That experiment implicated noradrenaline (NA) rather than dopamine (DA) in seizure suppression, but conclusive evidence was lacking. We report here that selective depletion of forebrain NA by use of intracerebral injections of the neurotoxin 6-hydroxydopamine produced a marked increase in the duration and intensity of metrazol-induced seizures in rats. Depletion of NA did not alter the latencies to onset of either the first myoclonic jerk or the fully generalized seizure, suggesting that the observed potentiation was not the result of a nonspecific effect such as increased penetration of Metrazol into the brain. In addition, more than half of the NA-depleted rats had two seizures each in a 1 hour session, whereas vehicle-treated control rats all had only one seizure each. Postmortem assay confirmed that severe and permanent depletion of NA had been achieved in the cortex-hippocampus and hypo-thalamus, with sparing of brain DA and noradrenergic systems to the cerebellum and spinal cord. These findings are consistent with the hypothesis that NA may act in the normal brain to suppress the intensity and duration of seizures and that deficits in noradrenergic activity may in some cases contribute to pathological epileptiform states.

EPILEPTIFORM SEIZURES IN DOMESTIC FOWL

D. D. Johnson, E. C. Crichlow, R. D. Crawford
Saskatoon

Crawford described a mutation in domestic fowl which produced a high seizure susceptibility. The seizure susceptibility is controlled by an autosomal recessive gene. Homozygotes are highly sensitive to stroboscopic stimulation and usually convulse within 30 sec whereas heterozygotes are unaffected. The type of seizure exhibited is best described as grand mal and will be illustrated by a film. The inter-ictal EEG of homozygotes is markedly different from that of heterozygotes and is characterized by slow-wave high-voltage activity with isolated spikes and spike and wave complexes. When epileptics are exposed to photic stimulation at 14 fps the slow-wave high-voltage activity disappears and is replaced by following waves at the same frequency as the stimulus. These waves evolve into high voltage spikes and their appearance coincides with the onset of the overt motor seizure.

When compared to heterozygotes the brain of homozygotes are deficient in 5-Ht, dopamine (DA) and GABA. Repletion of 5-Ht and DA by administration of precursors or by pharmacological manipulations did not reduce seizure susceptibility and thus abnormalities in these amines do not appear to be involved in genesis of the high seizure susceptibility. The levels of brain GABA of homozygotes are lower than those of heterozygotes. Compounds which increase brain GABA levels prevent stroboscopic induced seizures, whereas substances which decrease the levels of brain GABA enhance seizure susceptibility. Despite the apparent relationship between seizure susceptibility and brain GABA levels the GAD and GABA-T enzyme activities showed no significant differences between homozygotes and heterozygotes.

Supported by the MRC of Canada.

THE CONCEPT OF ABNORMAL LIMBIC SYSTEM SENSITIVITY AS A SUBSTRATE FOR SEIZURE AND FOR EMOTIONAL/BEHAVIORAL DYSFUNCTION

K. Livingston, C. Stark-Adamec, R. Adamec
Toronto

Studies by Adamec using the limbic (subcortical) model of kindling provide evidence that concomitant with the spreading subcortical epileptiform activity which precedes the appearance of generalized motor seizure, there are significant and long-lasting changes in emotionality and behavior. These changes seen in the experimentally kindled animal provide an interesting parallel with the progressive and long-lasting changes in emotionality and behavior seen in some clinical cases of "temporal lobe" epilepsy. In the experimental model these changes are established before the appearance of motor seizure and will be stable over long periods in animals which have never experienced generalized seizure activity. This evidence from the experimental laboratory supports the clinical contention that seizures of temporal lobe origin and associated changes in emotionality and behavior are expressions of physiological disturbance in a common limbic substrate.

If reliable clinical indices of abnormal limbic system sensitivity were available it would be possible to examine this question not only in patients with clearly identifiable temporal lobe epilepsy, but also in populations of patients in whom epilepsy has not been identified or suspected, but whose emotional and/or behavioral change appears as recurrent, episodic disturbance that might reflect fluctuating abnormality in temporal lobe or limbic circuits. We have been developing a clinical protocol using multifaceted non-invasive techniques for detecting, displaying, and measuring abnormal limbic system sensitivity. This protocol provides quantitative indices for the clinical diagnosis of limbic system abnormality. Such indices are useful in therapeutic management of patients with known temporal lobe epilepsy as well as patients with behavioral abnormalities associated with previously undetected abnormal limbic system sensitivity.

THE EFFECTS OF FOREBRAIN BISECTION ON KINDLED AMYGDALOID SEIZURE IN CATS

T. Nakashima, J. A. Wada
Vancouver

In our previous studies, prior forebrain commissural bisection was shown to facilitate the rate of amygdaloid (AM) kindling. In this study the effects of forebrain bisection upon kindled AM seizures were examined in five cats.

The following observations were made: 1) Primary-site AM stimulations following the callosal bisection produced significant modification of seizure pattern, from bisymmetrical generalized convulsions to lateralized or incomplete convulsive seizures.

2) When these animals were subjected to secondary-site AM kindling, convulsive seizure was lateralized or asymmetrical. In addition there was no significant acceleration of the kindling rate. This is in contrast to the significantly faster rate of secondary site AM kindling in non-bisected animals.

This finding suggests that the phenomenon of transhemispheric "transfer" was dependent on functional integrity of the bisected structure.

3) Electrographically, afterdischarge became latalized to the stimulated hemisphere regardless of whether primary-site or secondary-site was stimulated.

4) Bisection of the anterior commissure produced no additional change in electroclinical seizure patterns.

Results of the present study suggest that the purpose of forebrain commissurotomy to restrict seizure propagation might be achieved without transection of the anterior commissure. The effect of selective anterior commissural bisection upon AM kindling and AM kindled seizure is currently being examined.

ABSENCE OF LESIONS IN AMMON'S HORN NEURONS FOLLOWING METRAZOL INDUCED SEIZURES IN THE HYPERTHERMIC RAT

A. Escobar, D. Nieto
Mexico City

It is now accepted that early uncontrolled febrile seizures in children may lead to Ammon's horn sclerosis and in turn this secondary lesion become an active epileptogenic focus in itself. This point of view refutes the earlier idea that tentorial herniation at birth led to ischemia of the hippocampal gyrus hence to sclerosis of the Ammon's horn.

In an attempt to reproduce neuronal damage in Ammon's horn, seizures were induced with Metrazol in rat ranging from 8 days to 3 months in age. In one group a "febrile" condition was created by means of subcutaneous injection of a vaccine for human use. In that group seizures were induced while the rats were hyperthermic. A second group was given Metrazol only. A third group was "protected" with Diazepam given prior to Metrazol. A fourth group served as control. At least one episode of several seizures was given to each animal. If they survived they usually recovered within 12 hours and then again subjected to seizures at intervals of 36 hours each. After the fourth episode the animals were sacrificed and perfused. No lesions of the neurons in the Ammon's horn were observed in any of the groups. The results suggest that "febrile" experimental seizures in the rat do not constitute a pathogenetic mechanism for Ammon's horn sclerosis.

EXPERIMENTAL POST-TRAUMATIC EPILEPSY: NEUROCHEMICAL MORPHOLOGIC AND ELECTROENCEPHALOGRAPHIC OBSERVATIONS

L. J. Willmore and G. W. Sypert
Gainesville

Intra-cortical injection of 5 μl of 100 mM ferrous or ferric chloride into rat sensorimotor isocortex will induce a focus of recurrent seizure discharge. In the present study, animals were prepared by cortical iron salts injection or by acidic saline injection. Electroencaphalograms recorded with platinum needle electrodes 6 weeks after injection confirmed the presence of active epileptiform discharges in the experimental animals. Animals selected for histologic observation were killed by transcardiac perfusion with neutral buffered formalin. Alternate 25 μ serial sections through the epileptic focus were strained with H&E, thionin, prussian blue, and PTAH. Light microscopial observations showed iron-containing macrophages and fibroblasts lining the cavity formed at the site of iron injection. Nissl stains showed moderate neuronal depopulation and astrogliosis surrounding the epileptic focus. Medium pyramidal neurons located in lamina V beneath the injection site were ferruginated, being covered with particles of iron-cyanate complex after staining with prussian blue. Assessment of protein synthesis in the cortical focus, the contralateral homotopic cortex and the cerebellum by [3H] lysine uptake showed increased uptake of [3H] in the actively discharging epileptic focus, but the relative incorporation of [3H] lysine into protein was decreased. Thus it would appear that active focal epileptiform discharge alters either blood-brain barrier and/or focal blood flow while inhibiting cellular protein synthesis.

The persistence of epileptiform discharges within the ferrous/ferric focus, and the histopathologic changes resembling those found in resected human post-traumatic epileptic lesions suggest that iron liberated from hemoglobin following cortical contusion or cerebral infarction may be important in post-traumatic epileptogenesis.

KINDLING IN THE SEIZURE-PRONE AND SEIZURE-RESISTANT MONGOLIAN GERBIL, MERIONES UNGUICULATUS

D. P. Cain, M. E. Corcoran, J. A. Wada
London and Vancouver

Previous studies of Senegalese baboons with a genetic predisposition to photically-induced seizures have indicated an essential independence between the mechanisms of these seizures and electrically kindled seizures (Wada & Osawa, *Neurology,* 1976, *26,* 273). To provide additional data concerning the relation between naturally occurring seizure states and electrically kindled seizures, we examined amygdaloid kindling in the seizure-prone and -resistant strains of gerbil bred at U.C.L.A. (Loskota et al., *Epilepsia,* 1974, *15,* 109). Kindling in both strains proceeded rapidly through a number of stages of convulsive seizure with associated afterdischarge (AD), culminating in a generalized bisymmetric convulsion after 4.8 ADs in the seizure-prone strain and 9.8 ADs in the seizure-resistant strain. Additional kindling stimulation resulted in the development of "running-hopping" seizures after 4.9 ADs in the seizure-prone strain and 14.3 ADs in the seizure-resistant strain. Post-kindling tests of stress-induced seizure susceptibility (Loskota et al., 1974) indicated that most animals showed more frequent and stronger convulsions after kindling than before. In most cases there was a change in the convulsion manifestations as a result of kindling such that the stress-induced convulsions strongly resembled the kindled convulsions where they had not done so prior to kindling. These results suggest that the naturally occurring and kindled seizure states may depend in part on a common neural mechanism in this species.

DC POTENTIAL SHIFTS ASSOCIATED WITH PRIMARY AND TRANSFER KINDLING CONVULSION IN RABBITS

H. Kumashiro, E. Ohno, T. Aono, S. Nakanishi, S. Uemura, N. Mori, T. Fukatsu, Y. Kaneko
Fukushima

We caused epileptogenecity in 15 rabbit's amygdala (AMG) by the kindling method and recorded the DC potential shift of cortex, EEG of AMG and EEG of motor cortex for investigation of the relationship between these records and the development of epileptogenecity.

The results were as follows:
1) The DC shift was not seen at the subthreshold-stimulation which didn't cause the after-discharge (AD) in stimulating the AMG.
2) The negative DC shift was seen accompanied with the motor cortex AD in a latency of about 20 seconds after stimulation, when the motor cortex AD was generalized by repetitive threshold-stimulation of AMG.
3) At the final kindling stage, there was an obvious negative DC shift, which followed the conspicuous cortical AD, and the generalized convulsion (primary kindling convulsion).
4) When the transfer phenomenon was confirmed in contralateral AMG stimulation, the negative DC shift pertaining to the cortical AD and generalized convulsion, occurred earlier than in the case of primary kindling convulsion.

These results suggest that the DC shift is related to the development of the epileptogenesis.

DYNAMICS OF OLFACTORY CORTEX NEURONAL POPULATIONS DURING KINDLING IN DOG

K. van Hulten, F. H. Lopes da Silva, J. ten Veen and R. Acohen
Utrecht

Kindling of the olfactory cortex (prepyriform or PPC) was carried out in dogs (beagles) with 36 chronically indwelling electrodes in several brain areas mainly in limbic structures. EEG recordings were carried out by means of a 16-channel radiotelemetry system with the freely moving animals in a standard behavioural condition. In the course of PPC kindling (daily stimulation with a 1 sec train: 60 pulses/sec, pulses of 70-100 μA and 1 msec) characteristic changes in EEG-ongoing activity were found and quantified by spectral analysis; the occurrence of epileptiform paroxysmal activity was detected and quantified by automatic methods. Electro-clinical epileptic seizures were obtained after about 30-70 days of kindling; spontaneous seizures were also encountered after about 120 days. Before kindling procedure started and thereafter Evoked Potentials (EP's) to single pulse electrical stimulation (1/sec, 150-300 μA, 200μsec) of the lateral olfactory tract were recorded; the EP's of the PPC were studied quantitatively by way of a mathematical model. A significant change in amplitude, frequency of oscillation and decay rate of the PPC EP's was found in the course of kindling. This indicates that during kindling the dynamics of the PPC neuronal populations change in a significant way, namely the negative feedback gain of the closed loop constituted by the PPC's excitatory and inhibitory populations decreases.

SPECIFIC AND NON SPECIFIC MULTIPLE UNIT ACTIVITIES DURING PENTYLENETETRAZOL (PTZ) SEIZURES IN ACUTE "ENCEPHALE ISOLE" CATS

F. Velasco, M. Velasco and R. Romo
Mexico City, D.F.

The present report describes the sequence of activation and deactivation of central nervous structures and their relation with the muscular contractions during PTZ induced seizures in cats immobilized by a spinal transection (C1-C2). After the animals recovered from spinal shock, multiple unit activity (MUA) was recorded through stereotactically placed electrodes from mesencephalic and pontine reticular formation and pyramidal tract, EEG recorded from the motor cortex and EMG-MUA from the neck muscles innervated by nerve roots above the transection level. A threshold I.V. dose of PTZ (20 mg/kg) was injected and the following events recorded: 1) An initial increment in mesencephalic reticular MUA followed by increase in pontine and EMG-MUA 4 seconds (± 2) later, while EEG and pyramidal tract remained unchanged. 2) Further increase in mesencephalic MUA occurred 7 seconds ($\pm$ 2) later and accompanied by further increase in pontine and EMG-MUA as well as EEG and pyramidal tract tonic clonic discharges. 3) EEG and pyramidal tract MUA decreased to levels below the control period 23 seconds ($\pm$ 8) later, while mesencephalic, pontine and EMG-MUA remained very high. Quantitative evaluation of MUA demonstrated that these differences were statistically significant. The results suggest that PTZ seizure starts in mesencephalic reticular formation and reaches the muscles through at least two different pathways: pyramidal tract and possibly a reticulospinal pathway.

INHIBITION OF KINDLING AMYGDALOID SEIZURE AND TRANSFERENCE PHENOMENON BY THE COCAINE PRETREATMENT

N. Hikasa, M. Sato, S. Otsuki
Okayama

A series of our previous reports have shown the close relationship between brain catecholamine levels and kindling seizure susceptibility. There are, however, a few reports concerned with the functional role of receptor sensitivity of catecholaminergic neuron systems in epilepsy. In order to disclose this problem, the present investigation was intended to study the effects of cocaine-induced innervation supersensitivity of the dopamine neuron receptor on the amygdaloid seizure development in kindled cats. The animals in cocaine-pretreated group were sensitized to apomorphine after chronic repeated administration of cocaine (7.5-10 mg/kg/day; mean 30 day). The latency for developing generalized convulsions increased significantly in the cocaine-pretreated group ($p < 0.005$) and decreased in the haloperidol group ($p < 0.001$) than the untreated control group. Moreover, the transference phenomenon was also suppressed completely

in all cases of cocaine-pretreated group. It was concluded that dopamine neuron receptor sensitivity acted an important role in the kindling seizure development and its underlying trans-synaptic neural changes.

INTERICTAL SPIKING IN THE AWAKE KINDLED RAT: A MODEL FOR BIOCHEMICAL STUDY

J. G. Fitz and J. O. McNamara
Durham

Spontaneous interictal spiking (SIS) is the electroencephalographic (EEG) hallmark of partial epilepsy. Kindling is a recently developed animal model of epilepsy induced by periodic electrical stimulation of the brain. Detailed studies of SIS have been reported in kindled cats. The goal of this study was to systematically define the temporal spatial profile of SIS in kindled rats to provide a framework for biochemical studies. EEG recordings were obtained from eight kindled and four electrode implanted unstimulated control rats through electrodes stereotaxically implanted in the right septal nucleus and bilaterally in the neocortices, hippocampi, amygdalas, and reticular formation. Hourly stimulations were administered through a bipolar electrode in the right amygdala of male Sprague-Dawley rats until a single Class 5 motor seizure consisting of rearing and falling was elicited (kindled). A field effect transistor circuit eliminated movement artifact and permitted quantitation of SIS in awake, unrestrained rats. SIS: 1) did not occur in unstimulated rats; 2) developed and declined in a highly reproducible temporal and spatial pattern in all kindled rats; 3) occurred with maximal frequency (mean $\pm$ SEM of 23 $\pm$ 3 spikes/min) immediately following initially kindled seizures; 4) was less (mean $\pm$ SEM of 13 $\pm$ 2 spikes/min) immediately following the fully kindled seizures; 5) terminated completely by 5 days after kindling; 6) was confined mainly to limbic structures. This highly reproducible development and decline of SIS provides a model for biochemical study of the molecular mechanisms determining this pathophysiologic event.

FAILURE OF NALOXONE TO RETARD AMYGDALOID AND CAUDATE KINDLING

M. E. Corcoran, J. A. Wada
Vancouver

Repeated localized application of initially subconvulsant electrical stimulation can lead to the development of generalized convulsive seizures (kindling). Recent evidence suggests that endogenous opiate-like peptides (enkephalins and endorphins) have convulsant effects, and the question arose whether neurons containing these peptides might participate in kindling. To answer this question, we studied the effects on kindling of naloxone, an opiate antagonist that blocks the convulsant action of opiate peptides. Rats were kindled with a daily stimulation of the amygdala or caudate, two areas that are reportedly rich in opiate-binding sites. Ten minutes before each stimulation the rats received an IP injection of vehicle or naloxone at 20 or 40 mg/kg.

We were unable to detect a prophylactic effect of naloxone on either amygdaloid or caudate kindling. The threshold for local amygdaloid or caudate after-discharge did not differ between the naloxone-treated and control groups, and the rats receiving naloxone required no more stimulations than controls to develop generalized seizures. In fact, a slight *facilitation* in the rate of amygdaloid kindling occurred in the rats receiving 20 mg/kg of naloxone.

Insofar as the use of naloxone is a fair test of the function of central opiate-like peptides, these results indicate that the participation of enkephalinergic or endorphinergic neurons is not critical for the kindling of seizures.

ELECTROCLINICAL STUDY OF VISUAL SEARCHING BEHAVIOR IN PRIMATE AMYGDALOID KINDLING

S. Komai, J. A. Wada
Vancouver

Visual searching behavior (VSB) is not an uncommon ictal manifestation of human partial complex seizures. VSB is also the earliest ictal behavioral manifestation of amygdaloid (AM) kindling in Papio papio and Rhesus monkeys. It certainly precedes oral automatism. In view of this striking similarity, electrographic correlation of this particular clinical phenomenon was made in six Papio papio during AM kindling. The subjects carried multiple electrodes in limbic, thalamic and cortical structures.

The following observations were made: Clinically, VSB may appear as (1) the initial ictal pattern (4 animals), or 2) the ictal pattern following immobile staring (2 animals); Electrographically, 1) VSB was coincident with preferential afterdischarge (AD) propagation to the lateral geniculate body (GL) or GL + hippocampus (HIPP), and 2) VSB was coincident with initial AD propagation to HIPP and subsequent delayed propagation to GL.

When VSB was either the initial ictal pattern although short-lived, or the secondary ictal pattern, there was a considerable 3-7/sec slow wave discharge in the fronto-temporal cortices. No propagation to the medial geniculate body (GM) was observed until seizure became generalized.

The findings suggest that VSB is related to preferential AD propagation to GL but not GM and further suggest that this unique ictal behavior is likely due to visual perceptual disturbance associated with ictal interference of the visual pathway by seizure of AM origin.

HIPPOCAMPAL KINDLING EFFECT AND STATES OF ALERTNESS IN CATS. EFFECT OF ALPHA-METHYL-PARA-TYROSINE

G. Rondouin, P. Passouant
Montpellier, France

Daily low intensity electrical hippocampal stimulations induce progressive electroclinical seizures resulting in generalized convulsions. This phenomenon is called hippocampal kindling effect. Bipolar electrodes stereotaxically implanted into both ventral hippocampi, the right medial septal nucleus and both lateral geniculate nuclei, and classical electrodes for routine sleep recordings, were inserted into eight adult cats, separated into two groups.

The first group received a daily stimulation of 60 Hz. frequency, 2 sec. duration 1 msec. pulse duration with a mean intensity of 50 to 150 μA between 9:00 and 10:00 a.m. The second group received the same stimulation and 8 h 30 to 9 h after the stimulation an injection of alpha-methyl-para-tyrosine, methyl ester (50 mg/kg/IP) during three months, five days per week.

Hippocampal kindling can be subdivided into four stages according to electroclinical parameters. The first three stages represent the installation period or the kindling proper; the fourth one represents the kindled stage (generalized convulsions stage). The influence of hippocampal kindling on the states of alertness was researched in kindling and kindled cats. A marked decrease of rapid eye movement (REM) sleep appeared from stage 2 to stage 4 (mean percentage of the 24 hour period: Control : 12.1 $\pm$ 1.1%. Stage 2: 9.7 $\pm$ 1.1%. Stage 3: 8.8 $\pm$ 1.7%. Stage 4: 7.53 $\pm$ 2.14%). First REM sleep period latency increased from stage 1 to stage 4 (114 $\pm$ 56 min. in control recordings; 163 $\pm$ 61 min. in stage 4). REM sleep decrease remained even if stimulations were stopped (10.4 $\pm$ 3.4%). No significant modifications of waking and slow-waves-sleep occurred.

The role of sleep-waking cycle modifications on the kindling effect development was researched by means of alpha-methyl-para-tyrosine (AMPT), a catecholamine synthesis inhibitor known to modify the sleep-waking cyle in rats, cats, monkies and men. Two principal effects were found : 1°) An increase of REM sleep production during the six hours following AMPT injection. 2°) A blockade of kindling development associated with REM sleep increase.

The persistence of REM sleep decrease even if stimulations were stopped, the no-rebound phenomenon are in favour of the permanence of the kindling phenomenon and define the influence of kindling on sleep-waking cycle. Our results with AMPT shed light on an inhibiting effect of REM sleep increase upon kindling installation. They could be an argument for an hypothetic action of 5-hydroxytryptamine turnover on the development of kindling phenomenon.

INHIBITION OF AMYGDALOID KINDLING SEIZURE BY CHRONIC METHAMPHETAMINE PRETREATMENT IN CATS

M. Sato, T. Tomoda, S. Otsuki
Okayama

In order to investigate the relationship between epileptic seizure and psychotic state, the present study was intended to examine the influences of methamphetamine(MAP)-induced ''reverse tolerance phenomenon" (an experimental model of psychosis) on the seizure development of amygdaloid kindling (an experimental model of epilepsy) in cats. Cats in MAP-pretreated group were treated with daily administration of MAP(4-6 mg/kg/day) for nine days. After the treatment, all animals began to show marked stereotyped behavior by 1 mg/kg of MAP administration that was initially ineffective dose for inducing behavioral change. After confirming the sensitization to MAP, 1-dopa and apomorphine, daily electrical stimulation of the amygdala was commenced for establishing "kindling effect" in both the MAP-pretreated group and untreated control group.

Number of daily amygdaloid stimulation sufficient to develop generalized convulsions in MAP-pretreated group was significantly more than the control group (p < 0.01). Emergence of self-sustained afterdischarge and interictal spike discharge in the contralateral amygdala were also delayed in the MAP group. Together with our findings that amygdaloid seizure development was enhanced by the haloperidol treatment and suppressed by the chronic cocaine pretreatment, it was concluded that antagonistic relationship possibly via dopamine receptor sensitivity existed between these two experimental models of psychosis and epilepsy.

EFFECTS OF GONADAL HORMONES ON KINDLING

V. Jonec, W. A. Freckleton, C. G. Wasterlain
Sepulveda

A growing number of reports on catamenial epilepsy and related findings in animal experiments suggest that gonadal hormones may be intricately involved in the mechanism of epilepsy. We employed the kindling model of epilepsy to see whether physiological changes in the hormonal cycles affect the likelihood of developing an epileptic focus.

In our first experimental approach, regularly cycling female Holzman rats were kindled every fourth day, at a time when their morning vaginal smears exhibited either proestrus, and estrogen-dominated state (group PE), or diestrus, a presumably progesteron-dependent period of the cycle (D). Kindling involved subthreshold electrical stimulation through chronically implanted electrodes in the left basolateral amygdala. Development of kindled seizures was strikingly slower (P<0.001) in the D group than in the PE group, in which the rate of kindling was similar to that found in male rats stimulated at four-day intervals. The number of trials to the first stage 5 seizure was 5.7 $\pm$ 0.48 in the PE group, 8.5 $\pm$ 0.50 in the D group and 6.1 $\pm$ 0.82 in males (PE vs. D: P< 0.001). In the second series of experiments, ovariectomized rats bearing silastic implants filled with either 17β-estradiol (E) or progesterone (P) were kindled twice daily at three-hour intervals and compared with identically treated controls in which the implants contained no hormone (C). Significant facilitation of kindling by estrogen (P<0.05) and an opposite effect by progesterone was observed. The onset of stage 5 seizures in the respective groups required 7.1 $\pm$ 0.93 (E), 9.6 $\pm$ 0.54 (C) and 11.4 $\pm$ 1.05 (P) trials.

These studies show that physiological changes in the estrous cycle are associated with major variations in seizure susceptibility and perhaps in epileptogenesis. Our results in ovariectomized rats suggest that extradiol and progesterone have opposing effects on the propensity to develop kindled seizures and raise the possibility that hormonal effects may underly the lower incidence of seizures in females.

ANTIEPILEPTIC DRUG TREATMENT

Abstracts

MONOTHERAPY IN EPILEPSY

J. R. Hattab
Basle

One of the most unsatisfactory aspects of drug treatment of epilepsy is polypharmacy. In such a situation, the toxic effects of these drugs used in combination may be expected to increase or interact in other ways by impairing the biotransformation, distribution and excretion of the drugs.

The modern techniques for measuring serum levels of anticonvulsants and the establishment of optimal therapeutic ranges for the most effective control of seizures have made it easy and possible to use these drugs more efficiently and safely.

From the little available work done in the field of monotherapy, it seems that there is no methodologically sound evidence to show that two or more drugs are more effective than one and it is suggested that today most patients could be satisfactorily treated with one drug from the beginning, using as a guide plasma level monitoring. In this way, there could be a considerable reduction in chronic toxicity in addition to the lowering of the cost of treatment.

Further evidence to validate these findings is needed, especially in children, in whom polypharmacy may be even more dangerous than in adults. Polypharmacy, however, is generally still unavoidable when more than one type of epilepsy is present such as petit mal plus grand mal.

ONE DRUG FOR EPILEPSY

S. D. Shorvon, E. H. Reynolds, A. W. Gailbraith
London, U.K.

In the last 5 years we have investigated the potential for monotherapy and the necessity and effectiveness (if any) of polypharmacy in previously untreated new referrals with grand mal and/or partial seizures to a Neurological clinic.

In 26 patients on phenytoin (mean follow up 28.5 months) and 25 on carbamazepine (mean 12 months) only 12% on each drug have continued to have seizures despite an optimal blood level i.e. failure of monotherapy (Shorvon et al, British Medical Journal 1978, 1, 474). These trials are continuing and the results to date in over 80 patients will be presented.

The results will be discussed in relation to:
a. The avoidance of polypharmacy and chronic toxicity
b. The value of drug level monitoring from the start of treatment, and
c. The implications for long term prognosis.

PROSPECTIVE STUDY OF RELATIVE EFFICACY AND TOXICITY OF ANTIEPILEPTIC DRUGS ON WELL DEFINED TYPES OF SEIZURES

R. H. Mattson, et al.
West Haven

A prospective multicenter cooperative study of the relative efficacy and toxicity of antiepileptic drugs used to treat generalized tonic-clonic and partial seizures will be carried out. This information is not available despite world-wide usage of these drugs for many years. A population of 1680 patients will be treated with one or two of the 4 major antiepileptic drugs: phenytoin, phenobarbital, primidone or carbamazepine. The double-blind study will assign patients randomly, initially to a single drug, while later some patients may receive 2 drugs. Detailed assessment of efficacy and toxicity should allow conclusions at the end of the study as to which drug is optimal for treatment of each specific seizure type. A special composite rating scale will be used to quantitate combined drug efficacy and toxicity. The cooperative study is designed to answer the questions: which is the best first drug; the best second drug; and the optimum combination of 2 drugs for each type of seizure. The study will include three protocols.

Protocol 1: 480 patients with primary generalized, complex partial or elementary partial seizures who are newly diagnosed and/or currently receiving no antiepileptic medication will be assigned randomly to a sole drug therapy.

Protocol 2: 600 patients with complex partial or elementary partial seizures who are not controlled while receiving one drug will be changed randomly to a different single drug.

Protocol 3: 600 patients with one of the 4 seizure types who are not controlled while receiving one drug will be assigned randomly for a trial of two drugs in combination therapy.

MULTICENTRE THERAPEUTIC ASSESSMENT OF CARBAMAZEPINE IN EPILEPSY

J. Bernstein, K. Cartwright, R. A. Ellis,
C. K. Morrison, E. Macklam and H. Martin
Dorval

Carbamazepine (CBMZ) is an effective and well tolerated anticonvulsant which favorably influences not only epileptic seizures but also the associated behavioral and personality disorders. Although well controlled Phase II and III clinical trials have established CBMZ's anticonvulsant activity and safety, few data were available under conditions of office practice. Consequently a program of Phase IV testing of long-term efficacy and tolerability was implemented in 26 centres across Canada using an open-label non-comparative variable dose design. Male and female patients between the ages of 5-65 years with major epilepsy (excluding petit mal) and requiring either initiation or modification of anticonvulsant therapy were admitted. Patients were seen at 3-4 month intervals for up to 13 visits. A total of 317 patients entered the study, 87 of whom were followed for 2 years or more. The majority received 300-600 mg CBMZ daily. Physicians' global assessment revealed recovery in 6.5%, improvement in 60%, no change in 23%, and deterioration in 10.5%. The only serious adverse effect was a single case of mild leukopenia after 15 months of treatment with complete recovery after cessation of drug. No other laboratory abnormalities were reported. The results indicate excellent overall efficacy and safety.

COMPARATIVE TRIAL OF CARBAMAZEPINE-PHENOBARBITONE IN CHILDREN WITH MAJOR EPILEPSY

J. R. Roberts, A. E. McCandless, B. J. Horne, W. D. Harper
Liverpool

This paper describes a clinical trial comparing the use of carbamazepine and phenobarbitone in the treatment of major epilepsy in children between the ages of 5 and 15. 42 patients were each studied for a period of 2 years. At the outset every patient was assessed by clinical examination EEG, full blood tests and psychometric assessment. Reports were obtained from the schools and all assessments were repeated at regular intervals. The object was not only to control the epilepsy but to compare the effect of the drugs on behaviour and school performance. The trial illustrates problems of patient attendance and a high 'drop-out' rate. The results show carbamazapine to be superior to phenobarbitone in controlling epilepsy without interfering with school work or causing behaviour disturbance.

SERUM CONCENTRATIONS OF IMMUNOGLOBULINS IN EPILEPTIC PATIENTS ON CARBAMAZEPINE

R. E. Strandjord, S. I. Johannessen
Bergen
J. A. Aarli
Sandvika

Phenytoin has apparently a selective suppressive effect upon serum concentrations of IgA. Some patients develop IgA deficiency (IgA < 50 mg/l) which clinically may give an increased susceptibility to upper respiratory infections and perhaps also autoimmune diseases. It is not known whether carbamazepine has a similar effect.

The present study includes 47 adult patients with epilepsy treated with carbamazepine as the only drug. 29 patients (Group A) had formerly received phenytoin in combination with phenobarbitone

and/or primidone, while 18 patients (Group B) were given carbamazepine as the only drug from the beginning of the therapy. Serum concentration of IgG, IgA and IgM were determined by radial immunodiffusion. The mean concentration of serum IgA for all patients was 2100 mg/l. The mean IgA serum concentration was lower in Group A patients with the lowest concentrations observed in the males, than in Group B patients. For IgG and IgM serum levels no differences between the groups or sexes were detected. There were no differences between serum Ig concentrations in patients with carbamazepine level below 30 umol/l and those with a concentration above 30 umol/l.

Patients with low IgA serum levels were those who had previously used other antiepileptic drugs. The results indicate that carbamazepine does not suppress serum concentrations of immunoglobulins.

INTERLABORATORY VARIABILITY IN DETERMINATION OF SERUM ANTIEPILEPTIC DRUG CONCENTRATIONS IN JAPAN

K. Miyamoto, M. Seino
Tokyo

In an attempt to verify the interlaboratory reproducibility in determination of standardized serum antiepileptic drug concentrations, a survey was firstly conducted in Japan among 22 institutes in March, 1977.

The freeze-dried spiked specimens with four different concentrations of diphenylhydantoin (DPH), phenobarbital (PB) and primidone (PMD) were subjected to the study. The methods used were gas-chromatography, EMIT and heterogeneous enzyme immunoassay, ultra-violetspectrophotometry, radioimmunoassay and high pressure liquid chromatography. Some of the participating institutes employed more than two methods for each specimen to assess the intralaboratory reliability.

Twenty to 25% of the reported values were outside ± 1 standard deviation of the mean concentrations as a whole. The coefficients of variation ranged from minimum to maximum were: DPH 9.3-19.1, PB 11.7-28.1 and PMD 22.0-28.1%, respectively. The variability of the measured values was compared with those of that previously reported in North America and European countries.

Additional data from the second survey in May, 1978 participated by 49 laboratories are to be also reported on DPH, PB, PMD, carbamazepine and ethosuximide.

During the quality control program, it was found that efficient quantification by means of centrifugal autoanalyser using EMIT was practically applicable to clinical purpose.

COEFFICIENT OF VARIATION AS AN OBJECTIVE MEASURE OF COMPLIANCE

I. E. Leppik, J. Cloyd, R. Sawchuk, D. Fryd, CEP
Minneapolis

Although failure of adherence to prescribed medical regimens is a major obstacle to optimum seizure control, investigators in the field of patient behavior are hampered by the lack of a simple, objective measurement of drug ingestion behavior. During a study of the dose-dependent kinetics of phenytoin, 132 phenytoin steady state periods (SSP) were defined in 50 ambulatory patients. Each SSP consisted of three or more blood samples obtained at the same time on separate days, a minimum of eleven days after a change in dose. A coefficient of variation (CV) was calculated from the standard deviation (SD) and mean $\bar{x}$ of three or more plasma phenytoin concentrations by % CV = $100 \times SD/\bar{x}$. Compliance was determined by interviews (I) and capsule counts (CC); non-compliance was defined as failure to ingest one or more doses during the interval from dose change through blood sampling.

Nine patients not responsible for administration of their own medications because of age or institutionalization were compliant for all SSP and had a CV (mean $\pm$SD) of 5.3$\pm$2.7%. The CV for 84 SSP in 35 outpatients was 6.8 $\pm$3.9%. Values of CV calculated from SSP associated with non-compliance in 14 patients ranged from 73 to 95%, with a mean of 25.2$\pm$20.9%, significantly higher (p <.001) than for the compliant SSP. Eight patients were compliant for some and non-compliant during other SSP.

Thus, the contribution to CV by laboratory technique and pharmacokinetic factors is small, and calculation of CV from three plasma phenytoin concentrations at SSP provides an objective estimation of compliance.

(Supported by NINDS Contract #N01-NS-5-2327)

ANTICONVULSANT COMPLIANCE IN A PEDIATRIC SEIZURE CLINIC

J. T. Shope
Detroit

Noncompliance with prescribed anticonvulsant medication was studied in a comprehensive pediatric seizure clinic, testing the Health Belief Model, a theoretical framework used to explain health behavior. Mothers (N=200) were interviewed and anticonvulsant blood levels were done on their children. Levels more than 30% below those predicted from age-specific data were found in 25% of children taking phenobarbital and 46% of children taking phenytoin.

Variables in some components of the Health Belief Model were found (Pearson product-moment correlation) significantly related to the serum levels. The mothers' readiness to take prescribed action (health motivation and perceptions) was reflected in the following associations. Higher serum phenobarbital levels are seen in children of mothers who actively sought literature on seizures, do "a great deal" of special things to keep their children healthy, know the medication name and dosage, and feel seizures would recur early if medication were stopped. These children have a younger onset age, higher recent seizure frequency and have experienced seizures while off medication.

Several modifying factors are significant. Higher serum levels are found in younger children who have fewer siblings, fewer household members, but others who help remember the medication. These mothers have more recent contacts with the clinic, where they feel more satisfied with their care and respected by the physician, but also interact with other professionals.

Data analysis is ongoing. An experimental educational intervention and follow-up was also done.

Research supported by a grant from The Epilepsy Foundation of America.

TREATMENT OF EPILEPSY IN CHILDREN WITH NITRAZEPAM

M. Vanasse, G. Geoffroy
Montreal

During the last ten years, Nitrazepam was used as an anticonvulsant in 172 children in our neurology department. As a rule, it was utilized in refractory seizures and thus added to other anticonvulsant medications. Upon EEG and clinical criteria, we have included these patients in five groups: infantile spasms (18 patients), Lennox-Gastaut syndrome (21 patients), multifocal epilepsy (28 patients), focal and complex partial seizures (43 patients) - and generalized seizures — either Petit Mal, Grand Mal or both (62 patients). The addition of Nitrazepam enable us to have a 50% or greater reduction in seizure frequency in 72% of infantile spasm patients, 47.6% in Lennox-Gastaut syndrome, 53.6% in miltifocal epilepsy, 53.5% in focal and complex partial seizures and 64.4% in generalized epilepsies.

This last group was subdivised into grand mal or petit mal attacks or both and the results were essentially the same for each of these subgroups. Side effects were seen in 17.4% of the patients and were generally transient and rather benign. Posology was analyzed for each individual and seizure control does not seem to be directly related with the dose administered. However this is of limited value since no serum level determination could be done.

METHSUXIMIDE IN THE TREATMENT OF COMPLEX PARTIAL SEIZURES

B. J. Wilder,
Gainesville
R. A. Buchanan
Ann Arbor

Earlier studies have indicated that methsuximide (Celontin[R]) is clinically effective in managing psychomotor seizures (complex partial seizures). Methsuximide is metabolized to N-desmethylsuximide which has a long half-life and possesses anticonvulsant activity.

A clinical trial was conducted to test the efficacy of methsuximide in the management of complex-partial seizures in patients not controlled by phenytoin or carbamazepine plus phenobarbital or primidone. The study was non-blind, historically controlled, with patients receiving increasing doses of the drug. Other drugs were continued at the same or a lower daily dose. The seizure disorder had been present at least 6 months in all patients and each had been experiencing two or more attacks a month for 3 months following an adequate trial on phenytoin, carbamazepine, phenobarbital or primidone. Patients were men and women, 18 years of age or older, free of any metabolic defect which could interfere with metabolizing the drug. Patients were started on 300 mg. per day until seizures were controlled, adverse effects were observed, or the dose reached 1.2 g per day. The therapeutic dose was continued for 3 months. No dose increases were made in the patients who achieved seizure control at 300 mg/day.

Results showed that 11 of 20 patients studied responded to the addition of methsuximide to their regimens. The lowest dose at which effectiveness was observed was 300 mg/day with most achieving seizure control at 600 to 900 mg/day. The lowest dose at which adverse effects were noted was 600 mg/day and usually consisted of drowsiness. The plasma levels at which effectiveness was first observed ranged between 8 - 12 μg/ml. The plasma levels at which adverse effects were first noted were 20 - 25 μg/ml. One patient experienced sever photophobia with a plasma level of 9 μg/ml. Methsuximide should be considered in patients with complex-partial seizures who have not responded to customary therapy.

EPILEPSY: A CONSISTENTLY SUCCESSFUL TREATMENT REGIME (OVER 100 PATIENTS)

Moses Ilo
Kano

120 patients — all clinically diagnosed in a setting void of technological facilities and over 40% of whom were receiving therapy for the first time — were treated with a drug combination regime of sodium valproate (Epilim) and benzodiazepines (mainly diazepam and nitrazepam) over a period of one year. These patients embraced all forms except Jacksonians but for significance included a case complicated with hemi-athetosis. The barbiturates and conventional anticonvulsant drugs were completely stopped in previously treated patients and not used at all in the new patients. Only mild phenothiazines were incorporated in cases associated with psychosis. Results obtained were consistently good, void of side effects, and above all, gave encouragement for making the regime the choice in infants, children of school age, undergraduates and also the elderly. The author believes that the place of barbiturates in the management of epilepsy is due for a serious and critical review, and the use of the conventional anticonvulsants as also clonazepam be made more specific if not limited.

THE EFFECTIVENESS OF ANTICONVULSANTS ON IMMEDIATE POSTTRAUMATIC EPILEPSY — An Experimental Study

S. Manaka, H. Sugiyama, I. Kanazawa, T. Hori, T. Fuchinoue, and K. Sano
Tokyo

An experimental immediate posttraumatic epilepsy model was produced by a weight dropping technique in order to evaluate the effectiveness of anticonvulsants. Five-week-old male mice weighing about 20 gm were used. The ears of the mice were fixed by fingers on foamed polyethyrene pillow. The parietal region of the mice was struck with a cylinder (30 gm, 10 mm diam.) made of bakelite. A weight was allowed to fall 30 cm in height through a vertical plastic tube. This traumatic condition (900 gm, cm) produced typical immediate posttraumatic epilepsy in about 80% of the control group (n=143). Effectiveness of Diphenylhydantoin (DPH), Phenobarbital (PB), Carbamazepine (CBZ), Diazepam (DZP) and Dipropylacetate (DPA) of various doses was evaluated on the above mentioned epileptic model (n=293). PB, CBZ, DZP and DPA were significantly effective such 100% concentration at more than 15, 2.8, 1.0 and 400μg/ml respectively, but DPH had no anticonvulsant effect on this epileptic model. The clinical significance and application of these experimental results will be discussed.

ANTI-EPILEPTIC (AE) PROPHYLACTIC TREATMENT IN SEVERE HEAD INJURY RETROSPECTIVE ANALYSIS

N. Chiofaló, A. Sevilla, O. Olivares,
V. Armengol
Santiago

1,700 in-patients suffering severe head injuries during a period of 4 years were reviewed. Intra-hospitalary mortality rate was 30%, half of these patients dying after neurosurgical procedures due to different traumatic complications. Follow-up analysis of those available patients of both groups was made, during a minimal period of 18 months, in order to analyze patients with epileptic sequelae.

Emphasis was specially made to:
1. Head injury severity related with: traumatic mechanism; conscious impairment and neurological signs; localization, EEG findings, etc.
2. Neurosurgical conditions: procedure; type of complication; time elapsed between trauma-operation; post-operative evolution.
3. AE prophylactic treatment: rate of treated patients; onset; type of drug; administration period and treatment effectiveness.
4. Post-traumatic epilepsy: onset of seizures; type and frequency; EEG findings; other neurological sequelae.

Discussion will be done comparing the operated and non-operated groups and the AE prophylactic advantage of treated patients.

POST-TRAUMATIC EPILEPSY WITH SPECIAL EMPHASIS ON THE HEAD INJURY CHARACTERISTICS RETROSPECTIVE ANALYSIS

V. Armengol, O. Olivares, P. Vidal, P. Hernandez,
N. Chiófalo
Santiago

Ambulatory patients controlled for a period of 2 years suffering from epilepsy were analyzed. From a number of 2,100 epileptic patients, 320 were proved to have head injuries previous to the onset of seizures.

Review considered:
1. a) Type and frequency of seizures and EEG characteristics.
   b) Age of onset.
   c) Other neurological sequelae.
2. Correlation with:
   a) Severity of head injury.
   b) Localization.
   c) Neurosurgical complications and surgical procedures.
   d) Medical complications.
3. Anti-epileptic prophylactic treatment with special emphasis to: onset of treatment; type of drug; administration period and effect of the treatment.

Discussion will be done with the previous paper considering the way that epilepsy and prophylactic treatment is observed.

PLASMA CLEARANCE AND VOLUME OF DISTRIBUTION OF PHENYTOIN DURING PREGNANCY

E. Ramsay, I. Leppik, R. Strauss, B. J. Wilder, R. Sawchuck
Minneapolis

Changes in anticonvulsant plasma levels and dosage requirements, and seizure frequency has been reported to occur in some patients during pregnancy. Enzyme induction and accelerated metabolism has been suggested as the etiology for these changes. The following study was conducted in ten patients during and after pregnancy. Metabolic status, seizure frequency and anticonvulsant levels were monitored frequently. The patients were hospitalized three times (twice during and once after pregnancy) for drug kinetic studies. Following IV load of phenytoin, frequent plasma levels were determined over 24 hrs and the data were fitted by non-linear regression to both a two and three compartment model. A summary of results 1) The data conformed best to the two compartment model; 2) The T 1/2 of the Beta phase ranged from 6.3 to 73.6 hrs and was found to be dependent on the mean plasma concentration; 3) No relationship was found between evaluation period (pregnant or non pregnant) and the Beta phase T 1/2; 4) There was no difference in the T 1/2 of the α phase (.22±0.09) for the pre and post partum periods and was not related to dose or mean plasma level; 5) The volumes of distribution pre (.729 ± .197) and post-partum (.777 ± .169) were not significantly different; 6) The clearance ranged from .0099 to 0.0394 L/hr/kgm with no significant difference found between the evaluation periods and 7) The maximum weight difference was 15%; greatest in the 3rd trimester compared to post partum evaluation. The data indicate that for phenytoin 1) The placenta and fetus do not act as a sink 2) The metabolism is non-linear and dependent on the mean plasma level and 3) The plasma half life did not change with pregnancy; the variation in half life resulted from the effect of non-linear kinetics.

PHENYTOIN-THEOPHYLLINE INTERACTION: A CASE REPORT

R. W. Fincham, D. D. Schottelius, R. Wyatt, L. Hendeles and M. Weinberger
Iowa City

A thirty-three year old woman with life long epilepsy was treated with intravenous and later oral theophylline for status asthmaticus. The acute respiratory dysfunction was controlled but increasingly frequent seizures developed. Serum phenytoin levels were found to be decreased (5 to 8 mcg/ml) compared to a previous value (without concurrent theophylline) of 15.7 mcg/ml with the same dose (100 mg qid) of medication. Concurrent primidone and derived phenobarbital levels were unchanged from previous values. An increased oral dose of phenytoin (200 mg tid) was ineffective in bringing the serum levels to a therapeutic range (values ranged between 7 and 11 mcg/ml for 7 days) until the concurrent oral administration of theophylline and phenytoin was discontinued and these drugs were given separately, one to two hours apart. This change in dosage schedule actually led to a state of phenytoin toxicity in 10 days (32.8 mcg/ml) that was rectified by decreasing the daily oral dose of phenytoin to 450 mg. We suspected an absorptive interference of theophylline with phenytoin. This possibility has been investigated subsequently in four volunteers who on three separate occasions took single oral doses of 1) phenytoin (400 mg), 2) phenytoin (400 mg) with concurrent theophylline (7.5 mg/kg), and 3) theophylline (7.5 mg/kg) followed in two hours by phenytoin (400 mg). Serum levels of these drugs were closely monitored and the results will be presented. They are consonant with absorptive interference between the two drugs and indicate that an interval of two hours does indeed provide enhanced serum levels of both drugs when compared to the concurrent administration of theophylline and phenytoin.

INFLUENCE OF SMOKING ON PLASMA LEVELS OF DIPHENYLHYDANTOIN AND PHENOBARBITONE

H. M. Wiener, K. Fiedler, M. Herzberg, M. Streifler, D. F. Cohn
Tel-Aviv

A retrospective study was done on the influence of smoking on plasma levels of Diphenylhydantoin (DPH) and Phenobarbitone (PB). Repeated plasma DPH, PB, and Gamma-Glutamyltransferase (GGT) levels, and urinary Glucaric acid (GA) concentrations were determined in 80 epileptic patients. Of these 20 were smokers. All epileptic patients received 100-300 mg DPH and 100-200 mg PB daily. GGT and GA concentrations were established in order to measure the degree of enzyme induction and its effect on drug metabolism. The mean blood levels of the anticonvulsants in smokers were found to be appreciably lower than those of nonsmokers. Enzyme induction of oxydative and conjugative enzyme of these anticonvulsants as indicated by increased GGT and GA respectively was significantly higher in smokers. However induction of conjugation (Glucoronidation) was 3 to 6 times higher than of oxidation.

It seems that smoking markedly lowers the blood levels of DPH and PB and therefore their therapeutic effect, by increasing their rate of metabolism via the conjugation pathway in liver microsomes.

This effect is additive to the effect of PB on lowering DPH levels but of a markedly higher degree. Smoking should therefore be discouraged in epileptic patients taking anticonvulsants.

DIURNAL VARIATION OF DIPHENYLHYDANTOIN AND PHENOBARBITAL SERUM LEVELS IN JAPANESE EPILEPTIC INPATIENTS

H. Kazamatsuri, O. Kanno, K. Hanada
Tokyo

Serum levels of diphenylhydantoin (DPH) and phenobarbital (PB) were determined by UV spectrophotometry at four hour intervals during 24 hours in seventeen Japanese epileptic inpatients.

All patients took DPH and/or PB for more than five years in divided t.i.d. dosage schedule under the supervision of nursing staff.

1) The highest value of serum DPH level was obtained at 21:00 p.m., and the lowest value at 9:00 a.m. There was approximately 20% difference between the maximal and minimal serum DPH level in a day.
2) Serum PB levels showed little fluctuation throughout 24 hour period.
3) Serum level (μg/ml) / dose (mg/kg/day) ratio found in this study was 2.35 for DPH and 9.73 for PB respectively.
4) Continuous EEG telemetry recordings were performed simultaneously with the serum level study in 6 patients. There was little correlation between serum level of anticonvulsants and incidence of paroxysmal discharges in EEG.

THE DIRECT LINEAR PLOT: USE IN ESTIMATING MICHAELIS-MENTEN PARAMETERS AND INDIVIDUALIZING PHENYTOIN DOSAGE REGIMENS IN EPILEPTIC PATIENTS

J. C. Cloyd, R. J. Sawchuk, I. E. Leppik, S. M. Pepin
Minneapolis

The apparent saturable metabolism of phenytoin complicates the adjustment of phenytoin dosage. Furthermore, the variability in kinetic parameters among patients dictates the need for individualizing this adjustment. Phenytoin elimination parameters were calculated in thirty epileptic patients monitored during two or more steady states. At least three phenytoin plasma levels (Cp_{ss}) were measured at each dose. The parameters were estimated for each patient by: 1) regression analysis of the Hofstee transformation(H) of the Michaelis-Menten equation, and 2) a direct linear plot (DLP) which involves calculating coordinates of intersection for lines generated by (Cp_{ss}, dose) pairs. Parameter estimates ($\bar{X}\pm SD$) for the apparent V_{max}(mg/day)

were 8.6 ± 2.2(H) and 8.3 ± 1.7 (DLP). The mean values for the apparent K_m (mg/L) were 6.7 ± 5.4 and 6.0 ± 3.1, respectively. Twenty-three of the patients underwent one or more dosage adjustments based on their own parameters resulting in fifty-seven predictions of subsequent steady-state plasma levels. Using the DLP generated estimates, predictions were comparable to those obtained with regression analysis(H). Where the change in daily dose was ≤ 60 mg or > 60 mg, the observed level was within 3mg/L of that predicted in 64% or 33% of the predictions, respectively. Thus, the direct linear plot appears to be a reasonable guide for phenytoin dosage adjustment.

Supported by NINCDS #N01-NS-5-2327

ASSESSMENT OF CONCENTRATION-DEPENDENT KINETICS OF PHENYTOIN IN CHILDREN

W. E. Dodson
St. Louis

Previous methods for assessing nonlinear kinetics of phenytoin elimination required computerized parameter estimation, multiple blood samples, and were not readily applied to patient management or comparative pharmacokinetic studies. By measuring phenytoin concentrations under steady state conditions at varying doses, one can use these values to predict the levels produced by different doses in the individual patient.

Because low ebb concentrations correlate well ($r = .99$) with average concentrations at steady state when phenytoin is given orally every 12 hours, the low ebb concentrations at steady state can be related to dose by Lineweaver-Burke plots and an apparent Km and Vmax can be calculated. Data from children aged 4 months to 14 years indicate that phenytoin elimination is concentration-dependent and that large changes occur during childhood. In the age groups ≤ 1 yr, $1\le 3$, $3\le 9$, and $9\le 14$, average apparent Vmax's were 15.0 mg$\cdot$kg$^{-1}\cdot$day^{-1}, 11.7, 14.7 and 8.6, respectively, and Km's varied between .43 and 6.0 mg$\cdot$liter^{-1}. Using this method one can calculate the dose necessary to achieve a desired phenytoin level for an individual patient.

SEIZURES AND ALTERED PHENYTOIN METABOLISM IN MONONUCLEOSIS

I. E. Leppik, V. Ramani, R. J. Sawchuk, R. J. Gumnit
St. Paul

Seizures may be precipitated by intercurrent infections in patients receiving antiepileptic medication, but the role of altered pharmacokinetics during illness has not been well studied.

A 22-year-old woman was hospitalized for evaluation and treatment of seizures and psychiatric problems associated with epilepsy. During the first two weeks of hospitalization, her phenytoin dose was 5.5 mg per kg per day, and plasma concentrations were 13, 15 and 12 μg per ml. She then developed pharyngitis, lymphadenopathy, temperature of

39.5°C. Laboratory tests confirmed the diagnosis of infectious mononucleosis (IM). Approximately two weeks after the onset of IM, when her fever had subsided, she had two generalized tonic-clonic seizures, the first in many years. Plasma phenytoin concentration was low, and her dose was increased to 6.3 mg per kg per day. No further seizures occurred and plasma phenytoin concentrations were 5, 6, 5, 7, and 6 μg per ml over the next four weeks. After discharge, on the same dose, levels were 28, 26, and 30 μg per ml. Phenytoin binding was normal (free = 10.0% of total) during and after (10.3%) IM. During IM, 87% of the daily phenytoin dose was recovered in the urine as metabolites. Apparent clearance of phenytoin was 0.41 ± 0.05 before, 1.10 ± 0.14 during, and 0.22 ± 0.02 liters per kg per day after IM.

Exacerbation of seizures was not associated with fever but, rather, decreased phenytoin concentration due to increased clearance of this drug during IM. Antiepileptic drug concentrations must be measured during intercurrent illnesses, as dosages may need to be temporarily readjusted to prevent seizures. (Supported by NINDS Contract #N01-NS-5-2327)

PRIMIDONE PHARMACOKINETICS: EFFECT OF CONCOMITANT ANTICONVULSANT DRUGS AND DURATION OF THERAPY

K. W. Miller, J. C. Cloyd, I. E. Leppik
Minneapolis

Primidone (PRM) pharmacokinetics were investigated in two groups of seizure patients: 1) Nine patients who had not received other anticonvulsant therapy, and 2) Eight patients who were receiving one or more anticonvulsants. All patients received an initial PRM dose (250 mg po) and 24 hours later were placed on a PRM maintenance regimen. PRM plasma levels were measured following the initial dose and half-life (t½) and apparent total body clearance (ATBC) were calculated. ATBC was subsequently determined in a number of patients after they had reached steady state on one or more maintenance regimens. There was a significantly slower rate of PRM elimination after the initial dose in group 1 patients as indicated by t½ (15.2 vs 8.7 hours) and ATBC (35.5 vs 50.4 ml/hr/kg). There was also a longer delay between the start of PRM therapy and the appearance of its metabolites, phenobarbital and phenylethylmalonamide, in group 1 patients. Continued PRM therapy in group 1 patients was accompanied by either an increase in ATBC, suggesting an increased rate of elimination, or no change in ATBC. In several group 2 patients who discontinued other anticonvulsants, there was a decrease in ATBC suggesting a decreased rate of elimination. It thus appears that PRM pharmacokinetics and possibly clinical effect are significantly influenced both by concomitant anticonvulsant drugs and duration of therapy. (Supported in part by Comprehensive Epilepsy Program Contract N01 NS 5 2327).

SIMULTANEOUS ANALYSIS OF PRIMIDONE, PHENOBARBITAL AND PHENYLETHYLMALONAMIDE

K. Leal and A. J. Wilensky
Seattle

The therapeutic monitoring of certain anticonvulsant drugs is complicated by the presence of pharmacologically active metabolites that accumulate in chronic dosing. Work in our laboratory with primidone in humans and laboratory animals suggests that the metabolites, phenobarbital and phenyethylmalonamide, contribute significantly to the anticonvulsant and toxic effects. With the presence of two active metabolites, therapeutic monitoring of primidone is more complex and demands more thorough consideration than currently given. Presently, the phenylethylmalonamide component is receiving more attention as a source of primidone toxicity. Although numerous methods exist for the determination of primidone and phenobarbital, few incorporate phenylethylmalonamide and assay all three drugs at the same time.

The GLC method we have developed analyzes all three primidone components simultaneously with the use of a modified Supelco SP 2510-DA column and a flame-ionization detector. Extraction and analysis is applicable to both plasma and brain samples. The drugs are quantitated underivatized from a single sample. Extraction efficiency exceeded 92% for all components in both plasma and brain. Day-to-day variability for phenylethylmalonamide, phenobarbital, and primidone was measured and the coefficient of variation was 11, 12, and 7% respectively. Comparison of human plasma samples with the GLC derivatization technique of our laboratory showed correlations of 0.948 for phenobarbital and 0.975 for primidone by linear regression. Mean levels for all patients analyzed were 6.2 mcg/ml for phenylethylmalonamide, 26.1 mcg/ml for phenobarbital, and 8.6 mcg/ml for primidone.

PHARMACOKINETICS AND ANTICONVULSANT EFFICACY OF PRIMIDONE IN MICE

R. L. Rapport, K. W. Leal, A. J. Wilensky, P. N. Friel
Seattle

A new gas-liquid chromatographic method has been developed to evaluate simultaneously the pharmacokinetics of the anticonvulsant primidone (PRM) and its biologically active metabolites after a single dose in mice. The parent compound was isolated from its metabolites phenobarbital (PB) and phenylethylmalonamide (PEMA) by use of the inhibitor SKF 525-A, and the kinetics of each compound studied separately and in combination. The anticonvulsant properties of each molecular species were likewise studied independently against maximal electroshock (MES). Compared on a molar basis, PB is more effective than PRM alone, PRM and metabolites or PEMA. PRM is rapidly converted to PB and PEMA in the mouse following a single dose and has an apparent t1/2 in brain of 2.61 hours. The peak anticonvulsant effects, effective dose curves and half-lives of these compounds all indicate that the major anticonvulsant effect of oral PRM is from the derived PB; comparison of the linear regression of the dose-response curves for each component is highly significant only for PB. This study supports the argument that, while PRM and PEMA do have minor independent anticonvulsant properties, the major anticonvulsant effect of orally delivered PRM in the mouse is from derived PB.

This research was supported by NIH Research Grant #NS 04053 awarded by the NINCDS, PHS/DHEW.

SIDE EFFECTS OF DRUGS

Advances in Epileptology:
The Xth Epilepsy International Symposium,
edited by J. A. Wada and J. K. Penry.
Raven Press, New York © 1980.

A Collaborative Study of the Teratogenicity and Fetal Toxicity of Antiepileptic Drugs in Japan

*Teruo Okuma, **Ryo Takahashi, †Toyoji Wada,
††Yorio Sato, and **Yoshibumi Nakane

*Department of Psychiatry, Tohoku University School of Medicine,
1-1 Seiryo, Sendai, Japan; **Department of Neuropsychiatry, Nagasaki University
School of Medicine, 7-1 Sakamoto, Nagasaki, Japan; † National Epilepsy Center,
Shizuoka-Higashi Hospital, 886 Urushiyama, Shizuoka, Japan;
††Department of Mental Hygiene, Tokyo University School of Medicine,
7-3-1 Hongo, Bunkyo, Tokyo, Japan*

Several instances of the teratogenicity of antiepileptic drugs have been reported not only in Europe and America, but also in Japan. However, little research with a sufficient number of cases has been done even in Europe and America. In Japan, particularly, only a very limited number of data have been reported.

Consequently, we have carried out a wide scale investigation of this problem with multi-institutional collaboration throughout the country and the results obtained will be briefly summarized and discussed in this chapter.

PATIENTS AND METHODS

Subjects admitted to this study were pregnant epileptic persons who had been seen at the neuropsychiatric departments of nine university hospitals, the National Epilepsy Center (Shizuoka), and the National Research Institute for Mental and Nervous Diseases (Tokyo). The study began in 1974, and pregnancies that commenced in and after 1974 were studied progressively until the end of July 1977. A retrospective investigation of pregnancies occurring before 1974 was also conducted and the results are included in this study.

The information on the pregnancy cases was recorded on special forms by neuropsychiatrists at each institution.

RESULTS

The total number of pregnancies collected was 948, of which 46 were excluded because of pregnancy prior to the onset of epilepsy. The remaining

902 cases were evaluated. The pregnancies occurred in 453 female epileptic patients.

The 902 pregnancies were classified according to the presence or absence of medication during the first trimester of pregnancy; 657 (73%) were treated, 162 (18%) untreated, and in 83 (9.2%) details of the prescription were unknown.

Analysis of Background Factors in the Treated and Untreated Groups

There was no significant difference between the treated and untreated groups regarding age at marriage (mean: 23.5 years old), the age of the first pregnancy, or the age of the pregnancy under the present investigation. The age of the onset of epilepsy was a little earlier in the treated group than in the untreated group (mean: 15 years old) and the duration of the disease in the treated group was slightly longer than that in the untreated group (mean: 12.8 years). These differences were not statistically significant.

With regard to the clinical types of epileptic seizure, 55% of the treated patients had generalized seizures and 33% had partial seizures. The figures for the untreated patients were 41% and 51%, respectively, suggesting a significantly higher incidence of partial seizures in the untreated patients. Of all the pregnant epileptic women studied, 44% had seizures during pregnancy; the figure for treated patients was 43% and that for the untreated was 50%. Of 227 pregnancies for which reliable information pertaining to the frequency of seizures was obtained, pregnancy produced no change in seizure frequency in 133 cases (59%), an increase in 33%, and a decrease in the remaining 9%. When figures were compared between the treated and untreated groups, the percentage of patients with unchanged seizure frequency during pregnancy was lower and the percentage of patients with increased frequency was higher in the treated group than in the untreated group.

Ten (2.3%) of 432 epileptic women for whom data concerning malformations were confirmed had malformations in themselves. The percentage of patients with malformations was 1.8 in the treated group and 3.7 in the untreated.

Outcome of Pregnancy

Of the total 902 pregnancies, 638 (71%) terminated in live births including 54 cases (6%) of premature birth and 580 cases (64%) of fullterm birth, 94 (10%) terminated in spontaneous abortion, 11 (1%) in stillbirth, and 155 (17%) in artificial abortion.

In the treated group, 73% of patients had a live birth, 14% had an abortion or a stillbirth, and 13% underwent an artificial abortion. The figures for the untreated group were 80%, 4%, and 15%, respectively. The results suggest that treated patients developed much higher incidence of abortion or stillbirth than did the untreated patients.

Malformations in Infants

Various types of fetal malformation (Table 1) were encountered in 65 of the total 902 pregnancies (7.2%). The incidence of malformations was 57/675 (8.7%) in the treated group and 3/162 (1.9%) in the untreated group. As far as live-birth babies are concerned 63 of the total 638 live-birth babies (9.9%) were born with congenital defects including 55 cases (11.5%) in the treated group and three cases (2.3%) in the untreated group. The incidence of malformed babies in the former group was five times as high as that in the latter, with a difference evidently statistically significant.

In the treated group, the total number of malformations was 71, including multiple malformations in 13 babies. Various types of malformation were observed, concentrating on cleft-lip and/or palate (15 of the total 478 live-birth babies, 3.14%) and cardiovascular defect (14/478, 2.95%). On the other hand, as can be seen from Table 1, the above two types of malformation were not observed in the untreated group.

Statistical analysis of the data obtained in the treated group revealed that the age of pregnancy of the epileptic woman, the duration of her epilepsy, and the duration of medication did not correlate with the incidence rate of malformations. It was suggested, however, that the occurrence of partial seizures, congenital defects in the mother, and a last pregnancy terminating in abortion of stillbirth were correlated with the malformation rate.

In the untreated group, the factors in the causation of fetal malformations appear to be an organic etiology of the mother's epilepsy and a history of medication for epilepsy, especially for more than 5 years.

Analysis of the relationships between the presence of seizures and/or medication during pregnancy and the incidence of malformations revealed the lowest incidence of malformations in the untreated patients without seizures (1/54, 1.8%), higher incidence in the untreated patients without seizures (3/57, 2.6%) and in the treated patients without seizures (29/223, 11.5%), and the highest rate in the treated patients with seizures (28/192, 12.7%).

The incidence rate of malformations rose sharply with increasing numbers of drugs used in combination. The rate with three drugs (11.0%) was twice as high as that with two drugs (5.5%), and when four drugs were used jointly, the rate increased to 23.0%. It is evident from the findings that the combined use of more than three drugs produces a marked increase in the incidence of malformations.

For convenience in processing data by computers, we counted the minimum usual daily dose as 1 unit. Equivalent doses of representative

TABLE 1. *Details of malformations among 902 pregnancies according to the presence of antiepileptic medication*

	Treated group	Untreated group	Unknown group	Total	Code of Anomaly S[a]	R[b]	ICD-8
Anencephalus	2			2	1	A	740
Spinal meningocele	1	1		2	1	B	741.9
Microcephaly			1	1	1	D	743.1
Blephaloptosis and nystagmus	2			2	2	D	744.8
Strabism	4			4	2	E	373
Hyperterolism	3			3	2	C	756
Hypoplasia of nose	1			1	2	D	748.1
Preauricular fistura	1			1	2	D	745.4
Congenital dentition	1			1	2	E	520.6
Cleft palate	1		1	2	1	C	749.0
Cleft lip	7			7	1	A	749.1
Cleft lip and palate	7		2	9	1	B	749.2
Torticollis	4			4	2	D	756.8
Ventricular septal defect	4		1	5	1	D	746.3
Atrial septal defect	1			1	1	D	746.4
Other congenital heart disease	1			1	1	C	746.8
Other congenital heart anomaly	6			6	1	C	746.9
Patent ductus arteriosus	2			2	1	D	747.0
Talipes equines and valgus	1		1	2	1	C	754
Polydactyly	1			1	2	B	755.0
Syndactyly		1		1	1	B	755.2
Brachydactyly	1			1	1	B	755.3
Contraction of arm			1	1	2	C	755.5
Hypoplasia of nail	2			2	1	C	757.4
Congenital dis-location of hip	6			6	1	D	755.6
Undescended testis	1			1	2	D	752.1
Hypospadias	1			1	1	C	752.2
Hydrotestis	1			1	2	D	752.4
Inguinal hernia	4			4	2	D	550
Nevus	2			2	3	C	757.1
Melanosis	1			1	2	B	709
Hypertrichosis	1			1	2	E	757.3
Down's syndrome		1		1	1	C	759.3
Stomach tumor	1			1	1	D	195
Total	71	3	7	81			

[a]Severity of malformations: 1, major malformations; 2, minor malformations; 3, insignificant malformations.
[b]Ease of recognition: A, cannot be missed; B, seldom missed; C, easily found if searched for; D, requires thorough examination; E, requires unusual alertness, diagnostic aids.
[From Macheprang, M., et al. (1972): HSMHA Health Reports 87:43–49.]

drugs to 1 unit are as follows: phenobarbital (PB), 100 mg; mephobarbital (MB), 100 mg; methalbital, 100 mg; primidone (PMD), 500 mg; diphenylhydantoin (DPH), 100 mg; trimethadione (TMD), 1,000 mg; carbamazepine (CBZ), 200 mg; dipropylacetate (DPA), 200 mg; and diazepam, 4 mg.

Analysis of the relationship between the incidence of malformations and the magnitude of the dose administered revealed that the incidence of malformations increased significantly when the total dose administered in the first trimester of pregnancy exceeded 400 units and when the maximum daily dose exceeded 5 units.

The possible risk of occurrence of malformations when various antiepileptic drugs were used in the early stage of pregnancy was studied. Application of the χ^2 test with respect to the use of each drug and the occurrence of malformation yielded a 5% risk of malformations with TMD, PB, PMD, MB, pheneturide, and acetazolamide but no risk wth DPH, phenacemide, CBZ, and DPA.

Many patients received single therapy with DPH without any risk of malformations.

PB was given singly to 36 cases and malformation occurred in one of them. An increasing tendency of the teratogenic effect was noted with increasing doses of PB. This suggests that the maximum daily dose of PB should not exceed 1.5 units (150 mg) and that those of MB and PMB should be under 150 mg and 750 mg, respectively, for a similar reason.

TMD per se was found to be strongly related to the teratogenicity independently of the magnitude of the dose administered. In the only case of single therapy with TMD, malformation occurred at the minimum usual daily dose.

We have endeavored to determine the perilous combinations of these drugs, but in vain as yet. As examples of combinations of three or four drugs which were associated with high incidences of malformations, we can cite PB + DPH + TMD, DPH + TMD + ethosuximide and PB + PMD + acetylpheneturide and PB + PMD + DPH + TMD.

Premature Birth

We shall use the term "premature infant" to denote an infant weighing under 2,500 g at birth. Of 580 newborn infants in which information pertaining to the weight at birth was obtained, 49 (8.4%) were premature infants. In mothers receiving medication, 31 of 478 (6.5%) had premature babies, as compared to 12 of 129 (9.3%) in those who took no drugs.

DISCUSSION

The teratogenic effects of antiepileptic drugs have been known since the work of Meadow (1968), and instances of harelip, cleft palate, congenital facial abnormalities, hypoplasia of fingers and nails, and other multiple malformations have been reported. However, considering the etiology and the severity of epilepsy, and the incidence of malformations in epileptic women, it is not easy to elucidate the direct causal relationship.

In the present investigation, we have studied the incidence of malformations by detailed analysis of a large number of collected cases of pregnancy in epileptic patients.

According to Janz's report (1964) and 11 other papers that have appeared in the literature, the incidence of malformed baby in pregnant epileptic patients who received no medication is calculated as 3.64% (32/877). The rate for treated patients calculated on the basis of 27 statistically available reports is 7.2% (253 malformed in 3,475 live-birth babies in total).

The figures obtained in our study were 2.3% for untreated patients and 11.5% for treated patients. The difference in the incidence between the treated and untreated groups among our patients is more marked than those differences reported so far. There have been several papers which have reported an incidence of malformations of more than 10%; however, these reports are concerned with a relatively small number of cases. The high incidence in our series of patients may reflect the severity of their epilepsies.

Our findings in regard to the variety of malformations are in good agreement with those observed by other authors and it was confirmed that much attention should be directed to this.

We have proposed concrete recommendations for the safe use of antiepileptic drugs in respect of teratogenicity. We think it is thoughtless to jump to the conclusion that medication should be discontinued during pregnancy only because there is a possibility of teratogenicity in the use of antiepileptic drugs. The most important problem before us is to work out safer usages of these drugs in pregnancy.

SUMMARY

The abnormal developments in the course of pregnancy and its outcome and fetal abnormalities were examined in pregnant women: 657 cases receiving medication of antiepileptic drugs and 162 untreated cases.

In the treated group, the rate of live birth was 73% and that of natural abortions and stillbirths was 14% as compared with 80% and 4%, respectively, in the untreated group. The incidence of abortions and stillbirths was higher in the former group.

The incidence of malformations in live-birth babies was 11.5% (57 cases) in the treated group as compared with 2.3% (3 cases) in the untreated group, five times as high as that in the latter group. In the treated group, malformations occurred predominantly as cleft lip and/or palate and cardiovascular defects.

General background factors involved in the etiology of the malformed baby in epileptic patients were analyzed as well as whether or not anti-epileptic drugs were taken. As a result, it was found that treated patients who had seizures during pregnancy developed the highest incidence of mal-formations whereas treated patients who had no seizures had an incidence markedly higher than those with no treatment.

Taking the problem of teratogenicity of antiepileptic drugs into considera-tion, recommendations for safe use of these drugs during pregnancy are made with respect to the dosage, number of drugs used in combination, and maximum daily dose.

Investigators collaborating in the present work included: T. Sato, M.D. and Y. Fukushima, M.D.: Hirosaki University Hospital; H. Kumashiro, M.D.: Fukushima Prefectural Medical College Hospital; H. Kazamatsuri, M.D.: Teikyo University Hospital; T. Hara, M.D. and M. Inami, M.D.: Kitazato University Hospital; T. Onuma, M.D.: National Musashi Research Institute for Mental and Nervous Disease; M. Seino, M.D. and M. Miyakoshi, M.D.: National Epilepsy Center Shizuoka-Higashi Hospital; H. Hazama, M.D. and C. Ogura, M.D.: Tottori University Hospital; S. Ohtsuki, M.D. and K. Hosokawa, M.D.: Okayama University Hospital; K. Inanaga, M.D. and K. Kotorii, M.D.: Kurume University Hospital; Y. Fukuyama, M.D.: Tokyo Women's Medical College Hospital; T. Tanimura, M.D.: Kyoto University School of Medicine (Department of Anatomy).

ACKNOWLEDGMENTS

This investigation was supported by grants from the Ministry of Health and Welfare and the Ministry of Education.

We are grateful to Kyowa Hakko Kogyo Co., Ltd. and Dainippon Phar-maceutical Co., Ltd. for their support.

REFERENCES

Janz, D., and Fuchs, D. (1964): Sind antiepileptische Medikamente während der Schwangerschaft schädlich? *Deutsch Med Wochenschr.*, 89:241–243.

Meadow, S. R. (1968): Anticonvulsant drugs and congenital abnormalities. *Lancet*, ii: 1296.

Abstracts

THE PURKINJE CELL IN DILANTIN INTOXICATION, ULTRASTRUCTURAL AND GOLGI STUDIES: PRELIMINARY REPORT

H. Alcala, K. Lertratatanangkoon, W. Stenbach, P. Kellaway, A. G. Horning
Houston

Three male Sprague-Dawly rats, seven weeks of age, weighing 180-200 grams, received daily oral dosages of Phentoin (Dilantin^R) varying from 20 to 55 mg. The drug was administered in biscuits prepared with purina Rat Chow, gelatin, water and Dilantin^R. One rat of similar age, sex and weight was used as a control. Rat 1, 2 and 3 received total Dilantin dosages of 250, 850 and 1755 mg over a 10, 20 and 55 day period respectively. Throughout the study they were in good health and showed no neurologic signs. The cerebellum was removed under minimal chloroform anesthesia and a small sample immediately placed in 3% gluteraldehyde for electron microscopy. Another fragment was placed in a mixture of solution A and B (potassium dichromate and mercuric chloride — and potassium chromate and sodium tungstate) for the Golgi-Cox impregnation. The remaining tissue was placed in 10% formalin for light microscopy studies. When compared with the normal control light microscopy findings showed minimal Purkinje cell loss in rat 3. Ultra-structural changes in rat 1 and 2 showed markedly swollen mitochondria, with disrupted cristae and whorling arrangement of the rough endoplasmic reticulum. In addition, rat 3 showed numerous lipofucsin granules. Golgi studies did not show significant changes in rats 1 and 2. Rat 3 showed scattered dendritic spines with swollen terminals. Concentration of Dilantin metabolites in urine and serum are being determined in each animal. (Supported in part by grant #NS11535 NINCDS)

DRUG MONITORING AND CLINICAL EVALUATION OF PREGNANT EPILEPTIC WOMEN AND THEIR NEWBORNS. PRELIMINARY RESULTS OF A PROSPECTIVE STUDY

L. Bossi, G. Porro, G. Tognoni, R. Spreafico, R. Canger, L. Como, G. Pifarotti, M. De Giambattista, B. M. Assael, E. Caccamo, G. Pardi
Milan

This study was started on January 1977 in Milan, Italy. 25 epileptic women entered the study in early pregnancy; 15 had partial seizures, 10 had generalized seizures. Three patients underwent therapeutic abortion. Spontaneous abortion occurred in 1. Up to now there were 14 deliveries. 24 patients were on antiepileptic medication, mostly including barbiturates (20/24) or diphenylhydantoin (6/24).

1. Antiepileptic drug plasma levels were determined at regular monthly intervals. Phenobarbital (PB) and diphenylhydantoin (DPH) plasma clearance definitely increased during pregnancy; no significant changes were observed for ethosuximide and carbamazepine (1 patient each).
2. Seizure frequency did not differ significantly during pregnancy in respect to the 9 months before. In individual patients an increase in seizure frequency was observed in relation to a drop in drug plasma levels.
3. Newborns were evaluated for body weight, length, head circumference and malformations. One child was premature. No other significant alterations were found. Prospective evaluation is in progress.
4. PB and DPH blood levels were determined during delivery (mother and cord) and in the newborns up to 4-12 days. A slower disposition pattern was confirmed. Two newborns with high phenobarbital blood levels showed clinical features of the barbiturate withdrawal syndrome.

CONGENITAL MALFORMATIONS IN OFFSPRING OF EPILEPTIC WOMEN: CORRELATION WITH PLASMA ANTICONVULSANT LEVELS DURING PREGNANCY

L. Dansky, E. Andermann, A. L. Sherwin, F. Andermann, R. A. Kinch
Montreal

Plasma anticonvulsant levels were monitored during 31 pregnancies of 28 epileptic women. For each trimester, mean levels of diphenylhydantoin, phenobarbital, primidone and ethosuximide were compared between women who subsequently had normal or malformed offspring. Seven of the 31 pregnancies (22.6%) resulted in malformed offspring: three congenital heart disease, one cleft lip, one clubfoot, one polycystic kidney, and one child with multiple congenital anomalies.

For diphenylhydantoin, both the mean dosage (5.2±0.3 mg/kg) and mean plasma level (8.8±1.3 μg/ml) were significantly higher in mothers of malformed offspring, compared to mother who had normal children (4.3±0.3 mg/kg and 5.3±0.9 μg/ml, respectively). The mean plasma levels of phenobarbital and of ethosuximide were also higher in the malformed group, whereas mean levels of primidone were similar for the two groups.

In all patients, mean anticonvulsant plasma levels tended to be near the lower limit of the therapeutic range and to remain relatively constant throughout gestation. Cord blood anticonvulsant levels were almost identical to maternal levels at term.

These results demonstrate a markedly increased frequency of congenital malformations in offspring of epileptic women who took anticonvulsant medication during pregnancy, despite mean plasma levels at the lower limit of the therapeutic range. Furthermore, there is a positive correlation between the risk of malformation and plasma anticonvulsant levels.

EFFECTS OF ANTICONVULSANT DRUGS ON CHROMOSOMES IN MAN

Y. Matsusima, R. Kawahara, H. Hazama
Tottori

Toni et al. (1966) first showed the high ratio of abnormal chromosomes in lymphocytes from infants born from mothers having received anticonvulsants; since then there have been several reports about chromosomal aberrations caused by anticonvulsant medications. Nevertheless, no characteristic abnormality of chromosomes was found.

In the present study, we investigated effects of anticonvulsants on chromosomes in children born from epileptic mothers having received or not received anticonvulsant therapy. Chromosomes were examined by means of the analyses of lymphocytes cultured from the peripheral blood. In addition to the number of chromosomes, observations were made on the number of acrocentric chromosomes with satellite associations, breaks, gaps and other structural aberrations of chromosomes.

In mother group, tetraploid and heteroploid cells, and also structural abnormalities such as gaps, breaks and others were found. Nonramdom grouping of acrocentric chromosomes, apparently held together at their satellited ends, occurred most often in cells. In children group, chromosome abnormalities were observed more often than those of mother group. Effects of anticonvulsant drugs on chromosomes of children were recognized even in the 5th year after birth. We consider that the chromosomal abnormalities induced by anticonvulsant drugs are caused by interfering with the normal development of mitosis.

PRELIMINARY FINDINGS OF THE FETAL HYDANTOIN SYNDROME IN A MOUSE MODEL

R. H. Finnell, G. F. Chernoff
Vancouver

To separate the teratogenic effect of epilepsy from diphenylhydantoin (DPH) treatment, an animal model closely approximating the human condition was developed to meet the following criteria:
1. Test animals to have spontaneous seizures that are controlled by orally administered DPH;
2. DPH serum concentrations to fall within the

optimal human therapeutic range;
3. DPH treatment to begin prior to mating and be continued throughout gestation to control seizures.
4. The offspring of treated animals to exhibit the spectrum of malformations observed in the offspring of epileptic women.

To meet this criteria, mutant quaking (C57B1/6J, *gk/gk*) mice and the appropriate controls were administered DPH orally. Seizure activity was reduced by DPH. Monitored DPH serum levels indicated serum concentrations within the human therapeutic range at 40 and 60 mg/kg body weight dosages.

A preliminary application of this model indicates that it is the drug and not the maternal seizure disorder that causes the malformations. Further, the anomalies observed in this model represent the mouse equivalent of the fetal hydantoin syndrome. Similarities with the human syndrome include growth deficiency, neural, cardiac, ocular, orofacial and urinary defects.

DIPHENYLHYDANTOIN AND ITS EFFECT ON THE FERTILITY OF MALE RATS

D. F. Cohn, G. Paz, Z. T. Hommonai, M. Streifler
P. F. Kraicer
Tel-Aviv

This experiment was designed to study the effect of extended diphenylhydantoin (DPH) treatment during a period roughly equal to one complete spermatogenic cycle. Male rats were injected s.c. with 20, 40, and 80 mg/Kg body weight DPH daily for 2 months. The treated males were caged for 5 days with cyclic females. The number of impregnations was significantly reduced but only in the high dose group. Thereafter the males were autopsied, the organs of their genital tract examined and weighed and were found unaffected. The epididymal content and the motility of spermatozoa were normal. Blood testosterone concentrations and Leydig cell counts were normal. An assessment of the accumulation of DPH in the seminal secretion was made by analysis of the post-coital uterine fluid. DPH levels were undetectably low. Behaviourally the treated males seemed less excitable and made fewer mounting attempts. Thus the observed reduction of fertility was probably the result of a loss of libido. It should be stressed that no androgen deficiency was found. Changes in copulating activity are presumably due to behavioural responses to DPH.

THE EFFECTS OF DIPHENYLHYDANTOIN (DPH) ON MAN'S IMMUNITY

J. D. Gabourel, G. H. Davies, E. J. Bardana, Jr.
and D. M. Dordevich
Portland

DPH may cause serious side effects by alteration of the immune system. DPH effects on humoral and cellular immunity were prospectively studied in 104 patients. Sequential analysis of serum immunoglobulins, C3, C4, antinuclear antibodies and blastogenic responses to mitogens were carried out. Patients were classifed into 3 groups; I) 46 patients with idiopathic epilepsy (IE); II) 25 patients with secondary epilepsy (SE); III) 32 patients without seizures (WS) given DPH prophylactically post neurosurgery or for neuropathic pain. Before DPH treatment, 17% of IE, 8% of SE and 6% of WS had depressed serum IgA levels (< 60 mg%). Sixty-three patients (28, 16 and 19 from each group, respectively) were evaluated at least once after starting DPH. After 6 months of DPH therapy each patient's serum immunoglobulin levels were compared to his or her own pre-drug levels; DPH depressed IgA, IgM and IgG (p. < .001); complement components were not significantly altered. Similar individual pre/post DPH comparisons were made for lymphocyte responses to nonspecific mitogens (34 patients GP I, II and III combined). Results indicated more reductions than elevations for all 3 mitogens following DPH therapy (p < 0.02). This effect was greatest for two T-cell specific mitogens, phytohemagglutinin and concanavalin A when compared to pokeweed. Five IE, 2 SE and 1 WS developed de novo antinuclear antibodies without symptoms after 6 months of treatment. Our data are consistent with indications from retrospective studies in that: 1) patients with IE have a high incidence of serum IgA deficiency prior to starting DPH; 2) DPH has a definite suppressive effect on both humoral and cell mediated immunity; 3) patients on DPH can be expected to develop de novo antinuclear antibodies.

Supported by NINCDS contract N01-NS-5-2328 to Oregon Epilepsy Center.

AXOPLASMIC FLOW OF CEREBRAL GLYCO-PROTEINS AFTER DILANTIN

W. W. Hofmann
Palo Alto

To understand better the mechanisms by which diphenylhydantoin (DPH) controls seizures without producing consistent EEG changes, a study was made of its effects on axoplasmic flow in the rat brain. Using ocular injections of tracer and monitoring uptake in contralateral geniculate and occipital cortex it was found that DPH increases the radioactivity remaining in both areas at 5 days. It is assumed that the drug enhances movement of glycoproteins or precursors between sources of synthesis and distant neurones synaptically connected. To eliminate the possibility that the increased radioactivity accumulation was the result of a DPH-induced reduction in turn-over, the same studies were repeated with tracer and DPH both given intraocularly. Again there was an increase of radioactivity in neurones connected to the injected retina. These results suggest that the CNS-stabilizing effects of DPH arise partly from enhanced replenishment of neuronal membrane components. Elements "downstream" from the focus may thus have a higher threshold.

EFFECTS OF TREATMENT WITH PHENOBARBITAL AND PHENYTOIN ON SLEEP ORGANISATION IN EPILEPTIC PATIENTS

P. Wolf, U. U. Röder
Berlin

Changes in the sleep organisation of patients with epilepsy could be responsible for part of both therapeutic and untoward (e.g. behavioural) effects of antiepileptic drug treatment.

It is well known that the immediate effect of barbiturates is reduction of REM and, less pronouncedly, stage IV sleep. There is some evidence that with their continuous use sleep tends to return to its individual pre-treatment organisation. This, however, has not been investigated in epileptic patients, and much less is known about possible immediate and longterm effects of other antiepileptic drugs.

In a prospective study at our institute, the sleep of hitherto untreated epileptic patients is investigated polygraphically, and controlled with placebo, first drug exposition, after adjustment to a therapeutic steady state serum level, and after 6 months of treatment. Phenobarbital and phenytoin as sole agents are given to each patient in a cross-over design.

Preliminary results with about 25 patients are presented. Immediate reaction to phenobarbital resembles closely that seen in other probands, whereas phenytoin has much less spectacular effects. Adjustment to a steady state medication seems to have heterogenous consequences which could depend on the serum level.

EPILEPSY, MENTAL RETARDATION, AND INAPPROPRIATE ANTICONVULSANT THERAPY

K. Kaufman and L. Katz-Garris
Pittsburgh

Few studies are directed at the medical and financial aspects of inappropriate anticonvulsant drug therapy in patients without epilepsy. Preliminary findings from a survey of state institutions for mental retardation, a population noted to have increased seizure frequency, are presented. Of 127 patients reviewed, 81 were diagnosed as mentally retarded, 60 as schizophrenic, and 17 as epileptic. Anticonvulsants were taken by 41 patients — 17 with and 24 without epilepsy. Thus 58.5% of those patients on anticonvulsants did not have the appropriate diagnosis. None of the charts reviewed contained anticonvulsant blood levels or EEG reports. This lack of laboratory examinations precluded the determination of therapeutic blood levels and clinical neurophysiologic confirmation of diagnosis. Since toxicity to anticonvulsants is increased in mental retardation populations, appropriate diagnosis and minimum blood levels are essential, especially with an increased number of daily drugs. The mean number of daily drugs/patient on anticonvulsants was 4.88 compared to 2.33 for patients not on anticonvulsants. The 24 patients without epilepsy inappropriately received 50,000 anticonvulsant dosages annually costing $1412.

The authors suggest that inappropriate usage of anticonvulsants may be commonplace in state institutions for mental retardation. Specialized inservice training for those physicians treating this population is recommended.

METABOLIC BONE DISTURBANCE IN CHILDREN TREATED WITH PHENOBARBITAL

M. Kriz, E. Paucic-Kirincic
Rijeka

There is an increasing number of reports indicating that anticonvulsant drugs (phenobarbital, diphenylhydantoin) may interfere with vitamin D metabolism and cause metabolic bone disease.

The aim of this study was to elucidate in our own material the possible influence of a long term antiepileptic treatment on some biochemical parameters concerning bone metabolism (serum levels of calcium, phosphate and alkaline phosphatase), and to ascertain the eventual risks of clinical and radiological evidence of rickets in these patients. For that purpose, a group of fifteen children with febrile convulsions (age: 2-5 years) treated with phenobarbital for at least one year (serum levels ranging 15-25 μg/ml), was examined and compared with a control group (fifteen children of same age).

The results could be summarized as follows:

a. *Calcium:* Normal serum levels were found in both groups.

b. *Phosphate:* Significantly lower phosphate levels were found in the group treated with phenobarbital ($\bar{x}_1 = 4,5$ mg%, $\bar{x}_2 = 5,2$ mg%, t = 2,5, p < 0.02).

c. *Alkaline phosphatase:* A striking elevation of serum alkaline phosphatase was noted in children treated with phenobarbital in contrast to the normal values encountered in the control group. ($\bar{x}_1 = 156,7$ I.U., $\bar{x}_2 = 68,2$ I.U., t = 3,35, p < 0.01). As it could be seen the difference between two groups is highly significant.

d. *Clinical and radiological evidence of rickets:* In the group treated with phenobarbital two children developed clinical and radiological signs of rickets.

Conclusion: On the basis of this pilot study it appears rather possible that long-term treatment with phenobarbital may cause metabolic bone disturbance.

ANIMAL STUDIES ON THE BEHAVIORAL TOXICITY OF ANTIEPILEPTIC DRUGS

B. Kulig, H. Meinardi
Heemstede and Leiden

Although changes in cognitive functioning have been described in epileptic patients, the relative contribution of antiepileptic drugs in producing behavioral changes is not well understood. Animal studies were carried out to examine the dose-related effects of phenobarbital, sodium valproate and

phenytoin on learned and unlearned behavior in rats. At dose levels at or exceeding the MES anticonvulsant ED50, the behavioral toxicity of these compounds was reflected in changes in motor function, apparent as either sedation and/or incoordination. With operant learning techniques, behavioral changes could be detected at lower dose levels. In a fixed ratio task requiring a high response output (FR20), phenytoin produced a dose-dependent decrease in response rate. In contrast, treatment with phenobarbital or sodium valproate increased behavioral output at low doses and decreased response rates at high doses. The rate-increasing properties of these compounds was further studied in a timing task in which animals were required to space individual responses on a low rate schedule of reinforcement (DRL 12 sec). Both compounds exhibited disinhibitory effects, increasing both perseverative and anticipatory responses. These studies indicate that antiepileptic drugs produce heterogeneous behavioral effects which can be measured with operant techniques at dose levels at or below the anticonvulsant ED50.

INFLUENCE OF ANTIEPILEPTIC DRUGS ON PUPIL CYCLE TIME

D. Schottelius, R. Fincham, R. Zahoruk and
H. S. Thompson
Iowa City

Prolonged pupil cycle time (PCT) was noted in a few patients taking antiepileptic medications when examined in the neuro-ophthalmology clinic which suggested this prospective study. PCT is the time required for the constriction and redilation of the pupil, and these oscillations are a property of the pupillary light reflex arc. Speed, frequency, and intensity of afferent nerve impulses reaching the mid-brain, synaptic delays, the efferent nerve delays, and any structural slowness of the iris musculature are factors which could delay this arc. Simultaneous measurement of PCT and serum levels of antiepileptic drugs were made on a random sample of patients seen in the neurology clinic. These were separated into two groups: individuals whose only medication was phenytoin and individuals taking phenytoin plus other antiepileptic drugs. In addition, patients who were just beginning phenytoin therapy were followed from 0 dose to therapeutic serum levels. Individuals whose phenytoin serum levels were within the therapeutic range demonstrated no increase in PCT when compared to normals; however patients followed from initiation of phenytoin therapy showed increasing PCT with increasing serum levels. Individuals taking multiple antiepileptic drugs (with levels within therapeutic range) demonstrated an increased PCT when compared to normals. Patients with serum levels above the usual therapeutic range also had increased PCT. Utilization of pupil cycle time in treatment and relationship to seizure control will be discussed.

ANTICONVULSANT MEDICATION AND THYROID HORMONES

H. Fichsel
Bonn

During anticonvulsive long-term treatment we studied 150 epileptic children and juveniles under valproate monotherapy, phenytoin monotherapy, primidone monotherapy, carbamazepine monotherapy, and combination therapy. In all investigated children the concentration of serum PBI, T4, FT4, T3, basic TSH, T3-in vitro test, thyroxin-binding globulin, and the total cholesterol were measured. We carried out TRH-tests in an additional 70 patients.

Results: Combined anticonvulsant treatment caused the most marked decrease in PBI, T4, and FT4, while in contrast the concentration of serum cholesterol rises statistically. Carbamazepine monotherapy decreased statistically the concentration of PBI, T4, FT4, and T3 and resulted in a significant increase in serum cholesterol. These changes were dosage-dependent. Primidone monotherapy produced a significant decrease of PBI, T4, and FT4 without a significant elevation of serum cholesterol. There was no dosage-dependency. Phenytoin monotherapy decreased significantly PBI, T4, and T3 without elevation of cholesterol. There was a dose-dependency. Also valproate produced a slight, but significant decrease of T4 and T3 without an increase of cholesterol in a dosage-dependent manner. Basic TSH showed slightly higher values only in about 5% of patients, but in TRH-tests 8% of patients showed a markedly elevated TSH after stimulation. In 3 patients there was a secondary hypothalamic hypothyroidism. In another patient changes in the thyroid hormone system must be interpreted as a primary hypothyroidism.

The described effects of anticonvulsive drugs may be caused by a competitive displacement of thyroxin and possibly triiodothyronine from their plasma protein-binding sites. Another factor could be a more rapid metabolism of T4 and finally a possible inhibition of hypothalamic TRH release.

BEHAVIOR, PERFORMANCE, AND SEIZURES

Abstracts

RAPID STIMULATION IN CONTINUOUS PERFORMANCE TASKS UNDER EEG MONITORING

G. Erba, V. Cavazzuti
Boston

Subtle variations in vigilance and cognitive processes during ictal and interictal periods may be very relevant to explain certain behavioral patterns. A series of acoustically and visually mediated stimuli of very brief duration to match exactly concomitant EEG events are delivered. The difficulty of the task consists in the ability to process very simple information presented at near threshold level. Scoring is based on objective measurements of stimulus-response latency, variability of latency from trial to trial, length of presentation required for stimuli to be perceived and degree of correctness.

It has become apparent that fluctuations of performance in Generalized Epilepsies and complex seizure states vary greatly from retained to partially or completely abolished consciousness during spike-wave discharges whereas comparable changes can be detected during subtle EEG changes such as simple slowing of the background activity.

Correlation of these variables with concomitant EEG analysis is proposed as a way to classify epileptic syndromes and to differentiate abnormal performance due to interference of electrical paroxysms from impairment due to underlying pathology.

MENTAL ASPECTS IN DRUG-RESISTANT TEMPORAL LOBE EPILEPSY

I. Jensen, J. K. Larsen
Copenhagen

The psychiatric disorders in 74 patients with drug-resistant temporal lobe epilepsy were investigated. In all an anterior temporal lobectomy had been performed during the period 1960-1969 at Rigshospitalet. No tumor or gross vascular malformation had been recognized before or during the operation. At follow-up 45 patients were free from any seizures, while 15 had obtained a substantial reduction in their seizure frequencies. There were four postoperative deaths. Only six patients had never been psychiatrically abnormal. Behavioural disturbances were observed in 55 patients. Half the adult patients suffered from a diminished sexual drive. Fourteen patients attempted suicide one or more times. Preoperatively eleven patients displayed schizophrenia-like psychoses, and a further nine became psychotic during the follow-up period, six of them even after having been cured of their epilepsy. In 10 patients the interval between onset of epilepsy and onset of psychosis was more than 15 years. Eighty per cent of the psychotic patients were bright or normally gifted as compared to 60 per cent of the other patients. The psychoses were the only psychiatric disorder which presented differences in laterality, as comparatively more non righthanded than right-handed patients were psychotic, and furthermore more females than males were psychotic. Improvement in psychiatric conditions were found clearly correlated to a therapeutic success regarding relief from seizures. The postoperative psychiatric status of patients with no or only few seizures determined their social rehabilitation.

MECHANISMS OF AGGRESSIVE BEHAVIOR IN PATIENTS WITH TEMPORO-LIMBIC EPILEPSY

S. M. Ferguson, M. Rayport, W. S. Corrie
Toledo

Previous investigators have sought parsimony in their explanations of aggressive behavior in temporo-limbic epilepsy (TLE). Our data suggest the necessity of a multifactorial conceptualization under which aggressive behavior is subdivided into primary and secondary.

Data supporting the proposed hypothesis of 1° and 2° aggression in TLE have been gathered from 1) structured psychiatric interviews with patients and families; 2) neuropsychiatric examination and observations; 3) reports from nurses; 4) direct personal observations of seizures and of aggressive behavior occurring spontaneously and in response to pharmacologic activation or to electrical stimulation during chronic implantation of depth electrodes.

Patients with *1° aggressive behavior* have a dysfunction of brain circuits mediating aggression. The aggressive behavior may occur continuously as chronic irritability or intermittently during the prodrome or during a seizure.

Secondary aggression results from a complex intersect of ictal mental content, intrapsychic dynamics and external stimuli. Post-ictally, aggression may result from impaired cortical integration leading to misperceptions and diminished censoring and control of feelings.

More complex and frequently unrecognized is an ictal basis for aggressive symptomatology in the so-called "interictal period" in which aggressive behavior may follow one or several unrecognized minimal seizures. Undetected episodic higher function impairments due to minimal seizures may also account for aggressive behavior.

BEHAVIORAL CONSEQUENCES OF CEREBRAL HEMISPHERIC LOCATION OF SEIZURE DISORDER

S. Berent, T. J. Boll, B. Giordani, V. Jones
Charlottesville, Virginia

This work represents part of an overall project currently funded by a contract (#N01-NS-5-2329) from the National Institute of Neurological and Communicative Disorders and Stroke. This support is gratefully acknowledged.

In these studies, epileptic patients were examined in the investigator's laboratory at the Highlands Center for Epilepsy and Related Disorders.

Patients were administered a set of learning tasks that are believed to reflect differential processing between the two cerebral hemispheres. Heart rate and other peripheral physiological functions were monitored continuously during patient's performance.

Employing a "blind" procedure, patients were assigned to groups according to the nature of their seizure disorder—i.e. lateralized to the left cerebral hemisphere, lateralized right, etc. Determination of seizure location was based upon findings from clinical interview, electroenchephalogram, radiologic studies, and direct observation of onset of seizure.

Statistical comparisons were made between groups in terms of their performance on the learning and physiological measures. This presentation summarizes these results. In the discussion particular attention is paid to the interaction between location of seizure, task demand and subsequent physiological reactivity.

PATTERNS OF NEUROPSYCHOLOGICAL FUNCTIONING IN TEMPORAL LOBE AND PSYCHIATRIC PATIENTS

D. Crockett, C. Nemetz, J.A. Wada, P. Termansen
Vancouver

Most instances of neuropsychological functioning have focussed on patients who have been categorized into groups based on a priori descriptions of their psychiatric, epileptic, and mixed affective disorders (Heaton, et. al., 1978). This approach, while useful to validate neuropsychological tests, does little to tell us what pre-existing patterns of difficulties can be identified in these patients, and how these disorders relate to their neuropsychological and personality functioning.

In this study, the performance of sixty patients with mixed diagnoses was examined. The following tests were used: Wechsler Adult Intelligence Scale; Benton Visual Retention Test; Dichotic Listening Test; Word Fluency Test; Speech Perception Test; Sentence Repetition Test; Seashore Tonal & Rhythm Test; Categories Test; Dynamometer and Tapping Test; Trail Making Test; and MMPI. This test battery was factor analyzed to obtain a smaller set of more reliable scores which still reflected in the major dimensions of this test battery. These factor scores were then submitted to a cluster analysis programme to derive groups based on the salient features of their neuropsychological functioning. Once these groups were empirically derived they were compared with one another to define what particular patterns of difficulty identified each group. These groups were also examined to determine the relative frequency of epileptic or psychiatric disorders in each group.

THE MEASUREMENT OF INTERICTAL SPEECH AND LANGUAGE DISTURBANCES IN COMPLEX PARTIAL SEIZURES

S. Porrazzo, A. Mayersdorf
Minneapolis

Although disturbances in speech and language are a frequent concomitant of complex partial seizures (CPS), studies concerning these mechanisms and cognitive behavior in patients with an epileptogenic temporal lobe focus have been sparse and almost exclusively limited to subjects with temporal lobectomy. Paroxysmal speech disturbances are of considerable significance in CPS, often constituting either the crisis itself or one of its elements. It is also known that impairments in memory, retention, and learning, as well as aphasia, may accompany temporal lobe destructive lesions. However, no extensive exploitation of the correlation between the irritative lesions and speech and language disturbances has been carried out.

In a recent study, fifteen patients suffering from CPS were examined and subjected to a standardized speech and language test battery (the Porch Index of Communicative Ability, the Token Test, and the Word Fluency Test) in order to correlate their performances on these tests with their subjective speech and language difficulties and with location of the involved areas of the brain. The results showed that although none of the patients had clinical evidence of a destructive organic lesion in the temporal lobe areas, abnormal patterns in certain interictal speech and language abilities occurred, demonstrating that these subtle changes are related to irritative lesions and abnormal electrical discharges within the temporal lobes.

Address correspondence to: Assa Mayersdorf, M.D., Epilepsy Treatment Center (127C), Veterans Administration Hospital, 54th Street and 48th Avenue South, Minneapolis, Minnesota 55417

BEHAVIORAL CONCOMMITANTS OF BACKGROUND AND PAROXYSMAL EEG DISCHARGE

R. G. Bickford, C. B. McCutchen, K. R. Hanson, J. Cuchiara, V. Rochowansky
La Jolla

Optimal use of the EEG test requires that neurologic function associated with paroxysmal discharge and background activity should be measured during recording since this index is important in assessing such factors as work capactiy, activity restriction and anticonvulsant effectiveness in epileptic patients.

To provide this information, we have introduced a

response timing device into the routine clinical EEG lab which enables the technician to initiate a signal (click, word, flash, shock) to which the subject responds from switches held in left and right hand. The response time reads out in milliseconds and is marked on the record with appropriate coding of stimulus and response. Stimuli are applied both during background and paroxysmal activity. Words are generated electronically.

The device is useful to assess: 1) "Psychoparalytic" effects produced by a large variety of generalized or focal paroxysmal discharges (thus the report might read "generalized spike wave with 70% psychoparalytic component"). 2) Clinical significance of paroxysmal discharge during hyperventilation, photic stimulus and drowsiness states.

3) Effectiveness of anticonvulsant treatment by measurement during background (toxic effects) and paroxysmal discharge (anticonvulsant effects). 4) Mechanisms relating to the "seizure gating hypothesis" of EEG event behavior interaction (Bickford, R.G. The concept of a seizure gating mechanism in epilepsy. Electroencheph. clin. Neurophysiol., 38:551-552, 1975).

CLINICAL AND ELECTROGRAPHIC ASPECTS OF EPILEPSY

Abstracts

PROBLEMS OF DIAGNOSIS AND TREATMENT OF MYOCLONIC EPILEPSIES OF CHILDHOOD AND ADOLESCENCE

P. Jeavons
Birmingham, England

There are seven types of myoclonic epilepsy. *West and Lennox syndromes* are probably the same, arising at different ages. Both respond to corticosteroids or benzodiazepines, but Lennox syndrome is best treated with sodium valproate alone or with nitrazepam or acetazolamide. *Myoclonic epilepsy of childhood* starts before 9 years, *myoclonic epilepsy of adolescence* around puberty. In both the jerks mainly involve the upper part of the body: mentality is normal. Both respond to sodium valproate. Jerks are commoner after waking and during menstruation, often disappearing during pregnancy. Waking EEG often normal but 3 c/s spike and wave occurs with drowsiness. In *myoclonic absence* a generalized jerk occurs with each spike of the 3 c/s spike wave complex, with immediate return of consciousness at the end. Sodium valproate and ethosuximide combined are effective. There are two photomyoclonias, both with spike and wave on photic stimulation. In one there are myoclonic jerks with rare tonic-clonic fits, and response is to sodium valproate. In eyelid myoclonia jerking of the eyelids occurs on eyeclosure, absences are common and sodium valproate may need to be combined with ethosuximide. Considerable problems arise in the manipulation of antiepileptic drugs in the management of myoclonic epilepsies and these are discussed.

Results of therapy with sodium valproate

| | Total | Improved by: | | |
		100%	80%	50%
Lennox syndrome	35	8	4	7
Myoclonic of childhood	18	11	4	1
Myoclonic absence	5	3	1	1
Myoclonic of adolescence	26	17	3	1
Photosensitive myoclonic	9	8		1
Eyelid myoclonia	10	7	3	
Totals	103	54	15	11

UNILATERAL BLINKING AS A LATERALIZING SIGN OF PARTIAL COMPLEX SEIZURE OF TEMPORAL LOBE ORIGIN

J. A. Wada
Vancouver

Among disturbances of higher function during partial complex seizure, dysphasia, dysarthria, speech automatism and conceptual illusion such as deja-vu, have all been claimed to have some lateralizing values. Head-turning has little lateralizing significance in general, unless it is associated with conjugate eye deviation, mouth corner retraction and tonic eyelid closure, all to the same side. There has been no report of lateralizing motor ictal manifestations in man when there is no development of secondary motor seizures.

We now report a subtle but clearly lateralizing ictal clinical sign in five patients with partial complex seizures. All these patients were subjected to metrazol-megimide activation for identification of the side of origin of their seizures as preliminary evaluation for possible surgical treatment. Their habitual seizure pattern was secondary generalized convulsion in one patient and partial complex seizure in four patients. Three out of five patients had bilateral independent foci of interictal sphenoidal discharge. Induced clinical seizures, which were judged to be identical to their habitual seizures, showed 3-6/sec unilateral blinking ipsilateral to the side of ictal sphenoidal build-up. Although this particular ictal clinical sign was not described by any witnesses, subsequent warning of this sign enabled this particular manifestation to be noticed as an integral part of their habitual seizure in three cases.

It is therefore worth stressing the value of unilateral blinking to potential witnesses of habitual seizure since its recognition could help lateralize the origin of clinical ictal events.

DISORDERED TEMPORAL PERCEPTION FOLLOWING TEMPORAL LOBECTOMY FOR EPILEPSY

I. Sherwin
Boston

Temporal Perception and ordering is a central problem in the psychophysiology of cognition.

Earlier studies involving both visual and auditory modalities in patients with brain damage from trauma, strokes and tumors suggested a possible critical role for the temporal lobes. Since those lesions undoubtedly extended beyond the anatomical confines of the temporal lobe, we investigated this possibility by studying it in patients with lesions restricted to the temporal lobes, i.e.: anterior temporal resections for intractable epilepsy.

Five patients with left and six with right temporal lobe resections (all with normal pure tone audiometry) and eight controls were studied. They were tested monaurally for their ability to identify the order of presentation of pairs of brief, discriminable pure tones. The 80% correct level (inter-tone) interval for each ear in each subject was determined using the "transformed up-down rule". Nine of the eleven patients revealed significantly (p<0.01) poorer performance in the ear contralateral to the resected temporal lobe. No ear differences were noted in the controls.

The results suggest that the application of such techniques might have lateralizing diagnostic value in patients with lesions of the temporal lobes. Several possible mechanisms accounting for this contralateral monaural effect are discussed.

HEMISPHERIC PROCESSING AND CALLOSAL MECHANISMS IN PATIENTS WITH EPILEPSY

D. M. Daly, J. A. Wada, D. D. Daly
Vancouver

Synthetic, speech-like, sparse acoustic stimuli (SAS) can be used to evaluate cortical auditory processing; patients classify sets of SAS presented monaurally and binaurally, indicating responses by a motor act (e.g., pointing). Two patients with excision or extensive destruction of one hemisphere randomly classified SAS presented to contralateral ear. Patients with focal lesions involving auditory cortex have altered perceptions and aberrant classifications, more so in contralateral ear. Seizures occuring in auditory cortex alter perception of SAS; focal seizures elsewhere do not.

Two patients with mesial frontal lesions. 1 involving right and the other left hemisphere, had greater difficulty indicating classes of SAS presented to contralateral ear when using ipsilateral hand. This occurred only with certain types of stimuli and, thus, did not result from apraxia. Study of a patient with hemispheric disconnection syndrome after hemorrhagic infarct of anterior corpus callosum corroborated these findings.

Thus, this type of testing can provide measures of intra-hemispheric processing and hemispheric interactions. Our findings provide a rationale for using this test in the pre-operative evaluation of patients with intractable epilepsy who are candidates for callosal section and in the post-operative evaluation of the therapeutic effects of such surgery.

SEXUAL AURA IN SEIZURES WITH PARTIAL COMPLEX SYMPTOMATOLOGY

G. M. Rémillard, G. Testa, F. Andermann,
W. Feindel, P. Gloor, J. B. Martin
Montreal

A sexual aura was described by five female patients who had partial seizures with complex symptomatology. The descriptions ranged from a low abdominal or perineal sensation to a feeling of intromission and were likened to a sensation of sexual arousal, as in masturbation, intercourse or orgasm. Four of the five patients had other subjective manifestations suggesting localization in the temporal lobe, and all patients had infrequent generalized attacks. Onset was somewhat later than expected in patients with this type of partial seizures. So far a gross lesion (an angiomatous malformation) was found in only one case. These patients had no sexual automatisms, although the latter have been described by others, and have also been observed by us in other patients.

In one patient, the sexual aura was reproduced by amygdaloid stimulation at operation. No partial complex seizures recurred during the six years following her temporal lobectomy.

No males with this type of aura were encountered by our group. In the literature, a few female patients with sexual auras are described, but no convincing descriptions of such auras have been noted in males, although they may have various ictal sexual manifestations. This suggests that the limbic representation of sexual mechanisms may be different in the male and the female. This observation may correlate with the recognized hyposexuality of male patients with partial seizures with complex symptomatology, who also appear to have a higher incidence of homosexuality and other sexual deviations.

THE SIGNIFICANCE OF WATER DRINKING IN SEIZURES WITH PARTIAL COMPLEX SYMPTOMATOLOGY: A STUDY OF TWENTY PATIENTS

G. M. Remillard, F. Andermann, P. Gloor,
J. B. Martin, A. Olivier
Montreal

The urge to demand, pour and drink water was encountered in twenty patients with other manifestations of seizures with partial complex symptomatology. Fifteen patients were aware and five were unaware of their desire to drink. None of the patients described this urge as an awareness of thirst, and four interpreted it as a means of arresting the attack. The amount consumed rarely exceeded one glass, and only occasionally other liquids were substituted. Usually, drinking was appropriate, but one patient attempted to drink perfume.

One patient with bilateral independent interictal discharges from both temporal lobes was studied with bitemporal implanted electrodes to determine whether seizures originated only on one side. Drinking was associated with electrographic and clinical seizures starting in the left amygdala and hippocampus. Sometimes, this was the only clinical manifestation of such attacks, and its significance would have been missed in the absence of depth recording.

Ictal drinking is not a reflex related to disturbed water homeostasis; it is an activation of a motivating mechanism not triggered by oropharyngeal cues. It represents the execution of a basic drive initiated by the abnormal stimulus of temporal epileptic activity.

Drinking was never encountered in seizures other than those originating in temporal lobe structures, and therefore has localizing significance.

STARTLE DISEASE IN TWO FAMILIES: ITS THERAPEUTIC RESPONSE, RELATIONSHIP TO EPILEPSY AND THE JUMPERS OF MAINE

D. Keene, E. Andermann, F. Andermann, L. Quesney
Montreal

Two sisters and an unrelated boy were misdiagnosed as having spastic quadriplegia during infancy. Prolonged nocturnal jerking most noticeable in lower extremities with retained consciousness was interpreted as clonic seizures. Excessive startle due to unsuspected stimuli was very striking; but particularly strong stimuli led to falling without protective movements or loss of consciousness, frequent injuries, and occasional fractures.

The patients were markedly hyperreflexic, but had no pathological reflexes. Withdrawal of medications resulted in a timorous hesitant unsteady gait, holding onto the walls, and a reluctance to walk. One sister had congenital nystagmus.

One sister showed generalized, irregular spike and wave discharges. In the sibling, a prolonged jerking attack was recorded; it was impossible to decide whether the electrographic accompaniment consisted of generalized epileptic discharge or artifact. She had no inter-ictal epileptogenic discharges. The boy had a sharp wave focus at the parietal vertex.

The mother of the two girls startled excessively; two children of the older sister had excessive startle with febrile episodes, but no hypertonia. No abnormal startle was described in members of the second family.

The echopraxia and echolalia exhibited by the Jumpers of Maine were conspicuously absent in our kindreds.

Phenobarbital, diphenylhydantoin and primidone are effective in greatly reducing the clinical manifestations and improving the gait, but clonazepam is the drug of choice.

PARTIAL EPILEPSY OF SUPPLEMENTARY MOTOR AREA ORIGIN

J. R. Green, J. C. White Jr., A. D. Edes, and R. D. Smith
Phoenix

The functional significance of the supplementary motor area was defined in monkey and man by Penfield and Welch in 1949. Located on the mesial surface of each cerebral hemisphere, this area lies just anterior to the upper end of the sensori-motor strip, occasionally involves the superior convexity adjacent to the leg area of the motor cortex, usually is limited by the cingulate sulcus below, and may be separated from the Rolandic zone by a narrow strip which, at times, occupies a small vertical convolution.

Epileptic discharge, or electrical stimulation, in this area may create a variety of movements involved with the assumption and maintenance of posture,

maneuvers, rhythmic movements, and fragments, general or isolated movements of an extremity. Other responses include vocalization, slow or incomplete inhibition of voluntary movement (including speech), as well as perception of generalized body sensations and alterations of the pupils and heart rate. Cortical excision creates minimal, if any, permanent neurologic deficits.

The description of a patient with partial epilepsy (postural seizures) of supplementary motor area origin associated with an otherwise asymptomatic but large porencephalic cyst and a review of the relatively sparse literature on this subject comprise the basis for this presentation.

CT SCAN FINDINGS IN FOCAL EPILEPSY

E. Kobayashi, T. Mihara, K. Yamamoto, T. Asakura
Kagoshima

In 80 cases of focal epilepsy excluding such cases as late onset after 30 years old and traumatic and organic lesions, the epileptogenic foci have been studied comparing CT findings with seizure types and EEG findings. The results were as follows:

1) Abnormal CT findings were observed in 36% of the patients.
2) These findings were classified into four large groups: localized cerebral atrophy, localized low density, localized high density with contrast enhancement and diffuse cerebral atrophy.
3) The incidence of CT abnormality was higher in the cases with continuous and localized EEG abnormality than in the cases with other types of EEG abnormality.
   In 48% of the cases, location of abnormal CT findings were coincided with their EEG foci.
4) In the cases of temporal lobe epilepsy without abnormal CT images, print-out data were compared with the bilateral promised temporal regions, before and after contrast enhancement. EMI-No. of the medial temporal focus had increased more than that of the contralateral side in three out of four cases after contrast media injection.
5) Moreover, for the purpose of comparing the CT findings in general seizures with those in focal seizures, we studied 80 cases of general seizures. In the cases of general seizures, abnormal CT findings were observed in only 16%.
   These abnormal findings were diffuse in five cases, localized in five cases and combined in three cases.

COMPUTERIZED AXIAL TOMOGRAPHY IN TEMPORAL LOBE EPILEPSY

K. Yamamoto, T. Mihara, E. Kobayashi, K. Uetsuhara, and T. Asakura
Kagoshima

Computerized axial tomography (CT) of the brain has been used, as well as electroencephalography

(EEG), to study 56 patients with temporal lobe epilepsy from September 1976 to March 1978.

The results of the CT findings were as follows:

1) Thirty-three patients showed abnormal CT findings which corresponded to EEG abnormality.
2) Abnormal CT findings were: 11 cases (33%) of diffuse or focal cortical atrophy; 8 cases (24%) of localized low density in the temporal lobe; 5 cases (15%) of symmetrical or asymmetrical ventricular dilatation; 3 cases (9%) of arachinoid cyst in the temporal lobe; another 3 cases (9%) of middle cranial fossa asymmetry; one case (3%) of multiple calcification with ventricular dilatation; one case (3%) showed occipital lobe low density.

On correlation of CT findings with clinical seizure, 26% of patients with cortical atrophy showed automatism, while 21% of cases with localized low density of the temporal lobe had impaired consciousness.

3) In 6 out of 23 patients with normal CT findings, the difference of contrast enhancement in the amygdalo-hippocampal region was studied. Five out of 6 patients showed greater enhancement corresponding to the side of spike discharge in the EEG.

Although it is difficult to state a direct cause-and-effect relationship between CT findings and epileptic symptoms, a more precise diagnosis of epilepsy will be expected by CT scan.

IDENTIFYING EPILEPTIC FOCI ON CONTRAST ENHANCED COMPUTERIZED TOMOGRAPHIC (CT) SCANS

J. Oakley, G. Ojemann, L. Cromwell
Seattle

This study was directed at determining if there is a CT scan correlate of an interictal epileptic focus. All CT scans on patients at the University of Washington Comprehensive Epilepsy Centre were reviewed. Those showing grossly evident hemispheral lesions, a frequent finding in a population of severe epileptics as others have noted, were excluded. Only CT scans on 26 patients read as "normal" were further considered. Ten of these patients had highly focal EEG and clinical seizure patterns so that they had epileptic foci sufficiently localized to meet criteria for cortical resection. The change in number of CT scan "pixels" at each attenuation value between contrast enhanced and unenhanced scans, was computed for an area in the region of the focus and a same sized homologus area in the opposite cerebral hemisphere. More pixels with high attenuation values (greater than 40 New Hounsfield units) remained in the area of the focus, than in the homologus area of opposite brain in nine of the ten cases (p=.01). Whether this increased contrast enhancement of the area of the focus is due to a local increase in blood flow, structural change in the focus, such as gliosis, or altered blood-brain barrier is unknown. But this subtle increase in relative contrast enhancement, evident only on the histograms of contrast-no contrast difference in CT attenuation values, marks the focus from the homologus area of the opposite hemisphere.

This technique should be of value in resolving such problems as side of focus in patients with complex partial seizures and bitemporal spiking or without localizing EEG changes. Of ten patients in our series with this question, five showed clearly increased contrast enhancement on one side. And some patients with clinical and EEG generalized seizure patterns may have foci — three of five patients in this category showed lateralized increases in frontal contrast enhancement; whether these represent "false positives" or previously undetected foci requires further evaluation.

Supported by NIH Grant NS 04053 and NIH Contract N01-NS-6-2341.

AN EPILEPTOLOGICAL ASPECT OF THE EEG-CT CORRELATIVE INVESTIGATION

S. Ishida, K. Yagi, T. Fujiwara, T. Higashi,
S. Moriyama, T. Wada
Shizuoka

In order to make a precise correlation between EEG and CT, 700 patients were selected and subjected to both examination; 34 cases with primary generalized epilepsy (PGE), 181 with secondary generalized epilepsy (SGE), 61 with the Lennox-Gastaut Syndrome, 413 with partial epilepsy (PE) and 72 with undetermined and unclassifiable epilepsies. CT detected positive findings in 67% of all patients. It is surprising that the positive findings were found almost equally in 69% of SGE and PE. Patients with cerebral atrophy were more than 80% of patients who were CT positive.

A comparison was made between CT positive findings and EEG paroxysmal discharges and their relative spatial distribution, by comparing diffuse with focal. Consequently, the assumption that SGE without the Lennox-Gastaut Syndrome may be situated between PE and the Lennox-Gastaut Syndrome from the pathogenic point of view was derived. Although there was a low percent of interhemispheric disagreement between EEG and CT, an abnormality was disclosed. Namely, discrete organic lesion in one hemisphere and epileptogenic focal abnormality in the opposite hemisphere were found. The focal epileptogenesity was clinically exemplified by focal seizure which was ipsilateral to the organic lesion. Denervation hypersensitization is the most plausible explanation for this.

CLINICAL EVALUATION OF EPILEPTIC PATIENTS WITH COMPUTED TOMOGRAPHY

K. Amano, M. Notani, T. Miyazaki, H. Iseki,
H. Kawabatake, T. Tanikawa, H. Kawamura,
K. Matsumori and K. Kitamura, Tokyo

Since September 1975, a total of 6858 patients had computed tomograms, (CT scan) in our Institute. Of these, 842 cases (12.3%) were patients with epilepsy, the largest series in Japan of epileptic patients evaluated with CT scan. These 842 epileptic cases included 73 patients (8.7%) with organic brain disorders demonstrated on CT (brain tumor 26 cases, septal cyst 19 cases, cerebral infraction 10 cases, arteriovenous malformation 6 cases, porencephaly 5 cases, hydrocephalus 4 cases and subdural effusion 3 cases). Excluding these 73 cases with organic brain damage, 769 cases out of 842 epileptic patients were analyzed with CT scan according to clinical type of seizure. 511 cases of grand mal type (66.4%) showed normal CT in 255 cases (49.9%), diffuse CT abnormality in 171 cases (33.5%) and focal CT abnormality in 85 cases (16.6%). 118 cases of focal epilepsy (15.3%) demonstrated normal CT in 54 cases (45.8%), focal CT abnormality in 46 cases (39.0%) and diffuse CT abnormality in 18 cases (15.2%). 77 cases of petit mal type (10.0%) revealed normal CT in 38 cases (49.4%), diffuse CT abnormality in 28 cases (36.4%) and focal CT abnormality in 11 cases (14.2%). 42 patients with psychomotor seizure (5.5%) had normal CT in 22 cases (52.4%), diffuse CT abnormality in 11 cases (26.2%) and focal CT abnormality in 9 cases (21.4%). On the other hand, 18 cases (85.7%) out of 21 patients with infantile spasm showed abnormal CT scan. Based on these clinical results with CT scan, the authors investigated the present limits of CT scan for epileptic patients as well as future perspectives in this field of neuroscience.

COMPUTERIZED TOMOGRAPHICAL FINDINGS OF EPILEPTIC PATIENTS

I. Moriuchi, H. Kaiya, H. Kato, Y. Kawamura, T. Mori, T. Iwata, T. Iwato, M. Namba
Gifu City

Sixty-three epileptic patients were examined with COMPUTERIZED TOMOGRAPHY (CT, EMI-1000). The relationship between the type of epilepsy and the CT and EEG findings was studied. Seizure types were designated according to the International Classification. CT findings were analysed by measuring the area of the anterior horn and the whole lateral ventricles, from which the volume of the lateral ventricles was worked out by the LAGRANGE method. This study is suggestive of the following: 1) CT could differentiate primary brain diseases with seizures from epilepsy. 2) In most cases, primary generalized epilepsy showed fewer localized lesions that did other types of epilepsy. 3) The laterality of focal lesions in the CT findings is not always consistent with that in EEGs. 4) HUCKMAN numbering was found to be useful in evaluating anterior horn size. 5) The anterior horn size and the lateral ventricular volume in epileptic patients does not seem to be related to the aging process but appears to depend on the total number of past generalized seizures.

PSEUDOHYPOPARATHYROIDISM AND EPILEPSY: DIAGNOSTIC VALUE OF COMPUTERIZED CRANIAL TOMOGRAPHY

A. Guberman
Ottawa

Seizures occur in two-thirds of patients with idiopathic hypoparathyroidism (IHP) or pseudohypoparathyroidism (PHP) and are as common a manifestation as tetany in these disorders. We have studied a girl aged 12 and an unrelated boy aged 13 who presented with seizures of unapparent etiology. Both of these patients had a variety of seizures, some with focal features, and the first patient had poor seizure control over a seven-year period. Computerized cranial tomography (CCT scan) unexpectedly showed bilateral symmetrical intracerebral calcifications of the basal ganglia as well as other areas. Subsequent testing revealed hypocalcemia and other biochemical and radiological features of PHP despite a lack of the usual phenotypic features, tetanic symptoms or family history.

In epileptics with PHP or IHP, computerized cranial tomography can lead to a specific and unexpected etiological diagnosis when the commonly seen typical intracranial calcifications are present. When routine serum calcium determinations are overlooked, the CCT scan may offer the first clue of an underlying hypocalcemic disorder. Early detection of this metabolic condition is essential since persistent hypocalcemia can lead to permanent brain damage and poor seizure control. The CCT scan is also a useful means of accurately following the changes in the intracranial calcifications resulting from treatment.

ON THE POSSIBLE MECHANISM OF ORIGIN OF PERIODIC LATERIALIZED EPILEPTIFORM DISCHARGES (PLEDs)

A. Terao, T. Shirabe, N. Nomura, K. Morimoto, H. Fukunaga, E. Matsuda
Okayama

Electroencephalographical and clinicopathological findings were studied in order to examine the possible mechanism of origin of periodic lateralized epileptiform discharges (PLEDs). In a series of 10 cases with PLEDs, 6 cases were fatal and postmortem examinations were done in 4 cases, including 2 cases of metastatic brain tumor, one case of cerebral hemorrhage, and one case with subacute meningoencephalitis.

PLEDs were observed on the lesioned hemisphere in all cases. Of the 2 cases with metastatic brain tumor, one case with the right pairetooccipital mass lesion revealed diffusely edematous and demyelinating changes of the white matter on the affected hemisphere, through the cortical structures were relatively preserved. In another case with a right precentral mass lesion, the subcortical white matter was almost intact histopathologically, but the thalamus in that hemisphere was totally replaced with metastatic mass. Diffuse subcortical white matter hemorrhage and chronic necrotizing encephalitic pictures on the affected hemisphere was observed in each case of cerebral hemorrhage and of subacute meningo-encephalitis.

PLEDs may result from an anatomical or functional severence of normal connections between the cortical and the deeper structures including the thalamus.

"SMALL SHARP SPIKES" ("BENIGN EPILEPTI-FORM TRANSIENTS"). EEG RECORDINGS FROM THE SCALP AND THE AMYGDALOID NUCLEI OF A HUMAN SUBJECT

V. Fernandes de Lima, G. E. Chatrian,
G. A. Ojemann, E. Lettich
Seattle

A 27-year-old man with a long history of partial complex seizures uncontrolled by medications and typical "small sharp spikes" (SSS, Gibbs and Gibbs 1951) in his EEG had multi-electrode leads stereotactically implanted into the amygdaloid nuclei of both sides in anticipation of surgery. Recordings over one week demonstrated the following.

1) Spikes having the morphological features of SSS occurred in the amygdala of either side and showed gradual amplitude decrement towards the cortex.
2) Only 21% of amygdaloid spikes also appeared on the scalp, in all instances with the morphological and topographic characteristics of SSS.
3) Although the amygdaloid spikes were unilateral, their scalp distribution was bilateral in 63% of cases and unilateral (ipsilateral) in 37%.
4) Scalp and/or amygdaloid spikes were not detected by naso-pharyngeal electrodes.
5) Rapid intravenous injection of methohexital (1 mg/Kg) produced prominent slow and fast activity in depth and surface leads without obliterating the SSS in the amygdala.
6) Electrical stimulation of either the right or the left amygdala elicted electrical seizures involving depth and scalp leads. The associated clinical changes closely resembled the patient's spontaneous attacks.

The possibility is discussed that SSS might originate in medial temporal structures including the amygdala and be volume-conducted to the surface of the scalp. This isolated study contributes no conclusive information on the relationships between SSS and epilepsy.

TO DETECT A SPIKE AUTOMATICALLY BY COMPUTER

S. P. Ninomija
Tokyo

Purpose: To detect automatically by computer all spikes from a long period recorded EEG.

Data: Recorded from 7 year old female traumatic epilepsy.

Method: The analogue recorded EEG were converted by an IBM-1800 computer into digital data at 100 samples per second and proceeded by a larger general computer. To detect the spikes we used a *Computer Defined Spike,* that is if
1) the absolute value of the slope of the moving linear regression line for the digital data is calculated by using the method of the least-squares is larger than 20 micro-volts / 10 milli-seconds,
2) in the next interval (3/100 5/100 seconds) there

is also a slope larger than 20, but the sign of this slope is reversible,
3) the variance for the line between those acute slopes is larger than 150 (micro-volts)^2/10 milliseconds and for those lines are smaller than 70. Only if the wave satisfies those 3 conditions, may it be called a *Computer Defined Spike.*

Results: 90% of the spikes detected by this method were real spikes, the remaining 10% were sharp waves and noises. However 1% of the spikes which were detected by a specialist could not be detected using this method.

Conclusions: We could detect most of the spikes from any EEG. To use *Computer Defined Spike* is the outstanding point of this method. This definition is very simple and the program also, moreover the time to execute this program by a computer is considerably reduced.

The author owes thanks to Professor J. A. Wada, Dr. H. Iwasa and Dr. N. Itihara for submitting their Important data and helpful discussions.

DETECTION AND QUANTIFICATION OF PAROXYSMAL EEG ABNORMALITIES: AN ANALOG CIRCUIT METHOD

J. W. Whisler, W. J. ReMine, I. E. Leppik,
R. J. Gumnit
Minneapolis

Seizure monitoring is a useful tool in medication adjustment, surgical evaluation, and research. Two recurring problems in seizure monitoring are: 1) Determining when a seizure has occurred in the many patients who are unable to anticipate or report their seizures; and 2) Quantifying intermittant EEG abnormalities in records that are too long for visual inspection. This paper describes clinical experience with a special purpose analog circuit which detects any combination or sequence of spike and wave, polyspike or runs of spikes, and generalized 3 Hz waves.

A multi-level decision algorithm combining power spectrum, wave-shape, and interchannel comparisons is used. The decision logic can be altered according to the patient's abnormality and the information sought from the device. Preliminary results from a double blind statistical comparison of the device with certified electroencephalographers indicates that detection reliability exceeds 80% with fewer than 3 false positive detections per hour of EEG. Complete results of the evaluation will be presented.

The circuit described above has three advantages over the digital computer approach to the problem. First, the circuit's small size makes it readily portable. Second, time scaling the circuit allows it to operate at speeds in excess of 100 times real time and its speed is unchanged as algorithm complexity increases. Third, the circuit contains approximately $US300 in materials and has no continuing programming costs. This work was supported by NINDS contract #Nol-NS-5-2327.

THE RELATIVE VALUE OF CERTAIN EEG PARAMETERS AS INDICATORS OF INTELLECTUAL PERFORMANCE OF EPILEPTIC PATIENTS

C. B. Dodrill, R. J. Wilkus
Seattle

Visual analysis of conventional EEG recordings has allowed us to identify the relative potencies of certain EEG parameters in differentiating intellectual performances of 111 adult epileptic patients. The EEG variables evaluated were 1) dominant posterior ("alpha") rhythm frequency, 2) topographic distribution of epileptiform discharges, and 3) extent of generalized non-epileptiform abnormalities. The Wechsler Adult Intelligence Scale (WAIS) was administered within a median of 2.5 days of the EEG studies.

All EEG variables studied bore statistically significant relationships with intellectual performance. However, all were more closely related to the Performance Scale of the WAIS than the Verbal Scale. Furthermore, the EEG variable demonstrating the most potent relationship with intelligence pertained to generalized non-epileptiform abnormalities, topographic distribution of discharges was intermediate, and frequency of the dominant posterior rhythm was weakest. A simultaneous consideration of the first two variables further enhanced the correlations. These results have direct research and clinical applications. It is apparent that previous investigators have overemphasized the importance of the "alpha" rhythm in behavioral studies with insufficient attention to more broadly disbursed non-epileptiform abnormalities. Finally, maximal correlations are achieved when epileptiform and non-epileptiform EEG variables are simultaneously considered.

This project was supported by NIH Contracts N01-NS-0-2281 and N01-NS-6-2341, National Institutes of Neurological and Communicative Disorders and Stroke, PHS/DHEW, USA.

CHANGES OF EEG PAROXYSMAL ACTIVITIES DURING NOCTURNAL SLEEP IN PATIENTS OF MYOCLONUS EPILEPSY AND DYSSYNERGIA CEREBELLARIS MYOCLONICA

S. Niwa, H. Yamada, N. Anzai, Y. Saito, M. Jimbo
Tokyo

Five patients with myoclonus epilepsy of two families (A and S) and one patient with dyssynergia cerebellaris myoclonica were examined polygraphically during two successive nights. Ages of patients ranged from 24 to 66 years.

The second night's records were studied with special reference to the changes of EEG paroxysms during sleep.

All patients of families A and S were thought to be suffering from myoclonus epilepsy of degenerative type.

Results:

1. The characteristics of paroxysms during the waking resting state are summarized as follows:
Three patients of family A showed slow wave bursts dominating anteriorly and spikes appearing predominantly in occipital regions, and two patients of family S showed high amplitude spike & wave complexes in occipital regions. One patient with dyssynergia cerebellaris myoclonica showed high amplitude sharp waves in central region.

2. During orthosleep, the spikes declined in occipital regions and dominated in central regions. Paroxysms appeared less frequently during orthosleep except in one, in whom paroxysms appeared most frequently during sleep stage II.

3. During REM-sleep, paroxysms were observed similar to those during wakefulness but with lower amplitudes. They did not seem to change in their appearing frequencies compared with those during wakefulness in most patients. Further investigations will bring more details concerning this point.

ANALYSIS OF EEG'S OF EPILEPTIC SEIZURES: A COMPARISON OF METHODS.

N. J. I. Mars
Enschede
F. H. Lopes da Silva
Utrecht

A special purpose system for continuous epileptic seizure monitoring has been built around a PDP11/04 central processor using specially developed hardware for 16-channel EEG recordings with little inconvenience for the patients. The objective is to record reliably the EEG of epileptic patients immediately before, during and shortly after a seizure. This is done by continuously storing the EEG of the last few minutes in a temporary digital memory (a disk), and retaining in permanent storage only recordings prior to and during a seizure.

The voluminous amount of data acquired in this way (and the need for objective analysis) requires computer aided analysis of the recordings. As a necessary preliminary to the eventual development of a new method, a comparison of different already applied or proposed methods has been undertaken.

These methods range from the simple methods for showing the change with time of the spectral contents of the EEG (like the compressed spectral array) to the sophisticated ones for showing the relationships between different channels (by estimating time relationships from phase curves or by computing "causal driving" from partial coherences) or the amount of "structure" or "regularity" in single channels (like texture analysis or bispectral analysis).

In this way the relative merits of these methods for assisting the EEG'er in the diagnosis of a "primary focus" have been assessed.

DIFFERENCES BY SEX IN EEG FINDINGS OF EPILEPTICS

A. Mori
Tokyo

The differences by sex in EEG findings in 2899 cases of epilepsy (1640 males and 1259 females) were statistically observed.

The incidence of EEG abnormalities in females (85.8%) was significantly higher than that in males (77.4%). This tendency was found throughout all ages and the significant differences were more apparent in the 15-24 and the 30-49 age groups. Paroxysmal waves in females (55.4%) were significantly higher than those in males (41.4%). The incidence of spike or sharp waves was not related to age and was higher in females than in males. Paroxysmal high-voltage slow waves appeared more frequently in younger groups and was significantly higher in females aged 15-19 years. In the basic activity, the incidence of irregular, dysrhythmic and diffuse slow-wave patterns was observed to be higher in females than in males.

The differences by sex in prognosis for epilepsy were also observed clinically and electroencephalographically. As to the improvement of clincial seizures, differences by sex were not seen. But, as to EEG, the improvement of paroxysmal waves was significantly higher in males (60.0%) than in females (37.3%).

It is assumed that the cause of these differences by sex in EEG of epileptics is influenced by physiological and endocrine factors.

MULTIPLE CHANNEL, MULTIMODALITY EVOKED POTENTIALS IN PATIENTS WITH UNILATERAL EXTRATEMPORAL AND UNILATERAL TEMPORAL EPILEPTIC FOCI

J. A. Messenheimer, J. J. Brickley,
R. N. Johnson, and S. I. Lee
Charlottesville

There are few systematic studies of evoked potentials in epileptics which are not compromised by limitations on the number of EEG channels simultaneously averaged, by the use of only one or two stimulus modalities or by the clinical heterogeneity of the epileptic group studied. We are engaged in a detailed, systematic analysis of alterations of visual (VEP), auditory (AEP) and somatosensory (SEP) evoked potentials in relatively homogeneous subsets of a large population of epileptic patients, using a system permitting simultaneous averaging of 8 channels of EEG data.

Previous reports documenting focal augmentation of various components of the SEP in cases of focal epileptic lesions have not been spared the limitations outlined above. We have examined 8 channel VEP, AEP and SEP in patients with unilateral extratemporal foci (14), in patients with unilateral temporal foci (14) and in normal controls.

Although the most consistent alterations of SEP in patients with extratemporal foci were noted in the area of the epileptic focus, over 25% also demonstrated more widespread, even bihemispheric altera-

tions of these potentials. Asymmetries of VEP and AEP were noted in some cases. Focal changes were not evident in patients with temporal foci. It is suggested that altered neuronal excitability in both specific and nonspecific or diffuse projection systems may be involved in these changes and that this differential involvement may be demonstrated by evoked potential studies.
(Supported by NIH Contract #N01-NS-5-2329)

BRAINSTEM AUDITORY-EVOKED RESPONSES (BAERs) IN GENERALIZED PENICILLIN AND ENFLURANE EPILEPSY: CORRELATION WITH SPONTANEOUS MIDBRAIN RETICULAR AND CORTICAL EEG ACTIVITY

J. J. Stockard
Rochester, Minnesota
T. A. Jones
Davis, California

The generalized EEG spike-wave activity produced by both inspired enflurane and parenteral penicillin can be modulated by alterations in reticulocortical desynchronizing drive. Manipulations in the cat which depress spontaneous tonic neuronal activity in the midbrain reticular formation (MRF) increase the prevalence of ECoG spike-wave discharges produced by both agents (Electroencephalogr clin Neurophysiol 36: 517, 1974, and 41: 651, 1976).

In MRF multiple unit activity recordings from six cats, it was seen that enflurane had its own brainstem-depressant properties — which enhanced its epileptogenicity — while penicillin did not. The differing effects of these two drugs on spontaneous brainstem activity were paralleled by their differing effects on evoked brainstem activity. Concentrations of eflurane producing generalized ECoG spike-wave activity prolonged (p 0.001) the latencies of BAER components generated in the rostral brainstem. In contrast, epileptogenic concentrations of penicillin did not prolong the latencies of any BAER components; the BAER amplitude changes previously reported to occur with generalized penicillin epilepsy (Epilepsia 17: 293, 1976) were not reproducible.

The correlation between development of enflurane-induced epileptiform ECoG activity and BAER abnormalities suggests that the latter may indirectly reflect the role of brainstem depression in the epileptogenicity of this drug. BAERs might prove useful in distinguishing and identifying other forms of "corticoreticular" epilepsy, including clinical ones.

TRANSIENT ABOLITION OF GENERALIZED PHOTOSENSITIVE EPILEPSY IN MAN BY APOMORPHINE, A DOPAMINE AGONIST

L. F. Quesney, F. Andermann, S. Prelevic, S. Lal
Montreal

Previous investigations have demonstrated that Apomorphine reduces photically induced seizures in the baboon.

The effect of Apomorphine was studied in eight patients with active generalized photosensitive epilepsy (6 females, 2 males) whose mean age was 17.8 years. All patients except one were on anticonvulsant medication.

Apomorphine hydrochloride (1.125 - 1.5 mgs.) was administered subcutaneously and the response to I.P.S. was tested every 3 to 15 minutes during 1-1½ hours. The effect of normal saline (placebo) on photosensitivity was studied in five patients. Photically induced VER's were done in four patients prior to and after Apomorphine administration.

Results: Apomorphine abolished photically induced generalized epileptic activity in seven patients. This effect started 10-19 minutes after the drug injection and its mean duration was 32 minutes. The remaining patient exhibited a partial reduction of photosensitivity. Nausea and/or vomiting of transient duration (5-10 minutes) developed in 3 patients. Normal saline injection, did not alter the response to I.P.S. VER's were not significantly changed after Apomorphine administration.

These results suggest involvement of a dopaminergic system in generalized photosensitive epilepsy in man, which however does not seem to operate in the genesis of photically induced VER's.

THE SIGNIFICANCE OF THE CENTRO-TEMPORAL EEG PAROXYSMS AND THE NATURAL HISTORY OF THE BENIGN EPILEPSY OF CHILDHOOD

J. M. Martinez-Lage and G. Morales
Pamplona

Among 10,000 consecutive EEG records taken during the period of 1970-77 corresponding to the same number of new out-patients, centro-temporal paroxysms (CTP) were found in 170 cases (1.7%) whose age ranged between 2 and 18 years. Thirty children suffered from Benign Epilepsy (BE) diagnosed according to the well known and established criteria for it.

The significance of CTP, its circumstances of appearance and prognosis were analyzed. They are more correlated with genetic factors and abnormal perinatal history than with other factors.

We completely agree with the Heijbel's conclusions that BE did not influence the children's intelligence and the medical treatment ought to be able to be discontinued in all cases at the age of about 16. We prefer the use of sodium valproate than other antiepileptic drugs.

FREE AMINO ACIDS IN CEREBROSPINAL FLUID AND SERUM OF THE PATIENTS WITH INFANTILE SPASMS

C. Ohtsuka, H. Takahashi, Y. Minowa, H. Iwasaki, K. Takahashi
Tokyo

Several amino acids are well known as neurotransmitters and their precursors. The amino acids imbalance in the brain of animals during convulsion and of epileptic patients have been reported. The levels of free amino acids in CSF and serum of epileptic patients were measured by an amino acid autoanalyzer and the changes of several amino acid levels were found.

The object of this report is to demonstrate the specific changes of free amino acids in CSF and serum of the patients with infantile spasms. The levels of free amino acids in CSF and serum of 10 patients with infantile spasms were measured by an amino acid autoanalyzer. The results were compared with those of normal subjects and of 10 patients with the other types of epilepsy.

The following results were obtained.

1) In CSF of the patients with infantile spasms, histidine, arginine, lysine, glutamine and phenylalanine were slightly low level while valine was slightly high level, but the free amino acids in serum were normal level.

2) The glutamine levels in CSF of the uncontrolled patients with the other types of epilepsy were high, but those of infantile spasms were normal.

The amino acids imbalance in CSF of the patients with infantile spasms was different from that of the patients with the other types of epilepsy.

UNCONTROLLABLE CASES OF ABSENCE

I. Kawai
Kyoto

K. Shingu
Ohtsu

S. Fujii
Osaka

The "absence" here mentioned refers to the combination of an abrupt loss of consciousness and diffuse 3 Hz Sp-W-C patterns on the interval EEG. In spite of adequate use of anticonvulsant drugs for more than five years, several cases are left with minor attacks. In these cases, some of the following findings can be pointed out;

1) The onset is at the adult age, often preceded by grand mal seizures.

2) The attack is accompanied by retropulsive, sucking or chewing movements.

3) Gross brain damage can be presumed in the past history, in the anamnesis or during the course.

4) Mental retardation is found already as the onset, or mental deterioration develops during the course.

5) Already at the onset, the patient's character shows circumstantiality (or the character proposed by Janz as that of the sleep grand mal epilepsy in his typology).

6) The seizure pattern undergoes such changes as follows; An abrupt loss of consciousness is replaced by a gradual alteration of consciousness, which is accompanied by an automatism during the latter half of the seizure. In that case, the EEG will show pseudorhythmic slow Sp-W-C patterns or a temporal spike focus.

7) Psychotic state may be observed (different form petit mal status).

EPIDEMIOLOGICAL RESEARCHES ON THE EPILEPTIC DISCHARGES OF EEG RECORDS

Y. Fujiya, C. Haruhara
Tokyo

EEG records of three healthy groups were examined by the same method. Group A comprised applicants for automobile driver's license with an average age of twenty years, Group B consisted of bus drivers with over five years experience whose ages ranged from 27 to 45 years, and Group C consisted of females in nurses training whose average age was twenty years.

The results of our research follow:

EEG findings	normal	paroxysmal	(epileptic)
Group A 700 cases	618	82	(31)
Group B 280 cases	265	15	(3)
Group C 66 cases	37	29	(7)
Total cases 1,046	920 (88.0%)	126 (12.1%)	(41) 3.9%

There was significant statistical difference (under 1% by X sq. test) between each group. Spike and wave complex of typical epileptiform discharges was revealed in only four cases of Group A. We examined the mild transient symptoms (car sickness, attack of headache, dizzyness and cerebral anemia, etc.) in Group C. They revealed nine cases of normal EEG records, 21 cases of paroxysmal findings and all cases of epileptic revealed the symptoms.

On the basis of these data, we conclude that cases of epileptic EEG findings have been the subclinical and/or preliminary group of epilepsy.

DARK-ACTIVATED COMPLEX THANATOPHO-BIC SEIZURES

F. Sharbrough, B. Westmoreland, B. Mokri
Rochester, Minnesota

A rare case of complex seizures activated by darkness is presented. A 74-year-old man gave a 4-year history of an overwhelming fear of dying, which occurred after eye closure. Each time the patient experienced the thanatophobia with eye closure, there was an associated paroxysmal rhythmic fast-seizure discharge widespread in distribution and maximum in the central midline. The discharge and the sensation of fear occurred in 90% of the epochs after eye closure. In the 10% of the epochs free of the discharge, the patient experienced no fear. The seizures could also be activated with eyes open by placing the patient in total darkness. Eye opening in a lighted room always aborted the seizure, as did the shining of a bright light through closed eyelids. The interictal wake and sleep recordings were normal. The origin of the seizure discharge cannot be determined with certainty, but the widespread distribution without alteration of consciousness suggests that the seizure discharge may arise from the midline limbic system.

EYE CLOSURE SEIZURES

B. Sharf, E. Bental
Haifa

Two young adults with a history of premature birth and some convulsive generalized seizures were investigated because of numerous attacks of prolonged periods of eye closure, lasting sometimes a whole day, associated with gross electroenchephalographic abnormalities. During the eye closure periods a certain degree of impairment of consciousness could be observed. They did respond, however when spoken to and could voluntarily open their eyes whereupon the EEG turned immediately to normal. The act of eye closure seems to be induced through a central mechanism, presumably in analogy to what occurs during a petit mal status, manifesting itself in the EEG by spikes and slow wave activity. This can be instantly interrupted by eye opening, although the patients tended to fall back to the eye closure state. This phenomenon is discussed in the light of similar descriptions in the literature.

TWO RARE TYPES OF SENSORY INDUCED EPILEPSY

T. Ishiguro, K. Yui
Tochigi

Two rare types of sensory induced epilepsy were studied. The 1st case is a 41-year-old female with epileptic attack induced only by cooling. The attacks, which began as an adversive seizure and developed into a grand mal seizure, have been induced after several minutes cooling without any special emotion, although sometimes preceded by an aura of cold sensation like ice in her left foot. When her hands were cooled by ice water, the EEG revealed focal spikes at the right central, parietal and temporal areas, and then diffuse spike & wave complexes. The 2nd case is a 47-year-old male with grand mal attack induced only by playing Japanese chess, *go*. The grand mal attack often occurred after 4 to 10 hours of playing *go*. The EEG revealed focal spikes at the left central and parietal areas at resting record. After playing *go* for more than 19 hours with serial EEG recording, the EEG showed diffuse spikes with grand mal seizure. Both cases are considered to be reflex epilepsy in essence, but the 2nd case differs from ordinary reflex epilepsy in that 1) the latency of induced attack is longer, and 2) the exciting causes are multiple. Therefore, we believe that the 2nd case should be considered different from an ordinary one.

MYOCLONIC ATTACKS INDUCED BY L-DOPA AND BROMOCRYPTIN IN PARKINSONIAN PATIENTS. A SLEEP EEG STUDY

J. Vardi, J. M. Rabey, H. Glaubman,
and M. Streifler
Tel Aviv

Six patients with Parkinson's disease developed nocturnal myoclonic attacks after prolonged treatment with L-Dopa which were electroencephalographically recorded. These attacks were described as abnormal movements occurring during sleep and consisting of repetitive abrupt jerks of the extremities, the body and neck. The attacks occurred throughout the entire sleeping period and were sometimes more pronounced during drowsiness. These symptoms persisted after treatment with 2 bromo-alpha-ergocryptin (Bromocryptin) a dopamine receptor agonist, which was substituted for L-Dopa. Bromocryptin is known to have no pre- or postsynaptic effect on serotonin metabolism. It is proposed that these myoclonic phenomena are the expression of the hypersensitivity of denervated catecholamine receptors in the brainstem to the stimulation of L-Dopa and Bromocryptin. This thesis differs with previous suggestions that serotonin plays a major role in the genesis of myoclonic seizures in Parkinsonian patients treated with L-Dopa.

SEIZURES IN HYPERTHYROIDISM

B. Jabbari, A. D. Huott, F. A. Tavassoli
Washington

Two patients without prior history of convulsions or hyperthyroidism developed seizures while in acute thyrotoxicosis.

The first patient, a 19-year-old male, following a few days of tremulousness and irritability, developed a cluster of seven closely spaced generalized tonic-clonic seizures each one preceded by increased tone and adversive posturing of the right upper extremity. The laboratory findings were diagnostic of thyrotoxicosis. His seizures and epileptiform EEG findings ceased after correction of hyperthyroidism.

The second patient, a 54-year-old woman, developed acute thyrotoxicosis one month after treatment for a mild hypothyroid state. She presented with progressive confusion and several tonic-clonic seizures. An EEG showed a low voltage fast background with scattered sharp waves. Her mental confusion and seizures disappeared within a week after discontinuing treatment with thyroid extract.

Epileptic seizures related to hyperthyroidism are rare and only five such cases have been reported. Focal or generalized, these seizures are reversible and occur during a rapidly established thyrotoxic state. Changes in cerebral oxygen consumption or hypoglycemia have been postulated as etiologic factors. The exact cause of thyrotoxic seizures, however, still remains obscure and deserves further investigation.

EPILEPSY AND EXERCISE, ELECTROENCEPH-ALOGRAPHICAL AND BIOCHEMICAL STUDIES

A. Kuijer
Heeze

Observations of people who took part in sport learned that there is an increase in attacks in the period following exercise and besides that the increase after intermittent exercise is less than after continuous exercise. Some laboratory experiments were carried out during which an EEG was made while exercise was performed on a bicycle ergometer.

Investigated were: the incidence of epileptic activity in the EEG before and after the exercise, the biochemical changes regarding the acid-base equilibrium of the blood, the relationships between the EEG-findings and the biochemical changes, the type of epilepsy and the anti-epileptic medication that was used.

Main conclusions:

— There is a tendency towards an increase of epileptic activity in the EEG during the recovery phase after exercise, the degree of increase being different for different persons.

— The degree of increase is independent of the type of epilepsy and the type of medication used.

— The lower the values of the pH and Base-Excess after the exercise and during the recovery phase, the greater the increase of epileptic activity. The increase of the chemical variables during the recovery phase, lags behind in those subjects who show a distinct increase of epileptic activity after exercise.

A hypothesis is proposed to find an explanation for these phenomena.

FUKUYAMA TYPE CONGENITAL MUSCULAR DYSTROPHY (FCMD) AS ONE OF THE CAUSATIVE DISORDERS OF CHILDHOOD EPILEPSY

M. Segawa, Y. Nomura, K. Hachimori,
N. Shinomiya, A. Hosaka, and Y. Mizuno
Tokyo

FCMD, inherited autosomal-recessively, is characterized by muscular dystrophy associated with severe mental retardation and epileptic convulsions.

By examining 56 cases, followed more than 3 years, 75 EEG records on them, and autopsied materials (two personal and eight from the literature), the authors have aimed at clarifying the causative relationship between congenital CNS lesions and childhood epilepsy.

In 36/56 cases diffuse epileptic seizures were observed with onset at 1.64±1.0 years average. In 32/56 cases seizures developed before 3 years of age. In 51/75 EEGs and 55/56 cases, focal paroxysmal discharges (FPD), centro-parietal in younger and fronto-central in older cases, were observed. Abnormal basic activities (ABA), diffuse ∝ -activity and/or abundant or extreme spindles, were observed more often in older than younger cases. The incidence of FPD was similar between convulsive and non-convulsive cases, but ABA predominated in the former. CNS pathology revealed cerebral and cerebellar gyral abnormalities and a hypoplastic corticospinal tract probably occurred in the second trimester. The gyral lesions (verrucous polymicrogyria with adhesions of adjacent gyri and cellular disarrangement) were thought to be causative lesions for epilepsy.

Cortical non-progressive gyral lesions occurring around the second trimester could cause FPD and clinical diffuse epileptic seizures develop with other factors concerned with ABA.

ELECTROENCEPHALOGRAPHIC FINDINGS IN PETIT MAL EPILEPSY

S. N. Hamid, N. Khagani
Tabriz

Critical study of the EEG in the initial period of two years in this province of Azarbijan is reviewed with respect to the various electroencephalographic findings met with.

The following observations are recorded in 64 petit mal cases.

1) Ninety-eight per cent showed spike and wave pattern. Only 52% manifested classical 3/sec. spike and wave, the rest showed spike and wave but not 3/sec.

2) Forty-seven per cent showed slow wave. Out of these 14% had paroxysmal disturbance. Thirty-two per cent had sharp waves; 12.5% showed isolated spike; 10% had mixed discharge and 25% had high voltage disturbance only.

3) Discharge was more frequent in onset in occipital, equal in tempro-parietal and least in frontal regions. Localization of discharge was possible only in 28% of cases, in occipital region 8% as against 10% in fronto-temporal sites. Twenty-five percent of cases had bilateral disturbance.

4) Twenty-five per cent of the record showed abnormal background activity. Superimposed to 75% Alpha activity was 20% of Beta and Delta rhythm and 45% Theta disturbance.

5) Overbreathing in 67% provocated petit mal discharge. Only in 8% photic stimulation was helpful. Twenty-five per cent of cases failed to be confirmed with provocative procedures.

The observed findings are compared with the available literature favourably.

FUKUYAMA TYPE CONGENITAL MUSCULAR DYSTROPHY (FCMD) AS ONE OF THE CAUSATIVE DISORDERS OF CHILDHOOD EPILEPSY

M. Segawa, Y. Nomura, K. Hachimori, N. Shinomiya, A. Hosaka, and Y. Mizuno
Tokyo

FCMD, inherited autosomal-recessively, is characterized by muscular dystrophy associated with severe mental retardation and epileptic convulsions.

By examining 56 cases, followed more than 3 years, 75 EEG records on them, and autopsied materials (two personal and eight from the literature), the authors have aimed at clarifying the causative relationship between congenital CNS lesions and childhood epilepsy.

In 36/56 cases diffuse epileptic seizures were observed with onset at 1.64 ± 1.0 years average. In 32/56 cases seizures developed before 3 years of age. In 51/75 EEGs and 55/56 cases, focal paroxysmal discharges (FPD), centro-parietal in younger and fronto-central in older cases, were observed. Abnormal basic activities (ABA), diffuse $\propto$-activity and/or abundant or extreme spindles, were observed more often in older than younger cases. The incidence of FPD was similar between convulsive and non-convulsive cases, but ABA predominated in the former. CNS pathology revealed cerebral and cerebellar gyral abnormalities and a hypoplastic corticospinal tract probably occurred in the second trimester. The gyral lesions (verrucous polymicrogyria with adhesions of adjacent gyri and cellular disarrangement) were thought to be causative lesions for epilepsy.

Cortical non-progressive gyral lesions occurring around the second trimester could cause FPD and clinical diffuse epileptic seizures develop with other factors concerned with ABA.

IgM IN NASAL BIOLOGICAL SECRETIONS FROM DPH-TREATED IgA DEFICIENT EPILEPTIC PATIENTS — A COMPENSATORY MECHANISM?

J. A. Aarli, T. Haldorsen, S. Mørner
Bergen

Phenytoin treatment may induce an IgA deficiency. Recent data indicate that IgA-deficient epileptic patients have an increased susceptibility to upper respiratory infections. IgA, IgG and IgM concentrations were therefore determined in nasal washing from such patients. Earlier reports on Ig-concentrations have mainly been based upon studies of frozen nasal washings. In the present report, determination of Ig-concentrations was performed on fresh nasal washings. The mean concentration of IgA in normal human nasal secretions collected by lavage of the nasal cavities with isotonic salf solution was approximately 100 mg/l, as estimated by radial immuno-diffusion of fresh, non-lyophilized smaples. The calculation was based upon the assumption that IgA present in nasal secretions is mainly of secretory type. The results of ultracentrifugation experiments corroborated this hypothesis. Mean IgA concentration in nasal washings from epileptic patients was not significantly reduced, but 4 patients had undetectable IgA. These patients had also serum IgA < 50 mg/l.

The mean IgG-concentration in normal nasal washings was 18 mg/l in the normal group and 80 mg/l in the epilepsy group. IgM was not detected in any sample of nasal washing from healthy individuals, while mean IgM in the epileptic patients was 17.8 mg/l. All patients with undetectable IgA had also IgM present in nasal washings. This may be caused by a biological compensatory mechanism. However, IgM is not so resistant against proteolytic enzymes as secretory IgA.

EPILEPSY, IgA DEFICIENCY, HISTOCOMPATIBILITY ANTIGENS AND ANTI-ACETYLCHOLINE RECEPTOR ANTIBODIES

A. Fontana, B. W. Fulpius
Geneva

Serum levels of IgA were found to be reduced significantly in up to 12% of epileptics. On one side some studies have shown that serum IgA concentrations decreased throughout the course of hydantoin treatment. On the other hand, there are evidences of a drug independent humoral immunodeficiency state. They were obtained by the detection of IgA deficiency in untreated patients and the observed accumulation of IgA deficiency in some families with clustered epilepsy.

The data presented now, show the presence of

antibodies to muscle and brain nicotinic acetylcholine receptors (nAcChR) in three untreated patients with primary generalized seizures, IgA deficiency, HLA-A1 and B8 antigens and a positive family history in the instance of both, the seizure disorder and the humoral immunodeficiency disease. The HLA-A1 and B8 antigens were not detected in 16 other hydantoin treated IgA deficient epileptics lacking the anti-nAcChR antibodies. The genetic (HLA-A1 and B8) and immunological (IgA deficiency) characteristics of the patients with anti-receptor antibodies were also detected in the epileptic mothers of two patients. Both mothers had longterm hydantoin treatment, no signs of active disease for years, and no anti-nAcChR antibodies.

It is suggested that at least in some IgA deficient epileptics auto-immune reactions to brain receptors may play an important role in the development of the seizure disorder.

FEBRILE CONVULSIONS AND CSF IMMUNOLOGY

O. Eeg-Olofsson, H. Link, A. Wigertz
Linköping

A prospective study was performed during one year 1977-1978 on all children admitted to the hospital due to febrile convulsions. One of the aims of the study was to examine the cerebrospinal fluid (CSF) constituents.

The study comprises 88 children, 38 girls and 50 boys aged from 6 months to 5 years.

On admittance a lumbar puncture was performed and CSF analysed in the usual way. A portion was freezed for analysis together with another CSF sample taken about three weeks later.

The following analytical parameters of the CSF were examined: Albumin, alpha-2-macroglobulin, IgG, IgA, IgM, complement C_3 and C_4 and light chains of type kappa and lambda.

In 42 children a complete set of the two samples was received.

Preliminary results show that in about 20 per cent there is a synthesis of immunoglobulins from the CNS, this synthesis being related to lower ages. There was no complement consumption, and normal kappa/lambda quotients were found.

The results will probably give prognostic information as regards recurring febrile convulsions, later development of epilepsy, and will also be used as correlates to any future neurologic disturbance.

HLA AND EPILEPSY

O. Eeg-Olofsson, J. Safwenberg, A. Wigertz
Uppsala

Thirty-one families with primary epilepsy were HLA typed. The families included 62 parents and 76 children of which 31 were probands and 45 were sibs. Only 7 children were older than 15 years. Seventeen of the families had heredity epilepsy. The probands showed the following types of seizures: 16 with benign epilepsy of childhood (i.e. usually nocturnal, partial or generalized seizures in children

aged 5 to 11 years with EEG findings of spikes or sharp waves with central location), 8 grand mal and 7 petit mal.

The HLA pattern of the probands did not deviate from that among the controls, neither when analysed all together nor when divided according to the type of seizure. If the HLA haplotype pattern of the parents was compared to that among Scandinavian controls, a significant decrease of the A1, B8 haplotype was found ($X^2 = 5.84$ after Yates' correction, $p < 0.015$). We found two A1, B8 haplotypes where 11 was to be expected. The phenotype frequency of A1 was half that of the controls and the B8 frequency was normal. Generally, an association between HLA and a disease has involved one allele within one focus and not several linked loci. The question is asked, therefore, if the A1, B8 haplotype is usually associated to genes that protect us from some kind of cerebral damage that can provoke seizures?

CHILDHOOD EPILEPSY AND LOW SERUM IgA

M. Ariizumi, A. Baba, A. Osawa, N. Kuromori,
T. Ogawa, H. Shiihara
Tokyo

IgA deficiency or low IgA level of epileptics has been presumed to be a side-effect of DPH. However, it has been suggested also that patients with constitutional epilepsy might have a predisposition to the reduced levels of serum IgA. The purpose of this paper was to examine the serum IgA levels of epileptic children who have never been given any anticonvulsants.

The study consisted of 48 patients without anticonvulsant medication, in ages ranging from 1 to 14 years. Twelve out of 15 patients with primary generalized seizure had abnormal IgA levels below 2 SD limit and six of them had low IgA (under 20% of the mean IgA value in each age). In the other seizure types none of the patients had low IgA, although abnormal IgA levels were observed in three of 5 patients with psychomotor seizure, in one of 5 patients with secondary generalized seizure, in one of 11 patients with focal seizure, in one of 4 patients with infantile spasms, and in one with Lennox's syndrome.

It was concluded that low IgA observed in some seizure types might be based on a predisposition to reduced levels of serum IgA.

DERMATOGLYPHICS IN EPILEPSY

B. Schaumann, A. Mayersdorf, C. Hansen
Minneapolis

In recent years, associations have been demonstrated between various medical disorders and specific variations of dermatoglyphics (i.e. configurations of the epidermal ridges on the digital, palmar and plantar surfaces). The development of dermatoglyphic configurations is genetically predisposed. As it has also been assumed that genetic factors have a predisposing effect on the development of seizures in man, the present dermatoglyphic study was carried out on patients with epilepsy in order to determine whether characteristic deviations of dermatoglyphic traits exist in patients suffering from seizure disorders of different etiology and whether such traits can be used for diagnostic purposes.

The patients were considered in groups according to the presumed etiology, i.e., patients with post-traumatic seizures, seizures related to alcohol, idiopathic seizures and patients with a family history of seizures.

Statistical analysis demonstrated deviations in frequency of several dermatoglyphic traits such as fingertip pattern types, total finger ridge count, a-b ridge count, palmar patterns, and termination of mainline C in patients with epilepsy when compared to controls. Interestingly, these dermatoglyphic deviations were not limited to the types of seizure disorders with a known genetic predisposition (i.e. familial and idiopathic epilepsy) but were observed even in symptomatic (post-traumatic and alcohol-related) epilepsy, suggesting a possible genetic predisposition in the origin of even these types of seizure disorders.

Subject Index

President
J. KIFFIN PENRY
Bowman Gray School of Medicine
Wake Forest University
300 South Hawthorne Road
Winston-Salem. N.C. 27103 U.S.A.

Past-President
D. D. DALY
Dallas

1st Vice-President
D. JANZ
Berlin

2nd Vice-President
T. WADA
Shizuoka

Secretary-General
F. RUBIO-DONNADIEU
Instituto Nacional de Neurologia
Insurgentes Sur 3877
Mexico 22, D.F., Mexico

Treasurer
K.-A. MELIN
Stora Sköndals sjukhus
S-123 85 Farsta, Sweden
Account No. 5233-20 001 27
Skandinaviska Enskilda Banken
Office 5233
S-123 47 Farsta, Sweden

Editor-in-Chief of Epilepsia
A. A. WARD, JR.
Seattle

Dear Colleague:

The primary goal of the International League Against
Epilepsy is "the advancement and dissemination throughout
the world of knowledge concerning the epilepsies". It is,
therefore, with great pleasure that we present to you the
enclosed volume, Advances in Epileptology: The Xth
Epilepsy International Symposium.

The publication of this volume has been made possible by
a grant from Geigy Pharmaceuticals, a division of Ciba—
Geigy Corporation.

Sincerely yours,

J. Kiffin Penry, M. D.